THE CORNEA
Scientific Foundations and
Clinical Practice

THE CORNEA

Scientific Foundations and Clinical Practice

Edited by

Gilbert Smolin, M.D.

Clinical Professor of Ophthalmology, University of California, San Francisco, School of Medicine; Research Ophthalmologist, Francis I. Proctor Foundation, San Francisco

Richard A. Thoft, M.D.

Associate Professor of Ophthalmology, Harvard Medical School; Associate Chief of Ophthalmology, Massachusetts Eye and Ear Infirmary, Boston

With 29 Contributing Authors

Little, Brown and Company
Boston/Toronto

DEDICATION

This textbook has been written in its entirety by some of the present staff and former fellows of two centers of academic ophthalmology, the Massachusetts Eye and Ear Infirmary (Corneal Service) in Boston and the Francis I. Proctor Foundation for Research in Ophthalmology in San Francisco. The editors and contributors enthusiastically dedicate this book to two great contributors to ophthalmology in general and to our knowledge of the cornea and external eye disease in particular, Phillips Thygeson and Claes Dohlman. As is well known, Dr. Thygeson is closely associated with the Proctor Foundation and Dr. Dohlman with the Massachusetts Eye and Ear Infirmary.

Phillips Thygeson

The contributions of a man cannot be measured only in such tangibles as his position, his research, or his publications. There are subtler but often more important influences a great man can exert as a human being, as a teacher, or just as an example. In all of these ways, Dr. Thygeson stands tall.

First of all, he was a pioneer in the field of ocular microbiology. In 1926, during his early medical school days at Stanford University, his liking for medical microbiology in general was sharpened by his professor, Dr. Edwin W. Schultz. This interest continued to grow during his internship at the University of Colorado's General Hospital in Denver. There he took care of many patients with pulmonary tuberculosis and learned about ocular tuberculosis from Dr. William D. Finnoff. He also learned a great deal, especially about anaerobic bacteria, from Dr. Ivan C. Hall, Chief of the Department of Bacteriology.

During the Denver years, Dr. Thygeson also became interested in trachoma and published a preliminary report of his efforts to confirm Hideyo Noguchi's work on what he (Noguchi) believed to be a causal relationship between *Bacterium granulosis* and trachoma. This article attracted the attention of Dr. Francis I. Proctor, an eminent Boston eye surgeon who had retired and was living in New Mexico. In Santa Fe Dr. Proctor became deeply interested in trachoma among the American Indians, and he found Dr. Thygeson ready to share this interest with him. Eventually, in 1934, these two performed a decisive experiment on a human volunteer that established the agent of trachoma as a filterable agent, intermediate in size between the true viruses and the classic bacteria, that was later named *Chlamydia trachomatis*.

Meanwhile, Dr. Thygeson had joined the staff of the eye department at the University of Iowa and was teaching external diseases of the eye and conducting research. He developed an external disease program for the residents and continued his work on trachoma and related infectious diseases. He was a superb teacher and inspired his students. Drs. Alson E. Braley and James H. Allen are two such students who came to share his great interest in external disease. The high quality of the external disease program he established in Iowa became traditional and continues to the present day.

In 1936 Dr. Thygeson joined the staff of the Department of Ophthalmology of the College of Physicians and Surgeons of Columbia University in New York as Director of Research. In doing so, he assumed the duties of one of the country's first full-time university appointments in ophthalmology. At Columbia he continued his teaching and extended his trachoma studies to include related chlamydia diseases, staphylococcal eye disease, and viral eye disease.

At 36 years of age, Dr. Thygeson and Dr. John H. Dunnington were named co-chairmen of the Department of Ophthalmology at Columbia, a position he held until, as a volunteer Army Medical Corps officer, Dr. Thygeson joined up to serve the Colors.

Dr. Proctor died unexpectedly in 1936. After the war, and at Dr. Thygeson's suggestion and with his advice, Mrs. Proctor decided to establish an eye research center in her husband's memory. The Francis I. Proctor Foundation for Research in Ophthalmology was established in 1947 at the University of California Medical Center in San Francisco by the joint action of Mrs. Proctor and the Regents of the University. Dr. Michael J. Hogan was its first director, and Dr. Thygeson was named by Mrs. Proctor to serve as her representative on its three-man Board of Governors for the rest of his life.

At the Foundation, Dr. Thygeson gradually built up a highly sophisticated ocular microbiology laboratory, and, by virtue of his long-standing appointment as Consultant to the Division of Indian Health, the Foundation became the base of operations for an exhaustive study of trachoma and related diseases of the American Indian. Throughout these years, Dr. Thygeson also worked tirelessly for the World Health Organization Expert Committee on Trachoma, traveling extensively and never refusing a request for his services from either WHO or the U.S. Public Health Service.

During the Proctor Foundation's early years, Dr. Thygeson published prolifically. Many of his articles remain illuminating classics in the field of ocular microbiology. He encouraged the referral of patients with external disease and uveitis to the Proctor Foundation, establishing it in this way as a major referral center. Above all, he fostered the training of young ophthalmologists. Feeling that this could best be accomplished with trainees who had completed their ophthalmology residencies, he regularly accepted several postgraduate fellows for a year or more of clinical training in external disease, supplemented by laboratory training and training in ocular research methods. More than 100 fellows have now been so trained.

In 1959 Dr. Thygeson became the second director of the Proctor Foundation and continued his efforts on all fronts. As Director he also engineered the accession of a great deal of new space and many new facilities. In addition to many other benefits of this program of growth he made the Proctor Foundation available for the establishment of the WHO International Reference Centre for Trachoma.

After 50 extremely busy years, Dr. Thygeson at last retired. He continues to be a very active member of the Foundation's Board of Governors, however, and contributes generously to the teaching program of the Foundation's steady stream of research-oriented fellows. The success of his efforts in this important program is attested by the professional records of his trainees, some of whom have contributed to this volume.

Despite his impressive achievements and the many honors bestowed on him, Dr. Thygeson has retained his characteristic humility, accessibility, consideration for his fellow man, and keen interest in his students. He remains, indeed, the paragon of a physician dedicated to the service of mankind and an inspiring example to us all. His high standards of modesty, devotion to truth, and dedication to our profession are traditions we strive for at the Proctor Foundation.

Rarely in our lifetime does such a fine, gentle man grace our journey, and this volume is our collective, humble way of saying we care about him more than we can say.

Gilbert Smolin

Rarely in ophthalmology has the combination of industry, ability, and humanity been centered in one individual as it is in the case of Claes Henrik Dohlman. These attributes are responsible for what has been an extraordinary impact on the course of corneal research and training during the past 25 years. To enumerate those individuals who have trained with Dr. Dohlman is to list many of the outstanding experimentalists, clinicians, and administrators in ophthalmology throughout the world. Some of these individuals have contributed to this volume and in so doing express their gratitude to Dr. Dohlman for his preceptorship. Many others in the course of their daily activities frequently think of Dr. Dohlman and their time with him as critical in their professional maturation, and are equally grateful.

A native of Sweden, Dr. Dohlman received the Medicine Licentiat (the equivalent of an M.D. degree) in 1950 and the Medicine Doktor degree (the equivalent of the Ph.D. degree) in 1958 from the University of Lund, Sweden, where he undertook ophthalmology specialty training. He furthered his training in France at centers in Lyon and Paris. In 1952 he served as a Research Fellow in Ophthalmology at Johns Hopkins Hospital and in 1953 held a similar appointment at Stanford University and at the Retina Foundation in Boston.

Dr. Dohlman came to Boston in 1958 to join the Retina Foundation and the staff and faculty of medicine at Harvard and the Massachusetts Eye and Ear Infirmary. From 1961 to 1966 he served as Director of the New England Eye Bank and continues on its Board of Directors. In 1962 he became director of the Department of Cornea Research at the Retina Foundation and from 1964 to 1974 was Director of the Cornea Service at the Massachusetts Eye and Ear Infirmary. The Cornea Service was instituted by Dr. Dohlman in 1964—the first such subspecialty clinic in the world. The early days of the clinic were characterized by Dr. Dohlman's stimulating discussions of patients whose disease processes were explained using the basic observations that he and his colleagues made in the laboratory. His research into the synthesis of corneal stromal glycosaminoglycans, the function of the endothelium, and the complex processes involved in maintaining the normal hydration of the cornea brought rational therapeutic advances to patients suffering from corneal edema secondary to a variety of disease processes.

In January, 1974, Dr. Dohlman was named Professor of Ophthalmology and Chairman of the Department at Harvard Medical School, Chief of the Department of Ophthalmology at the Massachusetts Eye and Ear Infirmary, and Director of Harvard's Howe Laboratory of Ophthalmology, located also at the Infirmary. Since becoming Chairman at Harvard, Dr. Dohlman has continued to be active in corneal research, teaching, and clinical care. He continues to be committed to the teaching of future corneal subspecialists and is justifiably proud of being the academic "grandfather" of many clinical fellows training outside of Boston, whose preceptors were themselves taught earlier by Dr. Dohlman.

In great measure, therefore, this volume represents the extension not only of Dr. Dohlman's thinking but of his warm and generous personality. All of us trained by Dr. Dohlman hope that he will view this book as a sincere "thank-you" for the remarkable professional opportunities which he created for us.

Richard A. Thoft

CONTENTS

DEDICATION   v

PREFACE   xi

ACKNOWLEDGMENTS   xiii

CONTRIBUTING AUTHORS   xv

I. BASIC SCIENCE ASPECTS

1. PHYSIOLOGY   3

   Physiology of the Cornea
   CORNEAL EDEMA   3
   Claes H. Dohlman

   METABOLISM AND BIOCHEMISTRY   17
   Judith Friend

   Physiology of the Tear Film   31
   David W. Lamberts

2. MORPHOLOGY AND PATHOLOGIC RESPONSES OF THE CORNEA TO DISEASE   43
   Kenneth R. Kenyon

3. IMMUNOLOGY   77
   Gilbert Smolin

4. MICROBIOLOGY   105

   Infectious Agents
   BACTERIA   105
   Masao Okumoto

   VIRUSES   115
   Jang O. Oh

   FUNGI   127
   Masao Okumoto

   Antibiotic Mechanisms   134
   Jules Baum

II. CLINICAL ASPECTS

5. INFECTIOUS DISEASES   147

   Bacterial Diseases   147
   Robert A. Hyndiuk, Kamal F. Nassif, and Eileen M. Burd

   Fungal Diseases   168
   Richard K. Forster

Viral Diseases
   HERPETIC DISEASES   178
   Deborah Pavan-Langston

   ADENOVIRUS AND MISCELLANEOUS VIRAL INFECTIONS   196
   David W. Vastine

   Chlamydial Diseases   210
   John P. Whitcher

   Suspected Infectious Etiology   221
   H. Bruce Ostler

6. IMMUNOLOGIC DISEASES   231

   Ocular Allergies   231
   Mathea R. Allansmith and Mark B. Abelson

   Mooren's Ulceration   244
   David J. Schanzlin

   Rheumatoid Diseases   249
   Ronald E. Smith and David J. Schanzlin

   Ocular Manifestations of the Nonrheumatic Acquired Collagen Vascular Diseases   264
   C. Stephen Foster

   Corneal Manifestations of Dermatologic Disorders   284
   G. Richard O'Connor

7. DRY EYES   293

   Keratoconjunctivitis Sicca   293
   David W. Lamberts

   Sjögren's Syndrome   309
   Khalid F. Tabbara

8. CORNEAL MANIFESTATIONS OF NEUROLOGIC DISEASES   315
   C. Stephen Foster

9. DYSTROPHIES AND DEGENERATIONS   329
   Gilbert Smolin

10. CONGENITAL ANOMALIES   355
    Fred M. Wilson II

11. METABOLIC DISEASES   371
    Mitchell H. Friedlaender

12. CORNEAL TUMORS   391
    Devron H. Char

13. DIETARY DEFICIENCY   401
    Richard A. Thoft

14. CORNEAL INJURIES   413
    Trauma   413
    Robert G. Webster, Jr.

    Chemical Injuries   422
    James P. McCulley

15. KERATOPLASTY   437
    Therapeutic Keratoplasty   437
    S. Arthur Boruchoff

    Refractive Keratoplasty   453
    David J. Schanzlin and Anthony B. Nesburn

16. CONJUNCTIVAL SURGERY FOR CORNEAL
    DISEASE   465
    Richard A. Thoft

17. THERAPEUTIC SOFT CONTACT LENSES   477
    Richard A. Thoft

INDEX   491

PREFACE

The exponential growth of basic and clinical scientific research on the cornea has created a concomitant growth of information dissemination in the literature and necessitated the increased number of corneal subspecialists. Nearly two years ago the idea for this book began to take shape when it became apparent that there existed no readily accessible textbook that covered in sufficient detail the basic science and clinical information relating to corneal and external disease to warrant purchase by ophthalmic residents, fellows, and clinicians alike. We have addressed this need by preparing a book that is current and provides ready access in one source not only to current diagnosis and treatment but also to basic science fundamentals, to facilitate fuller comprehension of the pathogenesis and etiology of corneal disease, and to encourage thoughtful evaluation of future research findings and new therapies.

Combining the expertise of the faculty and former fellows of the Massachusetts Eye and Ear Infirmary and the Francis I. Proctor Foundation has permitted the editors to select contributors from a large pool of respected specialists whose areas of expertise are complementary. These specialists, despite many other obligations, have committed a great deal of their time and effort to producing their respective chapters. They have selected, from the abundance of materials available, the most relevant and important information in their areas of specialization.

We agree with the diagnostic and therapeutic recommendations made by our contributors in nearly all cases. When we did not concur with them (or, more likely, when we could not agree with one another) the statement is now preceded by "I believe." Such statements are few in number, and we are sure that our readers will agree that they concern issues that are controversial.

Our goal as editors of the book will be met if many of those faced with corneal and external disease problems find this book sufficiently detailed, authoritative, and readable to serve as the primary reference for study and treatment of these disorders.

Gilbert Smolin, M.D.
Richard A. Thoft, M.D.

ACKNOWLEDGMENTS

In addition to our contributors, we wish to express particular thanks to several individuals whose efforts and encouragement have been especially important. On the West Coast, we thank Ruth Lee Thygeson, who assisted in the editing of the book, and Rosalie DeChristopher, who typed the manuscript.

On the East Coast, our thanks go to Judith Friend, who managed to impose order on an otherwise chronically chaotic editorial process, and to Leslie Shepherd, whose work in typing (and retyping) the manuscripts was essential to shaping the Boston contributions.

Finally, we have been extraordinarily lucky in having Kathy O'Brien at Little, Brown as our editor. She has participated enthusiastically in every stage of the book's development, from initial outline preparation to final chapter organization, content, and style. Not only has she refereed discussions wherein firmly held convictions were modified, but she often determined what, in fact, we were trying to say and in so doing helped us to say it better. Kathy has kept this effort on course and we gratefully acknowledge her skill and commitment to this project.

CONTRIBUTING AUTHORS

Mark B. Abelson, M.D.

Assistant Clinical Professor, Department of Ophthalmology, Harvard Medical School; Attending Staff, Cornea Service, Massachusetts Eye and Ear Infirmary, Boston

Mathea R. Allansmith, M.D.

Associate Professor of Ophthalmology, Harvard Medical School; Senior Scientist, Eye Research Institute of Retina Foundation, Boston

Jules Baum

Professor of Ophthalmology, Tufts University School of Medicine; Senior Surgeon in Ophthalmology, New England Medical Center, Boston

S. Arthur Boruchoff, M.D.

Associate Clinical Professor of Ophthalmology, Harvard Medical School; Surgeon in Ophthalmology, Massachusetts Eye and Ear Infirmary, Boston

Eileen M. Burd, B.A.

Director, Ocular Microbiology Laboratory, The Medical College of Wisconsin, Milwaukee

Devron H. Char, M.D.

Associate Professor of Ophthalmology, University of California, San Francisco, School of Medicine; Director, Ocular Oncology Unit, Francis I. Proctor Foundation, San Francisco

Claes H. Dohlman, M.D.

Professor and Chairman, Department of Ophthalmology, Harvard Medical School; Chief of Ophthalmology, Massachusetts Eye and Ear Infirmary, Boston

Richard K. Forster, M.D.

Associate Professor of Ophthalmology, Bascom Palmer Eye Institute, University of Miami School of Medicine, Miami

C. Stephen Foster, M.D.

Associate Professor of Ophthalmology, Harvard Medical School; Director, Immunopathology Laboratory, Eye Research Institute of Retina Foundation; Director, Immunology and Uveitis Unit, Massachusetts Eye and Ear Infirmary, Boston

Mitchell H. Friedlaender, M.D.

Associate Clinical Professor of Ophthalmology, University of California, San Francisco, School of Medicine; Associate Research Ophthalmologist, Francis I. Proctor Foundation, San Francisco

Judith Friend, M.A.

Associate in Ophthalmology, Harvard Medical School; Assistant Scientist, Eye Research Institute of Retina Foundation, Boston

Robert A. Hyndiuk, M.D.

Professor of Ophthalmology, Eye Institute, The Medical College of Wisconsin; Director, Cornea External Unit, Milwaukee County Medical Complex, Milwaukee

Kenneth R. Kenyon, M.D.

Associate Professor of Ophthalmology, Harvard Medical School; Director, Cornea Service, Massachusetts Eye and Ear Infirmary, Boston

David W. Lamberts, M.D.

Associate Professor of Ophthalmology, Texas Tech University School of Medicine; Director of Cornea Service, Department of Ophthalmology and Visual Sciences, Lubbock General Hospital, Lubbock

James P. McCulley, M.D.

Professor and Chairman, Department of Ophthalmology, University of Texas Health Science Center at Dallas Southwestern Medical School; Chief of Service, Parkland Memorial Hospital, Dallas

Kamal F. Nassif, M.D.

Visiting Professor of Ophthalmology, The Medical College of Wisconsin, Milwaukee; Part-time Staff Physician, Department of Ophthalmology, Veterans Administration Hospital, Woods

Anthony B. Nesburn, M.D.

Associate Clinical Professor of Ophthalmology, University of Southern California School of Medicine; Director, Cornea and External Disease Unit, Estelle Doheny Eye Foundation, Los Angeles

G. Richard O'Connor, M.D.

Professor of Ophthalmology, University of California, San Francisco, School of Medicine; Director, Francis I. Proctor Foundation, San Francisco

Jang O. Oh, M.D., Ph.D.

Research Microbiologist, Francis I. Proctor Foundation, San Francisco

Masao Okumoto, M.A.

Specialist, Ophthalmic Microbiology, Francis I. Proctor Foundation, San Francisco

H. Bruce Ostler, M.D.

Clinical Professor of Ophthalmology, University of California, San Francisco, School of Medicine and Francis I. Proctor Foundation, San Francisco

Deborah Pavan-Langston, M.D.

Associate Clinical Professor of Ophthalmology, Harvard Medical School; Associate Surgeon in Ophthalmology, Massachusetts Eye and Ear Infirmary, Boston

David J. Schanzlin, M.D.

Assistant Professor of Ophthalmology, University of Southern California School of Medicine and Estelle Doheny Eye Foundation, Los Angeles

Ronald E. Smith, M.D.

Professor of Ophthalmology, University of Southern California School of Medicine and Estelle Doheny Eye Foundation, Los Angeles

Gilbert Smolin, M.D.

Clinical Professor of Ophthalmology, University of California, San Francisco, School of Medicine; Research Ophthalmologist, Francis I. Proctor Foundation, San Francisco

Khalid F. Tabbara, M.D.

Associate Professor of Ophthalmology, University of California, San Francisco, School of Medicine; Associate Research Ophthalmologist and Director, Heintz Laboratory, Francis I. Proctor Foundation, San Francisco

Richard A. Thoft, M.D.

Associate Professor of Ophthalmology, Harvard Medical School; Associate Chief of Ophthalmology, Massachusetts Eye and Ear Infirmary, Boston

David W. Vastine, M.D.

Chief of Ophthalmology, Highland General Hospital, Oakland; Department of Ophthalmology, Pacific Medical Center, San Francisco

Robert G. Webster, Jr., M.D.

Associate Clinical Professor of Ophthalmology, Pacific Medical Center, San Francisco

John P. Whitcher, M.D.

Assistant Clinical Professor of Ophthalmology, University of California Medical Center; Assistant Research Ophthalmologist, Francis I. Proctor Foundation, San Francisco

Fred M. Wilson II, M.D.

Professor of Ophthalmology and Codirector, Corneal and External Ocular Disease Service, Department of Ophthalmology, Indiana University School of Medicine, Indiana

THE CORNEA

Scientific Foundations and
Clinical Practice

NOTICE

The indications and dosages of all drugs in this book have been recommended in the medical literature and conform to the practices of the general medical community. The medications described do not necessarily have specific approval by the Food and Drug Administration for use in the diseases and dosages for which they are recommended. The package insert for each drug should be consulted for use and dosage as approved by the FDA. Because standards for usage change, it is advisable to keep abreast of revised recommendations, particularly those concerning new drugs.

I. BASIC SCIENCE ASPECTS

1. PHYSIOLOGY

Physiology of the Cornea: CORNEAL EDEMA

Claes H. Dohlman

Edema of the cornea is a major problem in ophthalmology. Only moderately common in occurrence, it can very quickly result in discomfort and marked reduction of vision, and it is frequently bilateral. Fortunately, in the last few decades great therapeutic advances have been made in treating corneal edema as a result of increased understanding of the basic physiology of the regulation of corneal water content, as well as the development of sophisticated diagnostic and therapeutic methods.

Edema of the cornea is the result of excess water in the epithelium, in the stroma, or in both of these layers simultaneously. It is important to consider epithelial edema and stromal edema separately since they arise from somewhat different pathophysiologic mechanisms and have different clinical effects. This section will discuss the normal regulation of corneal hydration, the pathophysiology of a variety of abnormalities that cause edema, and the medical and surgical approaches to the treatment of edema.

REGULATION OF STROMAL HYDRATION

For convenience, the term *stromal hydration* (H) has been used to quantitate the water content of the stroma. Hydration is defined as the weight of water in the stroma, divided by the stroma's dry weight (gm H_2O/gm dry weight). This value is about 3.4 in human and rabbit corneas.

The water content can also be expressed as percentage of water. The normal cornea is 78 percent water. However, a cornea of double normal thickness is about 87 percent water, whereas the H values have gone from 3.4 to 6.8 in the edematous cornea. The advantage of using H is that increases or decreases in hydration are linearly related to the thickness of the cornea, which can be measured clinically.

Regulation of corneal water content depends upon a variety of factors. These include the swelling pressure of the stroma, the barrier function of the epithelium and endothelium, and the water pumping mechanism located in the endothelium. Of lesser importance are the roles of evaporation from the corneal surface and the intraocular pressure. In Figure 1-1, these factors are shown in schematic fashion to indicate that all of them have an influence on the resultant corneal stromal thickness.

STROMAL SWELLING PRESSURE

The corneal stroma normally has a higher water content than most connective tissue elsewhere in the body. This relatively high hydration is ascribed to the water-binding capacity of the proteoglycans that fill the space between the collagen fibrils. The glycosaminoglycans characteristic of the cornea are keratan sulfate and chondroitin sulfate (of varying degrees of sulfation). Together they constitute about 1 percent of the corneal wet weight. These proteoglycans are thought to be responsible for the swelling of the corneal stroma when the endothelium and epithelium are absent. The degree of swelling is related to the parallel and poorly cross-linked configuration of the collagen fibrils, which allows swelling to several times normal thickness.

This tendency to swell has been called the *stromal swelling pressure*. It can be measured by using a manometer to determine the pressure the stroma can overcome yet still imbibe water. A more accurate method of measuring the stromal swelling pressure is to clamp isolated stroma between two glass filters and immerse it in saline. The force generated against the clamps can be converted into the swelling pressure. The swelling pressure has been measured in rabbit, bovine, and human corneal stroma and has been found to be 40 to 50 mm Hg at normal corneal thickness [15, 19, 28]. Although there are other constraints that help determine the ultimate thickness of a swollen cornea, the swelling pressure decreases as the cornea swells (Fig. 1-2). Thus when the stroma has swelled by 50 percent, its swelling pressure has dropped to about a third of its normal value. It is clear that, in vivo, the stromal swelling pressure and the dehydrating mechanism are in constant equilibrium. If dehydration becomes less effective because of trauma or disease, the stroma swells until a new equilibrium is found.

Also apparent from Figure 1-2 is the fact that compression of the stroma is associated with a greatly increased tendency to imbibe water, a feature that

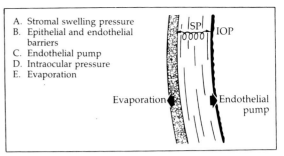

A. Stromal swelling pressure
B. Epithelial and endothelial barriers
C. Endothelial pump
D. Intraocular pressure
E. Evaporation

FIGURE 1-1. *Factors affecting hydration of the cornea. The tendency of the stroma to swell (swelling pressure [SP]) is balanced by the barriers imposed by the epithelium and endothelium, as well as by endothelial pumping. Evaporation plays a minor role, and intraocular pressure (IOP) has almost no effect over a wide range of pressures.*

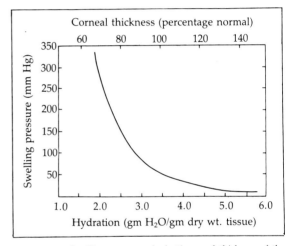

FIGURE 1-2. *Swelling pressure, hydration, and thickness of the cornea. As corneal thickness and hydration increase, the tendency to swell decreases.*

works against the thinning of the cornea by mechanical or physiologic means. The swelling pressure of the stroma therefore tends to set a limit on the minimum thickness of the cornea, while at the same time it tends to swell the cornea beyond its normal thickness.

The swelling pressure is due primarily to the glycosaminoglycans, which have a great tendency to expand their molecular volume [27]. As polyelectrolytes, their fixed negative charges repel each other, causing stretching of the molecules, which thereby occupy a larger volume than uncharged molecules would. In addition, the colloid-osmotic pressure of the tissue also contributes to the swelling pressure to a small degree.

EPITHELIAL AND ENDOTHELIAL BARRIERS

The tendency of the stroma to absorb water and swell must be constantly counteracted to keep the tissue dehydrated and transparent. It is well established that both the epithelium and the endothelium act as barriers to rapid fluid movement [43, 46, 51]. This is accomplished primarily by the high resistance to diffusion of electrolytes rather than by the resistance to water flow across these layers. The resistance of the epithelium to ions is about 2000 times that of the total stroma, and since the movement of ions is therefore restricted, the resulting osmotic pressure tends to retain water in the stroma. The relative thickness of epithelium, stroma, and endothelium is 0.1 : 1.0 : 0.01; the relative resistance to diffusion of electrolytes of these structures is 2,000 : 1.0 : 10.0 [43, 46, 51]. More recently, it has been shown that the barrier properties lie primarily at the level of the surface cells of the epithelium [35]. Thus, the epithelium constitutes an almost perfect semipermeable membrane but one that is quite vulnerable to trauma, inflammatory products, drug toxicity, and contact lens overwear. The single-cell endothelial layer is only slightly more leaky than the epithelium, its resistance to ions being about 10 times higher than that of the total stroma [46].

ENDOTHELIAL PUMP

Eventually the limiting cellular layers could not resist the stromal swelling pressure simply by their impermeability to solutes. In addition, some fluid undoubtedly enters the stroma across the limbus. A constant removal of a small volume of water from the stroma must therefore be postulated, but the mechanism for this dehydration is not entirely clear. The classic temperature reversal experiments showed that corneas will swell at low temperature but will again dehydrate if body temperature is restored [12, 26]. This metabolically related dehydration is blocked by inhibitors of anaerobic glycolysis such as iodoacetate, inhibitors of the respiratory chain of enzymes such as cyanide, inhibitors of Na-K ATPase such as ouabain, and deficiencies of essential nutrients such as oxygen and glucose [46].

Current information clearly identifies the endothelium as the layer across which the water transport takes place. Experimental demonstration of a fluid transport ability of great magnitude clearly implicates the endothelium as the layer responsible for the active dehydration of the cornea [45, 52]. Thus, the endothelium is capable of transporting at least 6.5 ml/cm^2/hour against normal hydrostatic pressure [45]. However, the mechanism by which this metabolic pump operates is not entirely clear. Of several hypotheses, the concept of a bicarbonate

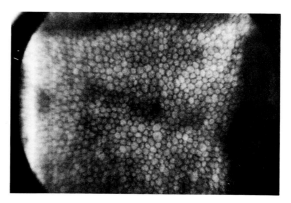

FIGURE 1-3. *Wide-angle specular microscopy showing normal endothelial mosaic. (Courtesy Calvin W. Roberts, M.D.)*

pump is presently in favor. An active transport of bicarbonate by the endothelium has been demonstrated [29, 31], and it may provide the missing link between cell metabolism and endothelial fluid transport. Whatever the exact mechanism, the cornea is definitely dependent on an intact, viable endothelial layer to keep the stroma from swelling excessively (Fig. 1-3).

Transport of certain ions has also been shown to occur across the epithelium. For example, chloride is transported from the stroma to the tear film; this transport is modulated by adenosine 3',5'-cyclic phosphate (cAMP) and stimulated by beta-adrenergic agonists [36]. However, the amount of water transported by this mechanism would be far too small compared with what leaks in to maintain normal hydration [37].

INTRAOCULAR PRESSURE

Intraocular pressure cannot be ignored in considering the fluid dynamics of the cornea. However, in the normal eye, variations in pressure from almost zero to 40 to 50 mm Hg have virtually no influence on stromal thickness and do not create any epithelial edema [63]. On the other hand, when endothelial abnormalities are present, intraocular pressure is an important causal factor in the development of epithelial edema.

EVAPORATION

Evaporation of water from the corneal surface occurs constantly between blinks. The resulting hypertonicity of the tear film causes water to move forward through the cornea to make up for the loss. This evaporation and tear film hypertonicity can have disastrous consequences in the diseased eye, especially if corneal sensation is reduced. In the normal eye, evaporation has no other influence than causing a slight thinning of the cornea during daytime compared with the night when the lids are closed [41]. The healthy cornea with intact innervation protects itself against evaporative damage by registering tear hypertonicity as a slight sting, which in turn elicits a blink to restore isotonicity.

DEVELOPMENT OF EDEMA

TYPES OF EDEMA

As mentioned earlier, epithelial and stromal edema deserve to be discussed separately since their pathophysiology and their influence on vision differ. In most situations, stromal edema precedes epithelial edema but stromal edema is usually symptom-free until epithelial edema occurs. It is only when epithelial edema ensues that vision, and sometimes patient comfort, become severely affected. Understanding of the causal factors involved and the sequence of events is important for clinicians in diagnosis, prognostication, and treatment of corneal edema.

STROMAL EDEMA

Stromal edema results in a thickening of the tissue in proportion to the increase in stromal hydration. The diameter of the collagen fibrils seems to remain the same; the additional fluid accumulates in the interfibrillar space. On swelling, corneal diameter does not change, and no anteriorly directed swelling takes place, as evidenced by the lack of change in the outer corneal radius. Swelling is directed posteriorly, with shortening and folding of Descemet's membrane, producing striae of the posterior surface, for which the clinical term is *striate keratitis*. In later stages a varying degree of scarring can develop in the stroma, particularly in the posterior folds (see Chapter 2, Morphology and Pathologic Response of the Cornea to Disease).

Stromal edema is always caused by the malfunctioning of one or both of the limiting cellular layers. If the epithelium is damaged or removed, tears are imbibed, but the resulting stromal thickening is slight and usually restricted to the tissue just beneath the area of damage. On the other hand, if corresponding damage occurs to the endothelium, the resulting stromal edema is much greater. Injury or disease of the endothelium has two adverse consequences: the loss of the barrier function and interference with the active pump mechanism. This combination of effects accounts for the profound effect of endothelial dysfunction on stromal hydration.

EPITHELIAL EDEMA

In most clinical conditions associated with stromal edema, the endothelium is the site of the primary abnormality. Nevertheless, epithelial involvement can develop nearly immediately; this involvement generally alarms the patient because of decreased vision or pain. Intercellular epithelial edema begins as fluid accumulation between the cells, particularly between the basal cells (Fig. 1-4). Depending on the degree of edema, the size and form of these accumulations vary, in advanced stages developing into blisters typical of bullous keratopathy. As distortion and elevation of the epithelial cells proceeds, interference with maintenance of normal cell permeability may lead to abnormalities of cation pumping, with subsequent development of intracellular edema (Fig. 1-5). This chain of events is quite different from that seen in the metabolic edema found after inappropriate contact lens wear, in which anoxia leads first to a failure of cation pumping and intracellular edema, with virtually no extracellular edema or bullae formation (see Chapter 17, Therapeutic Soft Contact Lenses).

The pathophysiology of epithelial edema differs to some extent from that of stromal edema. Epithelial edema is not only related to the state of the endothelium, but is also dependent upon intraocular pressure [63]. In fact, fluid accumulates in the epithelium only when the intraocular pressure has overcome the endothelial pump pressure and there is a forward bulk flow of fluid toward the epithelium. Owing to the great resistance to the movement of water across the anterior portion of the epithelium, the fluid is trapped primarily in the posterior or midportion of this layer, resulting in the clinical signs of epithelial edema. Thus, epithelial edema can occur with normal endothelial function but very high intraocular pressure (e.g., in acute glaucoma), with poorly functioning endothelium but normal pressure (e.g., Fuchs' dystrophy), or with a combination of both factors. Under any circumstance, intraocular pressure is the driving force; in phthisis with pressure near zero, no matter how damaged the endothelium is, epithelial edema never occurs.

Evaporation can have a considerable influence on epithelial edema, with almost no effect on stromal edema. It is a well-known clinical phenomenon that, in the early stages of epithelial edema, vision is worst in the morning after a night's lid closure and absence of evaporation from the ocular surface. As the day goes on, however, fluid is extracted from the epithelium because the tear film is intermittently made hyperosmotic by evaporation between blinks, and vision gradually clears. Sometimes epithelial edema is visible only in the upper part of the

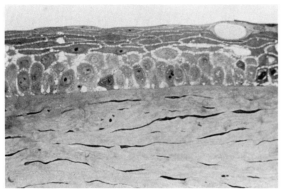

FIGURE 1-4. *Intercellular edema. This accumulation of fluid between the cells is frequently the result of endothelial damage.* (×500.)

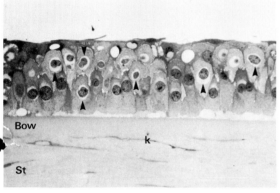

FIGURE 1-5. *Intracellular edema* (arrows) *occurs as the result of distortion of cell walls by edema fluid or by abnormalities of cation pumping.* (×500.) (Bow = Bowman's layer, St = stroma, k = keratocyte) (Courtesy Yasuo Ishii, M.D.)

cornea, where the upper lid permanently prevents evaporation. In more advanced edema, however, fluid flows into the epithelial layers so fast that evaporation does not clear the epithelium of excess fluid.

EFFECT ON VISUAL ACUITY

The transparency of the normal cornea is not readily explained in terms of geometric optics [47]. Rather, it has been proposed that the fluctuations in refractive index across the stroma and the cellular layers are so small that scattering of light is kept to a minimum. It is known from the field of optics that if such refractive index heterogeneities are distanced less than half the wavelength of light (about 2000 Å) apart, transparency is preserved. Normally, the collagen fibrils of the cornea are closer together than half the wavelength of light, satisfying this criterion for transparency. However, theoretically, abnormal

fluid accumulation between the fibrils should increase light scattering and decrease transparency. In support of this theory, such fluid accumulations with dimensions far greater than the wavelength of light can be seen in edema, not only in the corneal epithelium but also in the stroma, where irregular collections can form, especially around the keratocytes [22].

Epithelial and stromal edema differ in their effect on visual acuity, as already mentioned, with stromal edema far less important. A moderate swelling of the stroma without epithelial involvement has little influence on vision. For example, when bovine stroma is excised and evenly hydrated, a transparency equivalent to 20/30 vision still persists at a 60 percent increase in thickness [64]. However, later in the development of chronic edema, stromal scarring and posterior irregular astigmatism from the Descemet's folds result in more marked reduction of vision.

Epithelial edema, in contrast, affects vision early. The patient may report either colored haloes around lights or decreased acuity even though the edema can be seen only with the slit lamp. The reasons for this early and profound effect on vision are twofold: increased light scattering within and between the epithelial cells themselves, and, even more important, the microscopic irregularity of the surface. This latter effect can be thought of as conversion of the optically smooth epithelium into a mosaic of fine irregularities, each of which tends to refract the light rays that impinge on it in a different direction. The retinal image produced by such multiple refracting surface elements is not only blurred but is also characterized by color separation because of prismatic effects.

PATHOLOGIC PROCESSES LEADING TO EDEMA

Most causes of corneal edema have a direct adverse effect on the endothelial layer. These causes include inflammation, endothelial dystrophies, keratoconus, and trauma. Elevated intraocular pressure alone can also lead to edema, although the stromal component is much less prominent than the epithelial portion in this case. The basic pathophysiology of each of these conditions is described in the following paragraphs.

INFLAMMATION

Corneal edema can accompany any severe inflammation of the anterior segment. Unidentified inflammatory mediators or inflammatory cells seem to interfere with endothelial cell function in a manner that can be localized or generalized, reversible or irreversible. Certainly, the presence of keratitic precipitates (KP) on the surface of the endothelium would be expected to interfere with the metabolically active fluid pump. Even in herpetic keratouveitis the endothelium might be expected to suffer by being covered in part by inflammatory cells. This adverse influence of inflammatory cells and possible mediators of inflammation is probably the cause of corneal edema in acute herpes zoster or herpes simplex, bacterial and fungal infection, and some forms of uveitis.

However, the relationship of corneal edema to uveitis is a peculiar one. Chronic uveitis (e.g., rheumatic or idiopathic) can exist for years or decades without corneal damage, despite the intermittent presence of abundant KP on the back of the cornea. One can postulate that there are inflammatory mediators whose adverse effect on the endothelium is greater than that of the physical presence of KP.

The mechanism by which disciform edema in herpes simplex occurs may also depend in some way on humoral influences. Certainly, the development of such edema appears to be secondary to immunologic processes. Observations supporting such a pathogenesis include the presence in the stroma of remnants of herpes virus that might serve as antigens, the presence of lymphocytes, and the remarkable therapeutic effect of steroids. How this immunologic process leads to dysfunction of the endothelium is unknown. The development of stromal edema is so common in herpes simplex infection that the finding of edema with or without uveitis in one eye, the other being normal, must always lead to the consideration of herpes as the cause, even in the absence of a history of epithelial or stromal disease.

CORNEAL GRAFT REACTION

Immunologic graft rejection is a form of inflammation. After the recipient's immune system is triggered, lymphocytes can find their way to the corneal graft and attack its cells. Although rejection of both epithelial and stromal cells can occur, involvement of these two cell layers does not produce corneal edema. Rather, it is the damage to the endothelium that leads to edema of the graft (but not of the surrounding host cornea) and reduced vision [42]. In the early massive rejection of a graft in a vascularized recipient cornea, the lymphocytes appear to escape from the graft wound and migrate to the posterior surface, forming a line that slowly ad-

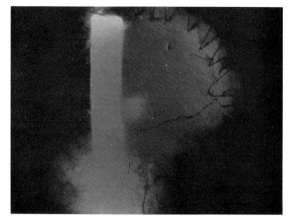

FIGURE 1-6. *Immunologic graft reaction showing a line of keratitic precipitates (Khodadoust line) on the endothelial surface.*

vances toward the center of the cornea, destroying the endothelium in the process [34] (Fig. 1-6). Edema is initially localized to the overlying area. Later (about 3 months after surgery) a rejection line is rarely seen, and damage takes a more diffuse form, with numerous KP and uniform graft edema. Presumably the lymphocytes derive from the iris via the aqueous in this form (see Chapter 3, Immunology).

ENDOTHELIAL DYSTROPHIES

FUCHS' DYSTROPHY

In 1910 Ernst Fuchs described the dystrophy that bears his name [21]. At that time only the epithelial manifestations of the advanced stage were recognized. Decades later it was realized that this form of dystrophy stems from a primary malfunction of the endothelium rather than of the epithelium (see Chapter 9, Dystrophies and Degenerations).

The first clinical sign of Fuchs' dystrophy is the appearance of guttata in the slit lamp when using specular reflection of the Descemet's membrane region (Fig. 1-7). The appearance, which has been likened to beaten silver or orange peel, begins centrally in both corneas. Sometimes a diffuse, golden brown pigmentation of the central posterior surface is also seen. Specular microscopy reveals decreased cell density, irregular-sized cells, and dark spots that presumably correspond to the guttate lesions [2]. Histologically the endothelial cells show degeneration and deposition of abnormal Descemet's membrane material to form the wartlike excrescences on the posterior surface of that membrane. The cells gradually thin over these prominences, and, on further deterioration, the apical junctions break up, which readily explains the concomitant decline in the barrier function of the endothelial layer.

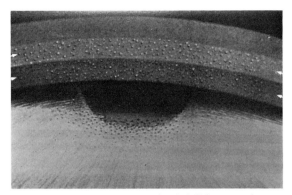

FIGURE 1-7. *Artist's conception of endothelial guttate changes. Posterior corneal surface shows the guttate changes seen in Fuchs' dystrophy* (white arrows).

The guttata often appear in early middle life and progress very slowly. In early stages there is no epithelial edema, and visual acuity is usually 20/30 or better. It is difficult to predict the rate of development of edema based merely on the guttate appearance in the slit lamp. Large and widespread guttate lesions may be compatible with many years of good vision. Thus, there can be a considerable discrepancy between the anatomic appearance (extent of guttata) and endothelial function. The degree of stromal edema (measured by pachometry) is the most reliable indicator of how close the cornea has come to the stage of epithelial edema. Such measurements are particularly important if surgery (e.g., cataract extraction) may be needed in the future.

Sooner or later, often decades after the guttate appearance was first observed, epithelial edema gradually develops, first as a fine bedewing and later as frank bullae. The edema begins centrally in the optical zone, and vision fails rapidly. Characteristically, vision is worse in the morning owing to the lack of evaporation from the tear film during sleep. Eventually the benefit of better vision late in the day is lost, the epithelium becomes more bullous, and photophobia or pain develops. Finally, in long-standing severe edema, connective tissue is formed between epithelium and stroma; at this point discomfort has disappeared, but vision has dropped to hand movements. This end stage is now less commonly encountered, since the natural history of the disease is usually interrupted by therapeutic measures.

Fuchs' dystrophy with epithelial edema is a relatively rare disease, although firm epidemiologic data on its frequency are lacking. Familial transmission of the disease is rare, but a dominant inheritance pattern has been reported [10]. Cataract and glaucoma are slightly more common in patients with Fuchs' dystrophy than in the general population, but there are no known systemic abnormalities.

CONGENITAL HEREDITARY ENDOTHELIAL DYSTROPHY

Congenital hereditary endothelial dystrophy (CHED) is an entity distinctly different from Fuchs' dystrophy. In CHED, the corneas are already hazy at birth. They are often extremely swollen, but epithelial edema is minimal. Keratoplasty specimens show markedly degenerated endothelium; sometimes this layer is almost absent. There is no vascularization or other signs of inflammation. Since the disease is already present at birth, deep amblyopia, nystagmus, and esotropia commonly occur. Also, glaucoma is not uncommon in severe cases (see Chapter 10, Congenital Anomalies).

CHED is autosomally hereditary, and both dominant and recessive forms have been reported. In the dominant form, the corneas are often less cloudy at birth, but the disease is still progressive. Because of the severity of this disease and the limited success of therapy for it, genetic counseling is advised.

CHANDLER'S SYNDROME

Chandler's syndrome is a rare ocular disease manifested by essential iris atrophy (often with distortion of the pupil), glaucoma, and corneal edema [8]. The condition is always unilateral and easy to diagnose. Fine guttata are visible early in the course of the disease, and peripheral anterior synechiae develop from an abnormal endothelial membrane that grows over the angle and the iris [6]. The corneal stroma is not very swollen, and the epithelial edema characteristically appears as a fine bedewing of the whole cornea (in contrast to Fuchs' dystrophy, in which the edema begins centrally). There is no evidence of a genetic basis in Chandler's syndrome. The Cogan-Reese syndrome seems to be a variant of Chandler's syndrome in that it exhibits similar characteristics, plus nevi, heterochromia, and ectropion uveae (see Chapter 9, Dystrophies and Degenerations).

KERATOCONUS

In a minority of patients with keratoconus, usually in those with advanced thinning, Descemet's membrane can suddenly break centrally. The edges roll up and aqueous enters the area, which is now devoid of endothelium, thus creating massive edema. The endothelium soon heals, presumably by cells sliding in and covering the defect, and the edema is cleared within 2 months. The edema usually leaves a small stromal scar, which is often located slightly eccentric to the visual axis. There is no treatment of this temporary edema, although a soft lens may ameliorate discomfort. Frequently the patient regains the vision he had before the episode.

TRAUMA

INTRAOCULAR SURGERY

Cataract extraction is the most frequent type of surgery associated with corneal endothelial cell damage. Currently, more than 400,000 cataract extractions are performed annually in the United States. In about a quarter of them, an intraocular lens is also inserted. The incidence of irreversible corneal edema after cataract surgery is not known with certainty; however, recent data compiled by the Food and Drug Administration have indicated an incidence of about 1 percent [62]. Also, many patients who developed edema postoperatively show guttate changes in the other eye, which suggests the presence of preoperative endothelial dystrophy in the edematous eye. This also explains why so many patients develop edema in both eyes after bilateral surgery.

It is often hard to pinpoint in retrospect what maneuver has damaged the endothelium during a seemingly uneventful and successful cataract extraction. Some damage is probably unavoidable and can be detected only by sophisticated methods such as specular microscopy. The average postoperative cell loss in clinically successful cases, as measured by specular microscopy, is less than 20 percent [60]. In less experienced hands, cataract surgery commonly results in some permanent increase in stromal thickness as well, but usually short of epithelial edema and without interference with vision [48]. When a polymethylmethacrylate intraocular lens is inserted, flat contact between the plastic material and the endothelium can result in surface adhesion and subsequent rupture of the posterior cell walls, resulting in widespread damage [4].

In the postoperative period, vitreous touch to the cornea can be another cause of edema. If the vitreous is solid and adhering to the corneal back surface, stromal swelling over the affected area, followed by total decompensation, can occur. On the other hand, loose vitreous, even filling the whole anterior chamber, is not likely to cause corneal decompensation. In fact, the role of vitreous contact in causing corneal edema seems to have been overestimated [3].

OTHER TRAUMA

Any injury, if severe enough, can cause either immediate or delayed corneal edema. In perforating injuries, permanent edema is common. Of interest is the slit lamp appearance of the eye after blunt trauma. The posterior surface can show temporary guttata indistinguishable from the permanent guttata of Fuchs' dystrophy [39]. After a few days these temporary guttata usually disappear, and there are no further consequences. However, this phenomenon raises questions about the exact anatomic nature of what is seen in the slit lamp as guttata.

ELEVATED INTRAOCULAR PRESSURE

In contrast to the clinical conditions described above, increased intraocular pressure does not directly injure the endothelium. However, elevation of pressure, especially acutely, may overwhelm the fluid transport mechanism of the endothelium, resulting in a bulk flow of aqueous into the stroma. The fluid separates and elevates the epithelial cells, giving rise to epithelial edema very soon after the pressure elevation.

The most striking condition producing corneal changes as a result of intraocular pressure elevation is acute glaucoma. A patient with epithelial edema, normal stromal thickness, pain, narrow chamber angles, and a fixed, semidilated pupil does not pose any diagnostic difficulties. Usually a pressure of more than 60 mm Hg is found. On normalization of the pressure, the epithelial edema clears very rapidly. However, in rare circumstances with longstanding high pressure, irreversible endothelial damage can occur and result in chronic edema.

Even mild elevation of pressure can lead to corneal edema in the presence of preexistent endothelial damage. Such vulnerability of the cornea can occur after cataract extraction or trauma or as a result of partial endothelial loss following endothelial graft reaction. Lowering the intraocular pressure usually eliminates the edema. However, in the long run, progressive deterioration of the endothelium often gradually lowers the pressure level above which epithelial edema occurs. Finally the edema becomes irreversible, even when ocular pressure is normal.

Even in open-angle glaucoma, stromal thickness is slightly increased, although it does not produce clinically detectable edema [13].

CLINICAL EVALUATION OF THE ENDOTHELIUM

Until recently, evaluation of the corneal endothelium was limited to biomicroscopic examination for guttata, folds, or KP. Such limited observation made it difficult to evaluate endothelial function and functional reserve, to predict the future course of a disease, or to determine the eye's ability to withstand surgery. It is also difficult by mere slit lamp examination to compare the relative merits of different surgical procedures or to diagnose drug toxicity in terms of endothelial damage. More recently, however, better techniques for in vivo evaluation of the endothelium have been introduced or simplified. These include specular microscopy, pachometry, and fluorophotometry. Endothelial morphology, pump function, and permeability characteristics can be quantitated with these aids, although there are still problems with accuracy, simplicity, and interpretation.

SPECULAR MICROSCOPY

The introduction of specular microscopy made possible the direct visual inspection of the endothelium [44] (see Fig. 1-3). Further development of the instrumentation [4, 40] has made in vivo observation relatively easy and permitted valuable clinical correlations. Noncontact and wide-angle instruments (encompassing a field of over 1 mm^2) have added versatility to this technique [30, 38].

The cells of the human corneal endothelium seem to have no ability to divide after birth. Therefore, any injury, mechanical or inflammatory, to this cellular layer heals only by the sliding, rearrangement, and enlargement of existing cells (see Chapter 2, Morphology and Pathologic Response of the Cornea to Disease). A large number of cells in the area around the defect are affected by this migration. Finally, new cell junctions are formed, and the dehydrating function of the endothelium regains its full efficiency. If the total cell loss is too great, however, irreversible corneal edema may result, although the critical cell density below which edema occurs is not well known.

The normal endothelial cell count is 3000 to 3500 cells per square millimeter in the young adult, decreasing to about two-thirds of that value in old age. This decrease in number is coupled with increased cell size and pleomorphism [4]. Drastic cell loss, to less than 400 cells per square millimeter, has been observed with clear corneal grafts. On the other hand, many cases of edema have a much higher cell count. In general, it has proved impossible to predict physiologic function merely on the basis of endothelial cell density and morphology [57].

Endothelial disease and trauma can be followed quite accurately with specular microscopy. Thus, in early Fuchs' dystrophy, endothelial abnormalities and Descemet's membrane excrescences can be diagnosed by specular microscopy before they be-

come visible by slit lamp observation [2]. The guttate excrescenses are seen as irregular dark areas where the endothelial cell contours cannot be distinguished (Fig. 1-8). Similarly, larger or smaller KP deposited on the endothelium can be readily observed by specular microscopy, and any gradual cell loss can be followed [54].

Specular microscopy has its greatest value in determining the relative trauma to the endothelium resulting from various surgical procedures, particularly cataract extraction techniques, intraocular lens implantations, and penetrating keratoplasty. Most studies indicate that uncomplicated intracapsular cataract extraction causes only minor cell loss (4–21 percent) [60]. Phacoemulsification is more traumatic, according to most accounts, and intraocular lens implantation can result in a very marked cell loss. These observations have led to substantial improvements in surgical technique and greater care in treating the endothelium. For instance, specular microscopy has proven the protective value of introducing sodium hyaluronate into the anterior chamber during intraocular lens implantation [49].

Using specular microscopy, corneal transplantation can also be evaluated in terms of endothelial cell loss during and after the surgery. Several studies have reported mean cell counts in clear grafts to be about 1000 to 2000 cells per square millimeter. As would be expected, a graft into a recipient with abnormal endothelium in edema undergoes greater cell loss than does a graft into a cornea with normal endothelium (e.g., in keratoconus) [11]. Specular microscopy may also find routine use in the in vitro evaluation of endothelial quality in donor tissue for keratoplasty [54, 55]. In general, this valuable technique will undoubtedly continue to be applied to studies of surgical procedures, corneal dystrophies and inflammations, and drug toxicity. In addition, specular microscopy may be a useful clinical tool for the routine evaluation of many patients.

PACHOMETRY

Since corneal swelling occurs only in the posterior direction, and since stromal hydration is regulated by the endothelium, it follows that measurement of corneal thickness should be an accurate indicator of endothelial function. Corneal (or stromal) thickness can be measured with an optical device called a pachometer, using a technique that was made practical after World War II [50]. In spite of later simplifications and marketing of slit lamp–attached

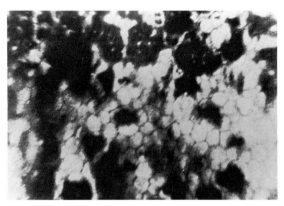

FIGURE 1-8. *Fuchs' dystrophy. The presence of guttata interferes with the normal imaging of the endothelial cells overlying the guttata. In advanced cases of Fuchs' dystrophy, the endothelial cells may be absent over the guttata. (Courtesy Calvin W. Roberts, M.D.)*

units, the technique is not as frequently used in routine ophthalmology as it should be, mainly because a good deal of practice is required to obtain reliable readings. With skill, the reading error is about ± 2 percent. New devices based on ultrasound and specular microscopy principles may eventually surpass the present split-image optical pachometer in accuracy. Such accuracy is of great importance in the performance of radial keratotomy, in which the depth of the corneal incision is determined by pachometry before the operation (see Refractive Keratoplasty in Chapter 15, Keratoplasty).

Measuring corneal thickness is often a useful maneuver when subclinical edema is suspected in the presence of guttata or after disease or surgery. The normal thickness is about 0.50 mm; a higher value indicates some endothelial dysfunction. Epithelial edema, with consequent decrease in vision, usually does not occur until the cornea has swelled to a thickness of 0.65 to 0.75 mm, provided the intraocular pressure is normal. If the pressure is elevated, epithelial edema occurs at lesser thicknesses [63]. The value of pachometry lies in estimating the functional reserve of the endothelium in a clear cornea: A reading close to 0.50 mm is reassuring for the future, whereas one around 0.70 mm means borderline decompensation and risk of imminent epithelial edema.

FLUOROPHOTOMETRY
A technique that allows measurements of fluorescein exchange between cornea and aqueous humor

can be utilized to determine endothelial permeability [53]. The fluorescein can be ingested, injected intravenously, or driven into the corneal stroma from the surface by means of iontophoresis, and the diffusion across the endothelium can be followed. In this way it has been shown that patients with guttata and some corneal thickness increase also have increased permeability to fluorescein, suggesting that in early Fuchs' dystrophy swelling is due to a breakdown of the barrier function rather than to a low endothelial pump rate [5]. Fluorophotometry definitely offers promise for the future as a useful diagnostic tool.

MEDICAL TREATMENT OF EDEMA
Nonsurgical treatment of corneal edema can be directed toward improving endothelial function itself, or toward either reducing epithelial edema or making such edema less troublesome for the patient. Reduction of stromal or anterior chamber inflammation, for example, is thought to reestablish more normal endothelial function. On the other hand, the use of hypertonic agents for epithelial dehydration and the application of a soft contact lens both serve to overcome the adverse consequences of epithelial edema. Depending upon the particular underlying disease state, any of these maneuvers may serve to make more complex surgical therapy unnecessary.

SUPPRESSION OF INFLAMMATION
When endothelial function is compromised as a result of inflammation in the cornea itself or in the anterior chamber, the use of topical corticosteroids may be considered. Corneal edema secondary to a variety of diseases, including traumatic keratouveitis, infectious keratouveitis as seen in herpes simplex, and immunologic corneal graft reaction, frequently responds to such therapy. Most practitioners feel that severe keratouveitis in the presence of known herpes simplex is an indication for the use of corticosteroids. However, active viral proliferation is usually a contraindication for topical steroid use, although systemic steroids may still be used when severe uveitis is present [32] (see Herpetic Diseases in Chapter 5, Infectious Diseases).

In obscure cases without a clear history of herpetic infections, a trial of topical steroids (e.g., 0.1% dexamethasone drops 5 times daily) may be carried out for 2 weeks, which should be enough time to indicate whether the edema is reversible or not. Smaller doses of antivirals and antibiotics may be added prophylactically.

REDUCTION OF INTRAOCULAR PRESSURE
Since it is intraocular pressure that pushes fluid into the epithelium, causing epithelial edema, it makes

sense to try to reduce the pressure. However, in most cases of chronic edema the pressure is normal and the usual antiglaucomatous medications have little effect.

The most effective use of pressure reduction is in the case of marginally compensated corneal grafts, where even mildly elevated pressure can cause epithelial edema. A parallel condition is that seen in the endothelial dystrophies, such as Chandler's syndrome, in which a very modest reduction in pressure can restore good visual acuity.

The reduction of high pressure in acute glaucoma is also followed by prompt reduction of epithelial edema. In this case, of course, the endothelium may not be at fault, except that it cannot transport the much greater bulk of fluid that is forced across the posterior boundary.

To date, there are no known medications or maneuvers that can directly stimulate the rate of endothelial fluid transport. However, some attention is being given to determining whether or not the endothelium has a variable rate of pumping and whether or not this rate can be accelerated by cellular stimulation.

HYPERTONIC AGENTS

Since epithelial edema is reduced somewhat by evaporation during waking hours, it is not surprising that hypertonic solutions instilled in the eye have similar effects. This treatment was introduced in 1942 [9]. Since that time, 5% sodium chloride drops 3 or 4 times per day and sodium chloride ointment of the same strength at night has been the therapeutic mainstay. The exact dosage regimen can be determined by the patient himself according to the severity of his symptoms. Anhydrous glycerol is useful for clearing the cornea of epithelial edema before gonioscopy but is too painful for routine use.

Other methods can be used to dehydrate the epithelium. Hot, dry air from a hair dryer held at arm's length can be quite helpful in clearing early morning epithelial edema, although care must be taken not to irritate the ocular surface by overdoing the treatment. Regardless of which technique is chosen to render the precorneal tear film hypertonic and thereby extract water from the epithelium, many patients with irreversible epithelial edema benefit from this type of osmotherapy for months or even years.

Hypertonic agents are not useful in reducing stromal edema. The reason is that stromal water volume is quite large compared with the tear volume, so that hypertonicity of the tear film can extract only a small amount of stromal fluid, which is readily replenished from the aqueous across the leaky endothelium.

SOFT CONTACT LENSES

As mentioned earlier, advanced corneal edema with large bullae can be quite painful, and hypertonic agents may have no ameliorating effect. If comfort, rather than vision, is the objective in such cases, a hydrophilic soft contact lens can be tried (see Chapter 17, Therapeutic Soft Contact Lenses). Thus, for an elderly person with good vision in the other eye, there is no need for keratoplasty, and a soft lens in the uncomfortable edematous eye can be quite successful. The lens should not be too thin and flimsy but rather rigid, and it should be left in the eye around the clock. Vision may become slightly worse, but the objective of comfort is achieved in about three-quarters of the cases [14]. Topical antibiotics (e.g., 0.5% chloramphenicol drops 1–3 times daily) may be given during the first few weeks, although the value of this prophylaxis is not proven. The lenses can remain in place for months without cleaning. The incidence of infection is very small, less than 1 percent (Fig. 1-9).

SURGICAL TREATMENT OF EDEMA

PENETRATING KERATOPLASTY

When corneal edema has reached an irreversible state with markedly reduced vision and perhaps pain, keratoplasty is often the treatment of choice. It was not always so, with the first successful transplants in edema reported only in 1952 [59]. Since that time progress has been rapid, owing to the use of larger grafts, greater attention to the endothelium, the availability of corticosteroids, and finer suture material [1]. Today the majority of people with severe corneal edema uncomplicated by other disease can be helped by surgery (see Chapter 15, Keratoplasty). However, some specific features of corneal edema warrant special consideration when keratoplasty is contemplated.

The indications for keratoplasty in edema cannot be stated with complete precision. However, in a patient with bilateral edema and visual acuity between 20/80 and 20/200, it is reasonable to graft the worse eye, especially if the condition has been rapidly deteriorating. If the visual acuity in the better eye is still 20/50 or better, surgery in the opposite eye can be postponed. If the better eye is completely normal, no surgery is indicated, especially if the patient is elderly and would not be expected to tolerate a contact lens or aniseikonia well. If the edematous cornea is painful, a permanent soft contact lens is usually a less complicated therapy than keratoplasty. Finally, if the patient has only one remaining eye, it is prudent to postpone keratoplasty until vi-

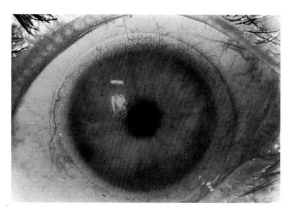

FIGURE 1-9. *A large soft contact lens can improve comfort in bullous keratopathy but does not improve vision in most cases.*

sion has fallen to 20/200 to 20/400. Needless to say, the patient's age and occupation, as well as any extracorneal pathologic conditions, will influence the decision concerning if and when to operate.

The presence of a significant cataract in addition to the corneal edema is normally an indication for the combined procedure of keratoplasty and cataract extraction. If the cornea exhibits only guttata and stromal swelling but no epithelial edema, standard intracapsular cataract extraction without transplantation is recommended. Even a borderline decompensated cornea often shows an unexpected resiliency and can remain clear for many years. Intraocular lens implantation in combination with keratoplasty for edema and cataract extraction (triple procedure) must be expected to entail a larger risk of damage to the graft endothelium, although several studies have disclosed remarkably good short-term results [61]. At present, it seems reasonable to reserve this procedure for situations in which preoperative hyperopia in combination with the aphakia would otherwise require an unacceptably high plus correction in glasses or contact lenses.

The keratoplasty technique for edema is the same as for other corneal diseases, except that a large graft (which carries a larger number of donor endothelial cells) is of greater importance than in situations in which the recipient's endothelium is normal. My technique for edema uses an 8.2- or 8.5-mm donor button, punched from the endothelial side on a silicone block. An 8.0-mm trephine is used for the recipient. In the elderly aphakic patient with a deep anterior chamber and massive corneal edema, a 9.0-mm graft into an 8.5-mm recipient opening might be recommended.

Postoperatively, the treatment relies heavily on the use of topical steroids to prevent an immune graft reaction. A substantial number of patients with edema are also aphakic, providing the surgeon with the opportunity to use more corticosteroids without causing a cataract [18]. In aphakic edema cases, I prefer to give steroids (0.1% dexamethasone drops) topically at the conclusion of the surgery and every 2 to 3 hours for the first day, and then taper the dosage over a period of a month or so to once daily. Most important, this once-daily regimen should be continued for the rest of the patient's life. Eyes that have been inflamed in the past may require a more intense steroid regimen.

Keratoplasty in uncomplicated edema now achieves clear grafts in 70 to 90 percent of cases [20], although some cases exhibit late failure many years postoperatively. Vascularization of the recipient cornea worsens the prognosis moderately, whereas chronic uveitis has a drastically unfavorable influence. Grafts in aphakia have slightly better expectations than do grafts in phakic eyes, probably because in aphakia the endothelium is usually protected during suturing by loose vitreous whereas in phakic eyes it is rubbed against the bulging iris. Keratoplasty for edema in children has notoriously poor prognosis, although encouraging results have been presented recently [58].

OTHER SURGICAL PROCEDURES

With the rising success rate of keratoplasty in edema and with the introduction of soft contact lenses for comfort, other surgical techniques are being employed less frequently. A total conjunctival flap is effective in eliminating all pain caused by bullous keratopathy and still is occasionally indicated in an elderly patient with a good opposite eye and difficulty in tolerating a soft contact lens [24, 25] (see Chapter 16, Conjunctival Surgery for Corneal Disease). The disadvantages of a total conjunctival flap are poor vision (usually finger counting), a poor appearance, and difficulty in examining deeper structures postoperatively.

Cautery of the corneal surface is another procedure aimed at providing comfort in painful edema. A large number of mild diathermy burns are applied to the whole surface, resulting in subepithelial scarring and marked corneal anesthesia [56]. A drawback of such cautery is the persistent epithelial defect that frequently follows it.

Several experimental and surgical procedures of considerable theoretical interest have been suggested for the amelioration of massive corneal edema. One approach has been to remove the edematous epithelium and bond a large polymethylmethacrylate contact lens to the basement membrane with the aid of cyanoacrylate adhesive applied peripherally. This greatly improves vision; however, in the long run, the bond loosens and the epithelium finds an opening to grow back in and cause irritation and diminution of vision. Another procedure utilizes a transparent, water-impermeable membrane, implanted intrastromally or attached to the posterior surface, that acts as a barrier to aqueous inflow. The cornea anterior to the membrane dehydrates, but interference with the supply routes of nutrients from the aqueous to the cornea causes frequent complications [16]. Finally, through-and-through keratoprostheses have been tried in corneal edema [7]. They have usually consisted of a methylmethacrylate stem attached to a supporting plate that anchors the device in the stroma. The advantage of these techniques is rapid restoration of very good vision, but complications are frequent and often severe. Ulceration around the stem can cause leaks, extrusion, infection, and retinal detachment [17]. In general, the procedures described have remained experimental owing to the rapid advances of corneal allografting.

Recent research in the surgical treatment of corneal edema has taken a more biologic turn and has explored the possibility of replacing malfunctioning endothelium with new cells that have been grown in tissue culture [33]. Cultured endothelial cells can be made to adhere in vitro to the denuded Descemet's membrane of a graft, and the cells coalesce and rearrange themselves into a layer indistinguishable from normal endothelium. Such a graft can be transplanted in the normal way and remain clear, indicating satisfactory dehydrating function of the new endothelium [23]. It even seems possible to grow noncorneal cells (e.g., vascular endothelium) from the recipient and make them function as a new corneal endothelium, thus possibly bypassing the otherwise severely limiting transplantation immunity problem. Undoubtedly these interesting techniques have great potential for the future.

REFERENCES

1. Abbott, R. L., and Forster, R. K. Determinants of graft clarity in penetrating keratoplasty. *Arch. Ophthalmol.* 97:1071, 1979.
2. Bigar, F., Schimmelpfenning, B., and Hurzeler, R. Cornea guttata in donor material. *Arch. Ophthalmol.* 96:653, 1978.
3. Boruchoff, S. A. Keratoplasty. In G. Spaeth (Ed.), *Ophthalmic Surgery.* Philadelphia: Saunders, in press.
4. Bourne, W. M., and Kaufman, H. E. Specular microscopy of human corneal endothelium in vivo. *Am. J. Ophthalmol.* 81:319, 1976.
5. Burns, R. R., Bourne, W. M., and Brubaker, R. F. Endothelial function in patients with cornea guttata. *Invest. Ophthalmol. Vis. Sci.* 20:77, 1981.
6. Campbell, D. B., Shields, M. B., and Smith, T. R. The corneal endothelium and the spectrum of essential iris atrophy. *Am. J. Ophthalmol.* 86:317, 1978.
7. Castroviejo, R., Cardona, H., and DeVoe, A. G. Present status of prosthokeratoplasty. *Am. J. Ophthalmol.* 68:613, 1969.
8. Chandler, P. A. Atrophy of the stroma of the iris, endothelial dystrophy, corneal edema and glaucoma. *Am. J. Ophthalmol.* 41:607, 1956.
9. Cogan, D. G., and Kinsey, V. E. The cornea: V. Physiologic aspects. *Arch. Ophthalmol.* 28:661, 1942.
10. Cross, H. E., Maumenee, A. E., and Cantolino, S. J. Inheritance of Fuchs' endothelial dystrophy. *Arch. Ophthalmol.* 85:268, 1971.
11. Culbertson, W., Forster, R., and Abbott, R. Endothelial cell loss in penetrating keratoplasty. *Ophthalmology* (Rochester). In press.
12. Davson, H. The hydration of the cornea. *Biochem. J.* 59:24, 1955.
13. DeCevallos, E., Dohlman, C. H., and Reinhart, W. J. Corneal thickness in glaucoma. *Ann. Ophthalmol.* 8:177, 1976.
14. Dohlman, C. H., Boruchoff, S. A., and Mobilia, E. F. Complications in the use of soft contact lenses in corneal disease. *Arch. Ophthalmol.* 90:267, 1973.
15. Dohlman, C. H., Hedbys, B. O., and Mishima, S. The swelling pressure of the corneal stroma. *Invest. Ophthalmol.* 1:158, 1962.
16. Dohlman, C. H., Brown, S. I., and Martola, E. L. Replacement of endothelium with alloplastic materials: A new technique in corneal surgery. *Trans. Am. Acad. Ophthalmol. Otolaryngol.* 71:851, 1967.
17. Dohlman, C. H., Schneider, H. A., and Doane, M. G. Prosthokeratoplasty. *Am. J. Ophthalmol.* 77:694, 1974.
18. Donshik, P. C., et al. Posterior subcapsular cataracts induced by topical corticosteroids following keratoplasty for keratoconus. *Ann. Ophthalmol.* 12:29, 1981.
19. Fatt, I., and Goldstick, T. K. Dynamics of water transport in swelling membranes. *J. Colloidoidal Sci.* 20:434, 1965.
20. Fine, M., and West, C. E. Late results of keratoplasty for Fuchs' dystrophy. *Am. J. Ophthalmol.* 72:109, 1971.
21. Fuchs, E. Dystrophia epithelialis corneae. *Arch. f. Ophthalmol.* 76:478, 1910.
22. Goldman, J., et al. Structural alterations af-

fecting transparency in swollen human corneas. *Invest. Ophthalmol.* 1:501, 1968.

23. Gospodarowicz, D., and Greenburg, G. The coating of bovine and rabbit corneas denuded of their endothelium with bovine corneal endothelial cells. *Exp. Eye Res.* 28:249, 1979.

24. Gundersen, T. Conjunctival flaps in the treatment of corneal disease with reference to a new technique of application. *Arch. Ophthalmol.* 60:880, 1958.

25. Gundersen, T. Surgical treatment of bullous keratopathy. *Arch. Ophthalmol.* 64:260, 1960.

26. Harris, J. E., and Nordquist, L. T. The hydration of the cornea. *Am. J. Ophthalmol.* 40:100, 1955.

27. Hedbys, B. O. The role of polysaccharides in corneal swelling. *Exp. Eye Res.* 1:81, 1961.

28. Hedbys, B. O., and Dohlman, C. H. A new method for determination of the swelling pressure of the corneal stroma in vitro. *Exp. Eye Res.* 2:122, 1963.

29. Hodson, S., and Miller, F. The bicarbonate ion pump in the endothelium which regulates the hydration of the rabbit cornea. *J. Physiol.* (Lond.) 203:563, 1976.

30. Holm, O. High magnification photography of the anterior segment of the human eye. Transaction of the Swedish Ophthalmology Society. *Acta Ophthalmol.* (Copenh.) 56:473, 1977.

31. Hull, D. S., et al. Corneal endothelial bicarbonate transport and the effect of carbonic anhydrase inhibitors on endothelial permeability and fluxes and corneal thickness. *Invest. Ophthalmol.* 16:883, 1977.

32. Jones, B. R., et al. Objectives in therapy of herpetic eye disease (Symposium on Herpes Simplex Eye Disease.). *Trans. Ophthalmol. Soc. U.K.* 97:305, 1977.

33. Jumblatt, M. M., Maurice, D. M., and McCulley, J. P. Transplantation of tissue cultured corneal endothelium. *Invest. Ophthalmol. Vis. Sci.* 17:1135, 1978.

34. Khodadoust, A. A., and Silverstein, A. M. Transplantation and rejection of individual cell layers of the cornea. *Invest. Ophthalmol.* 8:180, 1969.

35. Klyce, S. D. Electrical profiles in the corneal epithelium. *J. Physiol.* (Lond.) 226:407, 1972.

36. Klyce, S. D., Neufeld, A. M., and Zadunaisky, J. The activation of chloride transport by epinephrine and Db cyclic-AMP in the cornea of the rabbit. *Invest. Ophthalmol.* 12:127, 1973.

37. Klyce, S. D. Enhancing fluid secretion by the corneal epithelium. *Invest. Ophthalmol.* 16:698, 1977.

38. Koester, C. J., et al. Wide field specular microscopy. *Ophthalmology* (Rochester) 87:849, 1980.

39. Krachmer, J. H., Schnitzer, J. I., and Fratkin, J. Cornea pseudoguttata: A clinical and histopathologic description of endothelial cell edema. *Arch. Ophthalmol.* 99:1377, 1981.

40. Laing, R. A., Sandstrom, M. M., and Leibowitz, H. M. In vivo photomicrography of the corneal endothelium. *Arch. Ophthalmol.* 93:143, 1975.

41. Manchester, P. T. Hydration of the cornea. *Trans. Am. Ophthalmol. Soc.* 68:425, 1970.

42. Maumenee, A. E. Clinical aspects of the corneal homograft reaction. *Invest. Ophthalmol.* 1:244, 1962.

43. Maurice, D. M. The permeability to sodium ions of the living rabbit's cornea. *J. Physiol.* (Lond.) 112:367, 1951.

44. Maurice, D. M. Cellular membrane activity in the corneal endothelium of the intact eye. *Experientia* (Basel) 24:1094, 1968.

45. Maurice, D. M. The location of the fluid pump in the cornea. *J. Physiol.* (Lond.) 221:43, 1972.

46. Maurice, D. M. Cornea and Sclera. In H. Davson (Ed.), *The Eye* (3rd ed.). New York: Academic, in press.

47. Miller, D., and Benedek, G. B. Intraocular Light Scattering. Springfield, Ill.: Thomas, 1973.

48. Miller, D., and Dohlman, C. H. Effect of cataract surgery on the cornea. *Trans. Am. Acad. Ophthalmol. Otolaryngol.* 74:369, 1970.

49. Miller, D., and Stegman, R. Use of sodium hyaluronate in human intraocular lens implantation. *Ann. Ophthalmol.* 13:811, 1981.

50. Mishima, S. Corneal thickness. *Surv. Ophthalmol.* 13:57, 1968.

51. Mishima, S., and Hedbys, B. O. The permeability of the corneal epithelium and endothelium. *Exp. Eye Res.* 6:10, 1967.

52. Mishima, S., and Kudo, T. In vitro incubation of rabbit cornea. *Invest. Ophthalmol.* 6:329, 1967.

53. Ota, Y., Mishima, S., and Maurice, D. M. Endothelial permeability of the living cornea to fluorescein. *Invest. Ophthalmol.* 13:945, 1974.

54. Roberts, C. W., and Koester, C. J. Video with wide-field specular microscopy. *Ophthalmology* (Rochester) 88:146, 1981.

55. Roberts, C. W., Rosskothen, M. D., and Koester, C. J. Wide-field specular microscopy of excised donor corneas. *Arch. Ophthalmol.* 99:881, 1981.

56. Salleras, A. Bullous Keratopathy. In J. H. King, Jr., and J. W. McTigue (Eds.), *The Cornea World Congress*. Washington. Butterworth, 1965. P. 292.

57. Sato, T. Studies on the endothelium of the corneal graft. *Jpn. J. Ophthalmol.* 22:114, 1978.

58. Schanzlin, D. J., Goldberg, D. B., and Brown, S. I. Transplantation of congenitally opaque

corneas. *Ophthalmology* (Rochester) 87:1253, 1980.

59. Stocker, F. W., and Irish, A. Fate of successful corneal graft in Fuchs' endothelial dystrophy. *Am. J. Ophthalmol.* 68:820, 1969.

60. Sugar, A. Clinical specular microscopy. *Surv. Ophthalmol.* 24:21, 1979.

61. Taylor, D. M., Kaliq, A., and Maxwell, R. Keratoplasty and intraocular lenses: Current status (Symposium on Intraocular Lenses). *Ophthalmology* (Rochester) 86:242, 1979.

62. Worthen, D. M., et al. Interim FDA report on intraocular lenses. *Ophthalmology* (Rochester) 87:267, 1980.

63. Ytteborg, J., and Dohlman, C. H. Corneal edema and intraocular pressure: II. Clinical results. *Arch. Ophthalmol.* 74:477, 1965.

64. Zucker, B. Hydration and transparency of corneal stroma. *Arch. Ophthalmol.* 75:228, 1966.

Physiology of the Cornea: METABOLISM AND BIOCHEMISTRY

Judith Friend

EPITHELIUM

The primary function of the corneal epithelium is, with the tear film, to provide a very smooth refracting surface at the front of the eye. Interference with this surface by drying, edema, or epithelial defects can have severe visual consequences. The epithelium is a relatively impermeable barrier to water soluble agents from the tear film and to bacterial and fungal infections, though perhaps not to virus. It is probably only minimally involved in active corneal dehydration, but its barrier function reduces evaporation and minimizes absorption of fluid from the tears, thus helping to maintain proper corneal hydration [15, 48–50].

METABOLISM

GLUCOSE AND GLYCOGEN

The principal substrates for energy production in the corneal epithelium are glucose and glycogen. Most of the glucose for the cornea, including the epithelium, comes from the aqueous humor. Only about 10 percent of the glucose required to support the epithelium diffuses from the limbus or comes from the tears. In addition to the free glucose available, epithelium has large glycogen stores that, under anaerobic conditions or in response to mild trauma, are rapidly reduced, which indicates prompt mobilization of glycogen in response to metabolic demands that cannot be met by free glucose alone [22, 76]. Table 1-1 shows levels of some human and rabbit anterior segment metabolites. It is interesting to note that, in general, rabbits have considerably more anterior segment glucose and glycogen than do humans.

Epithelial glucose utilization rates in rabbits, measured directly and calculated on the basis of lactate production, are approximately 16 $\mu g/cm^2$/hour in oxygen and 25 $\mu g/cm^2$/hour in nitrogen [67, 76]. Flux measurements have demonstrated that 110 $\mu g/cm^2$/hour of glucose are available, which shows that there is an ample glucose supply under normal conditions [76]. If humans use the same amount, but have only about half the supply from the aqueous, it

Supported by research grants R01-EY01830 and R01-EY03061 from the National Eye Institute.

is possible that nutritional deficiencies may occur more readily in humans than in rabbits.

In addition to anaerobic glycolysis—the breakdown of glucose to lactate in the absence of oxygen, which occurs in the cell cytosol—the corneal epithelium also uses two other metabolic pathways, the tricarboxylic acid cycle (TCA cycle, Krebs cycle) and the hexose monophosphate shunt (HMS) (Fig. 1-10). The shunt, also located in the cytosol, initially converts glucose-6-phosphate to ribulose-5-phosphate; it eventually releases carbon dioxide (CO_2) and forms nicotinamide adenine dinucleotide phosphate (NADPH), and some adenosine triphosphate (ATP), the high-energy compound. The shunt mechanism is quite active; at least in vitro, 35 percent of the glucose used by the epithelium goes through it.

The TCA cycle breaks down lactate and pyruvate to CO_2 and water, which leads to the release of large amounts of ATP by oxidative phosphorylation. These systems are located in cell mitochondria, and although their presence has been demonstrated in corneal epithelium, they are not very active there, as would be expected since mitochondria are relatively sparse in epithelium [41, 50].

A third pathway that has been identified in corneal epithelium is the sorbitol pathway, which converts glucose to sorbitol and fructose (Fig. 1-10). In the presence of excess glucose, excess sorbitol may be produced. Since cell walls are impermeable to sorbitol, that molecule may accumulate intracellularly, causing osmotic cell damage. This mechanism is believed to be involved in diabetic abnormalities in lens and nerve, but its role in corneal epithelial diabetic abnormalities is less clear [23, 42].

OXYGEN
Oxygen, also required by the corneal epithelium, is supplied by atmospheric oxygen dissolved in the tear film when the eye is open. When the eye is closed, the oxygen diffuses from the palpebral conjunctival blood vessels. Thus, the partial pressure of oxygen in the tears is about 155 mm Hg when the eye is open and falls to about 55 mm Hg on closure. Even this lower partial pressure is apparently adequate to supply the oxygen demand of the epithelium, which is about 3.5 µl/cm²/hour [50, 81].

AMINO ACIDS AND PROTEINS
For the rapid turnover of epithelium, estimated to be once every 7 days [26], substantial amounts of amino acids are used. These are probably supplied by the aqueous humor since tears have a very low amino acid content and the epithelium is impermeable to amino acids from the tear side. Corneal epithelial cells do, however, have the ability to concentrate amino acids supplied from the posterior side [77]. The mechanism of protein synthesis from amino acids in the epithelium is presumed to be the same as elsewhere in the body [50].

There is little evidence for the presence of collagen in normal adult corneal epithelium. There is, however, evidence that embryonic cells, regenerating epithelium, and epithelial cells in culture produce basement membrane, and epithelium may be routinely responsible for basement membrane formation and maintenance [31, 75].

Corneal epithelial cells are not normally keratinized. However, recent work has indicated that they contain certain specific keratin proteins [17]. Characterization of these proteins, in corneal and other stratified squamous epithelial cells, under various conditions in vivo and in vitro, is being used as a tool to study the mechanisms involved in epithelial differentiation [17].

CHOLINERGIC AND ADRENERGIC SYSTEMS
High levels of acetylcholine, choline acetylase, and cholinesterase exist in corneal epithelial cells [50]. These compounds do not seem to be strictly of neural origin since they remain if trigeminal inner-

TABLE 1-1. *Anterior Segment Glucose and Glycogen*

Tissue	Human		Rabbit	
	Glucose	Glycogen	Glucose	Glycogen
Tears[a]	0.2	—	—	—
Corneal epithelium[b]	5.6	100	15.0	240
Stroma[b]	8.8	—	16.0	—
Aqueous humor[a]	3.0	—	6.5	—

[a]Values are averages given as µMol/ml tissue water.
[b]Values are averages given as µMol/gm dry weight.
SOURCE: Data from J. Friend [22], M. Reim et al. [65], and R. A. Thoft and J. Friend [76, 79].

vation to the cornea is destroyed. Also, these substances are found in major quantities in isolated cultured cells. One kind of cholinergic receptor, muscarinic, has been shown in cultured cells but was not present in suspensions of cell membranes; the other, nicotinic, has not been demonstrated in any preparations [9, 59]. The function of the cholinergic system in epithelium remains a mystery, although many roles have been postulated [8, 50].

In corneal epithelium, alpha-adrenergic receptors have not been found, but beta-adrenergic receptors are present on the cell surfaces [7, 19]. "First messenger" compounds, such as the catecholamines (epinephrine, for example) work through beta-adrenergic receptors to cause the production (by the enzyme adenyl cyclase) of cyclic adenosine monophosphate (cAMP), a "second messenger" within the cell. cAMP, in turn, activates various enzymes to cause an eventual biochemical or physiologic response of cells. Other compounds, e.g., some prostaglandins and cholera toxin, cause increased pro-

duction of cAMP in cells, possibly by direct stimulation of adenyl cyclase. Compounds that block beta receptors (e.g., propranolol) or prostaglandin synthesis (e.g., aspirin) and compounds that activate phosphodiesterase (the enzyme responsible for the destruction of cAMP) all can reduce the levels of intracellular cAMP and therefore reduce the pharmacologic effects of increased levels of cAMP.

Currently, much research is aimed at achieving a more complete understanding of the role of cyclic nucleotides, prostaglandins, and adrenergic and cholinergic compounds in corneal epithelial metabolism and wound healing [7–9, 19, 37].

EFFECTS OF DENERVATION

Corneal innervation is from the ophthalmic branch of the trigeminal nerve (fifth cranial nerve). The

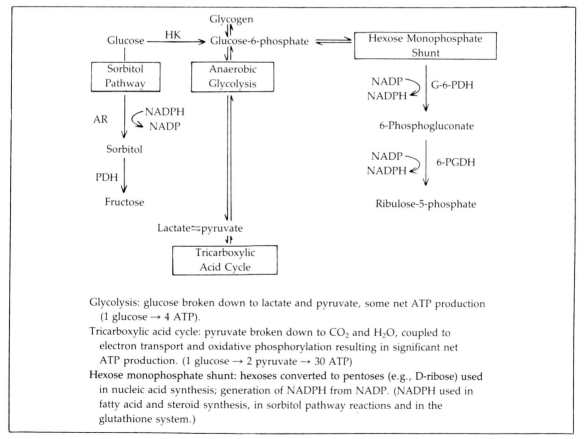

Glycolysis: glucose broken down to lactate and pyruvate, some net ATP production (1 glucose → 4 ATP).

Tricarboxylic acid cycle: pyruvate broken down to CO_2 and H_2O, coupled to electron transport and oxidative phosphorylation resulting in significant net ATP production. (1 glucose → 2 pyruvate → 30 ATP)

Hexose monophosphate shunt: hexoses converted to pentoses (e.g., D-ribose) used in nucleic acid synthesis; generation of NADPH from NADP. (NADPH used in fatty acid and steroid synthesis, in sorbitol pathway reactions and in the glutathione system.)

FIGURE 1-10. *Pathways of glucose metabolism. HK = hexokinase; AR = aldose reductase; PDH = polyol dehydrogenase; G-6-PDH = glucose-6-phosphate dehydrogenase; 6-PGDH = 6-phosphogluconate dehydrogenase; ATP = adenosine triphosphate; NADP = nicotine adenine dinucleotide phosphate (formerly known as TPN); NADPH = nicotine adenine dinucleotide phosphate, reduced form (formerly known as TPNH).*

other branches of the fifth nerve supply the rest of the globe and orbit.

Denervation of the corneal epithelium and ocular surface has been of laboratory and clinical interest for many years, but accomplishing such denervation has proved to be a problem. Fifth nerve ganglionectomy is surgically difficult, has a high rate of animal mortality, and may affect structures other than the cornea. A recently developed method, freezing around the limbus, avoids those problems [10]. If the usual criteria for denervation (loss of sensation and absence of histologically distinct nerves in corneal epithelium) are applied, denervation by freezing is seen to be of short duration. However, it does seem that certain morphologic changes, notably a thinning of the epithelium, do occur after denervation, that nerves are required for corneal mitotic activity, and that epithelial healing rates are decreased by denervation [10, 69].

BIOCHEMISTRY OF CONTACT LENS WEAR
The effect of contact lenses on corneal metabolism is caused by two factors, trauma and anoxia. Following are brief descriptions of the known separate effects of anoxia and trauma on the epithelium, as well as a discussion of the effects of contact lenses.

ANOXIA
Studies of corneal anoxia not using contact lenses are rare. Studies in which nitrogen gas is bubbled over the surface of the eye show that anoxia results in corneal haze and haloes [63, 72], which are presumably caused by epithelial edema. Some in vitro and in vivo work has demonstrated increased epithelial glucose utilization and lactate production in nitrogen [76]; glycogen, lactate dehydrogenase (LDH), and succinic dehydrogenase (SDH) are decreased under anoxic conditions [46, 78].

TRAUMA
Even rarer than studies on anoxia alone are studies of the effects of trauma alone. Burns and Roberts attempted to divide the anoxic effects from the trauma effects of lens wear by bubbling oxygen-free gas in a chamber over the eye and comparing the results with the results of lens wear [6]. They found that such trauma produced a glycogen drop comparable to that seen with lenses but a smaller rise in lactic acid. Thoft and Friend caused mild trauma to the cornea and found, within 30 minutes, increased epithelial hydration and decreased epithelial glycogen and ATP, all of which promptly returned to normal [78]. The edema thus produced was intracellular, indicating direct damage to the epithelial cells, rather than damage to the endothelium, which appears in the epithelium as intercellular edema.

CONTACT LENSES
Anoxia and trauma caused by contact lenses lead to epithelial damage such as increased thickness, corneal haze, and haloes (Fig. 1-11) [63, 72].

One of the biochemical changes secondary to lens wear is decreased glycogen [6, 72, 78]. Under unfitted hard contact lenses, for example, a depletion to 40 percent of normal within 6 hours was measured [78]. Since low levels of glycogen have been associated with the appearance of epithelial defects and ulceration [79], these decreases cannot be ignored. Lactate increases, glucose decreases, and decreases in some enzyme activities (e.g., LDH and hexokinase) have also been reported [6, 46, 72].

The mechanism for glycogen depletion secondary to the stress of contact lens wear or mild trauma is not clear. Measurements of glucose flux and utilization show that the glucose supply for the epithelium is adequate even for totally anoxic conditions [67, 76]. Therefore, no mobilization of glycogen should be necessary under lenses. Since it is mobilized, however, it seems that, under stress, the epithelial enzymes may not be able to utilize enough of the available glucose to meet possibly increased demands, and the tissue must then call on secondary supplies such as glycogen. It is an unproven possibility that an enzyme (e.g., hexokinase, the entry enzyme for glucose into glycolysis) is rate-limiting in the epithelium.

Soft lenses, in general, seem to be less disruptive than hard ones, producing less severe biochemical changes [6, 78]. However, soft lens wear, especially if prolonged, can result in striate keratopathy, a phenomenon seen in edematous corneas and believed to be caused by folds in Descemet's membrane. This is rarely seen in hard lens wear. This keratopathy may be caused by excessive corneal hydration, which may, in turn, be caused by lactic acid poisoning of the endothelium secondary to lactic acid buildup under soft lenses. Prolonged wear causes more severe lactate buildup than does short wear and is associated with correspondingly more keratopathy. However, greater lactate buildup has been measured, but no striate keratopathy observed, under hard lenses. It is possible that epithelial damage occurs before endothelial damage under hard lenses and that the lenses are therefore removed before the effects of lactic acid on the endothelium become apparent. That anoxia is a problem in lens wear is confirmed by the observation

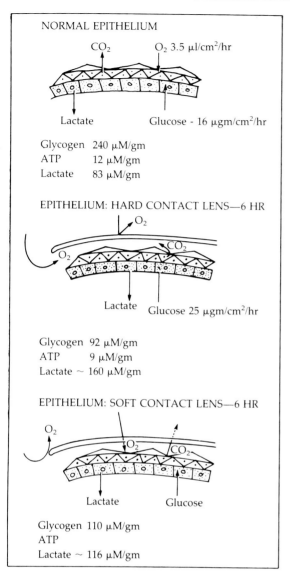

NORMAL EPITHELIUM

CO_2 O_2 3.5 μl/cm^2/hr

Lactate   Glucose - 16 μgm/cm^2/hr

Glycogen 240 μM/gm
ATP   12 μM/gm
Lactate   83 μM/gm

EPITHELIUM: HARD CONTACT LENS—6 HR

O_2

O_2 CO_2

Lactate   Glucose 25 μgm/cm^2/hr

Glycogen 92 μM/gm
ATP   9 μM/gm
Lactate ~ 160 μM/gm

EPITHELIUM: SOFT CONTACT LENS—6 HR

O_2

O_2 CO_2

Lactate   Glucose

Glycogen 110 μM/gm
ATP
Lactate ~ 116 μM/gm

FIGURE 1-11. *Epithelial metabolism under hard and soft contact lenses.*

that the oxygen flow across lenses is insufficient to meet epithelial demands even with some of the new gas-permeable lenses [34].

The specific route of oxygen supply for the cornea under contact lenses depends largely on the type of lens. With hard lenses, oxygen is supplied by "tear pumping" around the edges of the lens. With soft or gas-permeable lenses, oxygen is supplied primarily by diffusion of gas through the lens, with only a small contribution made by tear pumping. The exact percentages of oxygen supply from each source, of course, depends on the fit and the physical characteristics of the lens (e.g., material, thickness).

STROMA

COMPOSITION

TERMINOLOGY FOREWORD

There are two major classes of carbohydrate and protein–containing macromolecules, representatives of which are found in the corneal stroma: the glycoproteins and the proteoglycans. The terminology used to describe these molecules has caused some confusion, especially to nonexperts. This section attempts to clarify that terminology.

GLYCOPROTEINS

Glycoproteins are proteins containing one or more sugars covalently bound to a polypeptide (amino acid) chain. The sugar units may be single or double (disaccharides) or may contain several sugars (oligosaccharides), but the amount of sugar is low compared with the amount of protein, and there is no serially repeating sugar unit. Glycoproteins contain certain characteristic sugars, including D-galactose, D-mannose, L-fucose, D-xylose, N-acetyl-D-glucosamine, N-acetyl-D-galactosamine, and sialic acid. (N-acetyl-D-glucosamine is simply glucose with an amino group $[-NH_2]$, the nitrogen of which is attached to an acetyl group $[-CH_2]$.) The nature of the carbohydrate (e.g., the sugars, the linkages of the sugars to each other and to the peptide, branching, sulfation) and peptide chain composition are used to characterize the glycoproteins [71, 74].

The carbohydrate-peptide linkage between sugars and amino acids is one of the key structural features used to define different groups of glycoproteins. In animal tissues, there are three major linkages: the N-glycosidic linkage of N-acetyl-D-glucosamine to asparagine (the linkage found in immunoglobulin G [IgG] and many other compounds), the O-glycosidic linkage from N-acetyl-D-galactosamine or xylose to serine or threonine (the linkage found in mucins), and the O-glycosidic linkage from galactose to hydroxylysine (the linkage found in collagen and basement membrane). *O-glycosidic* and *N-glycosidic* refer to whether the linkage from the sugar to the amino acid is through a nitrogen molecule (N) or an oxygen molecule (O).

Glycoproteins are found in the body as enzymes, hormones, membrane constituents, and serum glycoproteins (e.g., IgG), but perhaps the best known single glycoprotein is collagen (see p. 23). One large class of glycoproteins important to the eye are the mucins (mucoids), which make up mucus. Mucus is the complex of proteins and glycoproteins that protects and lubricates epithelial surfaces (e.g., in the eye); mucins are the glycoprotein components of mucus. Mucins are characterized by oligosaccharide units of sialic acid, fucose, galactose, and N-acetylhexosamines (e.g., N-acetylglucosamine) linked to peptide chains by O-glycosidic bonds to serine or threonine [71, 74].

PROTEOGLYCANS

The second large class of macromolecules that contain carbohydrate and protein are the proteoglycans, which are characterized by the presence of a large polysaccharide moiety, frequently containing oligosaccharides or glycosaminoglycans, attached to a relatively small (proportional to the amount of carbohydrate) protein backbone. Glycosaminoglycans (GAGs), known in the older literature as mucopolysaccharides or acid mucopolysaccharides, are characterized by the presence of repeating disaccharide units forming a linear polymer, and are polyanionic (owing to the presence of many carboxyl [−COOH] and sulfate [−SO₄] groups). The disaccharide typically consists of a hexosamine (D-glucosamine or D-galactosamine) plus a uronic acid (D-glucuronic acid or L-iduronic acid). The hexosamines are frequently N-acetylated (have an acetyl group attached to the nitrogen) and in some cases may also be sulfated. Table 1-2 shows the components of the major GAGs. With the exception of hyaluronic acid, GAG in the native state is covalently linked to proteins to form proteoglycans, creating subunits that may

form very large proteoglycan aggregates (e.g., molecule weight 10^8). The term *chondroitin sulfate proteoglycan* thus refers to a proteoglycan whose carbohydrate moiety consists of the GAG chondroitin sulfate. Similar terms are used to describe keratan sulfate proteoglycan and the others [45].

Proteoglycans containing GAG, oligosaccharides, or both make up the ground substance (matrix) between the cells and collagen of connective tissue and are therefore structurally very important.

Glycoproteins and proteoglycans do share some features, e.g., sugars and peptide carbohydrate linkages. However, there are three features that permit differentiation between them: Proteoglycans have a much higher ratio of carbohydrate to protein, proteoglycans are characterized by the repeating disaccharide units of the GAG or oligosaccharide portion of the molecule, and hexuronic acid has not been identified in any glycoprotein [45, 71, 74].

CORNEAL PROTEOGLYCANS

In cornea, early histologic work with metachromatic toluidine blue and periodic acid–Schiff staining demonstrated the presence of GAGs within the stroma (see reference 50 for review). Subsequent biochemical analysis of the hexose, hexuronic acid, and hexosamine content of the GAGs, their amino acid composition, and the resistance of the proteoglycan molecules to selective enzymatic degradation have been used to define the type of GAG proteoglycan in the stroma. The bulk of the corneal GAG (ca. 65 percent) is keratan sulfate; most of the rest (ca. 30 percent) is chondroitin-4-sulfate, with smaller amounts of the other chondroitin-type GAGs. Chondroitin sulfate and keratan sulfate are

TABLE 1-2. *Glycosaminoglycans in Cornea*

Glycosaminoglycan	Amino Sugar	Uronic Acid	Sulfate	Present in Cornea
Hyaluronic acid	N-acetylglucosamine	Glucuronic	No	Embryologically, scars
Chondroitin	N-acetylgalactosamine	Glucuronic	No	Probably
Chondroitin-4-sulfate*	N-acetylgalactosamine	Glucuronic	Yes	Yes
Chondroitin-6-sulfate*	N-acetylgalactosamine	Glucuronic	Yes	Yes
Dermatan sulfate*	N-acetylgalactosamine	Glucuronic and iduronic	Yes	Yes
Keratan sulfate	N-acetylglucosamine and galactose	None	Yes	Yes
Heparin	Glucosamine and N-acetylglucosamine	Iduronic and glucuronic	Yes	No
Heparan sulfate	Glucosamine and N-acetylglucosamine	Iduronic and glucuronic	Yes	No

* Chondroitin-4-sulfate, chondroitin-6-sulfate, and dermatan sulfate are also known as chondroitin sulfate A, C, and B, respectively.
SOURCE. Data from Axelsson and Heingard [1], Hassell et al. [27–30], Lambert and Stoolmiller [45], and Maurice and Riley [50].

general classes of GAGs, within which there may be different molecular species, varying in degree and sites of sulfation, branching, and other features. For example, at least two keratan sulfates, I and II, have been isolated from corneal stroma. The proteoglycans apparently exist as two species: one protein core with keratan sulfate GAG and oligosaccharides attached, and a second protein core with the chondroitin sulfates and oligosaccharides attached [1, 27, 30] (see Table 1-2).

The funtion of the proteoglycans in the cornea is probably at least twofold: to be a filler between the cells and the collagen, thus contributing to the structure and transparency of the cornea [30], and to be involved in corneal hydration [32].

Early studies by Hedbys indicated that GAGs are primarily responsible for the imbibition pressure that draws water into the cornea, water that must then be removed by endothelial pump activity [32]. There is some evidence that maintenance of corneal hydration may be related to the characteristics of the different GAGs in the stroma [30].

During wound healing, the amount of keratan sulfate in corneal scar tissue is reduced relative to the amount of chondroitin sulfate, and corneas have increased water content [30]. The proteoglycans in opaque scar tissue are significantly larger than those in normal, nonopaque corneas; this increase in size may result in abnormally large separations of collagen fibrils. As the scars become less opaque, the corneal hydration and proteoglycan types and sizes return to normal, which support the concepts that the distance between collagen fibrils is the key to corneal transparency and that proteoglycans are important in corneal transparency [2, 18, 30].

Some recent studies have demonstrated that corneas from patients with macular corneal dystrophy synthesize an essentially normal chondroitin sulfate proteoglycan, but do not synthesize normal mature keratan sulfate or keratan sulfate proteoglycan. Instead, they may produce a slightly smaller glycoprotein with unusually large oligosaccharide side chains. This molecule is immunologically related to, and may be a precursor form of, mature keratan sulfate [28, 29]. This association of abnormal proteoglycan with corneal cloudiness further indicates that proteoglycans may play a major role in corneal transparency.

COLLAGEN

Collagen, which makes up 71 percent of the dry weight of the cornea [57], is the most abundant protein in the body. It provides the structural backbone of many tissues (e.g., cornea, cartilage, skin, and tendon) by making up, along with the proteoglycan matrix, the bulk of the connective tissue between

the cells. In cornea, collagen is present as the subepithelial basement membrane, the relatively unorganized fibrils of Bowman's layer, the lamellae of the stroma, and Descemet's membrane. Although a detailed discussion of collagen biochemistry is beyond the scope of this chapter, a summary of what collagen is, including a review of its biosynthesis and structure, may be useful.

COLLAGEN BIOCHEMISTRY AND SYNTHESIS
Collagen is a protein [5, 52, 62], but, because its peptide chains are glycosylated (have sugar molecules attached), it is also a glycoprotein. It is characterized by its high glycine (33 percent of the amino acid content) and proline and hydroxyproline (25 percent) content and major amounts of hydroxylysine.

Production of collagen begins intracellularly with synthesis of procollagen in the rough endoplasmic reticulum, followed by secretion from the cell, probably through the Golgi apparatus. The first step in collagen synthesis is the production of the primary subunits, the pro alpha chains, which are made up of a string of amino acids (Fig. 1-12). Pro alpha chains, like all protein molecules, are synthesized by polyribosomes following directions from DNA via RNA in a process called translation. The changes that occur in the molecule later, post-translational modifications, may play an important role in the final makeup of the collagen molecule, but its fundamental character is defined by the composition of the alpha chains. After translation (synthesis), the pro alpha chains are hydroxylated ($-$OH groups are added to some of the proline and lysine residues), and some glycosylation may occur (sugar residues may be added to some of the hydroxylysine residues). The pro alpha chains are folded into individual helices, and then combined in groups of three to form procollagen molecules (Fig. 1-12). Hydroxylation is believed to add stability to the ultimate collagen helix; glycosylation may be important in secretion, fibrillogenesis, or both. Procollagen is characterized then by three pro alpha chains in a helical structure. At each end of the procollagen molecule are nonhelical peptides, the registration peptides. It is possible, but not yet proved, that disulfide bonding between the nonhelical peptide portions of the procollagen molecules plays a role in helix formation. In addition, the presence of glycine as every third amino acid residue and the high proline and hydroxyproline content are also involved in directing the molecular configuration of collagen.

Procollagen is secreted from the cell, and subsequent development occurs extracellularly. First, the nonhelical peptide ends, the registration peptides, are enzymatically cleaved, leaving tropocollagen, the basic building block of collagen fibrils. The size of procollagen relative to tropocollagen is not known, but procollagen may be as much as 30 to 40 percent larger.

Collagen fibrils in the native state are made up of tropocollagen molecules (about 300 nm long) arranged in a staggered array. Study of laboratory products of collagen breakdown and reassembly has helped collagen biochemists determine this structure. By analysis of segment long-spacing (SLS) and fibrous long-spacing (FLS) collagens (both

of which are produced only by laboratory manipulations of collagen) and study of electron micrographs and x-ray diffraction patterns of collagen, it has been found that tropocollagen molecules typically line up with an approximately ¼-molecule overlap with each other (Fig. 1-12); this overlapping causes the banding pattern seen in electron micrographs of collagen. The molecules are staggered by the distance D (67 nm), which is also one of the typical band distances in native collagen. Assembly of collagen to form microfibrils, fibrils, and fibers is the subject of much current study, and the mechanisms are not well understood.

Thus, all collagenous tissues are made up of tropocollagen molecules, and the specific architecture of tissue results from the exact nature of the tropocollagen and the interactions among tropocol-

---

INTRACELLULAR

Translation: Synthesis by ribosomes of pro α chains

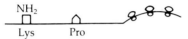

Hydroxylation: Addition of −OH to some proline and lysine residues

Glycosylation: Addition of galactosyl- or glucosyl-galactosyl- residues to some
    hydroxylysine residues

Formation of procollagen: Three pro α chains combine to form procollagen -
    a triple helix of α chains with non-helical terminal peptide groups, the registration
    peptides (R)

SECRETION OF PROCOLLAGEN FROM CELL INTO TISSUE: EXTRACELLULAR

Formation of tropocollagen: conversion of procollagen to collagen
    Cleavage of registration peptides from procollagen leaving tropocollagen with shorter
    non-helical terminal peptides, the teleopeptides (T)

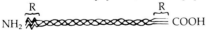

Fibrillogenesis: Formation of fibrils from tropocollagen. Tropocollagen molecules line
    up with ¼ stagger

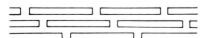

Fibrinogenesis: Combining of fibrils to form fibers

FIGURE 1-12. *Important steps in the formation of collagen. Lys = lysine; Pro = proline; hylys = hydroxylysine; hypro = hydroxyproline.*

lagen molecules and among tropocollagen and the glycoproteins and proteoglycans of the extracellular space [5, 52, 62].

COLLAGEN TYPES

The several types of collagen are defined by the kind of alpha chains present. There are four kinds of alpha chains, $\alpha 1$, $\alpha 2$, αA, and αB, chemically distinguished by their amino acid content and sequence (order in which the amino acids appear) and other physicochemical properties. Even within those basic kinds, there is heterogeneity, so that there is a type I $\alpha(1)$ chain found primarily in skin, and denoted $\alpha 1(I)$ in collagen terminology. Correspondingly, there is a type II $\alpha(1)$ chain ($\alpha 1[II]$) that is found primarily in cartilage.

Based on alpha chain composition, there are five types of collagen currently recognized by most experts. One is type I collagen, found in bone, tendon, and skin. It contains two $\alpha 1$ type I chains and one $\alpha 2$ chain and is therefore designated as $\alpha 1(I)_2 \alpha 2$. Type II collagen, found in cartilage, contains three $\alpha 1$ type II chains and is designated $\alpha 1(II)_3$. Type III, frequently found in association with type I in skin, blood vessels, and smooth muscle, consists of three $\alpha 1(III)$ chains and is designated $\alpha 1(III)_3$. In addition, basement membrane collagen (type IV collagen), whose alpha chain composition has not been defined, and type AB (type V), probably consisting of two αB chains and one αA chain, have been described [5, 52, 62].

CORNEAL COLLAGEN

STROMA. In cornea, the stromal collagen fibers (typically 250–300 Å), consisting mainly of types I and AB collagen, form a highly ordered lamellar array, which, because of its arrangement, is transparent [2, 18, 48]. It is a stable component with little turnover in the course of a year [73].

In vitro studies have indicated that type I collagen is the primary collagen of corneal stroma (about 80–90 percent of the total) and that keratocytes can secrete type I collagen, although this type of collagen is considerably more glycosylated than usual type I collagen. Solubility studies have shown that type AB (ca. 10 percent) and type III (1–2 percent) may also be present, and embryonic tissue may contain some type II collagen as well [12, 21, 31, 56, 57, 70].

BOWMAN'S LAYER. Bowman's layer is the collagen and ground substance lying immediately beneath the corneal epithelium in some eyes (e.g., human, primate, and avian), but not in others (e.g., rabbit). This area is microscopically distinguishable from the rest of the stroma by the random arrangement of the short collagen fibrils and by the lack of cells. The exact composition of the collagen types is not known, but they may be at least in part type I.

EPITHELIAL BASEMENT MEMBRANE. Biochemical studies on the epithelial basement membrane have, of course, been extremely difficult. In vitro studies indicate that the layer is produced by epithelial cells in culture [31, 75]. Recent studies comparing the hydroxylysine-lysine ratios in basement membrane from normal and diseased eyes may permit an evaluation of the changes in this tissue in some disease states [43].

DESCEMET'S MEMBRANE. Descemet's membrane, the 6 μm wide layer of collagen adjacent to the endothelium, is believed to be secreted by endothelium and to be the basement membrane of that cell layer. The larger amounts of material available and the relative ease of collecting it has permitted more detailed analyses of Descemet's than of other ocular basement membrane layers. Although characterized by the usual high hydroxyproline content and peptide helical features of collagen, it is unusual collagen in many respects, including a high carbohydrate content and an amorphous electron microscopic appearance. Its biochemical character is not yet fully defined [38], but it is in large part type IV collagen.

ABNORMALITIES OF COLLAGEN

Abnormalities of corneal collagen have not been specifically characterized in relation to corneal disease, but systemic connective tissue and collagen disease is frequently accompanied by ocular disease. Collagen abnormalities are visible morphologically in some diseases [39] (e.g., diabetes, in which thickened epithelial basement membranes may occur), and biochemical abnormalities of basement membranes have been found in keratoconus corneas [56]. Scarred corneal collagen is less soluble and less glycosylated and has wider and more variable fiber size than does fetal or normal adult corneal collagen [11]. The functional importance of these changes is unknown.

COLLAGENASE AND ULCERATION

Corneal ulceration—caused by infections, chemical and thermal injury, Vitamin A and protein deficiencies, exposure, and disease—is one of the most frequent causes of corneal vision loss. Actual perforation of the cornea, formation of opaque scar tissue, and vascular invasion are all possible blinding sequelae of corneal ulcerations, and none of these is easily correctable. Even corneal grafting after active ulceration and scarring have been quieted is frequently unsuccessful, in that the grafts themselves may ulcerate.

During ulceration, the extracellular structures of the cornea are destroyed. Degradation of collagen has been studied extensively since collagen is the major structural protein of the cornea, but destruction of associated proteoglycans and other glycoproteins of the matrix is undoubtedly also a problem in ulceration. Many factors are involved in causing corneal ulceration, but the ultimate destructive processes are enzymatic. Proteases, hydrolases, and collagenases destroy the cornea by destroying the macromolecules of which it is made.

Ulceration may be due either to the injurious agent itself or to the host response. Thus, in ulcerations caused by *Pseudomonas*, the organism itself produces a protease that degrades proteoglycans. On the other hand, the host inflammatory response to injury or disease may also contribute to ulceration since polymorphonuclear leukocytes (PMNs) or corneal fibroblasts themselves may release matrix-destroying enzymes. In addition, in disorders such as Mooren's ulcer and rheumatoid disease, there is increasing evidence that autoimmune phenomena underlie the production of destructive enzymes [20, 54]. The immunologic aspects of corneal ulceration are discussed in Chapter 3, Immunology, and Chapter 6, Immunologic Diseases. This chapter reviews the work on collagenase and efforts to treat ulceration by interfering with collagenase. For a more detailed discussion of this work, Berman's review [3] is invaluable.

COLLAGENASE

Collagenases are enzymes isolated from bacterial or mammalian tissue that are defined by their ability to cleave soluble, type I collagen, at exact sites on the alpha chains, into fragments three-fourths and one-fourth the length of the tropocollagen. These fragments can be accurately identified either by electron microscopy or by electrophoresis [3]. The role of collagenase is to split the helical collagen molecule, leaving the rest of the molecule vulnerable to attack and ultimate destruction by other proteases, e.g., trypsin, which cannot attack collagen itself [3].

In the eye, true collagenases have been isolated from ulcerating alkali-burned and thermal-burned corneas, and medium containing collagenase from ulcerating eyes can induce ulceration when injected into nonulcerated alkali-burned eyes. Depending on the methods of preparation used, at least two species of corneal collagenase seem to exist: one with a molecular weight of about 23,000; and the other with a molecular weight about 40,000. Aggregates of these two species also exist. In addition, a species with a molecular weight of 725,000 has been found, but this is probably a complex of one of the smaller species with macroglobulin. A latent form, activated by trypsin, plasmin, and mercurials, has also been found in ulcerating rabbit corneas and is produced by rabbit corneal fibroblasts in culture [3].

SOURCES OF CORNEAL COLLAGENASE: ROLE OF CELL TYPE

Several cell types may be involved in the production of collagenase in corneal ulceration: epithelium, PMNs, and fibroblasts.

Epithelium has been thought to be a source of collagenolytic activity because of the association of epithelial defects with ulceration and the ability of explants of epithelium from ulcerating eyes to lyse collagen gels in vitro [3]. In addition, if epithelium is prevented from covering an alkali-burned rabbit eye (by gluing on a hard contact lens), stromal ulceration is avoided, although it must be noted that such treatment prevents infiltration of PMNs and fibroblasts into corneal stroma as well as preventing epithelial regrowth [40]. However, collagenase has not been demonstrated in epithelium using immunologic methods [3].

Injured epithelium releases a compound called plasminogen activator. This compound converts plasminogen to plasmin, a component of blood plasma believed to be involved in the dissolution of fibrin and fibrin clots. Plasmin, through a complex series of steps involving the immunologic system, generates a factor that attracts PMNs into the stroma. In addition, plasmin activates latent collagenase and causes permeability changes in blood vessels. Thus, the role of epithelium in corneal ulceration may not be to produce collagenase directly, but rather indirectly by activating latent collagenase released from fibroblasts or PMNs and perhaps by generating factors that increase the inflammatory response and PMN population of injured eyes [3].

The exact role of PMNs in collagen destruction has not been defined. These cells may be involved through plasmin activation of latent collagenase or may release collagenase themselves [3].

Fibroblasts in culture produce latent soluble collagenase similar to that isolated from ulcerating corneas. It seems likely that this may be a normal part of repair and remodeling after injury. However, in the presence of large amounts of activator from other cell types, fibroblast collagenase may be important in corneal ulceration [3].

Inhibition of collagenase as a method of controlling ulceration has been extensively studied in vitro, using collagen gel lysis as a model, and in vivo, often using the alkali-burned rabbit eye as a model. In vitro, the amount of collagen destroyed by collagenase with or without inhibitors is measured. In vivo, the frequency and severity of ulceration in rabbit eyes after chemical (usually sodium hydroxide) injury is measured with and without inhibitors. In addition, a few controlled clinical trials of collagenase inhibitors have been undertaken.

Since collagenase requires Ca^{2+} and Zn^{2+}, it can be inhibited by metal-binding agents such as ethylene-diaminetetraacetic acid (EDTA) and thiols. CaEDTA, cysteine, and acetylcysteine are all effective in reducing ulceration of alkali-burned rabbit eyes. Clinically, CaEDTA has been effective in reducing ulceration, but it is relatively toxic; the efficacy of any agent used to inhibit must, of course, be weighed with regard to its toxicity and stability. Cysteine, acetylcysteine, and acetylcysteine with EDTA have been tried clinically and seem to be effective, but there have been no controlled, double-masked studies of these compounds [3].

Serum antiproteases (alpha-2-macroglobulin and alpha-1-antitrypsin) are also collagenase inhibitors. Alpha-1-antitrypsin does not inhibit rabbit corneal collagenase, but serum and alpha-2-macroglobulin do. These compounds seem to act by binding tightly with collagenase to form a complex that is taken up and destroyed by mononuclear cells. However, although increased levels of serum alpha-2-macroglobulin have been found in tears from ulcerating eyes (probably reflecting the increased vascular permeability of the eyes), ulceration is not blocked, possibly because the size of the antiproteases precludes their reaching the site of tissue damage [3, 4].

Collagen destruction can be halted, at least theoretically, by means other than blocking the tropocollagen-splitting activity of collagenase. For example, one can attempt to optimize repair processes by ensuring adequate amounts of materials needed for collagen synthesis. Thus, ascorbic acid, which is required for hydroxylation and secretion of collagen and which is abnormally low in alkali-burned eyes, has been useful in preventing ulceration. Recent work also indicates that citric acid, a compound similar to ascorbic acid, may be even more effective in treating severe burns [60, 61].

Interference with cell migration, e.g., prevention of the influx of potentially dangerous PMNs and fibroblasts by glued-on lenses or steroid treatment, may be helpful in injured eyes. Unfortunately, the role of steroids is not clear. Since corticosteroids

may suppress repair processes, their long-term use to treat the inflammation associated with ulceration may actually aggravate the ulcers, though the drugs may be useful in very early control of inflammation [16]. However, medroxyprogesterone, which decreases the inflammatory reaction, also decreases the collagenase content of corneas without interfering with collagen syntheses [55].

Thus, as this brief summary suggests, ulcers can be treated at many control points of the collagen-collagenase system.

SURFACE PROTEINS

Recently considerable attention has been focused on the role of certain surface proteins. These glycoproteins are present on the surface of cells, on connective tissue matrices, and in extracellular fluids. They may be involved in such important biologic functions as cell adhesion, malignant transformation, embryonic differentiation, and immunity. Among the surface proteins recognized in the cornea, and currently the subject of considerable study, are laminen and fibronectin. Laminen is believed to be a major structural component along with type IV collagen of the corneal basement membrane. Fibronectin, found both on cell surfaces and on noncellular surfaces, may be involved in cell binding to collagen and may be important in wound healing [24, 47, 80, 82].

CELLULAR METABOLISM

The cells of the stroma are primarily keratocytes, long flat cells with numerous processes. They are highly differentiated cells, able to produce the collagen and matrix of the stroma. Other cells, e.g., PMNs, lymphocytes, and plasma cells, are also normally found in corneal stroma.

The energy metabolism of these cells has not been studied because of the difficulty of isolation, although it is known that they have glycogen stores and require glucose and oxygen.

ENDOTHELIUM

The single layer of cells lining the inner surface of the cornea, the endothelium, performs several functions vital to the cornea. First, embryologically, it has important secretory functions such as production of hyaluronic acid, which may be important in the dramatic embryonic increase in corneal hydration [31]. Endothelium may also produce some of the chondroitin and keratan sulfates of the stromal proteoglycans, and it is responsible for the production of Descemet's membrane.

The primary function of the endothelium, however, is corneal dehydration. Acting against forces that tend to draw or force water into the corneal stroma, e.g., swelling and imbibition pressures, the correctly functioning endothelial pump keeps the corneal stroma hydration at about 3.5 mg water per milligram dry weight. Major increases in hydration can cause loss of transparency and, if prolonged or very large, scarring. After early investigators had firmly established that active endothelial metabolism played a major role in the control of corneal hydration, the existence of the endothelial pump was postulated [13, 48, 49, 50, 53]. After a long search, the active transport of bicarbonate by the endothelium was found [33, 36, 51]. Current research is directed at defining exactly how the pump regulates corneal hydration (see Physiology of the Cornea: Corneal Edema by C.H. Dohlman, above).

METABOLISM

GLUCOSE AND OXYGEN

The metabolic machinery providing energy for the endothelium has not been analyzed to the extent that that of the epithelium has, probably in part because of the limited amount of material available. However, since poisons to glycolytic metabolism or oxygen deprivation inhibit or stop the dehydrating activity of the pump [14, 48, 50], glucose metabolism must be important to the endothelium, as it is to most tissues. Analysis of endothelial metabolites and enzymes shows that the enzymes of the glycolytic pathway are present, but their activities are considerably lower in epithelium [64]. Similarly, shunt enzymes and metabolites are present in the endothelium but at lower levels than in epithelium, which suggests that the shunt may be less active in the endothelium than in epithelium. In humans, this lower activity may be associated with the endothelium's lack of regenerative capacity, but other endothelia (e.g., rabbit) with low enzyme activities are capable of regeneration.

Recent advances in measuring the natural fluorescence of reduced pyridine nucleotides (NADH and NADPH) and oxidized flavoproteins in different layers of the cornea in vivo may help overcome the difficulties of metabolite measurement in endothelium caused by the paucity of material. Although these methods are still experimental, future application may succeed in providing valuable information about the metabolic condition of diseased corneal layers [44].

The primary source of energy for the endothelium, as for the epithelium, is glucose derived from the aqueous humor; there may also be glycogen stores in the endothelium. The mechanism of glucose transfer from aqueous to endothelium is probably facilitated transfer, since passage is more rapid than would be expected on the basis of diffusion alone [25, 67].

Endothelial oxygen is also supplied by the aqueous humor, as has been demonstrated by experiments showing no change in endothelial oxygen with lid closure. If aqueous humor oxygen is elevated (by causing experimental subjects to breathe pure oxygen), there is no increased oxygen detected on the epithelial surface, which suggests that the endothelium, the stroma, or both may be capable of a far greater amount of aerobic glycolysis than they normally perform [81].

GLUTATHIONE

The tripeptide glutathione (glutamyl-L-cysteinylglycine) and its metabolism have been of considerable interest to students of the corneal endothelium since Dikstein and Maurice demonstrated that the substance is essential for normal endothelial function in vitro [14]. One possible role of the glutathione system is the elimination of toxic peroxides. This may occur when glutathione peroxidase (GSHPX) converts reduced glutathione (GSH) to its oxidized form (GSSG). Peroxides are formed in tissue by radiation (e.g., light), especially in the presence of oxygen, and some cell membrane lipids are oxidized to toxic peroxides. Glutathione reductase (GR), which converts GSSG to GSH, requires NADPH. Thus, the glutathione system is closely linked to the hexose monophosphate shunt (see Fig. 1-10). Or the glutathione system may be involved in regulation of ATPase activity, and therefore in endothelial pump activity [66].

The concentration of endothelial glutathione is about 776 ng per milligram tissue wet weight. Approximately 13 percent of endothelial glutathione is present in the oxidized form, a considerably higher percentage than in other tissues. This redox state of the glutathione system of the endothelium may reflect a relatively higher ration of GSHPX to GR, which may in turn indicate that the role of the glutathione is related to removal of toxic peroxides [35, 58, 66, 68].

ACKNOWLEDGMENT

The author wishes to thank Peter Mallen, who provided drawings for the figures.

REFERENCES

1. Axelsson, I., and Heinegard, D. Characterization of the keratan sulfate proteoglycans from bovine corneal stroma. *Biochem. J.*169:517, 1978.

2. Benedek, B. G.   Theory of transparency of the eye. *Appl. Optics* 10:459, 1971.

3. Berman, M. B.   Collagenase and Corneal Ulceration. In D. E. Wooley and J. M. Evanson (Eds.), *Collagenase in Normal and Pathological Connective Tissues*. New York: Wiley, 1980. Pp. 141–174.

4. Berman, M. B., et al.   Corneal ulceration and the serum antiproteases. *Exp. Eye Res.* 20:231, 1975.

5. Bornstein, P., and Sage, H.   Structurally distinct collagen types. *Annu. Rev. Biochem.* 49:957, 1980.

6. Burns, R. P., and Roberts, H.   Effect of contact lenses on corneal metabolism. In *Symp. Ocular Pharm. Therapeutics*. Trans. New Orleans Acad. Ophthal. St. Louis: Mosby, 1970. P. 73.

7. Candia, O. A., and Neufeld, A. H.   Topical epinephrine causes a decrease in density of β adrenergic receptors and catecholamine stimulated chloride transport on the rabbit cornea. *Biochim. Biophys. Acta* 543:403, 1978.

8. Cavanagh, H. D., et al.   The pathogenesis and treatment of persistent epithelial defects. *Trans. Am. Acad. Ophthalmol. Otolaryngol.* 81:745, 1976.

9. Cavanagh, H. D., and Colley, A. M.   β adrenergic and muscarinic binding in corneal epithelium. *Invest. Ophthalmol. Vis. Sci.* 20 (Suppl.):37, 1981.

10. Cintron, C., Kublin, C. L., and Friend, J.   Rabbit corneal denervation. Histological and biochemical analysis of the corneal epithelium. In preparation.

11. Cintron, C., Hong, B. S., and Kublin, C. L.   Quantitative analysis of the collagen from normal developing cornea and corneal scars. *Curr. Eye Res.* 1:1, 1981.

12. Davison, P. F., Hong, B. S., and Cannon, D. J.   Quantitative analysis of the collagens in the bovine cornea. *Exp. Eye Res.* 29:97, 1979.

13. Davson, H.   The hydration of the cornea. *Biochem. J.* 59:24, 1955.

14. Dikstein, S., and Maurice, D. M.   The metabolic basis to the fluid pump of the cornea. *J. Physiol.* (Lond.) 221:29, 1972.

15. Dohlman, C. H.   The function of the cornea in health and disease. *Invest. Ophthalmol.* 10:376, 1971.

16. Donshik, P. C., et al.   Effect of topical corticosteroids on ulceration in alkali burned corneas. *Arch. Ophthalmol.* 96:2117, 1978.

17. Doran, T. I., Vidrich, A., and Sun, T. T.   Intrinsic and extrinsic regulation of the differentiation of skin, cornea and esophageal cells. *Cell* 22:17, 1980.

18. Farrell, R. A., McCalley, R. L., and Tatham, P. E. R.   Wavelength dependencies of light scattering in normal and cold swollen corneas and their structural implications. *J. Physiol.* (Lond.) 233:589, 1976.

19. Fogle, J. A., and Neufeld, A. H.   The adrenergic and cholinergic corneal epithelium. *Invest. Ophthalmol. Vis. Sci.* 19:1212, 1979.

20. Foster, C. S.   Immunosuppressive therapy for external ocular inflammatory disease. *Ophthalmology* (Rochester) 87:140, 1980.

21. Freeman, I. L.   Collagen polymorphism in mature rabbit cornea. *Invest. Ophthalmol. Vis. Sci.* 17:171, 1978.

22. Friend, J.   Biochemistry of ocular surface epithelium. *Int. Ophthalmol. Clin.* 19(2):73, 1979.

23. Friend, J., Kiorpes, T. C., and Thoft, R. A.   Diabetes mellitus and rabbit corneal epithelium. *Invest. Ophthalmol. Vis. Sci.* 21:317, 1981.

24. Fujikawa, L. S., et al.   Fibronectin in healing rabbit corneal wounds. *Lab. Invest.* 45:120, 1981.

25. Hale, P. N., and Maurice, D. M.   Sugar transport across the corneal endothelium. *Exp. Eye Res.* 8:205, 1969.

26. Hanna, C., Bicknell, D. S., and O'Brien, J. E.   Cell turnover in the adult human eye. *Arch. Ophthalmol.* 65:695, 1961.

27. Hassell, J. R., Newsome, D. A., and Hascall, V. C.   Characterization and biosynthesis of proteoglycans of corneal stroma from rhesus monkey. *J. Biol. Chem.* 254:12346, 1979.

28. Hassell, J. R., et al.   Macular corneal dystrophy: Failure to synthesize a mature keratan sulfate proteoglycan. *Proc. Natl. Acad. Sci. U.S.A.* 77:3705, 1980.

29. Hassell, J. R., et al.   Deposits in macular corneal dystrophy contain abnormal proteoglycans. *Invest. Ophthalmol. Vis. Sci.* 20(Suppl.):115, 1981.

30. Hassell, J. R., et al.   Proteoglycan changes during restoration of transparency in corneal scars. *Biochem. J.*, in press.

31. Hay, E. D.   Development of the vertebrate cornea. *Int. Rev. Cytol.* 63:263, 1980.

32. Hedbys, B. O.   The role of polysaccharides in corneal swelling. *Exp. Eye Res.* 1:81, 1961.

33. Hodson, S., and Miller, F.   The bicarbonate ion pump in the endothelium which regulates the hydration of rabbit cornea. *J. Physiol.* (Lond.) 263:563, 1976.

34. Holly, F. J., and Refojo, M. F.   Oxygen permeability of hydrogel contact lenses. *J. Am. Optom. Assoc.* 43:11, 1972.

35. Hull, D. S., Strickland, E. C., and Green, K.   Photodynamically induced alteration of corneal endothelial cell function. *Invest. Ophthalmol. Vis. Sci.* 18:1226, 1979.

36. Hull, D. S., et al.   Corneal endothelial bicarbonate transport and the effect of carbonic anhydrase inhibitors on endothelial permeability

and fluxes and corneal thickness. *Invest. Ophthalmol.* 16:883, 1977.

37. Jumblatt, M. N., Fogle, J. A., and Neufeld, A. H. Cholera toxin stimulates adenosine 3',5'-monophosphate synthesis and epithelial wound closure in the rabbit. *Invest. Ophthalmol. Vis. Sci.* 19:1321, 1980.

38. Kefalides, N., Alper, R., and Clark, C. C. Biochemistry and metabolism of basement membranes. *Int. Rev. Cytol.* 61:167, 1979.

39. Kenyon, K. R. Recurrent corneal erosion: Pathogenesis and therapy. *Int. Ophthalmol. Clin.* 19(2):195, 1979.

40. Kenyon, K. R., et al. Prevention of stromal ulceration in the alkali burned rabbit cornea by glued on contact lens: Evidence for the role of polymorphonuclear leukocytes in collagen degradation. *Invest. Ophthalmol. Vis. Sci.* 18:570, 1979.

41. Kinoshita, J. H. Some aspects of the carbohydrate metabolism of the cornea. *Invest. Ophthalmol.* 1:178, 1962.

42. Kinoshita, J. H., et al. Aldose reductase in diabetic complications of the eye. *Metabolism* 28:462, 1979.

43. Kiorpes, T. C., et al. Determination of the hydroxylysine-lysine ratio of anterior stromal layers. *Invest. Ophthalmol. Vis. Sci.* 20(Suppl.):213, 1981.

44. Laing, R. A., Fishbarg, J., and Chance, B. Non-invasive measurements of pyridine nucleotide fluorescence from cornea. *Invest. Ophthalmol. Vis. Sci.* 19:96, 1980.

45. Lambert, S. I., and Stoolmiller, A. C. Glycosaminoglycans: A biochemical and clinical review. *J. Invest. Dermatol.* 63:433, 1974.

46. Lowther, G. E., and Hill, R. M. Corneal epithelium: Recovery from anoxia. *Arch. Ophthalmol.* 92:231, 1974.

47. Martin, G. R., et al. Regulation of Tissue Structure and Repair by Collagen and Fibronectin. In G. T. Shares and J. K. Dineer (Eds.), *Biology and Management of Surgical Wounds.* Philadelphia: Lea & Febiger, in press.

48. Maurice, D. M. The Cornea and Sclera. In H. Davson (Ed.), *The Eye* (2nd ed.). New York: Academic, 1969. Vol. 1, p. 489.

49. Maurice, D. M. The location of the fluid pump in the cornea. *J. Physiol.* (Lond.) 221:43, 1972.

50. Maurice, D. M., and Riley, M. V. The Cornea. In C. N. Graymore (Ed.), *Biochemistry of the Eye.* New York: Academic, 1970.

51. Mayes, K. R., and Hodson, S. An in vivo demonstration of the bicarbonate ion pump of rabbit corneal endothelium. *Exp. Eye Res.* 28:699, 1979.

52. Miller, E. J., and Gay, S. Collagen: an overview. *Methods Enzymol.* 82:3, 1982.

53. Mishima, S., and Hedbys, B. O. The permeability of the corneal epithelium and endothelium to water. *Exp. Eye Res.* 6:10, 1967.

54. Mondino, B., Brown, S. I., and Rabin, B. Cellular immunity in Mooren's ulcer. *Am. J. Ophthalmol.* 85:788, 1978.

55. Newsome, D. A., and Gross, J. Prevention by medroxyprogesterone of perforation in the alkali burned rabbit cornea: Inhibition of collagenolytic activity. *Invest. Ophthalmol.* 16:21, 1977.

56. Newsome, D. A., et al. Detection of specific collagen types in normal and keratoconus corneas. *Invest. Ophthalmol. Vis. Sci.* 20:738, 1981.

57. Newsome, D. A., Gross, J., and Hassell, J. R. Human corneal stroma contains three distinct collagens. *Invest. Ophthalmol. Vis. Sci.* 22:376, 1982.

58. Ng, M. C., and Riley, M. V. Relation of intracellular levels and redox state of reduced glutathione to endothelial function in the rabbit cornea. *Exp. Eye Res.* 30:511, 1980.

59. Olsen, J. S., and Neufeld, A. H. The rabbit cornea lacks cholinergic receptors. *Invest. Ophthalmol. Vis. Sci.* 19:1216, 1979.

60. Pfister, R. R., Nicolaro, M. L., and Paterson, C. A. Sodium citrate reduces the incidence of corneal ulcerations and perforations in extreme alkali-burned eyes. Acetylcysteine and ascorbate have no favorable effect. *Invest. Ophthalmol. Vis. Sci.* 21:486, 1981.

61. Pfister, R. R., et al. The efficacy of ascorbate after severe experimental alkali burns depends upon the route of administration. *Invest. Ophthalmol. Vis. Sci.* 19:1526, 1980.

62. Piez, K. A., and Miller, A. The structure of collagen fibrils. *J. Supramol. Struct.* 2:121, 1974.

63. Polse, K. A., and Decker, M. Oxygen tension under a contact lens. *Invest. Ophthalmol. Vis. Sci.* 18:108, 1979.

64. Reim, M., and Turss, R. R. Über Metabolitspiegel in Cornea-Endothel und Kammerwasser beim Rindern. *Albrecht Von Graefes Arch. Klin. Exp. Ophthalmol.* 176:252, 1968.

65. Reim, M., et al. Glucose levels in the different layers of the cornea, aqueous humor and tears. *Ophthalmologica* 154:39, 1967.

66. Reim, M., Heuvels, B., and Cattepoel, H. Glutathione peroxidase in some ocular tissues. *Ophthalmol. Res.* 6:228, 1974.

67. Riley, M. V. Glucose and oxygen utilization by the rabbit cornea. *Exp. Eye Res.* 8:193, 1969.

68. Riley, M. V., et al. Oxidized glutathione in the corneal endothelium. *Exp. Eye Res.* 30:607, 1980.

69. Schimmelpfennig, B., and Beuerman, R. Sensory deprivation of the rabbit cornea affects epithelial properties. *Exp. Neurol.* 69:196, 1980.

70. Schmut, O. The identification of type II collagen in calf and bovine cornea and sclera. *Exp. Eye Res.* 25:505, 1977.

71. Sharon, N., and Lis, H. Glycoproteins: Research booming on long ignored ubiquitous compounds. *Chemical and Engineering News,* March 30, 1981.

72. Smelser, G. K., and Chen, O. K. Physiological changes induced by contact lenses. *Arch. Ophthalmol.* 53:676, 1955.

73. Smelser, G. K., Pollock, F. M., and Ozaniks, V. Persistence of donor collagen in corneal transplants. *Exp. Eye Res.* 4:349, 1965.

74. Spiro, R. G. Glycoproteins: Their biochemistry, biology and role in human disease. *N. Engl. J. Med.* 281:991, 1043, 1969.

75. Sundar-Raj, C. V., Freeman, I. L., and Brown, S. I. Selective growth of rabbit corneal epithelial cells in culture and basement membrane synthesis. *Invest. Ophthalmol. Vis. Sci.* 19:1222, 1980.

76. Thoft, R. A., and Friend, J. Corneal epithelial glucose utilization. *Arch. Ophthalmol.* 88:58, 1971.

77. Thoft, R. A., and Friend, J. Corneal amino acid supply and distribution. *Invest. Ophthalmol.* 11:723, 1972.

78. Thoft, R. A., and Friend, J. Biochemical aspects of contact lens wear. *Am. J. Ophthalmol.* 80:139, 1975.

79. Thoft, R. A., and Friend, J. Biochemical transformation of regenerating ocular surface epithelium. *Invest. Ophthalmol.* 16:14, 1977.

80. Timple, R., et al. Laminen. *Methods Enzymol.* 82:831, 1982.

81. Weissman, B. A., Fatt, I., and Rasson, J. Diffusion of oxygen in human corneas *in vivo. Invest. Ophthalmol. Vis. Sci.* 20:123, 1981.

82. Yamada, K. M., and Olden, K. Fibronectins—Adhesive glycoproteins of cell surfaces and blood. *Nature* 275:179, 1978.

Physiology of the Tear Film

David W. Lamberts

This chapter will deal with the function, structure, and physiology of the tear film. The emphasis is on a scientific approach to tears, although the clinical testing of tear function is also discussed. Pathologic changes in the tear film and dry eye states are discussed in Chapter 7.

FUNCTION

The tear film fulfills several important functions in the eye:

1. Forms and maintains a smooth refracting surface over the cornea
2. Maintains a moist environment for the epithelial cells of the cornea and conjunctiva
3. Has bactericidal properties
4. Lubricates the lids
5. Transports metabolic products (primarily oxygen and carbon dioxide) to and from the epithelial cells and cornea
6. Provides a pathway for white blood cells in case of injury
7. Dilutes and washes away noxious stimuli

STRUCTURE

It is classically taught that the tear film is a three-layer structure composed of lipid, aqueous, and mucous layers from anterior to posterior. It is more accurate, in fact, to think of the tear film as a two-layer structure [34]: a thin lipid film floating on a large aqueous lake. The mucous layer, by virtue of its anatomy and physiology, belongs most appropriately to the corneal and conjunctival epithelium to which it is intimately attached. The entire tear film, including the mucous layer, is about 7μ thick (Fig. 1-13).

LIPID LAYER

The lipid layer is approximately 0.1μ thick. It is secreted primarily by the meibomian glands in the upper and lower lids and consists of esters, triacylglycerols, free sterols, sterol esters, and fatty acids [64]. The mixture melts at about 35°C and thus is always fluid in the living eye. The lipid layer was originally postulated by Wolf [96] and subsequently described, via interference patterns, by McDonald [58]. In 1972, Brauninger [8] and coworkers demonstrated directly the presence of a superficial lipid layer. They sprayed the surface of the human tear film with an atomizer containing either water or a lipid. They postulated that if the front layer of the tear film was truly a lipid, then minute particles of oil landing on such a film would spread on or merge with this oily layer. If, on the other hand, the front layer of the tear film was aqueous, then oil droplets would roll down the surface. The results were as expected and confirmed the presence of the anterior lipid layer.

It is important to understand that the lipid layer behaves as a film essentially independent of the aqueous layer underneath. It is anchored at the orifices of the meibomian glands above and below and does not take part in the flow of tears from lateral canthus to puncta. Debris and desquamated cells may be seen to flow along the "lacrimal river" at the junction of the lid with the globe, but this streaming occurs underneath the lipid layer. When the lids close during a blink, the lipid layer is compressed over the aqueous layer [34], the latter remaining in place on the cornea (Fig. 1-14). When the lids open, the lipid layer begins to spread again over the aqueous layer as oil spreads on water. The spreading front can move faster than the opening lid, and so the aqueous layer is never left exposed [34]. During lid closure, the lipid layer thickens; during opening, it thins. This phenomenon can be observed with the slit lamp as a subtle color change at the surface of the tear film [58]. One sees colors produced by interference patterns as light passes through an oily layer whose thickness is changing.

The function of the lipid layer is to inhibit evaporation of the tears, especially under conditions of low humidity and turbulent air flow [35]. It also protects the aqueous layer from polar lipid contamination that would tend to rupture the tear film prematurely [36]. Furthermore, the lipid present at the meibomian gland orifices acts as a hydrophobic barrier to prevent the overflow of tears. As the lipid spreads over the aqueous layer, it drags along with it additional fluid (the Marangoni effect), thus slightly thickening the tear film.

AQUEOUS LAYER

The bulk of the tear film consists of the aqueous layer, which is about 7 μ thick. It is here that the numerous solutes, electrolytes, proteins, enzymes, and other tear components are found. Table 1-3 lists the various components of the aqueous phase, concentrations when appropriate, and a reference on each component. Table 1-4 lists some of the physical characteristics of tears.

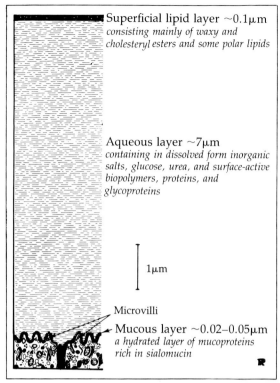

FIGURE 1-13. *Three layers of the tear film, drawn to scale. (From F. J. Holly and M. A. Lemp, Tear physiology and dry eyes.* Surv. Ophthalmol. *22:69, 1977.)*

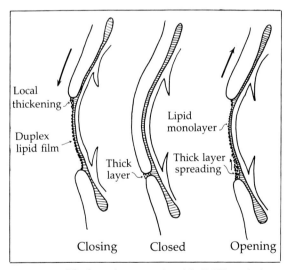

FIGURE 1-14. *The dynamic compression of the lipid layer during a blink. (From F. J. Holly, Tear film physiology.* Am. J. Optom. Physiol. Optics *57:252, 1980. Copyright 1980, The American Academy of Optometry.)*

Several of the components of tears are of particular interest and deserve individual comment.

1. PHYSIOLOGY 33

GLUCOSE

At one time it was felt that the nutrition for the
cornea was supplied by glucose in the tear film.
Thoft and Friend [82] have shown that this is not so.
The glucose concentration present in the tear film is
too low to satisfy the needs of the corneal
epithelium. Corneal glucose is obtained from the
aqueous.

Gassett and colleagues [27] found a correlation
between hyperglycemia and elevated glucose in
tears. They found that 96 percent of patients with a
diabetic glucose tolerance curve had a positive
Clinistix test for tear glucose 2 hours after the glucose load. In normal subjects, no change in the
Clinistix color was observed at 2 hours. They suggested that the tear Clinistix test offers a simple
screening procedure for diabetes mellitus.

OXYGEN

It is well substantiated that the oxygen in the tear
film is the major source of this metabolite for the
cornea and that oxygen is probably the only
metabolite that the cornea obtains from the tear
film. With eyes open, atmospheric oxygen is available to the tear film, so a partial pressure of 155 mm
Hg is maintained. With lids closed, an oxygen partial pressure of about 55 mm Hg is obtained from
diffusion of oxygen through the conjunctival capillary bed into the tear film. One of the major problems in designing a continuous wear contact lens
was to provide the cornea with an adequate oxygen
supply when the lids were closed.

LYSOZYME

Lysozyme in human eyes was first described by
Fleming in 1922 [21]. Lysozyme (muramidase) destroys bacterial cell membranes by breaking down
the N-acetylglucosamine-N-acetylneuraminic acid
polymer to tetrasaccharides [41]. It probably, therefore, plays a role in maintaining the sterility of the
tear film. Because the concentration of lysozyme is
much higher in tears than in serum, it has been
assumed that the lacrimal gland is able to synthesize
the enzyme. Gillette and colleagues [29], using immunohistochemical localization, did indeed demonstrate lysozyme in the acinar and ductal epithelial
cells of both main and accessory lacrimal gland. The
interstitial tissues of these glands did not stain.
These findings are highly supportive of the hypothesis that lysozyme is produced, or at least concentrated, by the lacrimal epithelial cells. Tear lysozyme levels have been shown to be decreased in
keratoconjunctivitis sicca [59], lupus erythematosus
[61], smog irritation [72], trachoma [76], and herpes
simplex [19]. The methods used to measure tear lysozyme are numerous. An excellent synopsis of

TABLE 1-3. *Composition of Tears*

Component	Concentration	Reference
Water	98.2%	Ridley and Sorsby [69]
Sodium	145 mEq/L	Iwata [41]
Potassium	20 mEq/L	Iwata [41]
Chloride	128 mEq/L	Iwata [41]
Bicarbonate	26 mEq/L	Thaysen and Thorn [81]
Calcium	2.11 mg/dL	Huth et al. [39]
Magnesium	Trace	Iwata [41]
Zinc	Trace	Iwata [41]
Glucose	3 mg/100 ml	Reim et al. [68]
Amino acids	8 mg/100 ml	Balik [5]
Urea	7–20 mg urea N/100 ml	Thaysen and Thorn [81]
Oxygen	155 mg Hg (eyes open)	Kwan et al. [49]
Total protein	$0.9 \pm 0.1\%$	Tsung [unpublished, 1981]
Lysozyme	1.3 ± 0.6 mg/ml	Sen and Sarin [76]
Complement	Present	Yamamoto and Allansmith [97]
Mucus secretory substance	Present	Franklin and Bang [24]
Lysosomal hydrolases	Present	van Haeringen and Glasius [89]
Lysosomal enzymes	Present	Tsung and Holly [85]
Lactate and Pyruvate	Present	van Haeringen and Glasius [88]

methods used and a bibliography are provided by Sen and Sarin [76]. Pitfalls and errors in the measurement of tear lysozyme are likewise numerous and explain in part the discrepancies in normal values that appear in the literature. Many of these difficulties are detailed in a recent publication by Copeland and others [13].

Other enzymes with antibacteria properties including lactoferrin [9] and betalysin [22] have been described in tears. Lactoferrin binds iron necessary in the metabolic pathway of many bacteria; betalysin attacks and ruptures cell membranes by an unknown mechanism.

IMMUNOGLOBULINS AND COMPLEMENT
All of the known immunoglobulins have been found in normal human tears, but only IgA is present in significant quantities (20–30 mg/100 ml). It has recently been shown by Yamamoto and Allansmith [97] that the entire complement pathway (both classic and alternate) is present in normal human tears. The complement system builds a cell membrane–bound protein chain that eventually lyses the victim bacterial cell.

In addition to containing the substances discussed above, the tears also contain specific antibodies [75]. These include antibodies to the influenza virus [93], herpes simplex virus [11], and trachoma virus [63]. Ironically these antibodies seem to have no effect upon their respective diseases. In the case of herpesvirus, both IgG and IgA can be found in tear samples from which live virus is cultured. After the development of trachoma in children, Mull and coworkers [63] found specific tear antibodies of IgA, IgG, and IgM in tear samples. These antibodies, however, do not seem to halt the progression of the disease. On the other hand, some investigators have found decreased IgA levels in certain diseases such as leprosy [71], trachoma [77], and ataxia-telangiectasia [80].

Very little is known regarding the role of tear antibodies in bacterial infections. Williams and Gibbons [95] have shown that IgA may inhibit the adherence of bacteria to mucous membrane, thereby preventing colonization of the conjunctival surface. Indeed, Reed and Cushing [67] were able to prevent shigella conjunctivitis in guinea pigs by precoating the organisms with IgA. Mestecky and coworkers [60] have shown that the ingestion of capsules containing killed *Streptococcus mutans* by four healthy subjects led to the production of specific antibodies (IgA) in the tears and other external secretions. No rise in serum antibody levels was observed.

It is clear from these observations that tear antibodies play a role in viral and bacterial infections, but a great deal remains to be learned about their specific functions.

An enormous amount of literature describes many other substances found in tears of patients with ocular or systemic disease. Table 1-5 lists these substances.

MUCOUS LAYER
The surface of the corneal epithelium is hydrophobic. Saline or tear placed on a freshly wiped rabbit cornea will bead up and not wet the surface. Mucus is extremely hydrophilic. Its primary function is to coat the surface of the corneal epithelium and thus render it wettable by the aqueous tears. The mucous layer is 0.02 to 0.05 μ thick and is secreted by the goblet cells of the conjunctiva, although some of it may be derived from the main lacrimal gland. The average goblet cell count in the normal human eye is 8.8 glands per square millimeter [66]. Mucus has another important function in the eye: that of maintaining the stability of the tear film. To understand this, one must have some knowledge of the dynamics of tear film formation. After a blink, the upper lid wipes the cornea and resurfaces it with a fresh, clean layer of mucus. The mucous layer is separated from the lipid layer by the aqueous phase of the tear film, but after a blink the lipid begins to diffuse throughout the aqueous layer, eventually reaching

TABLE 1-4. *Physical Characteristics of Aqueous Tears*

Characteristic	Value	Reference
pH	6.5–7.6	Abelson et al. [2]
Osmolarity	302 ± 6.3 mOsm/L	Gilbard et al. [28]
Volume	6.5 ± 0.3 μL	Scherz et al. [73]
Evaporation rate	10.1×10^{-7} gm/cm^{-2}/sec^{-1}	Iwata et al. [42]
Flow rate	1.2 μL/min^{-1}	Mishima et al. [62]
Refractive index	1.336	von Roth [94]
Surface tension	40.1 ± 1.5 dyne/cm	Holly et al. [37]

the mucus. This lipid contamination may increase until the mucus becomes hydrophobic, the tear film ruptures, and a dry spot forms on the surface of the cornea (Fig. 1-15). Enough mucus must be present to mask the lipid and maintain the tear film stability until the next blink occurs [36]. Indeed, this is what usually happens in a normal eye; i.e., a blink occurs before a dry spot forms.

NEUROGENIC CONTROL OF TEAR FILM FORMATION
That cholinergic agents increase the rate of lacrimal secretion is well accepted. Anatomically, one can trace the parasympathetic preganglionic fibers from their origin in the pons just above the superior salivary nucleus to their synapse in the sphenopalatine ganglion. The postsynaptic fiber then enters the lacrimal gland via the lacrimal nerve (see Fig. 8-4, p. 317). Blocking the sphenopalatine ganglion reduces the tear flow [31]. Additional evidence in support of parasympathetic innervation comes from pharmacologic observations. Parasympathomimetic drugs such as pilocarpine increase lacrimal flow. Parasympatholytic drugs such as atropine decrease lacrimal flow. The role of the sympathetic system in lacrimal flow is less well understood. Sympathetic fibers to the lacrimal gland originate in the hypothalamus, synapse in the superior cervical ganglion, and reach the gland in association with the vidian (deep petrosal branch) and lacrimal nerves. It

has been taught that the sympathetic fibers control tearing by influencing the flow of blood through the gland. Their actual role, however, is probably more complex than this. Maes [56] demonstrated that section of the superior cervical ganglion rendered the gland hypersensitive to *both* sympathomimetic and parasympathomimetic drugs. More recently Bromberg [10] has demonstrated that propranolol and phentolamine both inhibited the sympathetic initiation of protein secretion in rabbit lacrimal gland slices, thus implying the presence of both alpha- and beta-adrenergic receptors. Furthermore, he observed that the threshold for lacrimal secretion by isoproterenol (a beta agonist) is actually lower than that for secretion by carbachol (a cholinergic). In addition, synergism was shown between isoproterenol and carbachol. Because this study was done on sliced rabbit cornea, vascular effects could not be studied. It seems that the adrenergic, sympathetic system may be more important in lacrimal gland secretion than previously thought. What effect, if any, the autonomic system has on the accessory lacrimal glands remains a mystery.

EFFECT OF DRUGS ON TEAR FLOW
Except for the autonomic drugs mentioned above, little is known regarding systemic drugs and tear

TABLE 1-5. *Tear Components Associated with Diseases*

Substance	Associated Disease	Reference
Histamine	Vernal conjunctivitis	Abelson et al. [1]
Prostaglandins	Vernal conjunctivitis, trachoma	Dhir et al. [18]
Glucose	Diabetes	Gasset et al. [27]
Antitrypsin	External ocular inflammation	Anderson and Leopold [3], Zirm et al. [98]
Lactate dehydrogenase	None found in retinoblastoma	MacKay et al. [55]
Hepatitis B antigen	Hepatitis	Darrell and Jacob [15]
Blood	Factor VII deficiency	Slem and Kumi [78]
Salicylic acid	Aspirin ingestion	Valentic et al. [86]
"Orange tears"	Rifampin ingestion	Lyons [54]
Anticonvulsants	Seizure disorders	Tondi et al. [83]
Beta-hexosaminidase	Diabetic retinopathy in pregnancy (none found)	van Haeringen et al. [90]
Cerebrospinal fluid	Traumatic CSF fistula	Joshi and Crockard [45]
α-Mannosidase (decreased)	Mannosidosis	Libert et al. [53]
Catecholamines (decreased)	Glaucoma	Zubareva and Kiseleva [99]
Calcium and magnesium	None found in hypocalcemia or hypercalcemia	Avisar et al. [4]
Beta-galactosidase	G_{M1} gangliosidosis	Tsuboyama et al. [84]
Beta-hexosaminidase (decreased)	Tay-Sachs disease	Goldberg et al. [30]

secretion. A few authors have postulated that oral contraceptives may have a deleterious effect on tear production [70, 92]. However, in a study of 70 women (34 were using the pill, 36 were not) recently reported by Frankel and Ellis [23], no difference in tear production could be detected between the two groups by either Schirmer testing or tear breakup time.

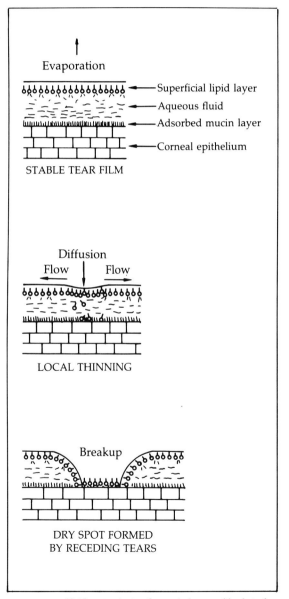

FIGURE 1-15. *Lipid contaminates the mucin layer and leads to dry spot formation. (From F. J. Holly, [34].)*

It is well known that antihistamines have some anticholinergic activity. Koffler and Lemp [47] studied the effect of a commonly used antihistamine, chlorpheniramine maleate, on normal volunteers. In their single-blind, crossover study of 17 people, they found that there was a decrease in aqueous production in all subjects on the days on which the antihistamine was administered.

Clinically it would be helpful to have a drug that could be used systemically or topically to stimulate patients' lacrimal glands to produce more tears. Although no such drug is currently available for use in this country, several have been described in the European literature. Bromhexine hydrochloride is a drug used to treat chronic bronchitis because of its ability to increase the amount of bronchial secretions while decreasing viscosity. At least one double-blind, controlled study on bromhexine hydrochloride in the eye has been reported. Frost-Larsen and colleagues [25], in 1978, studied 29 patients with Sjögren's syndrome. These authors found that when bromhexine hydrochloride was used in a dosage of 48 mg per day, a statistically significant increase in both tear breakup time and Schirmer test scores was observed in the test group. A different approach was described by Italian investigators using polypeptide kinins. One of these drugs, physalaemin, is a kinin extracted from the skin of a South American amphibian, *Physalaemus fuscumaculatus.* Bertaccini and coworkers [7] described the effects of physalaemin on lacrimal glands of dogs. They found that very small amounts of the extract were potent stimulators of lacrimal secretion. Pretreatment of the animals with sympatholytic and parasympatholytic drugs did not diminish the effect of physalaemin. Thus physalaemin apparently exerts its effect directly on the lacrimal gland and not via stimulation of the autonomic nervous system. Another kinin, eledoisin, is obtained from the salivary gland of the Mediterranean octopus (*Eledone moschata*). It is not quite as potent as physalaemin. Eledoisin was tested in humans by Impicciatore and others [40] in 1973. The drug was administered as an eye drop (20 μg/day) to ten normal subjects and ten dry eye patients. Although eledoisin was not effective in the normal subjects, the dry eye patients who received it showed an increase in tearing. None of these medications is currently approved for use in this country, although the potential for such a medication is great.

Many other drugs have been described as having an effect on lacrimation. To discuss them all is beyond the scope of this chapter. Table 1-6 lists many of these medications along with references on each. Much of this information appears in a comprehen-

TABLE 1-6. *Effect of Drugs on Human Tear Flow*

Drug	Reference
DRUGS THAT DECREASE LACRIMATION	
Atropine, scopolamine	Erickson [20]
Antihistamines	Chang [12]
Practolol	Garner and Rahi [26]
Nitrous oxide, halothane, enflurane	Krupin et al. [48]
DRUGS THAT INCREASE LACRIMATION	
Pilocarpine	Balik [6]
Methacholine	Erickson [20]
Neostigmine	DeHaas [17]
Bethanechol chloride	Grant [32]
Epinephrine	Erickson [20]
Ephedrine	Erickson [20]
Ketamine hydro-chloride	Kitamura and Ogli [46]
Marijuana	Dawson et al. [16]
Fluorouracil	Hamersley et al. [33]

sive review of the effect of systemic drugs on the tears by Crandall and Leopold [14]. Included in that review is an excellent synopsis of antibiotic levels in tears.

TEAR SECRETION RATE

Schirmer [74] first determined the rate of tear flow in humans in 1903. He calculated a flow rate of 0.6 to 0.8 μL per minute by measuring the quantity of tears overflowing the cul-de-sac in patients with extirpated lacrimal sacs. Since then, numerous estimates of tear flow have been made using fluorescein dye dilution techniques. These studies involve placing a small, known amount of fluorescein in the cul-de-sac, allowing it to mix with a known amount of tears, and measuring the dilution of the fluorescein by the tear flow, as manifested by decreasing fluorescence. In most cases, the fluorescence is measured using a fluorophotometer attached to a slit lamp [57]. Using this method, Mishima and coworkers [62] found a steady state tear volume of 7.0 ± 2.0 μL. They calculated tear flow at 1.2 μL per minute with a turnover rate of 16 percent per minute. In addition, they noted that tear volume increased with increasing tear flow rate. Sorenson [79], using a technetium-99 tracer and a gamma camera, determined a tear flow rate of 0.6 μL per minute.

The terms *basic secretion* and *reflex secretion* are in common usage today and deserve some comment. This division of tear flow was originally suggested by Jones [43] in 1966 to help explain some observa-

tions regarding tearing. The "basic secretors," he felt, were the eyelid glands of Kraus and Wolfring (the accessory lacrimal glands), which have no known innervation. The "reflex secretors" were the main lacrimal glands, possessing an autonomic innervation. Jones went on to say that the first 8- to 15-mm wetting of the Schirmer strip was produced by the basic secretors. His basic secretion test measured Schirmer wetting after topical anesthesia. Although firmly entrenched in the literature and the vocabulary of ophthalmology, the distinction between basic and reflex secretions is in fact rather arbitrary and has no sound physiologic basis. Jordan and Baum [44] have shown that as tear flow measurements are made less traumatic, the tear flow diminishes. When measured by the least invasive method, using fluorophotometry and topical anesthesia, flow rates fell to 0.3 μL per minute. Indeed, under general anesthesia, flow rates are almost zero [48]. Rather than dividing tear flow into reflex or basic, it is probably more accurate to think of tearing as a secretion dependent upon many psychogenic and sensory stimuli. If basic secretion (independent of external stimuli) does exist, it must be very low, below 0.3 μL per minute. Certainly it is not measured by the Schirmer test with topical anesthesia, because even this test is a strong lacrimal stimulus [44].

TEAR FILM DYNAMICS

The human tear film is a constantly changing fluid membrane. Many different forces come into play to determine its formation and renewal. Flow in the tear film only occurs in the aqueous layer. The lipid layer remains intact between blinks and the mucous layer remains adherent to the epithelium. Even then, the greatest amount of flow occurs in the meniscus adjacent to the upper and lower lid, the so-called lacrimal river. Negligible fluid movement occurs in the precorneal or preconjunctival tear film. After a blink, the three layers are intact and relatively discrete as described previously. Lipid, however, immediately begins to diffuse through the aqueous layer. When lipid strikes the mucous layer and contaminates it sufficiently, a hydrophobic spot that will not wet is formed on the cornea. This is the mechanism of tear breakup time as suggested by Holly [34] (see Fig. 1-15). As the eye remains open before the next blink, the aqueous layer begins to evaporate and thin, in effect bringing the lipid closer to the mucus. Thus the tear film will break up eventually, if the eye is held open long enough. If enough mucus is present, however, the lipid molecules initially can be masked by the mucus before the hydrophilic character of the surface changes and a dry spot forms. In addition, mucus dissolved in the aqueous layer (a normal finding in human tears) helps lower the interfacial tension of the aqueous layer and enables it to wet more readily [34]. Mucin thus plays three roles in maintaining a stable tear film. First, the mucin dissolved in the aqueous component increases the film pressure of the superficial lipid layer, thereby lowering the surface tension of the tear film and rendering it more stable. Second, adsorbed mucin renders the surface of the cornea wettable. Third, an adequate layer of mucin masks lipid molecules arriving at the corneal surface, thereby maintaining its hydrophilic character until the next blink.

During a blink, the lipid layer is compressed between the closing lids. Through shear forces across the aqueous layer, conjunctival mucin is spread over the epithelium, providing it with a fresh surface. Debris and lipid-contaminated mucous strands are brushed away into the lacrimal river eventually to find their ways into the upper and lower puncta.

CLINICAL MEASUREMENT OF TEAR FUNCTION

SCHIRMER TEST

Of the many ways to measure tear flow, only the Schirmer test is generally used in a clinical setting. With passing years the minimum accepted wetting value has dropped. Most reasonable is the suggestion of van Bijsterveld [87], who found that by using a cutoff value of 5.5-mm wetting in 5 minutes the correct diagnosis could be made in 83 percent of the dry eye patients tested. More recently, a similar study was done in normal subjects using the Schirmer test with and without topical proparacaine hydrochloride anesthesia [50]. Part of this study involved the concurrent measurement of the height of the lower lid meniscus (Fig. 1-16). The authors reached the following conclusions: (1) Proparacaine hydrochloride reduced mean Schirmer test values by 40 percent. (There were, however, wide individual variations.) (2) There was no statistically significant difference between men and women in tear production. (3) Tear production did not drop significantly with advancing age. (4) No correlation existed between meniscus height and subsequent Schirmer test scores, either with or without anesthesia. The authors also noted that if topical anesthesia was used for Schirmer testing, a lower cutoff value of 3-mm wetting would be found in only 15 percent of a normal population.

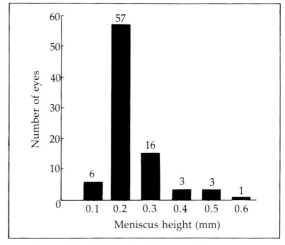

FIGURE 1-16. *The distribution of meniscus height in a normal population. (From D. W. Lamberts, C. S. Foster, and H. D. Perry, Schirmer Test after topical anesthesia and the tear meniscus height in normal eyes.* Arch. Ophthalmol. *97:1082, 1979. Copyright 1979, American Medical Association.)*

Another recent study was designed to determine the result of Schirmer testing on normal subjects with their eyes open or closed [51]. There was no statistically significant difference in wetting with eyes open or closed. There was a significant difference, however, depending on the *order* of the tests if they were done within a relatively short time. Whichever Schirmer test was done second (with the eyes open or closed) tended to yield lower values than the test done first. The reason for this is not certain. It may be partial exhaustion of tear flow, or possibly the subjects adapted to the discomfort of the Schirmer papers.

Although the Schirmer test is notoriously inaccurate, it remains the mainstay in the clinical diagnosis of dry eyes. It can be used with added confidence if repeated measurements give consistently low readings.

TEAR BREAKUP TIME

Breakup time (BUT) is a measure of the length of time the eye can be kept open before the tear film ruptures spontaneously. It is only a measure of the relative instability of the tear film, and results could have many causes. The test is performed by placing a drop of fluorescein in the cul-de-sac, asking the patient to blink several times, and then scanning the stained tear film with the cobalt blue light. The lids must not be touched nor elevated above their normal open position. The end point is recorded in seconds at the first appearance of a dry spot. A dry spot appears as a black area on the corneal surface where there is no wetting (no fluorescein), surrounded by the normal fluorescein-marked tear film. It is important to remember that any elevation on the corneal surface will cause almost instantaneous break up of the tear film. For this reason, dry spots must occur at random locations to be counted as accurate end points. The test should be repeated several times and an average taken. Since originally described by Lemp and coworkers [52], the BUT test has received a certain amount of criticism [65, 91]. Vanley and colleagues [91] pointed out several potential shortcomings of the BUT test, including uneven mixing of fluorescein in the tear film, partial blinking, unknown fluorescein concentration, and lag time between the appearance of a dry spot and its discovery by the observer. Recent work by Holly (unpublished data, 1981) has shown a heretofore undescribed variable in BUT measurement, namely, surface-active components in the fluorescein solutions or the fluids used to wet the fluorescein strips. He noted that when preservative-containing solutions were used to administer fluorescein for a BUT test, the results were erratic and often shortened. Even when sterile saline without preservatives was used to wet a paper fluorescein strip, similar results were obtained because of the surface-active preservatives leached from the paper strips. However, when sterile, nonpreserved fluorescein purified through a chromatography column was used, longer and reproducible results were obtained.

The BUT test has a great deal of potential as a useful clinical measurement. It is noninvasive and measures the common denominator of tear film abnormalities, i.e., loss of tear film stability. One hopes greater efforts will be made to standardize the test.

ROSE BENGAL STAIN
Rose bengal is a vital dye that stains injured epithelial cells. Fluorescein, on the other hand, stains areas where epithelium is absent, although it will pool in areas of epithelial irregularity. Rose bengal is helpful in studying tear problems in several different ways. First, it stains dry, desiccated epithelium while those cells are still in situ. Second, it stains corneal filaments a bright pink (fluorescein does not stain filaments). Third, rose bengal stains lipid-contaminated mucous strands, a common finding in dry eye states. Often the area on the top of a pterygium or pinguecula will stain with rose bengal, as will the epithelium in previous contact with a Schirmer strip. These are spurious findings and not indicative of abnormal tearing. Rose bengal staining secondary to dry eye states shows a specific pattern, so typical as to be pathognomonic. Two triangles are seen on the conjunctiva within the palpebral fissure, with their bases on the limbus. In more severe drying, a contiguous band of staining is seen across the cornea.

TEAR OSMOLALITY
Within the last few years a great deal of interest has been generated concerning tear osmolality and the role of tear osmolality in dry eye patients. Many workers use the term osmolarity (mOsm/L) rather than osmolality (mOsm/kg). Under most conditions the values are very similar. Gilbard and coworkers [28] have demonstrated an increase in tear osmolarity (usually above 310 mOsm/L) in patients with dry eyes. Whether this represents a primary defect in tear production or is a secondary effect from tear concentration after evaporation remains to be seen. The ability to alter the tear osmolality with drops is a controversial topic. Holly and I [38] have recently shown that tear osmolality can be reduced by using hyposmotic drops, but the effect is very transient. Normal osmolality is reestablished within 60 to 90 seconds.

REFERENCES
1. Abelson, M. B., et al. Histamine in human tears. *Am. J. Ophthalmol.* 83:417, 1977.
2. Abelson, M. B., Udell, I. J., and Weston, J. H. Normal human tear pH by direct measurement. *Arch. Ophthalmol.* 99:301, 1981.
3. Anderson, J. A., and Leopold, I. H. Antiproteolytic activities found in human tears. *Ophthalmology* (Rochester) 88:82, 1981.
4. Avisar, R., et al. Tear calcium and magnesium levels of normal subjects and patients with hypocalcemia or hypercalcemia. *Invest. Ophthalmol.* 16:1150, 1977.
5. Balik, J. Secretion of chloride ion in tears. *Cesk. Oftalmol.* 11:256, 1955.
6. Balik, J. Effect of atropine and pilocarpine on the secretion of chloride ion into the tears. *Cesk. Oftalmol.* 14:28, 1958.
7. Bertaccini, G., DeCaro, G., and Impicciatore, M. Effects of physalaemin on some exocrine secretions of dogs and cats. *J. Physiol.* (Lond.) 193:497, 1967.
8. Brauninger, G. E., Shah, D. O., Kaufman, H. E. Direct physical demonstration of oily layer on tear film surface. *Am. J. Ophthalmol.* 73:132, 1972.
9. Broekhuyse, R. M. Tear lactoferrin: A bacteriostatic and complexing protein. *Invest. Ophthalmol.* 13:550, 1974.
10. Bromberg, B. B. Autonomic control of lacrimal protein secretion. *Invest. Ophthalmol.* 20:110, 1981.

11. Centifanto, Y. M., and Kaufman, H. E. Secretory immunoglobulin A and herpes keratitis. *Infect. Immun.* 2:778, 1970.

12. Chang, F. W. The possible adverse effects of over-the-counter medications on the contact lens wearer. *J. Am. Optom. Assoc.* 48:319, 1977.

13. Copeland, J. R., Lamberts, D. W., and Holly, F. J. Investigation of the accuracy of tear lysozyme determination. *Invest. Ophthalmol. Vis. Sci.* 22:103, 1982.

14. Crandell, D. C., and Leopold, I. H. The influence of systemic drugs on tear constituents. *Ophthalmology* (Rochester) 86:115, 1979.

15. Darrell, R. W., and Jacob, G. B. Hepatitis B surface antigen in human tears. *Arch. Ophthalmol.* 96:674, 1978.

16. Dawson, W. W., et al. Marijuana and vision—After ten years' use in Costa Rica. *Invest. Ophthalmol.* 16:689, 1977.

17. DeHaas, E. B. H. Lacrimal gland response to parasympathomimetics after parasympathetic denervation. *Arch. Ophthalmol.* 64:34, 1960.

18. Dhir, S. P., et al. Prostaglandins in human tears. *Am. J. Ophthalmol.* 87:403, 1979.

19. Elyan, E., et al. Lysozyme tear level in patients with herpes simplex virus eye infections. *Invest. Ophthalmol.* 16:850, 1977.

20. Erickson, O. F. Drug influence on lacrimal lysozyme production. *Stanford Med. Bull.* 18:34, 1960.

21. Fleming, A. A. On a remarkable bacteriolytic element found in tissues and secretions. *Proc. R. Soc. Lond.* (Biol.). 93:306, 1922.

22. Ford, L. C., DeLange, R. J., and Petty, R. W. Identification of a non-lysozymal bactericidal factor (beta-lysin) in human tears and aqueous humor. *Am. J. Ophthalmol.* 81:30, 1976.

23. Frankel, S. H., and Ellis, P. P. Effect of oral contraceptives on tear production. *Ann. Ophthalmol.* 10:1585, 1978.

24. Franklin, R. M., and Bang, B. G. Mucus-stimulating factor in tears. *Invest. Ophthalmol. Vis. Sci.* 19:430, 1980.

25. Frost-Larsen, K., Isager, H., and Manthorpe, R. Sjögren's syndrome treated with bromhexine: A randomized clinical study. *Br. Med. J.* 1:1979, 1978.

26. Garner, A., and Rahi, A. H. S. Practolol and ocular toxicity: Antibodies in serum and tears. *Br. J. Ophthalmol.* 60:684, 1976.

27. Gasset, A. R., Braverman, L. E., and Fleming, M. C. Tear glucose detection of hyperglycemia. *Am. J. Ophthalmol.* 65:414, 1968.

28. Gilbard, J. P., Farris, R. L., and Santamaria, J., 2d. Osmolarity of tear microvolumes in keratoconjunctivitis sicca. *Arch. Ophthalmol.* 96:677, 1978.

29. Gillette, T. E., Greiner, J. V., and Allansmith, M. R. Immunohistochemical localization of human tear lysozyme. *Arch. Ophthalmol.* 99:298, 1981.

30. Goldberg, J. D., Truex, J. H., and Desnick, R. J. Tay-Sachs disease: An improved, fully automated method for heterozygote identification by tear beta-hexosaminidase assay. *Clin. Chim. Acta* 77:43, 1977.

31. Gottesfeld, B. H., and Leavitt, F. H. "Crocodile tears" treated by injection into the sphenopalatine ganglion. *Arch. Neurol.* 47:314, 1942.

32. Grant, W. M. *Toxicology of the Eye* (2nd ed.). Springfield, Ill.: Thomas, 1974.

33. Hamersley, J., et al. Excessive lacrimation from fluorouracil treatment. *JAMA* 225:747, 1973.

34. Holly, F. J. Formation and rupture of the tear film. *Exp. Eye Res.* 15:515, 1973.

35. Holly, F. J. Formation and stability of the tear film. *Int. Ophthalmol. Clin.* 13(1):73, 1973.

36. Holly, F. J. The precorneal tear film. *Contact Intraocular Lens Med. J.* 4:134, 1978.

37. Holly, F. J., Pattern, J. T., and Dohlman, C. H. Surface activity determination of aqueous tear components in dry eye patients and normals. *Exp. Eye Res.* 24:479, 1977.

38. Holly, F. J., and Lamberts, D. W. Effect of nonisotonic solutions on tear film osmolality. *Invest. Ophthalmol. Vis. Sci.* 20:236, 1981.

39. Huth, S. W., Hirano, P., and Leopold, I. H. Calcium in tears and contact lens wear. *Arch. Ophthalmol.* 98:122, 1980.

40. Impicciatore, M., Mariani, G., and Bertaccini, G. Action of eledoisin on human lacrimal secretion in normal and pathologic conditions. *Naunyn Schmiedebergs Arch. Pharmacol.* 279:127, 1973.

41. Iwata, S. Chemical composition of the aqueous phase. *Int. Ophthalmol. Clin.* 13(1):29, 1973.

42. Iwata, S., et al. Evaporation rate of water from the precorneal tear film and cornea in the rabbit. *Invest. Ophthalmol.* 8:613, 1969.

43. Jones, L. T. The lacrimal tear system and its treatment. *Am. J. Ophthalmol.* 62:47, 1966.

44. Jordan, A., and Baum, J. Basic tear flow: Does it exist? *Ophthalmology* (Rochester) 87:920, 1980.

45. Joshi, K. K., and Crockard, H. A. Traumatic cerebrospinal fluid fistula simulating tears: Case report. *J. Neurosurg.* 49:121, 1978.

46. Kitamura, S., and Ogli, K. The lacrimation under katamine anesthesia. *Jpn. J. Anesthesiol.* 20:749, 1971.

47. Koffler, B. H., and Lemp, M. A. The effect of an antihistamine (chlorpheniramine maleate) on tear production in humans. *Ann. Ophthalmol.* 12:217, 1980.

48. Krupin, T., Cross, D. A., and Becker, B. Decreased basal tear production associated with

general anesthesia. *Arch. Ophthalmol.* 95:107, 1977.

49. Kwan, J., Niinikoshi, J., and Hunt, T. In vivo measurement of oxygen tension in the cornea, aqueous humor and anterior lens of the open eye. *Invest. Ophthalmol.* 11:108, 1972.

50. Lamberts, D. W., Foster, C. S., and Perry, H. D. Schirmer test after topical anesthesia and the tear meniscus height in normal eye. *Arch. Ophthalmol.* 97:1082, 1979.

51. Lamberts, D. W., Perry, H. D., and Holly, F. J. Der Schirmer-Test bei offenen und geschlossenen Augen. *Contactologia* 2D:115, 1980.

52. Lemp, M. A., and Hamill, J. R. Factors affecting tear film break up in normal eyes. *Arch. Ophthalmol.* 89:103, 1975.

53. Libert, J., et al. Mannosidosis: Diagnosis by conjunctival biopsy and enzymatic analysis of the tears. *Bull. Mem. Soc. Fr. Ophtalmol.* 89:291, 1977.

54. Lyons, R. W. Orange contact lenses from rifampin. *N. Engl. J. Med.* 300:372, 1979.

55. MacKay, C., et al. Lactate dehydrogenase in tears. *Am. J. Ophthalmol.* 90:385, 1980.

56. Maes, J. The effect of removal of the superior cervical ganglion on lachrymal secretion. *Am. J. Physiol.* 123:359, 1938.

57. Maurice, D. M. New objective fluorophotometer. *Exp. Eye Res.* 2:33, 1963.

58. McDonald, J. E. Surface phenomena of the tear film. *Am. J. Ophthalmol.* 67:56, 1969.

59. McEwen, W. K., and Kimura, S. J. Filter paper electrophoresis of tears: I. Lysozyme and its correlation with keratoconjunctivitis sicca. *Am. J. Ophthalmol.* 39(Suppl.):200, 1955.

60. Mestecky, J., et al. Selective induction of immune response in human external secretions by ingestion of bacterial antigen. *J. Clin. Invest.* 61:731, 1978.

61. Minton, L. R. Paralimbal ring keratitis and absence of lysozyme in lupus erythematosus. *Am. J. Ophthalmol.* 60:532, 1965.

62. Mishima, S., et al. Determination of tear volume and tear flow. *Invest. Ophthalmol.* 5:264, 1966.

63. Mull, D. J., Peters, J. H., and Nichols, R. L. Immunoglobulins, secretory component, and transferrin in eye secretions of infants in regions with and without endemic trachoma. *Infect. Immun.* 2:489, 1970.

64. Nicolaides, N., et al. Meibomian gland studies: Comparison of steer and human lipids. *Invest. Ophthalmol. Vis. Sci.* 20:522, 1981.

65. Norn, M. S. Desiccation of the precorneal film: I. Corneal wetting time. *Acta Ophthalmol.* 47:865, 1969.

66. Ralph, R. A. Conjunctival goblet cell density in normal subjects and in dry eye syndromes. *Invest. Ophthalmol.* 14:299, 1975.

67. Reed, W. P., and Cushing, A. H. Role of immunoglobulins in protection against shigella-induced keratoconjunctivitis. *Infect. Immun.* 11:1265, 1975.

68. Reim, M., et al. Steady state levels of glucose in different layers of cornea, aqueous humor blood and tears in vivo. *Ophthalmologica* 154:39, 1967.

69. Ridley, F., and Sorsby, A. *Modern Trends in Ophthalmology.* New York: Hoeber, 1940.

70. Ruben, M. Contact lenses and oral contraceptives (letter to the editor). *Br. Med. J.* 1:1110, 1966.

71. Saha, K., et al. Ocular immunoglobulins in lepromatous leprosy. *Int. J. Lepr.* 4:338, 1977.

72. Sapse, A. T., et al. Human tear lysozyme: III. Preliminary study on lysozyme levels in subjects with smog irritation. *Am. J. Ophthalmol.* 66:76, 1968.

73. Scherz, W., Doane, M. G., and Dohlman, C. H. Tear volume in normal eyes and keratoconjunctivitis sicca. *Albrecht Von Graefes Arch. Klin. Exp. Ophthalmol.* 192:141, 1974.

74. Schirmer, O. Studien zur Physiologie und Pathologie der Tranenabsonderung und Tranenabfuhr. *Albrecht Von Graefes Arch. Ophthalmol.* 56:197, 1903.

75. Selinger, D. S., Selinger, R. C., and Reed, W. P. Resistance to infection of the external eye: The role of tears. *Surv. Ophthalmol.* 24:33, 1979.

76. Sen, D. K., and Sarin, G. S. Immunoassay of human tear lysozyme. *Am. J. Ophthalmol.* 90:715, 1980.

77. Sen, D. K., Sarin, G. S., and Saha, K. Immunoglobulins in tears in trachoma patients. *Br. J. Ophthalmol.* 61:218, 1977.

78. Slem, G., and Kumi, M. Bloody tears due to congenital factor III deficiency. *Ann. Ophthalmol.* 10:593, 1978.

79. Sorenson, T. Determination of tear flow using a radioactive tracer. *Acta Ophthalmol.* (Suppl.) 125:43, 1975.

80. South, M., et al. The IgA system. The clinical significance of IgA deficiency: Studies in patients with agammaglobulinemia and ataxiatelangiectasia. *Am. J. Med.* 44:168, 1968.

81. Thaysen, J. H., and Thorn, N. A. Excretion of urea, sodium, potassium and chloride in human tears. *Am. J. Physiol.* 178:160, 1954.

82. Thoft, R. A., and Friend, J. Corneal epithelial glucose utilization. *Arch. Ophthalmol.* 88:58, 1972.

83. Tondi, M., et al. Greater reliability of tear versus saliva anticonvulsant levels. *Ann. Neurol.* 4:154, 1978.

84. Tsuboyama, A., et al. The use of tears for diagnosis of GMI gangliosidosis. *Clin. Chim. Acta* 80:237, 1977.

85. Tsung, P. K., and Holly, F. J. Protease activities in human tears. *Curr. Eye Res.* 1:351, 1981.

86. Valentic, J. P., Leopold, I. H., and Dea, F. J. Excretion of salicylic acid into tears following oral administration of aspirin. *Ophthalmology* (Rochester) 87:817, 1979.

87. van Bijsterveld, O. P. Diagnostic tests in the sicca syndrome. *Arch. Ophthalmol.* 82:10, 1969.

88. van Haeringen, N. J., and Glasius, E. Collection method dependent concentration of some metabolites in human tear fluid with special reference to glucose in hyperglycemic conditions. *Albrecht Von Graefes Arch. Klin. Exp. Ophthalmol.* 202:1, 1977.

89. van Haeringen, N. J., and Glasius, E. Lysosomal hydrolases in tears and the lacrimal gland: Effect of acetylsalicylic acid on the release from the lacrimal gland. *Invest. Ophthalmol. Vis. Sci.* 19:826, 1980.

90. van Haeringen, N. J., Vrooland, J. L., and Glasius, E. Beta-hexosaminidase activities in tears and plasma diphosphoglycerate in blood of diabetic patients. *Clin. Chim. Acta* 86:333, 1978.

91. Vanley, G. T., Leopold, I. H., and Gregg, T. H. Interpretation of tear film breakup. *Arch. Ophthalmol.* 95:445, 1977.

92. Verbeck, B. Augenbefunde und Stoffwechselverhalten bei Einnahme von ovulationshemmern. *Klin. Monatsbl. Augenheilkd.* 162:612, 1973.

93. Vinogradova, V. L., and Basova, N. N. Micromethod of carrying out the passive hemagglutination reaction for detecting antibodies to influenza A2 virus in tears and aqueous humor. *Lab. Delo* 6:338, 1979.

94. von Roth, A. Uber die Tranenflussigkeit. *Klin. Monatsbl. Augenheilkd.* 68:589, 1922, cited by A. C. Krause, *The Biochemistry of the Eye.* Johns Hopkins Press, Baltimore, Maryland, 1934.

95. Williams, R. C., and Gibbons, R. J. Inhibition of bacterial adherence by secretory immunoglobulin A. A mechanism of antigen disposal. *Science* 177:697, 1972.

96. Wolf, E. *Anatomy of Eye and Orbit.* New York: Blakiston, 1954. Pp. 207–209.

97. Yamamoto, G. K., and Allansmith, M. R. Complement in tears from normal humans. *Am. J. Ophthalmol.* 88:758, 1979.

98. Zirm, M., Schmut, O., and Hofmann, H. Quantitative Bestimmung der Antiproteinasen in der menschlichen Tranenflussigkeit. *Albrecht Von Graefes Arch. Klin. Exp. Ophthalmol.* 198:89, 1976.

99. Zubareva, T. V., and Kiseleva, Z. M. Catecholamine content of the lacrimal fluid of healthy people and glaucoma patients. *Ophthalmologica* 175:339, 1977.

2. MORPHOLOGY AND PATHOLOGIC RESPONSES OF THE CORNEA TO DISEASE

Kenneth R. Kenyon

The constituents of the cornea are few, comprising only three distinct cell types (epithelium, keratocytes, and endothelium) and an extracellular matrix made up of collagen and glycosaminoglycans. It is convenient to consider corneal morphology and pathology in accord with the three major anatomically functional components that these cells and matrix form: the epithelium and its basement membrane, the keratocytes and stromal collagen, and the endothelium and Descemet's membrane. In this chapter, the discussion of these anatomic layers will be limited to general considerations of normal ultrastructural morphology, normal wound healing responses, reactions to specific insults (such as chemical injury or bacterial infection), and involvement in selected diseases.

NORMAL MORPHOLOGY

EPITHELIUM AND BASEMENT MEMBRANE

The cornea is surfaced by a nonkeratinized, squamous epithelium of five to seven cell layers; it is the most regularly arranged of all squamous epithelia in the body. The basal layer is composed of a single layer of columnar cells that are responsible for mitotic activity. Secreted by these cells and closely applied to their under surface is a thin (about 500 Å), uniform basement membrane that, together with its attendant hemidesmosomes and anchoring fibrils, composes the attachment complexes responsible for tight adhesion of the epithelium to the underlying Bowman's layer. A prominent cytoplasmic component of the basal cells are fine tonofilaments (keratofilaments) that converge on both the basal hemidesmosomes and the multiple desmosomes (maculae adherens) serving to attach adjacent cells focally along their interdigitated lateral plasma membranes (Fig. 2-1).

Multiple branches of the trigeminal nerve termi-

Supported in part by the James S. Adams Award from Research to Prevent Blindness, Inc., and by a grant-in-aid from Fight for Sight, Inc., New York City.

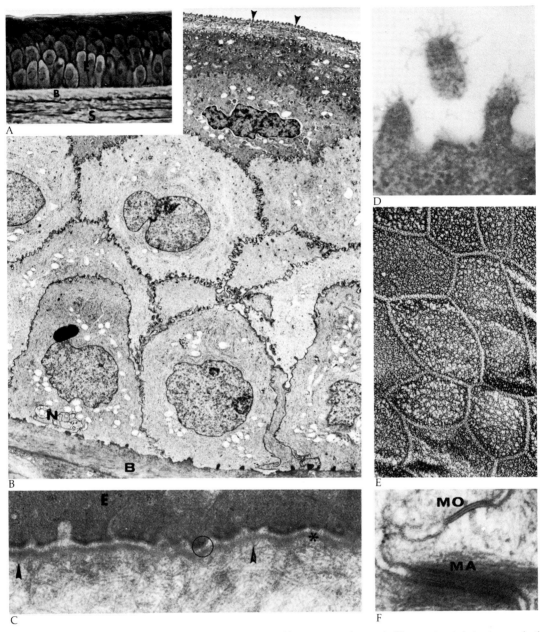

FIGURE 2-1. *Morphology of normal human cornea: epithelium and basement membrane. A. Phase-contrast photomicrograph of anterior corneal layers illustrates stratified, nonkeratinizing squamous epithelium (E) overlying a uniform Bowman's layer (B) and fibrocellular stroma (S). (Paraphenylenediamine, ×750.) B. Transmission EM of an area corresponding to A reveals flattened superficial epithelial cells with numerous surface microvilli (arrowheads), polygonal intermediate cells, and cuboidal basal cells closely apposed to Bowman's layer (B). A nonmyelinated sensory nerve ending (N) is seen among the basal cells. (×4000.) C. Transmission EM of interface between basal epithelial cells (E) and Bowman's layer resolves components of the basement membrane adhesion complex as hemidesmosomes (circled) of the basal cell membrane, a uniform continuous extracellular basement membrane (asterisk), and anchoring fibrils (arrowheads). Note uniform diameter collagen fibrils randomly arrayed as an acellular Bowman's layer. (×39,000.) D. High magnification transmission EM reveals cell membrane surface specializations as microvillous projections with fine glycoprotein material extending anteriorly into the tear film. (×95,000.) E. Scanning EM of superficial epithelial cells exhibits polygonal cell profiles and surface microvilli. (×2000.) F. High magnification transmission EM of junctional complex between superficial cells includes both macula occludens (tight junction, MO) and macula adherens (desmosome, MA). (×110,000.)*

44

nate as free, unmyelinated nerve endings between cells of the basal layer. Daughter cells of the basal layer are forced anteriorly to form the two or three intermediate layers of the wing or polygonal cells. These cells also contain diffusely distributed tonofilaments and a few small mitochondria. The two layers of superficial cells are extremely attenuated—they reach as much as 40 μ in length by about 4 μ in thickness. Junctional complexes are more numerous, and particularly important are the zonulae occludens or tight junctions between superficial cells, which form an important permeability barrier. The paucity of mitochondria and abundance of glycogen granules are consistent with low aerobic oxidation and greater dependence upon the pentose shunt. Although tonofilaments are abundant, no keratohyalin is normally formed in these cells. Another unique feature is the innumerable microplicae and microvilli of the anterior plasma membrane. By greatly augmenting the free surface area, these microprojections increase tear film retention and enhance diffusion and active transport processes. Fine filaments extending from the surface projections are probably absorbed mucopolysaccharides, or mucins, essential contributors to tear film stability.

The surface characteristics of these cells are best observed by scanning electron microscopy. The flat, polygonal epithelial cells are firmly attached to each other along relatively straight cell boundaries. In most species, microvilli and microplicae measuring 0.5 to 1.0 μ high and about 0.15 μ wide occur in a random reticular or corrugated pattern [50, 87], although the intricate fingerprintlike surface configurations found in marine teleosts are a striking contrast [46]. The relative density of surface elaborations accounts for the variable texture of these cells seen by scanning electron microscopy: "Light" cells have more microprojections; "dark" cells have fewer. This correlates well with cell age. The younger cells have the most elaborate reticulation, whereas the older, desquamating cells have lost this membrane specialization and with it the ability to hold the tear film [50].

KERATOCYTES AND STROMA

Immediately subjacent to the epithelium and basement membrane is Bowman's layer, an acellular area approximately 10 μ thick consisting of randomly oriented collagen fibrils of relatively small diameter (approximately 160–220 Å) within a glycosaminoglycan ground substance [55, 58]. The anterior surface of Bowman's layer is smooth where it faces the basement membrane, but posteriorly it merges indistinctly with the less densely compacted collagen of the stroma. In some species, Bowman's layer is thought to represent a remnant of the primary stroma deposited by the embryonic epithelium [48]; however, there is no evidence for this origin in higher species. Bowman's layer is considered to have no regenerative capacity when damaged, so that healing involves scarring (Fig. 2-2).

In the human, the corneal stroma is approximately 500 μ thick centrally and 1000 μ thick peripherally, thereby representing about 90 percent of the entire corneal thickness. There are 200 to 250 stromal lamellae, each about 2 μ thick and 9 to 260 μ wide. Individual collagen fibrils measure 240 to 300 Å in width, with larger fibrils more posterior. The relatively even spacing of collagen fibrils is promoted by the glycosaminoglycans surrounding them. The uniform diameter of the collagen fibrils, their parallelism within the layers, the relatively equal distances among them, and the even layering of the approximately orthogonally arrayed lamellae confer clarity on the cornea. Biochemically, the collagen fibrils are predominantly type I, with some types II and AB also present [47]; the glycosaminoglycans consist primarily of keratan sulfate and chondroitin sulfate in a ratio of about 3 : 1 [7].

The main cellular constituent of the stroma is the keratocyte, a mesenchymally derived cell with fibroblastic capabilities for synthesis and secretion of the stromal collagens and ground substances in both developmental and reparative states. Under normal conditions, the keratocytes are relatively few, accounting for only 5 percent of the corneal dry weight. Morphologically, these cells are fusiform with long cytoplasmic processes coursing between the planes of adjacent collagen lamellae. Their organelles are typical of a protein-secreting cell: free ribosomes, cisternae of rough-surfaced endoplasmic reticulum, Golgi apparatus, lysosomes, secretory vesicles, and mitochondria [45]. In addition to active participation in wound healing, the keratocytes are also involved in other pathologic processes, as evidenced by the intracellular accumulation of neutral and complex lipids, mucopolysaccharides, proteins (e.g., cysteine and myeloma proteins), and drug metabolites [60].

In addition to keratocytes, occasional polymorphonuclear leukocytes (PMNs), plasma cells, and macrophages are evident in the normal stroma. The sensory nerves that ultimately terminate in the basal epithelial layer also course radially from the limbus through the anterior stroma.

ENDOTHELIUM AND DESCEMET'S MEMBRANE

The endothelium is the most posterior corneal layer and consists of a monolayer of approximately 0.5 million hexagonal cells of mesenchymal origin (Fig. 2-3). Uniform cell size (about 20 μ in diameter and 5 μ thick) and regular spacing in early life gives way to irregular spacing and size in older adults as cells die and are not capable of mitotic replacement [53]. The normal endothelial cell is cuboidal and contains a large oblong nucleus and cytoplasmic organelles including rough- and smooth-surfaced endoplasmic reticulum, prominent Golgi apparatus, an apical terminal web, numerous pinocytotic and exocytotic vesicles, and myriad mitochondria, plus occasional phagocytosed melanin [54]. The lateral plasma membranes of adjacent cells are extensively interdigitated and have been shown to be the location of a Na-K ATPase–dependent pump [76]. Intercellular junctions along these same membranes near their apical borders are mainly composed of gap junctions with tight junctions evident in only some areas [75]. Thus, as a continuous monolayer of closely apposed, metabolically capable cells, the corneal endothelium is suited for its functions as a barrier to fluid flow and as an actively transporting ion pump.

Descemet's membrane is a true basement membrane derived from the endothelial cells, and is interposed between stroma and endothelium. It is initially evident during the fourth month of fetal development as single and then multiple basement membrane layers that become organized into the banded (ca. 1100-Å period) anterior portion of Descemet's membrane (ca. 3-μ thickness at birth). Subsequent endothelial cell secretion of Descemet's membrane consists of more homogeneous material that continues to thicken throughout life, attaining as much as 10 to 15 μ in the normal adult [15, 52]. Biochemical characterization of normal Descemet's membrane indicates that it is type IV collagen, whereas the abnormal posterior collagen layers secreted by distressed endothelium also contain type I collagen [59, 84]. Such thickenings of Descemet's membrane provide a morphologic record of the chronology of recurrent endothelial disease [66, 104].

PATHOLOGIC RESPONSES

EPITHELIUM AND BASEMENT MEMBRANE

NORMAL WOUND HEALING

Immediately after full-thickness wounding of the corneal epithelium, the damaged cells adjacent to the wound edge lose surface microvilli [45, 77]. Within 1 hour, the basal cells begin to flatten as intermediate and superficial cells reduce their des-

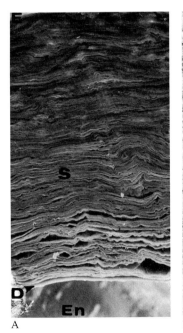
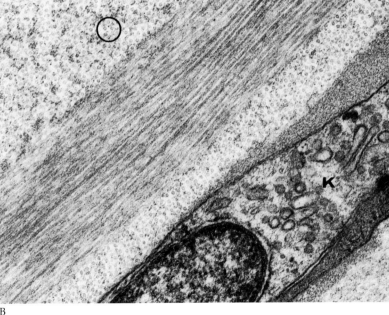

A   B

FIGURE 2-2. *Morphology of normal human cornea: keratocytes and stroma. A. Scanning EM of transversely sectioned cornea demonstrates epithelial cell layers (E), multilamellar stroma (S), uniform Descemet's membrane (D, arrowhead), and endothelial monolayer (En). (× 200.) B. Transmission EM of stroma shows adjacent lamellae to be composed of closely arrayed collagen fibrils (circled) with uniform 240- to 260-Å cross-sectional diameter organized as orthogonal plys with intervening fibrocytic keratocytes (K). (× 50,000.)*

mosomal junctions and glycogen storage, evidencing their impending movement. Fibronectin, the glycoprotein widely involved in cell-to-cell and cell-to-substrate interactions, is deposited on the denuded corneal surface, along with fibrinogen and fibrin [38]. PMNs arrive via the tear film and begin the process of debriding cellular remnants. At approximately 6 hours after wounding, the epithelial cells initiate wound closure by sliding into the area of defect at a rate of about 0.75 μ per minute [74, 86]. Basal cells distant from the wound begin to undergo mitosis. Epithelial sliding is quite active by 15 hours as the leading cells extend ruffled pseudopods whose motility depends upon the actin filaments of the cytoskeleton [40]. Actin filaments may also be involved in cell adhesion as they insert into the electron-dense inner aspect of the hemidesmosome attachment plaques. As the defect is closed, contact inhibition causes cessation of cell movement and alteration in cellular configuration as these migrating squamous cells again assume the cuboidal configuration of basal cells. At the same time, DNA synthesis begins. Between 24 and 48 hours after wounding, epithelial proliferation within the wound, now at its peak, forms an epithelial plug,

and all PMNs vanish. By 3 to 4 days after wounding, the epithelial plug regresses and mitotic figures first appear within the wound [5] (Fig. 2-4).

If the epithelial basement membrane has not been damaged by the abrasion, the recovering epithelial cells are able to utilize it for tight adhesion to the underlying stroma, as is evidenced both morphologically by the reappearance of hemidesmosomes on day 2 after injury, as well as clinically by tight adhesion shortly thereafter [72]. However, if the basement membrane has been damaged, then new basement membrane complexes, comprising short discontinuous segments of basement membrane material with associated hemidesmosomes and anchoring fibrils, begin to re-form within 5 to 7 days after injury. Depending upon the severity of basement membrane damage, as long as 6 to 8 weeks may be required for complete basement membrane reconstruction. This process is closely paralleled by delayed epithelium-to-stroma adhesion until the intact basement membrane has been restored [68].

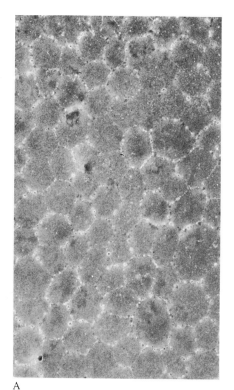
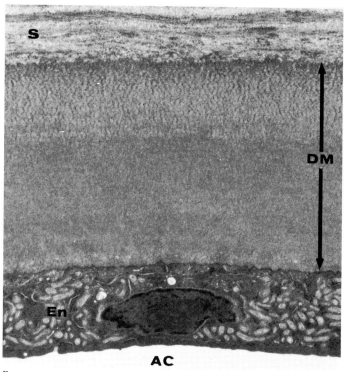

A   B

FIGURE 2-3. *Morphology of normal human cornea: endothelium and Descemet's membrane. A. Scanning EM best illustrates the closely contiguous monolayer of polygonal endothelial cells. (×500.) B. Transmission EM of posterior corneal layers includes the collagenous stroma (S), Descemet's membrane (DM) with anterior banded and posterior nonbanded portions, and mitochondria-rich endothelial cell (En) bordering the anterior chamber (AC). (×6,000.)*

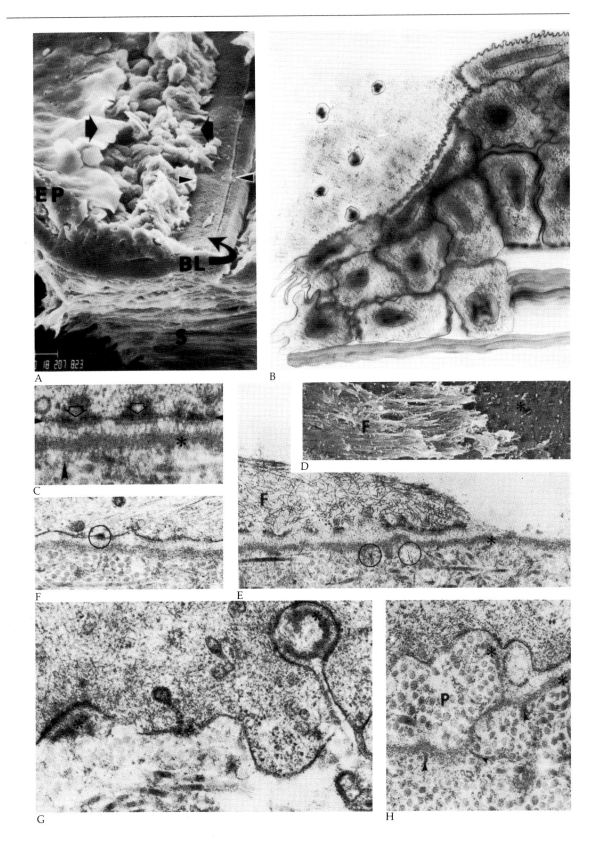

A

B

C

D

E

F

G

H

FIGURE 2-4. *Normal epithelial wound healing. A. Scanning EM immediately after trephine incision of epithelium and stroma, with wound margin seen at right. Immediately adjacent to the wound margin, an exposed zone of Bowman's layer (BL) appears intact (between arrowheads) but is devoid of epithelial cells. Farther from the wound margin, an area of disrupted epithelial cells is evident (between arrows), and more distant from the wound edge, the epithelium (EP) appears unaffected. (S = stroma.) (× 600.) B. Diagram of epithelium 15 to 72 hours after wounding. Epithelial sliding is active as filopodia extend from the crest and edges of ruffled epithelial cells into the defect area. Intracellular spaces are distended. As the base of the wound is covered, the cells increase in height and begin again to resemble basal cells. Cellular organelles increase in size and complexity, and villous specializations of the free surface membrane begin to reappear. (A and B from P. S. Binder, et al. Corneal anatomy and wound healing.* Trans. New Orleans Acad. Ophthalmol. St. Louis: Mosby, 1980.) *C. Transmission EM at high magnification shows basement membrane attachment complexes to comprise cytoplasmic filaments within basal epithelial cells, converging at hemidesmosomes (arrows), penetrating the plasma membrane (small arrowheads), bridging the lamina lucida between plasma membrane and basement membrane (asterisk), and establishing continuity with anchoring fibrils (large arrowhead) in Bowman's layer. (× 100,000.) D. Transmission EM of rabbit cornea immediately after mechanical scraping of epithelium. The basal cells have been ruptured transversely, leaving masses of filamentous debris (F) overlying an intact basement membrane (asterisk) with well-developed anchoring fibrils (circled). (× 30,000.) E. Scanning EM of preparation corresponding to D reveals filamentous cellular debris (F) adherent to exposed and intact basement membrane (asterisk). (× 1500.) F. Transmission EM of rabbit cornea 3 days after mechanical scraping of epithelium. Newly migrating epithelium has come to rest upon the original basement membrane, and few hemidesmosomal attachment sites (circled) have formed. (× 40,000.) G. Transmission EM of rabbit cornea 7 days after superficial keratectomy illustrates beginnings of attachment complex reconstruction as short discontinuous segments of basement membrane (asterisk) with attendant hemidesmosomes along infoldings of the basal cell membrane. (× 40,000.) H. Transmission EM of rabbit cornea 30 days after superficial keratectomy includes areas of irregularity and duplication of basement membrane (asterisk), separated from basal cell membrane by fibrillar collaginous pannus (P), as evidence of probable epithelial erosion or edema. Numerous anchoring fibrils (arrowheads) are evident. (× 40,000.)*

After regression of the epithelial plug, mitoses appear in the wound base, and soon the overlying new epithelium becomes even with the adjacent old epithelium. The regenerating epithelium is important in activating the underlying keratocytes, since they fail to transform into fibroblasts in the absence of overlying epithelium [21, 24]. The epithelium may also be involved in the recruitment of PMNs into the wound area.

Another important aspect of corneal epithelial wound healing is the effect of hormones, biochemical messengers, and pharmacologic agents. At present, however, data on the effects of these agents on epithelial proliferation are fragmentary and in some cases contradictory. For example, the classic studies of Friedenwald and Bushke indicated

that influences on the corneal epithelial healing were adrenergically mediated, since topically administered epinephrine reduced epithelial cell locomotion, mitosis, and wound healing [34]. Subsequently, however, it was demonstrated that partial autonomic denervation of the cornea by sympathetic ganglionectomy (which should *reduce* the amount of norepinephrine at the epithelial cells) also led to a substantial reduction of epithelial mitosis and severe neurotrophic keratitis [1, 9, 79]. Adding to the confusion is the fact that sympathetic fibers have not been traced into the human corneal epithelium, even though adrenergic receptors have been found on the epithelial cells [82].

Similar paradoxes are found in the parasympathetic-acetylcholine (Ach) system. The evidence for parasympathetic innervation of the cornea is circumstantial, and such innervation seems especially unlikely in the absence of demonstrable Ach receptors on the epithelial cells. The question regarding parasympathetic innervation exists despite the fact that the epithelial cells themselves contain very high levels of Ach, which may function in some yet-to-be-defined way to regulate cellular metabolism in a nonneuronal fashion [83].

So-called second messengers, including adenosine 3',5'-cyclic phosphate (cAMP) and guanosine 3',5'-cyclic phosphate (cGMP) have been implicated in corneal epithelial cell metabolic control by Cavanagh [12]. Although a direct, inverse relationship between the levels of these two substances no longer seems likely in the cornea, it is likely that regulation of cAMP by other messengers such as prostaglandins may well play an important role in corneal epithelial healing [27].

Another modulator of mitotic rate in corneal epithelium is epidermal growth factor (EGF). Frati and coworkers [33] and Savage and Cohen [90] have independently shown that EGF applied to wounded rabbit corneas stimulates re-epithelialization by a transient hyperplasia of epithelial cell layers. The mechanism by which EGF influences proliferation of corneal epithelium is unknown.

RESPONSE TO LIMITED OCULAR SURFACE INJURY
The course of healing of the ocular surface epithelium varies with the extent as well as the intensity of the injury (Fig. 2-5). Limited mechanical abrasions and mild chemical or thermal burns of the central cornea usually heal rapidly by the mechanism detailed in the previous section. In the rabbit, regenerated corneal epithelium shows restoration of its biochemical components, including glycogen

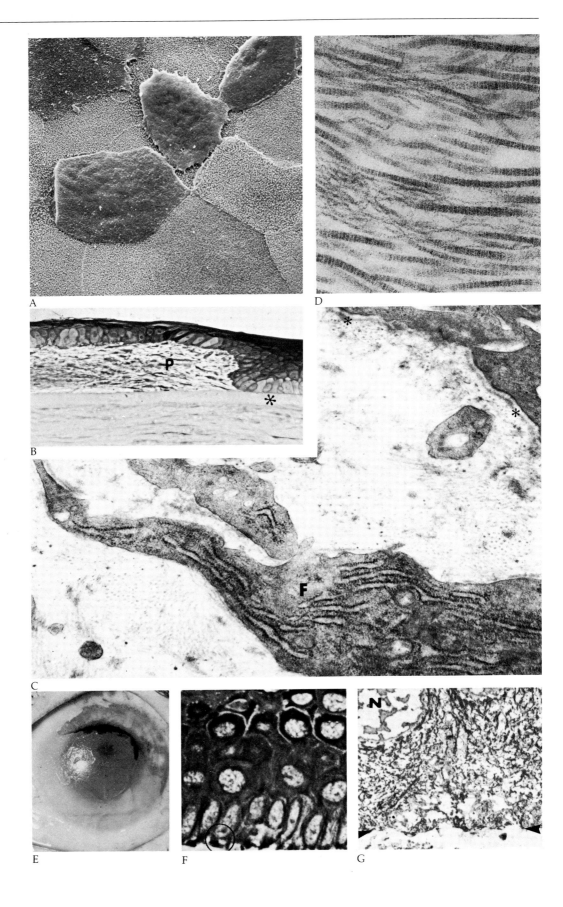

A

B

C

D

E

F

G

P

*

*

*

F

N

FIGURE 2-5. *Healing response to mild ocular surface injury. A. Scanning EM of monkey cornea after thermal cauterization illustrates morphology of superficial punctate keratitis as individual epithelial cells have lost surface membrane infoldings and are desquamating. Underlying and surrounding normal-appearing epithelium exhibits surface microplicae. (×1000.) B. Phase-contrast photomicrograph of human cornea 1 year after penetrating injury demonstrates proliferation of fibrocellular pannus (P) between epithelium and intact Bowman's layer (asterisk). (Paraphenylenediamine, × 500.) C. Transmission EM of corresponding area reveals basement membrane (asterisk) to be complete except for focal discontinuity. Multiple fibroblastic cells (F) within collagenous pannus appear synthetically active as evidenced by abundant rough endoplasmic reticulum. (×42,000.) D. At higher magnification, transmission EM reveals collagenous components of pannus to be randomly organized, banded fibrils of variable large diameter (up to 500 Å), with fine filaments interspersed. (×62,000.) E. This 33-year-old woman sustained an extensive burn by weak acid of nearly the total ocular surface epithelium. Anatomic and visual recovery were excellent after vigorous topical steroid and antibiotic therapy. F. Phase-contrast photomicrograph of debrided corneal epithelium (48 hours after injury) of eye shown in E demonstrates preservation of epithelial cell organization, despite cytoplasmic coagulation. (Paraphenylenediamine, ×1000.) G. Transmission EM of area circled in F shows nuclear (N) and cytoplasmic coagulation of basal epithelial cells. Basal plasma membrane (between arrowheads) is notably devoid of basement membrane, which is presumed to have remained attached to Bowman's layer. (×5000.)*

and glycolytic enzymes, as soon as healing is completed, and this corresponds to a normal clinical and morphologic appearance as well [35, 98]. With more severe injury of the corneal surface, involving damage to the basement membrane complexes of the basal epithelial cells and the anterior stroma, recovery may be slowed, however. For example, extreme chemical burns involving both the corneal and conjunctival epithelium heal slowly with recurrent epithelial erosions, scarring, and vascularization; this pattern of healing is related in part to the intrinsically different regenerative capacities of the corneal and conjunctival epithelial cells.

Compromise of the epithelial cells and their surface characteristics is clinically evident as surface irregularity and superficial punctate keratitis, which corresponds to microscopic epithelial defects, and also as loss of normal cell surface microplicae in the desquamating cells. Although basement membrane damage can also contribute to the formation of persistent epithelial defects or recurrent erosions, as will be described below, these problems are fortunately unusual. Thus, for example, even after a relatively extensive acid burn of the human cornea and bulbar conjunctiva, epithelial recovery is rapid and secure [100]. As shown in Figure 2-5, the denatured corneal epithelium demonstrates nuclear pyknosis and cytoplasmic shrinkage. However, transmission electron microscopy fails to disclose any basement membrane material adherent to these devitalized

basal epithelial cells, and the functional integrity of the original basement membrane is clinically attested by tight adhesion of the regenerated epithelium, which rapidly resurfaces the entire cornea and involved bulbar conjunctiva. Because of limited acid-induced denaturation of stromal collagen and ground substance, topical steroids can be liberally applied to inhibit inflammation.

Should, however, chemical penetration be more severe, then subepithelial fibroblastic proliferation may result in superficial stromal scarring in the form of a fibrocellular pannus with or without neovascularization. This pannus comprises randomly arrayed type II collagen fibrils of variable sizes and is the product of keratocytes that have been stimulated to transform into fibroblasts. Such a pannus may accumulate between the epithelium and Bowman's layer or, more commonly, may develop in the anterior stroma with minimal detriment to corneal clarity and vision.

RESPONSE TO EXTENSIVE OCULAR
SURFACE INJURY

Injuries involving larger areas of the ocular surface show a different pattern of healing (Fig. 2-6). If, for example, the wound involves the entire cornea and extends beyond the limbus, the corneal surface must be recovered with epithelium of conjunctival origin. In this situation, the obligate transformation of conjunctival cells into corneal epithelium is prolonged functionally, morphologically, and biochemically [35, 98, 100]. Such eyes face extended clinical morbidity as they are beset with chronic inflammation, persistent epithelial defects, recurrent erosions, stromal neovascularization, and sterile ulceration. Epithelial cells at the margin of persistent defects often display an elevated border, having undergone an arrest of both migratory and mitotic activity. Nor is there evidence of cellular synthesis of the basement membrane material that may have been chemically denatured by the injury [49].

The overgrowth of conjunctival epithelium onto the cornea is also marked by the presence of goblet cells. Such retention of goblet cells on the cornea has been observed to correspond very closely to areas where the stroma has become vascularized, which is perhaps indicative of the persistently altered biochemical state and metabolic needs of epithelial cells [91, 98]. Somewhat paradoxically, as has been recently observed in chemically burned human eyes, goblet cells are not only numerous and morphologically normal [26], but nongoblet epithelial cells appear to be increasingly involved in mucus

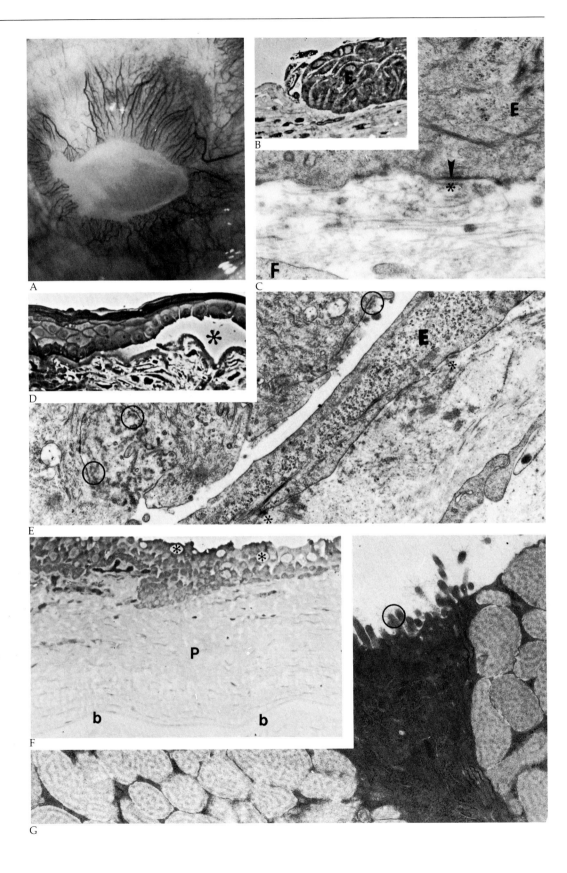

FIGURE 2-6. *Healing response to severe ocular surface injury. A. This 43-year-old industrial worker is seen 1 year after acid and alkali injury to the entire ocular surface, with central persistent epithelial defect surrounded by vascularized conjunctival overgrowth. B. Phase-contrast photomicrograph of monkey cornea 2 weeks after thermal cauterization shows multilayered, amitotic epithelium (E) at edge of a persistent epithelial defect. Severe inflammatory and fibrocytic cells appear in the superficial stroma. (Paraphenylenediamine; × 900.) C. Transmission EM of area in B discloses slowly advancing epithelium to have produced only rare basement membrane (asterisk) and hemidesmosomes (arrowhead). A fibroblast (F) has infiltrated Bowman's layer. (× 32,000.) D. Phase-contrast photomicrograph at 10 weeks after dilute sulfuric acid burn of rhesus monkey cornea shows irregular epithelial sheet separated (at asterisk) from scarred Bowman's layer and anterior stroma. (Paraphenylenediamine; × 600.) E. Transmission EM of corresponding area shows epithelium to have become elevated with adherent fragments of basement membrane material (circled), allowing insinuation of flattened epithelial cells (E) with limited basement membrane deposition (asterisk) (× 17,500.) F. Light photomicrograph of human cornea shown in A demonstrates characteristics of conjunctival overgrowth. Disorganized epithelium containing goblet cells (asterisk) overlies a thick fibrovascular pannus (P) that has developed anterior to the relatively intact Bowman's layer (b). (Paraphenylenediamine; × 250.) G. Transmission EM of area shown in F shows that epithelial surface cells have normal microvillous surface membrane specialization (circled) and adjacent goblet cells have normal-appearing mucin globules. (× 18,700.)*

secretion as well [44]. Hence, in contrast to previous interpretations, mucus deficiency need not be invoked as a significant contributor to the pathologic changes of the ocular surface of the chemically burned eye.

Epithelium derived from conjunctiva also has a dramatic effect on the response of the corneal stroma to subsequent wounding; a rabbit cornea covered by epithelium conjunctival origin demonstrates a marked stromal neovascular response to subsequent wounding [99].

SPECIFIC PATHOLOGIC REACTIONS

KERATINIZATION: XEROPHTHALMIA

Xerophthalmia is a highly clinically relevant example of ocular surface keratinization. *Xerophthalmia* is the term used to describe the irregular, lusterless, poorly wettable surface of the conjunctiva and cornea associated with vitamin A deficiency (see Chapter 13, Dietary Deficiency). Bitot's spots, the triangular, foamy, keratotic areas of interpalpebral bulbar conjunctiva adjacent to the limbus, are also sometimes correlated with vitamin A deficiency. In humans, biopsy specimens of xerotic conjunctiva and cornea show remarkable acanthosis and hyperkeratosis with a prominent granular cell layer containing keratofibrils and keratohyalin granules [94, 95] (Fig. 2-7). Frequently, pleomorphic gram-positive bacilli, presumably diphtheroids, are clustered about the superficial keratin debris. Electron

microscopy shows that the superficial cell layers appear cornified and have lost almost all recognizable organelles except extremely compacted keratofibrils. The surface plasma membrane has greatly reduced microplicae, as confirmed by scanning electron microscopy. If vitamin A therapy is effective, clinical and histologic normalization begins within 1 to 2 weeks, although conjunctival goblet cells are only initially evident at 1 month and may require 2 or 3 months or longer for complete restoration [94].

CICATRIZATION: PEMPHIGOID

Cicatricial pemphigoid is a slowly progressive, chronic condition primarily affecting the mucosa of the mouth, nose, pharynx, and conjunctiva with bullous formation, shrinkage, and scarring (see Corneal Manifestations of Dermatologic Disorders in Chapter 6, Immunologic Diseases). Cutaneous lesions may involve the face and scalp. These bullous lesions occur between the basal cells and basement membrane, and in a fully developed blister the basement membrane is usually destroyed. In many patients with clinically active disease, immunofluorescence studies disclose fixed immunoglobulins in the basement membrane zone of involved skin or mucosa as well as circulating basement membrane antibodies [39, 80]. With progression of the conjunctival involvement, connective tissue proliferation and symblepharon result. In extreme cases, xerosis, keratinization of the conjunctiva, and epidermidalization of the cornea develops (Fig. 2-7E–I).

Histologically, the conjunctival and corneal epithelium demonstrates surface keratinization with acanthosis and spongiosis. By transmission electron microscopy, keratohyalin granules are particularly visible in the thickened granular cell layer, as are increased desmosomes [11]. Although actual bullous lesions are not seen clinically in the conjunctiva, ultrastructural examinations disclose duplications of multilaminar basement membrane in the bulbar conjunctival epithelium, which may be related to the reformation of basement membrane complexes after resolution of an epithelial separation. These histologic and immunopathologic findings are similar to those in bullous pemphigoid, a nonocular bullous disease in which circulating antibodies react with a specific antigen localized to the lamina lucida portion of the basement membrane zone [32]. Because of these similarities, it may be appropriate to consider cicatricial mucous membrane pemphigoid and bullous pemphigoid as representing the same pathologic process.

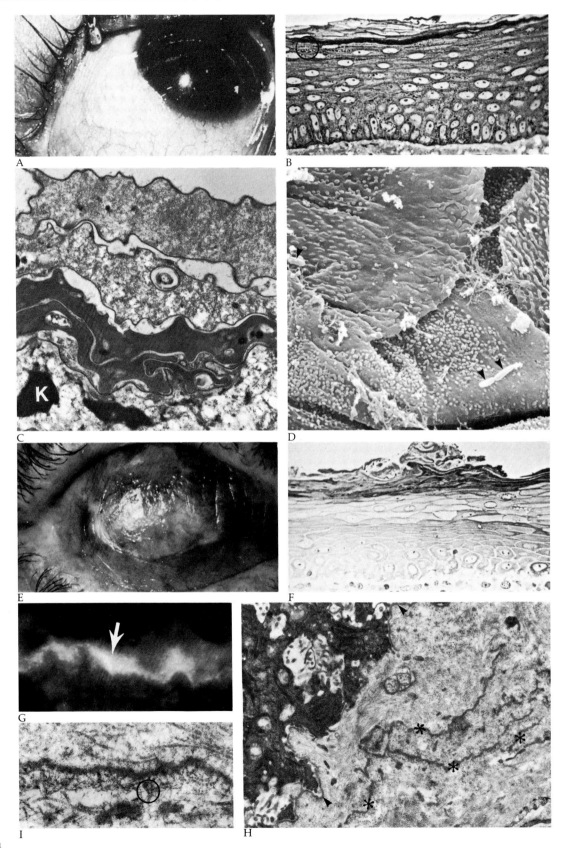

A

B

C

D

E

F

G

H

I

FIGURE 2-7. *Keratinization and cicatrization. A. In this patient with vitamin A deficiency, corneal xerosis and conjunctival Bitot's spot are evident. B. Phase-contrast photomicrograph of conjunctival epithelium from Bitot's spot discloses surface keratization, granulosa cell layer with numerous keratohyalin granules (circled), acanthosis, and disorganization of basal cells. (Paraphenylenediamine, ×700.) C. Transmission EM of area seen in B shows multiple cornified epithelial remnants, with granulosa cells containing keratohyalin (K). (×13,500.) D. Scanning EM of this specimen shows multiple laminations of keratinized cellular remnants with bacilli (arrowheads) adherent. (×5,000.) E. This advanced case of cicatricial mucous membrane pemphigoid shows total ankyloblepharon with an absolutely dry, vascularized, epidermidalized corneal surface. F. Phase-contrast microscopy of bulbar conjunctiva of eye in E shows surface keratinization, granulosa cell layer containing keratohyalin granules, and chronic inflammatory infiltrate of stroma. (Paraphenylenediamine, ×400.) G. Normal human conjunctiva stained by indirect immunofluorescent technique after exposure to serum from pemphigoid patient shows immunoglobulins localized along the basement membrane zone (arrow) of the epithelium. (Fluorescein-conjugated antihuman IgG; ×400.) (From R. M. Franklin [32].) H. Transmission electron microscopy of conjunctiva shows intracellular edema of basal cells and discontinuous basement membrane (arrowheads). Multiple laminations of basement membrane material (asterisk) are separated from the basal epithelium by scar collagen. (×6000.) I. Higher magnification of area indicated by asterisk in H shows duplication of entire basement membrane complexes, complete with anchoring fibrils (circled), and random arrangement of fibrillar collagen intervening between laminations. (×30,000.)*

RECURRENT EPITHELIAL EROSION: PRIMARY AND SECONDARY BASEMENT MEMBRANE DISORDERS

In the preceding sections it was emphasized that basement membrane complexes are responsible for the maintenance of tight adhesions between the corneal epithelium and stroma. Hence, any dystrophic or traumatic abnormality of the basement membrane complex would be expected to compromise the bond between epithelium and stroma and could then result in recurrent epithelial erosions [62]. In fact, when basement membrane is experimentally damaged by any technique, the consistent sequelae include irregularity and defects of the epithelial surface. Discontinuities and duplications of basement membrane complexes persist for 8 weeks or more, during which time the nonadherent epithelium is easily separable from the stroma [29, 68, 72]. These same studies also emphasize the importance of the anterior stromal collagen of Bowman's layer to which the basement membrane adheres. Although abnormalities of basement membrane complexes alone may explain poor adhesions and recurrent erosions in some situations, in others, damage to Bowman's layer and anterior stroma with the accumulation of cellular and extracellular debris may also confound adhesion, despite the presence of basement membrane that appears morphologically normal [49].

Many clinical conditions that affect the corneal surface are manifested by recurrent erosions and persistent defects of the epithelium. These conditions can be considered as either primary or secondary causes of erosion, depending on whether the defect in the epithelial basement membrane is intrinsic or acquired. Among the primary disorders, map-dot-fingerprint dystrophy is most common (Fig. 2-8A–G). This designation is based on the clinical morphologic finding of opaque intraepithelial cysts (dots), maplike geographic patterns, and whorled fingerprintlike ridges at the level of the epithelial basement membrane [16, 89]. Such changes have been noted in many people who are clinically asymptomatic, and in some families an apparent autosomal dominant inheritance has been determined [101] (see Chapter 9, Dystrophies and Degenerations). In symptomatic persons, the epithelium shows loose adhesion, and it may detach either spontaneously or after minor trauma. Thus, in patients presenting with recurrent erosion, slit lamp examination of the uninvolved eye and of asymptomatic family members may establish a diagnosis.

Light and electron microscopy studies have established that the microcystic areas correspond to intraepithelial pseudocysts containing cellular debris. Geographic configurations represent thickened subepithelial plaques composed of abnormal multiple laminations of basement membrane and fibrillar collagens; fingerprint lines consist of ridges of aberrant collagen and fibrous tissue [16, 28, 89]. In these conditions, it is possible that dystrophic abnormalities of basement membrane complexes or adjacent structures permit the loosely adherent epithelium to shift, which would account for the accumulation of these abnormal configurations and for the predisposition to symptomatic erosions.

In some patients, diabetes mellitus produces abnormalities of corneal epithelial adhesion. These corneal changes might also be considered a primary corneal basement membrane disorder. Ultrastructural studies of the human diabetic cornea have revealed an abnormality of the epithelial basement membrane that consists of thickening of the multilaminar basement membrane and duplications of anchoring fibrils [62] (Fig. 2-8H–J). These changes are identical to those of the primary epithelial dystrophies. Although diabetic patients apparently do not experience an increased incidence of spontaneous epithelial erosions, vitreoretinal surgeons know that the diabetic corneal epithelium becomes clouded very early during surgery and often

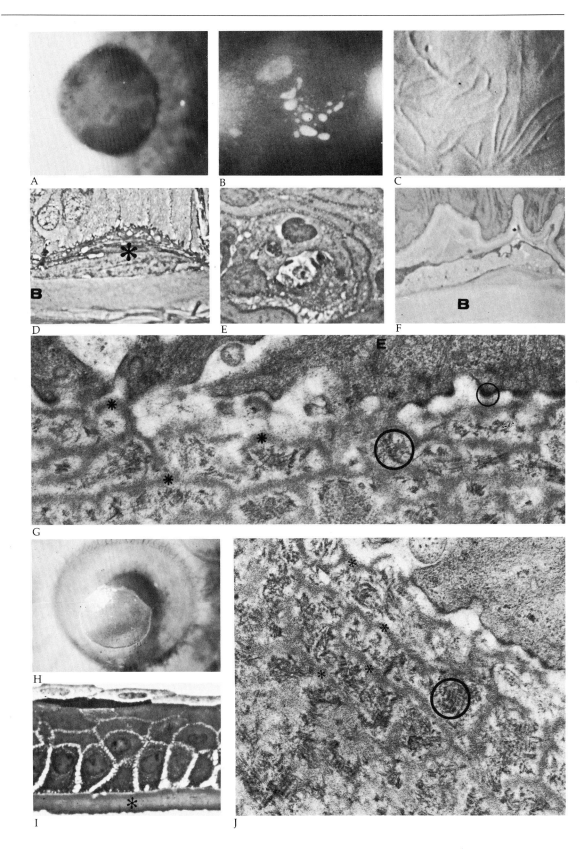

FIGURE 2-8. *Primary basement membrane disorder: recurrent corneal erosion. Map-dot-fingerprint dystrophy. A. Clinical photo of 37-year-old man with nontraumatic recurrent erosion shows characteristics of map dystrophy with superficial geographic haze interrupted by clear areas. B. In the dot form of microcystic dystrophy, superficial opaque cysts are evident within the epithelium. C. In fingerprint dystrophy, subepithelial ridges are particularly enhanced by retrolumination. (Slit lamp photo courtesy Lawrence Hirst, M.D.) D. Phase-contrast microscopy of map dystrophy shows fibrous tissue (asterisk) between epithelium and Bowman's layer (B). (Paraphenylenediamine, × 1000.) E. Phase-contrast microscopy of dot dystrophy shows an intraepithelial pseudocyst evolving from disintegration of desquamating cells. (Paraphenylenediamine; × 1200.) F. Phase-contrast photomicrograph of fingerprint dystrophy illustrates intraepithelial extensions of abnormal fibrocellular material anterior to the normal-appearing Bowman's layer (B). (Paraphenylenediamine; × 800.) G. Transmission EM in these disorders consistently finds multiple laminations of basement membrane material (asterisk) with reduced hemidesmosomes (small circle) and increased anchoring fibrils (large circle) beneath epithelium (E). (× 40,000.) Diabetes mellitus. H. Trophic-appearing epithelial defect in a diabetic patient after vitreous surgery. I. Phase-contrast photomicrograph of nonadherent epithelium removed during vitreous surgery reveals extensively thickened basement membrane material (asterisk) adherent to intact epithelial layer. (Paraphenylenediamine, × 1000.) J. Transmission EM of this specimen shows remarkable multilaminar configuration of basement membrane (asterisk) with aberrant anchoring fibrils (circled) interspersed (compare with G). (× 40,000.)*

sloughs as an intact epithelial sheet. Postoperatively, these corneas are slow to reepithelialize and can develop persistent defects [85]. In nondiabetic humans and animals, corneal epithelial scraping results in rupture of basal cells with maintenance of basement membrane attachment to Bowman's layer. In the diabetic cornea on the other hand, the entire epithelium separates as an intact sheet with the entire basement membrane remaining adherent to the basal cells [62]. This observation suggests that a major component of this erosive disorder is the lack of adhesion between the basement membrane complex and the underlying stroma.

Among secondary erosive disorders, stromal dystrophies of the cornea may also be clinically evident as surface problems, particularly in patients with lattice or granular dystrophy. Although lattice dystrophy, a dominantly inherited form of corneal amyloidosis, primarily involves the stroma, amyloid deposition also frequently occurs between the epithelium and Bowman's layer [28, 62] (see Chapter 9, Dystrophies and Degenerations). The resultant irregularity of basement membrane complexes interferes with epithelial adhesion, and erosive episodes are frequently the initial visual symptom in the young patient with lattice dystrophy (Fig. 2-9A, B).

Although intraepithelial herpes simplex virus does not produce erosive problems, the corneal epithelium frequently will not adhere to the stroma in metaherpetic keratitis because of damage to basement membrane complexes and the anterior stroma [57]. This may result from multiple recurrences of viral infection, from overly vigorous debridement using chemical cauterization, from toxic effects of antiviral drugs, or from collagenolytic enzymes. In metaherpetic keratitis, ultrastructural examination of debrided epithelium frequently discloses segmental basement membrane material remaining adherent to the cell along with other fine fibrillar debris (Fig. 2-9C, D). This finding again emphasizes the importance of the anterior stromal substrate in epithelial adhesion. Limited mechanical debridement of cellular and other remnants seems clinically appropriate as the means of providing a smooth substrate upon which regenerating epithelium may better adhere.

KERATOCYTES AND STROMA

NORMAL WOUND HEALING
After a penetrating injury of the stroma, keratocytes immediately adjacent to the wound margin are killed, and the defect soon fills with a fibrin clot (Fig. 2-10). The stromal lamellae become edematous, and the adjacent keratocytes withdraw their cytoplasmic processes [105]. Within 2 hours, these cells increase their RNA content and endoplasmic reticulum cisternae, and they begin protein synthesis [93]. PMNs appear in the wound within 2 to 6 hours and engage in the proteolytic debridement of necrotic cellular and extracellular debris. By 24 hours, DNA synthesis and tritiated thymidine uptake by the keratocytes are maximum. Within 3 days after wounding, these reactive keratocytes have reached the wound edge, are lined up parallel with the wound margins, and are secreting collagens, predominantly of type II, plus glycosaminoglycans, particularly keratan sulfate [2, 23, 88]. The initial PMNs reaching the stromal wound come from the limbal vasculature via the tear film; additional PMNs reach the wound by migration through the stroma.

By the end of the first week, fibroblasts and PMNs have invaded the fibrin plug. With increasing deposition of collagen the tensile strength of the wound slowly improves. This collagen is randomly organized, large-diameter extracellular fibrillar collagen. Subsequent wound healing largely involves additional collagen secretion. By the end of 8 weeks, there are virtually no inflammatory cellular components, but rather only numerous fibroblastic cells.

INFLAMMATION, VASCULARIZATION, AND SCARRING

The wound strength continues to increase for 3 to 6 months. Cintron and coworkers have found that after injury the adult rabbit cornea produces structural macromolecules and collagen cross-links similar to those in the developing cornea [14]. Although the scar tissue becomes more compact and eventually blends into the adjacent stroma, uniformity of fibrillar organization is never restored; however, the pattern of macromolecules and cross-links becomes more similar to that in normal transparent tissue.

INFLAMMATION

The classic experiments of Cohnheim provided the initial pathologic description of the recruitment of leukocytes from limbal vasculature into inflammatory corneal stromal lesions [17]. From this concept evolved the general recognition of several aspects of the inflammatory response. In the cornea, as in all other tissues, inflammation is a nonspecific result of tissue damage, however it may be caused. Corneal tissues can be directly damaged by foreign bodies and chemical or thermal burns. Among the several

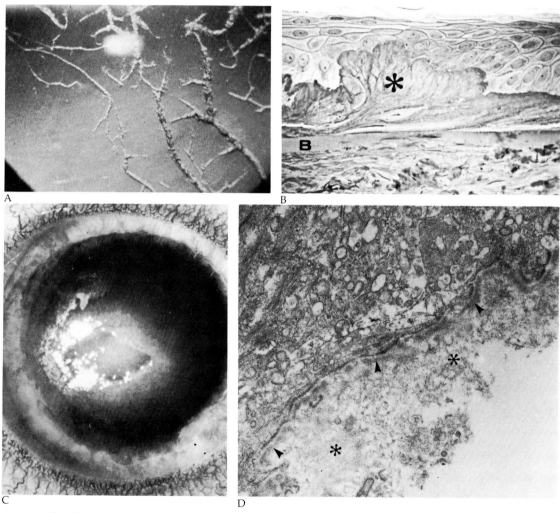

FIGURE 2-9. *Secondary basement membrane disorder: recurrent corneal erosion—Lattice corneal dystrophy. A. Clinical appearance of typical branching stromal lesions. (Slit lamp photograph courtesy W. J. Stark, M.D.) B. Phase-contrast photomicrograph shows subepithelial accumulation of fibrillar amyloid deposits (asterisk) causing distortion of basal epithelial contour. (B = Bowman's layer.) (Paraphenylenediamine, × 800.) Metaherpetic keratitis. C. Persistent epithelial defect and superficial stromal scarring are evident. D. Transmission EM of debrided loosely adherent epithelium shows fragmented segments of basement membrane material (arrowheads) with attached fibrillar debris (asterisks) that interferes with epithelial stromal adhesion. (× 22,000.)*

agents that can elicit an inflammatory response in the cornea, the two most common are microbial infections (either bacterial, viral, or fungal) and various immunologic conditions (including hypersensitivity, allergy, and autoimmunity) [19]. Antigens initiate the immune response with B- and T-lymphocytes responsible for antibody and cytotoxic components, respectively. Two other components are macrophages, which have an important role in processing antigens, and PMNs, whose proteolytic enzymes have extensive destructive potential. The complement system also plays a central role in inflammation activated characteristically by antigen-antibody interactions as, for example, in herpetic interstitial keratitis.

VASCULARIZATION

Corneal neovascularization is a sequel to numerous inflammatory diseases of the ocular anterior segment, including trachoma, luetic and viral interstitial keratitis, microbial keratoconjunctivitis, and the immune reaction elicited by corneal transplantation.

The vascular response to various noxious stimuli, including application of alloxan, thermal and chemical cautery, or intrastromal implantation of tumor angiogenesis factor, is the well-known sequence of limbal capillary and venule dilation followed by diapedesis of leukocytes into the stroma with extravasation of fibrin and other serum proteins (Fig. 2-11). Subsequent vascular endothelial migration and proliferation occurs in a pattern suggestive of directed growth toward the neovascular stimulus, possibly caused by a substance diffusing from the point of injury.

Although early studies incorrectly related the ingrowth of new blood vessels to stromal edema, Fromer and Klintworth more recently observed that stromal neovascularization was preceded by inflammation and postulated that the PMNs that produced a growth-stimulating substance were responsible for vascular proliferation [36, 37]. Further, they showed that leukopenic rats did not develop neovascularization of the cornea after silver nitrate burns. However, Eliason reported corneal vascularization resulting from chemical cautery in leukopenic rats and suggested that the regenerating corneal epithelium is the source of vasostimulating substances [25]. Sholley and associates have similarly shown that in leukopenic rats, corneal neovascularization does occur after thermal cautery, albeit at a slower rate than in nonleukopenic controls [92]. Thus, stromal inflammation appears to provide a sufficient but not altogether necessary stimulus for new blood vessel formation.

Other investigators have attempted to alter or inhibit the ingrowth of new blood vessels by various

agents. For example, intracorneal implantation of tumor angiogenesis factor, biogenic amines, acetylcholine, histamine, serotonin, and bradykinin have been shown to induce new blood vessel growth into the cornea [31, 78, 106]. Recently, BenEzra reported intrastromal implantation of polymers containing prostaglandin E_1 as a potent stimulator of vascular growth [3]. The role of prostaglandins in the sequence of neovascularization is further suggested by Deutsch and Hughes, who showed that topical indomethacin suppresses neovascularization after thermal cautery and that this suppression is associated with a decreased number of PMNs [20]. Inhibition of corneal vascularization has also been reported by Keutner and associates, who observed a proteinase inhibitor activity in the cornea, aorta, and cartilage [71]. This led others to show that purified extract of bovine aorta or cartilage injected subconjunctivally inhibited neovascularization of the cornea after chemical cautery [42].

SCARRING

Scarring is a particularly important consequence of external infectious diseases (such as trachoma), penetrating corneal injuries, and other cicatricial diseases (such as pemphigoid and erythema multiforme). As fibroblasts within the corneal and conjunctival tissues proliferate and elaborate collagens, their productive potential is greatly enhanced by the presence of inflammatory cells. The interaction and unfortunate synergism of primary inflammatory reactions and coincident bacterial infection is also known to enhance the cicatricial process.

Two factors have been hypothesized as necessary for stromal transparency: Individual stromal collagen fibers must be of small uniform diameter (ca. 240 Å), and the distances between adjacent fibrils must be less than half the wavelength of visible light (ca. 2000 Å) in order that fluctuations in refractive index do not result in light scattering [41]. Stromal scarring disturbs these important parameters in both respects, as the collagen fibrils that are produced vary markedly in cross-sectional diameter, from 200 to 1200 Å, and never become organized into the latticelike array with the elements less than 2000 Å apart characteristic of normal lamellar architecture. Stromal scar tissue differs from normal cornea in glycosaminoglycan content, and it is thought that these components of the interfibrillar matrix may be important determinants of collagen fibril size and spatial arrangement. In contrast, in any condition causing stromal edema alone (e.g., compromised endothelial function), loss of stromal

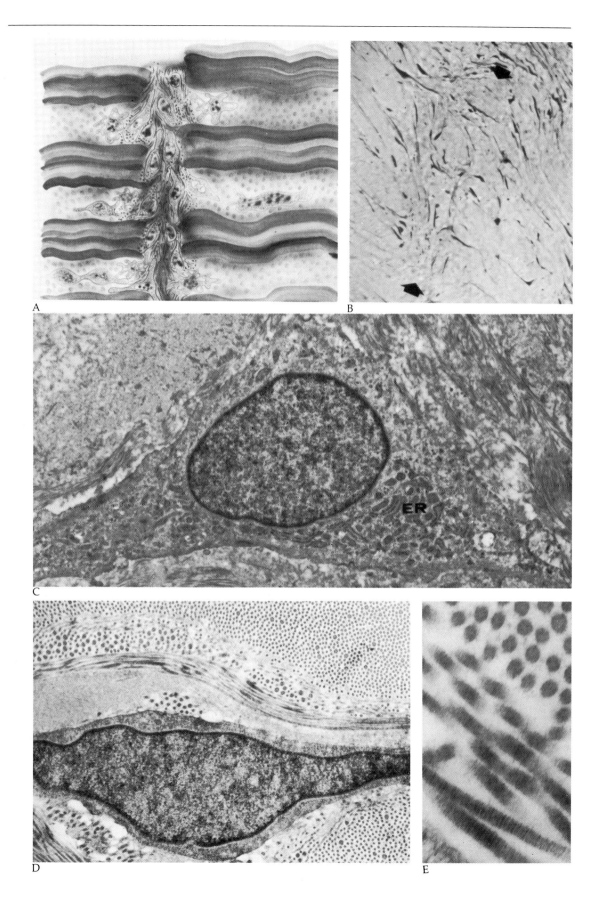

A

B

C

ER

D

E

FIGURE 2-10. *Normal stromal wound healing. A. Diagram of stroma 2 to 8 days after penetrating wound. The transformation of fibrocytes into fibroblasts continues until day 6. Fibroblasts and neutrophils invade the fibrin plug. The fibroblasts continue to produce primitive collagen and glycosaminoglycan. Mononuclear cells that have migrated through the stroma from the limbus arrive at the wound and are transformed into macrophages. Fibroblasts adjacent to the wound are actively dividing. (From P. S. Binder, et al., Corneal anatomy and wound healing. Trans. New Orleans Acad. Ophthalmol. St. Louis: Mosby, 1980.) B. Phase-contrast photomicrograph of human cornea, one year after perforating injury, shows hypercellularity of wound area with fibroblasts aligned along wound axis (arrowheads). (Paraphenylenediamine, × 500.) C. Transmission EM of area shown in B depicts reactive keratocytes with extensive endoplasmic reticulum cisternae (ER). The extracellular collagen is markedly disarrayed. (× 9000.) D. Transmission EM of stromal scar appearing several years after alkali injury shows collagen fibers of abnormally large diameter. Amorphous granular material is adjacent to a quiescent-appearing keratocyte. (× 8000.) E. Transmission EM at higher magnification resolves individual collagen fibrils of normal longitudinal macroperiodicity but cross-sectional diameters of more than twice normal. (× 80,000.)*

transparency occurs as the spaces among collagen fibrils become fluid-distended. No change, however, occurs in the individual fibril dimensions, and hence when the edema subsides, stromal transparency is restored, with return of the normal interfibrillar spatial relationships.

ULCERATION

Stromal ulceration is a particularly disastrous sequela of inflammation and infection of the external eye and cornea (Figs. 2-12 and 2-13). Bacterial toxins themselves are not directly capable of collagenolytic activity, although *Pseudomonas* species do produce a protease capable of glycosaminoglycan destruction [70]. Thus, it is likely that host cellular responses, particularly those of acute inflammation, are responsible for corneal destruction in infections and sterile injuries. Indeed, the pathogenesis of noninfectious stromal ulceration, or "melting," is of particular concern, because it is a frequent complication of chemical injury, herpetic keratitis, collagen vascular diseases, and nutritional deficiency (see Chemical Injuries in Chapter 14, Corneal Injuries) [63].

Whatever the cause, stromal melting is almost invariably preceded by a corneal epithelial defect and appears to be associated with an inappropriate inflammatory response. As Berman has stated, "Why the cornea ulcerates might be related to the trapping of wound healing in a phase of proteolytic debridement related to a persistent epithelial defect" [4]. Such ulceration is known to be secondary to the action of tissue collagenases, which perform the initial cleavage of stromal collagen fibril, with further

degradation of collagen and glycosaminoglycans involving proteases, peptidases, and cathepsins.

The cellular constituents responsible for ulceration and their interactions are subjects of extensive research interest. Although substantial evidence has implicated the actions and interactions of injured corneal epithelium and keratocytes, other pathologic and experimental studies have emphasized the role of acute inflammatory cells, particularly PMNs. These cells contain more than a dozen lytic enzymes (including collagenase, elastase, and cathepsin) within their primary lysosomes and are ubiquitous at the site of active ulceration and in the tear film of melting corneas [69]. In herpes simplex interstitial keratitis, for example, current pathogenetic concepts implicate immunologic efforts aimed at destroying stromal cells that have acquired herpes antigens, thereby resulting in an influx of PMNs and phagocytes that are the effectors of tissue destruction.

On the reparative side, the roles of keratocytes and blood vessels are essential. Reactive fibroblasts with dilated cisternae of rough endoplasmic reticulum participate in the secretion of new collagen for wound healing, although their presence within the central ulcerative areas is somewhat delayed. Equally apparent, however, from cell culture is that such fibroblasts can simultaneously synthesize both collagen and collagenase, thereby allowing the same cells to participate both in ulceration and repair. Conn and coworkers demonstrated the ability of stromal neovascularization to inhibit ulceration; corneas prevascularized by tumor angiogenesis factor were less likely to ulcerate after experimental thermal burns [18]. It is likely that both serum antiproteases (such as alpha-2-macroglobulin) and nutrients (including ascorbate) are delivered by vessels to the ulcerated area.

Tissue adhesives used to strengthen or seal ulcerating and perforated corneas appear to decrease the number of inflammatory cells in the surrounding corneal stroma. Recently it has been demonstrated that the application of tissue adhesive to sterile ulcers arrests further stromal loss in the same manner as does the glued-on hard contact lens, that is, by the exclusion of acute inflammatory cells from the involved stroma [65, 69]. This effect is undoubtedly due partly to denying PMNs from the tears access to the ulcer site. The adhesive may also interrupt the further chemotaxis of intrastromal or tearborne inflammatory cells. These findings have therefore prompted the earlier application of adhesive in either progressive stromal ulceration or impending perforation; the adhesive is easily applied at the slit lamp [30].

ENDOTHELIUM AND DESCEMET'S MEMBRANE

NORMAL WOUND HEALING

Since maintenance of a continuous endothelial cell monolayer is critical to stromal deturgescence and hence optical clarity, endothelial repair processes following a variety of inflammatory and mechanical insults are of great clinical concern. Immediately after a posterior corneal wound, the cut edges of Descemet's membrane retract and curl anteriorly toward the stroma (Fig. 2-14A–D). Adjacent endothelial cells are lost, and a fibrin clot is formed in the wound. Within hours, adjoining endothelial cells attenuate with extensive cytoplasmic processes and migrate into the wound [6, 13, 102]. In the adult human, virtually the entire healing effort occurs by means of cellular reorganization, enlargement, and migration to reconstitute an intact monolayer. In rabbits, the endothelium is capable of mitotic division; in cats and primates, the mitotic capabilities of the endothelium are limited; and in the human, endothelial cell division is an extremely minor component of the reparative response [10, 22, 103].

Depending on the size of the wound, the entire defect can be recovered within 1 or more weeks. Once Descemet's membrane has been resurfaced by a continuous endothelial monolayer, the cells become contact inhibited and form contiguous cellular junctions. The cells that have been involved in the

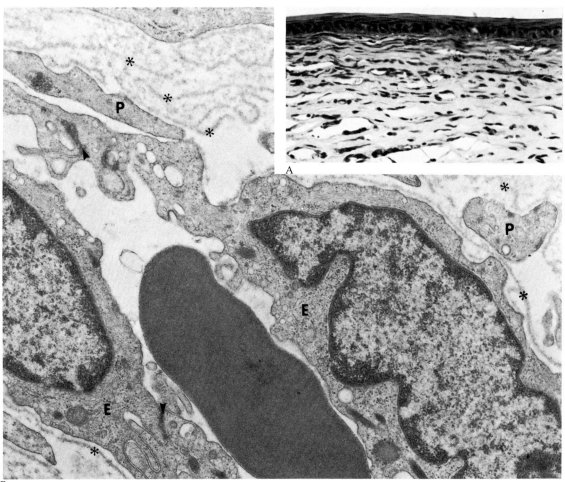

B

FIGURE 2-11. *Stromal vascularization. A. Light photomicrograph of peripheral rabbit cornea 2 months after mild chemical injury shows hypercellular stroma with a few chronic inflammatory cells and numerous small diameter blood vessels. (H&E, × 250.) B. Transmission EM of corresponding area demonstrates stromal vessels comprising mature-appearing endothelial cells (E) with well-developed intracellular junctions (arrowheads). Cytoplasmic processes of pericytes (P) are seen adjacent to the epithelium, and multiple laminations of basement material (asterisks) envelop both cell types. An erythrocyte is evident within the capillary lumen. (× 14,000.)*

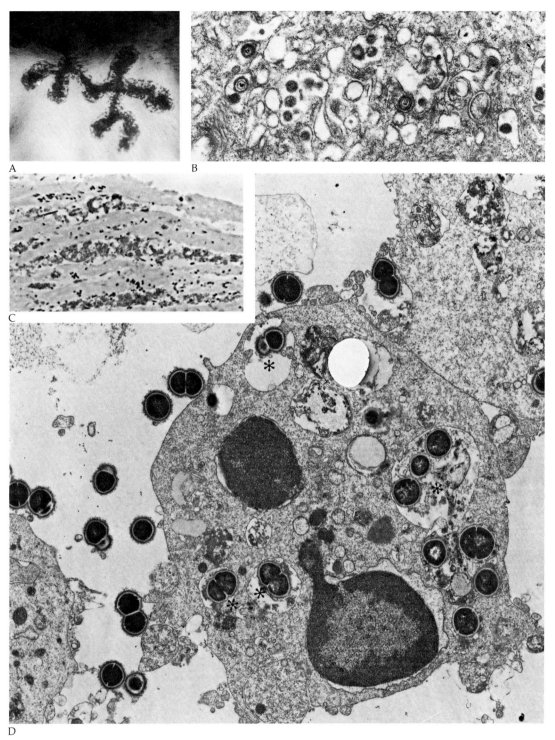

FIGURE 2-12. *Infectious ulceration. A. Slit lamp photo with rose bengal staining shows dendritic figure with balloon swelling of marginal epithelial cells in intraepithelial herpes simplex. (Courtesy L. Hirst, M.D.) B. Transmission EM of debrided epithelial cell shows numerous virus particles consisting of DNA-containing nucleoid surrounded by protein capsid. (×30,000.) C. Phase-contrast photomicrograph of bacterial corneal ulceration shows separation of disorganized stromal lamellae by inflammatory cell debris interspersed with myriad of bacterial forms. (Paraphenylenediamine, ×700.) D. Transmission EM of area corresponding to that shown in C shows a polymorphonuclear leukocyte containing several phagosomes (asterisks) with bacteria and extracellular debris content. The cell has discharged most of its primary lysosomal granules. Extracellularly, many other diplococcal bacterial profiles are evident. (×13,000.)*

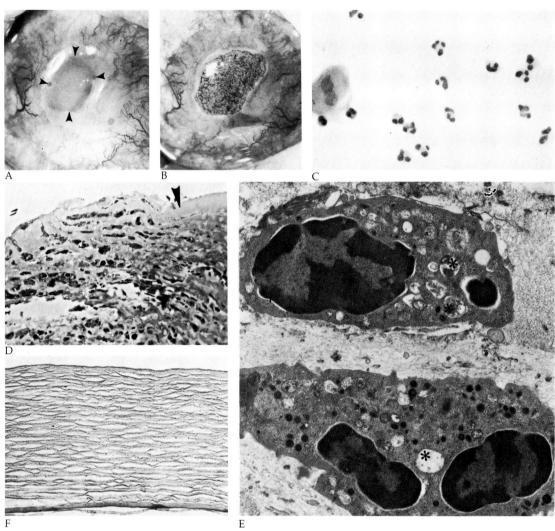

FIGURE 2-13. *Noninfectious ulceration. A. This patient with erythema multiforme, having undergone multiple penetrating kerato-plasties, developed a central epithelial defect with extensive stromal melting to a descemetocele (arrowheads). B. Treatment of this eye with cyanoacrylate tissue adhesive and therapeutic soft contact lens resulted in arrest of ulceration and stabilization of cornea. C. Tear samples taken from descemetocele disclosed numerous polymorphonuclear leukocytes. (Giemsa, × 1,000.) D. In a patient with severe alkali burn, two penetrating keratoplasties succumbed to sterile stromal melting. As shown by phase-contrast microscopy, the actively ulcerating stroma contained numerous polymorphonuclear leukocytes. Note termination of Bowman's layer at arrowhead. (Paraphenylenediamine, × 450.) E. Transmission EM of stromal areas shown in D demonstrates polymorphonuclear leukocytes appearing actively engaged in degranulation and phagocytosis (asterisks), indicating their involvement in the degradation of the melting stroma. (× 9000.) F. The effect of cyanoacrylate tissue adhesive is shown in this alkali-burned rabbit cornea several weeks after injury. Cornea has not undergone stromal degradation and maintains stromal acellularity after application of a glued-on contact lens. (× 100.)*

FIGURE 2-14. *Endothelial wound healing. A. Diagram of endothelium 5 to 72 hours after wounding. The endothelial cells adjacent to the wound are flattened and begin to slide into the defect. As they do so, they take on fibroblastlike characteristics. The cut edges of Descemet's membrane retract and curl anteriorly. The wound is filled with fibrin and cell remnants. B. Scanning EM of posterior corneal surface after posterior trephination. The edge (arrowheads) of the cut stroma (ST) is some distance away from the edge (arrows) of the remaining endothelial cells (CE). The intervening area of bare Descemet's membrane (DM) shows endothelial debris. (× 130.) (A and B from P. S. Binder, et al. Corneal anatomy and wound healing. Trans. New Orleans Acad. Ophthalmol. St. Louis: Mosby, 1980.) C. Scanning EM of posterior surface of human cornea 1 year after perforating injury shows areas of corrugated Descemet's membrane (asterisk) overlain by fibrillar collagen strands. Distended and disorganized endothelial cells have recovered part of this surface. (× 100.) D. Scanning EM of area bracketed in C discloses attenuated endothelial cells in multilayered configuration. These cells have extensive cytoplasmic processes interdigitating with fibrillar posterior collagen layer. (× 500.) E. In keratoconus with healed hydrops, slit lamp*

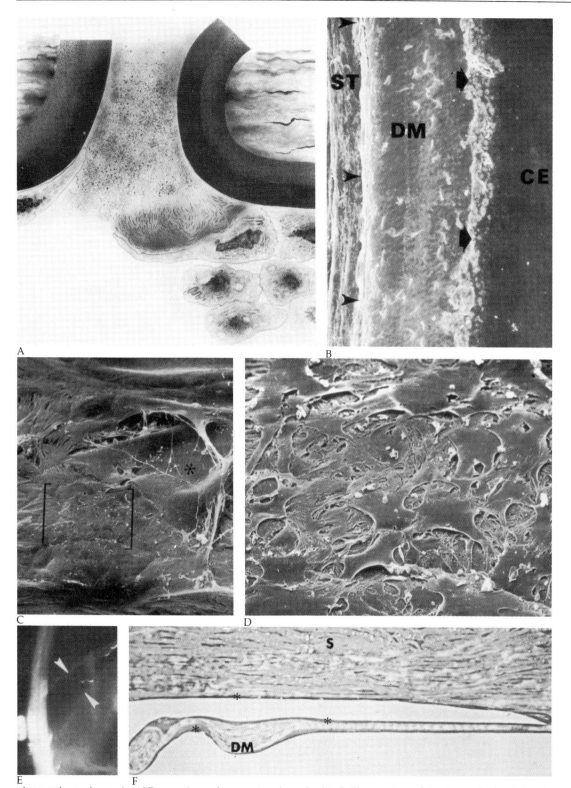

photograph reveals margins of Descemet's membrane rupture (arrowheads). F. Phase-contrast photomicrograph of posterior stroma in healed hydrops shows a ledge of Descemet's membrane (DM) with adherent collagen that has separated from the posterior stroma (S). Note that a continuous endothelial cell layer (asterisks) has migrated to resurface the anterior aspect of the ledge plus the entire denuded posterior surface of the stroma. (Paraphenylenediamine, ×250.)

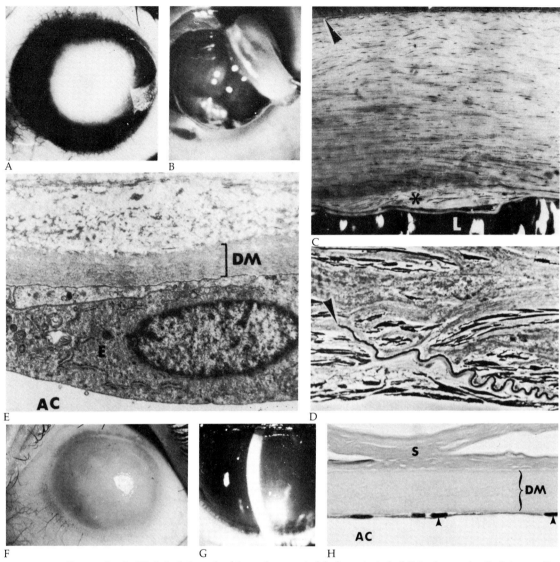

FIGURE 2-15. *Dysgenesis. A. Clinical photograph of large dense central leukoma typical of Peters' anomaly. B. Interoperative photograph of penetrating keratoplasty in Peters' anomaly shows adherence of clear lens (centrally) to the thickened cornea (grasped by forceps). C. Phase-contrast photomicrograph of cornea illustrated in C shows thickened central stroma with adherent lens (L). Bowman's layer terminates centrally (arrowhead). Descemet's membrane present peripherally, but ends centrally in a layer of retrocorneal fibrous tissue (asterisk) approximately 75 μ thick between lens and corneal stroma. (Paraphenylenediamine, ×60.) D. Phase-contrast photomicrograph of posterior cornea adjacent to central stromal defect shows termination (at arrowhead) of undulating Descemet's membrane within the posterior collagen layer. (Paraphenylenediamine, ×400.) E. Transmission EM in Peters' anomaly shows extremely thin Descemet's membrane (DM), abnormally laminated, with attenuated endothelium (E). (AC = anterior chamber.) (×7700.) F. Congenital hereditary endothelial dystrophy (CHED). In this severe case, there is diffuse ground-glass opacification of the stroma with edematous stippling of the epithelium. G. In this more mildly affected patient, the cornea has only moderate haze that obscures the iris and lens but nonetheless permits 20/200 vision. Note diffuse edematous thickening of the stroma revealed by slit lamp beam. H. Light photomicrograph of cornea of 6-year-old boy with CHED reveals enormous thickening of Descemet's membrane (DM) with dystrophic endothelial cells (arrowheads). (S = posterior stroma; AC = anterior chamber.) (H&E, ×600.)*

FIGURE 2-16. *Endothelial dystrophy (Fuchs'). A. Clinical photo illustrates epithelial bullae, scarring, and neovascularization resulting from long-standing stromal edema. B. Light photomicrograph of early bullous keratopathy shows intracellular and extracellular hydropic changes of basal epithelial cells, with duplication and thickening of basement membrane and subepithelial neovascularization (asterisk). (H&E, ×250.) C. Light photomicrograph of posterior cornea shows thickened Descemet's membrane with guttate excrescences (arrowheads) and dystrophic, attenuated endothelial cells. (H&E, ×250.) D. Scanning EM of area comparable to that shown in C shows extensive areas of exposed Descemet's membrane with numerous guttata (asterisks). The remaining endothelial cells (En) are severely*

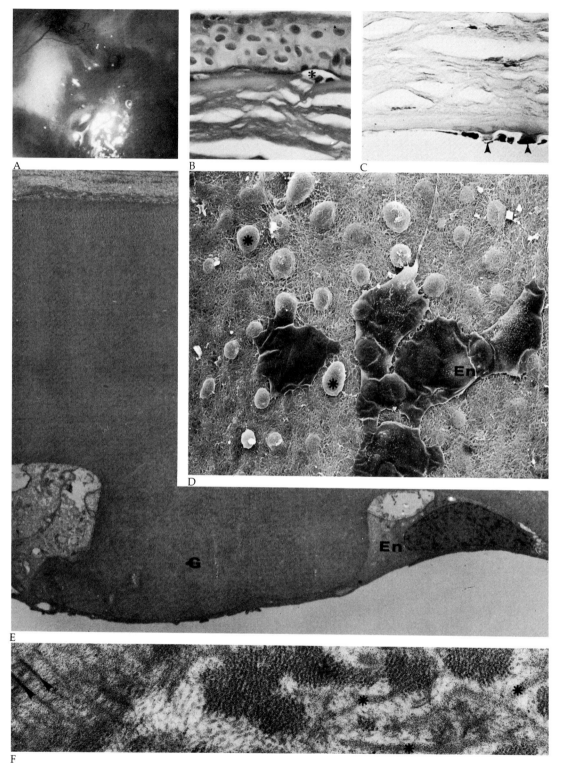

F

degenerated and attenuated. The exposed surface of the posterior collagen layer appears as a fibrous feltwork. (×300.) Transmission EM of posterior cornea shows unremarkable stroma and anterior Descemet's membrane but thickening of posterior Descemet's to 12 μ with additional superimposition of large guttata (G). The remaining endothelial cells (En) are extremely attenuated. (×5000.) F. High-magnification transmission EM of guttata resolves fine filaments, multiple segments of basement material (asterisk), and collagen in long-spacing configuration (arrowheads). (×50,000.)

67

healing process are now much larger than those in the uninvolved periphery of the cornea. Once the integrity of the endothelial cell layer has been restored, its pump and barrier functions soon begin to stabilize, as evidenced by stromal deturgescence, thinning, and increasing clarity.

As part of the wound healing response, and indeed as a nonspecific response to any form of endothelial trauma, the regenerating endothelium deposits new layers of Descemet's membrane material [104]. This is clearly evident, for example, in keratoconus cases with acute hydrops: The migrating endothelium that resurfaces the exposed posterior stroma secretes new Descemet's membrane (Fig. 2-14E, F) [96]. Where the wound is well apposed, a single endothelial layer appears and functions normally. Where there is poor wound apposition, endothelial cells are multilayered and undergo a fibroblastic transformation resulting in posterior collagen layers comprising fibrillar banded collagen, basement membrane material, and fine filaments. In time, these cells also appear capable of reverting to a more normal endothelial morphology. However, the chronology of posterior wound healing is prolonged—months to years may be required for transformation into endothelium with new Descemet's membrane of normal morphology and thickness.

SPECIFIC PATHOLOGIC REACTIONS

DYSGENESIS: PETERS' ANOMALY AND CONGENITAL HEREDITARY ENDOTHELIAL DYSTROPHY
The mesenchymal dysgeneses of the cornea are a spectrum of developmental disorders of the corneogenic mesenchyme, including posterior keratoconus, posterior central corneal opacity (Peters' anomaly), congenital hereditary endothelial dystrophy (CHED), sclerocornea, and the iridocorneal-endothelial (ICE) syndromes [61] (see Chapter 10, Congenital Anomalies).

Peters' anomaly is a congenital central corneal opacity with corresponding defects in the posterior stroma, Descemet's membrane, and endothelium. Strands of iris tissue often extend to the posterior border of the corneal leukoma, and central keratolenticular adherence sometimes occurs with shallowing of the anterior chamber. The peripheral cornea is usually clear but may be partially scleralized. Histopathologic changes are present in all layers of the cornea (Fig. 2-15A–E). Anterior changes, including disorganization of epithelium, pannus, and loss of Bowman's layer, are probably

FIGURE 2-17. *Endothelial degeneration: aphakic bullous keratopathy. A. Clinical photograph shows diffuse stromal edema. B. Phase-contrast photomicrograph shows normal Descemet's membrane (D) with associated posterior collagen layer (asterisks) anterior to the degenerating endothelial cells. (Paraphenylenediamine, ×700.) C. Scanning EM of posterior corneal surface reveals remaining endothelial cells to be extremely flattened and attenuated. Note the exposed surface of posterior collagenous layer (F) appearing as a randomly organized fibrous network. (×1000.) D. For direct comparison to C, normal adult human endothelium demonstrates uniformly hexagonal cells approximately 20 μ in diameter arranged in a continuous monolayered mosaic. (×1000.) E. Transmission EM in eye with aphakic bullous keratopathy discloses usual ultrastructure of banded and nonbanded portions of Descemet's membrane (DM) and loose fibrous composition of posterior collagen layer (F). The remaining endothelial cell (En) contains phagocytosed melanin. (×13,000.)*

secondary to the primary posterior abnormalities. The stroma is edematous in the affected region; ultrastructural studies of stromal collagen have disclosed fibrils as large as 600 Å. In peripheral, unaffected areas, the endothelium is continuous, and Descemet's membrane is of normal uniform thickness. In the area of the defect, however, endothelium and Descemet's membrane can terminate abruptly or be severely attenuated. The lens may be involved, which suggests a primary incomplete separation of the lens vesicle or a secondary anterior displacement of normally developed lens causing apposition between lens and cornea. Etiologically, although there may be multiple causes of this clinical entity, the probably incomplete central migration of mesenchymal cells destined to become keratocytes and endothelium accounts for concurrent posterior stromal and endothelial defects [81, 97].

Among dysgeneses appropriate for comparison with Peters' anomaly, CHED is pertinent, because this disorder is characterized clinically by diffuse bilaterally symmetric corneal edema in the presence of normal intraocular pressure. The degree of edematous corneal clouding varies from a mild haze to a milky ground-glass opacification (Fig. 2-15F–H). Histologic study reveals anterior and stromal changes consistent with long-standing secondary edema. It may be important that in some cases, greatly enlarged stromal collagen fibrils are evident ultrastructurally. Descemet's membrane is uniform, with no evidence of guttata. Although the thickness of Descemet's membrane is always uniform in a given specimen, it may range from less than 3 μ to more than 40 μ. In eyes with thin Descemet's membrane, it appears that complete endothelial loss occurred in utero, so that only the fetal anterior por-

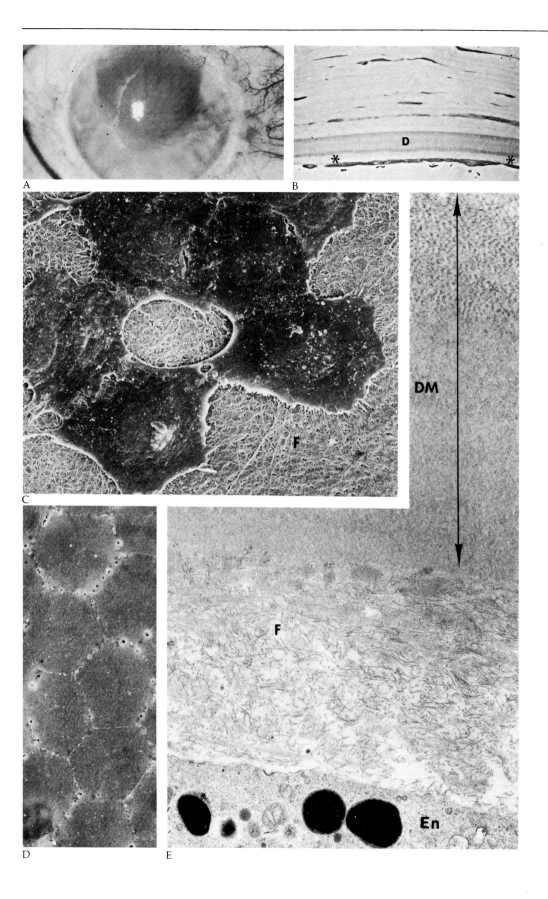

A

B

C

D

E

tion of Descemet's membrane was secreted [64]. In contrast, thickened Descemet's membrane is the result of dystrophic but persistent endothelium having secreted a hypertrophic posterior collagen layer. With the exception of the lack of guttata, these Descemet's membrane findings are similar to those in adult endothelial dystrophy (Fuchs') and thus represent another example of posterior collagenous layer formation by either primarily or secondarily abnormal endothelium [104].

DYSTROPHY: GUTTATA AND FUCHS' DYSTROPHY

Slit lamp examination of a patient with corneal guttata reveals focal excrescences of Descemet's membrane that represent abnormal basement membrane elaboration by aging or otherwise distressed endothelial cells.

Cornea guttata are often seen as a primary condition in patients of middle to older age. Progressive bilateral accumulation of corneal guttata, usually seen in the fifth or sixth decade and somewhat more commonly in women, is typical of late hereditary endothelial dystrophy of Fuchs (see Corneal Edema in Chapter 1, Physiology of the Cornea and Chapter 9, Dystrophies and Degenerations). As guttata become numerous and central, the endothelial cells are compromised to the extent that both their barrier and fluid transport functions become inefficient. Then stromal edema occurs, followed by bullous epithelial edema, and the condition may be justly termed Fuchs' dystrophy.

Secondary guttata are usually associated with degenerative corneal disease, trauma, or inflammation. The endothelial cells may be adversely affected by iritis, deep stromal inflammation (e.g., luetic interstitial keratitis), corneal ulcers, and anterior segment surgery. In severe inflammation, edema of the endothelial cells may resemble corneal guttata. However, upon removal of the causative agent, edema subsides, whereas true corneal guttata are permanent [73].

By light microscopy, corneal guttata indent the underlying endothelial cells and display a mushroom-shaped configuration (Figure 2-16). Descemet's membrane can become thickened to three or more times normal (20–40 μ). The endothelial cells undergo degeneration and alteration to fibroblastlike cells that become thin or focally absent beneath the excrescences. These abnormal cells produce the thickened Descemet's membrane in the form of guttata by laying down randomly organized collagen fibrils, small-diameter filaments (approximately 100 Å), and multiple laminations of basement membrane material on the posterior surface of the thickened Descemet's membrane [51].

DEGENERATION: APHAKIC BULLOUS KERATOPATHY

An example of endothelial degeneration having particular clinical relevance is aphakic bullous keratopathy (see Corneal Edema in Chapter 1, Physiology of the Cornea). This condition of persistent corneal edema is a clinically important complication in 4 to 6 percent of cataract extractions and has become an increasingly important indication for penetrating keratoplasty; keratoplasty for aphakic bullous keratopathy comprises 20 to 30 percent of corneal grafts performed. As a functional disturbance of the corneal endothelium, aphakic bullous keratopathy most often develops in eyes with preexisting endothelial dystrophy, with surgical complications, or with persistent vitreous-cornea contact (vitreous touch syndrome). Pathologically, aphakic bullous keratopathy consistently involves endothelial cell degeneration and proliferation of a posterior collagen layer between Descemet's membrane and the endothelial cells (Fig. 2-17). By scanning EM, focal discontinuities of the endothelial cell layer are seen to occur diffusely over the entire posterior corneal surface. The remaining endothelial cells become flat, attenuated, and enormously enlarged with numerous cytoplasmic extensions, often assuming elongated configurations in apparent effort to recover the bare surface of Descemet's membrane.

The posterior collagen layer appears by light microscopy as a cellular fibrous band extending uniformly across the entire posterior aspect of Descemet's membrane. Transmission EM shows this layer to be composed of randomly arrayed collagen fibrils, approximately 200 to 300 Å diameter, interspersed among multilaminar basement membrane segments and bundles of fine filaments. Similarly, on scanning EM, the exposed surface of the fibrous layer is a loosely fibrillar feltwork of a consistency different from that of the normally compact Descemet's membrane. In some cases, another pattern of a thicker fibrocellular layer is sometimes evident, presumably the result of fibrous ingrowth by stromal keratocytes [67]. In many specimens, definite histologic evidence of preexisting endothelial disease is often apparent—thickened Descemet's membrane along with typical central corneal guttata.

The collagenous tissue lining the posterior aspect of Descemet's membrane is a typical response of distressed endothelial cells. The ultrastructural composition of this posterior collagenous layer is identical to that found in many situations involving endothelial dysgenesis, dystrophy, trauma, or in-

epithelium or endothelium on the stromal keratocytes. *Invest. Ophthalmol.* 7:520, 1968.

22. Doughman, D. J., et al. Human corneal endothelial layer repair during organ culture. *Arch. Ophthalmol.* 94:1791, 1976.

23. Dunnington, J. H., and Smelser, G. K. Incorporation of S^{35} in healing wounds in normal and devitalized corneas. *Arch. Ophthalmol.* 60:116, 1958.

24. Dunnington, J. H., and Weimar, V. Influence of the epithelium on the healing of corneal incisions. *Am. J. Ophthalmol.* 45:89, 1958.

25. Eliason, J. A. Leukocytes and experimental corneal vascularization. *Invest. Ophthalmol. Vis. Sci.* 17:1087, 1978.

26. Faulkner, W., et al. Chemical burns of the human ocular surface: Clinicopathologic studies of 14 cases. *Invest. Ophthalmol. Vis. Sci.* 20(Suppl.):8, 1981.

27. Fogle, J. A., and Neufeld, R. H. The adrenergic and cholinergic corneal epithelium. *Invest. Ophthalmol. Vis. Sci.* 18:1212, 1979.

28. Fogle, J. A., et al. Defective epithelial adhesion in anterior corneal dystrophies. *Am. J. Ophthalmol.* 79:925, 1975.

29. Fogle, J. A., Kenyon, K. R., and Stark, W. J. Damage to epithelial basement membrane by thermokeratoplasty. *Am. J. Ophthalmol.* 83:392, 1977.

30. Fogle, J. A., Kenyon, K. R., and Foster, C. S. Tissue adhesive arrest, stromal melting in the human cornea. *Am. J. Ophthalmol.* 89:795, 1980.

31. Folkman, J. Tumor angiogenesis factor. *Cancer Res.* 34:2109, 1974.

32. Franklin, R. M., and Fitzmorris, C. T. Antibodies against conjunctival basement membrane zone in cicatricial pemphigoid. *Am. J. Ophthalmol.* In press.

33. Frati, L., et al. Selective binding of the epidermal growth factor and its specific effects on the epithelial cells of the cornea. *Exp. Eye Res.* 14:135, 1972.

34. Friedenwald, J. S., and Bushke, W. The effects of excitement, of epinephrine, and of sympathectomy on the mitotic activity of the corneal epithelium in rats. *Am. J. Physiol.* 141:689, 1944.

35. Friend, J., and Thoft, R. A. Functional competence of regenerating ocular surface epithelium. *Invest. Ophthalmol. Vis. Sci.* 17:134, 1978.

36. Fromer, C. H., and Klintworth, G. K. An evaluation of the role of leukocytes in the pathogenesis of experimentally induced corneal vascularization: I. Comparison of experimental models of corneal vascularization. *Am. J. Pathol.* 79:537, 1975.

37. Fromer, C. H., and Klintworth, G. K. An evaluation of the role of leukocytes and the pathogenesis of experimentally induced corneal vascularization: II. Studies on the effect of leukocyte elimination on corneal vascularization. *Am. J. Pathol.* 81:531, 1975.

38. Fujikawa, L. S., et al. Fibronectin in healing rabbit corneal wounds. *Lab. Invest.* 45:120, 1981.

39. Furey, N., et al. Immunofluorescent studies of ocular cicatricial pemphigoid. *Am. J. Ophthalmol.* 80:825, 1975.

40. Gipson, I. K., and Anderson, R. A. Actin filaments in normal and migrating corneal epithelial cells. *Invest. Ophthalmol. Vis. Sci.* 16:161, 1977.

41. Goldman, J. N., et al. Structural alterations affecting transparency in swollen human corneas. *Invest. Ophthalmol.* 7:501, 1968.

42. Goren, S. B., Eisenstein, R., and Choromokos, E. The inhibition of corneal neovascularization in rabbits. *Am. J. Ophthalmol.* 84:305, 1977.

43. Grayson, M. The nature of hereditary deep polymorphous dystrophy of the cornea: Its association with iris and anterior chamber dysgenesis. *Trans. Am. Ophthalmol. Soc.* 72:516, 1974.

44. Greiner, J. V., et al. Mucus secretory vesicles in conjunctival epithelial cells of wearers of contact lenses. *Arch. Ophthalmol.* 98:1843, 1980.

45. Haik, B. G., and Zimny, M. L. Scanning electron microscopy of corneal wound healing in the rabbit. *Invest. Ophthalmol. Vis. Sci.* 16:787, 1977.

46. Harding, C., et al. A comparative study of corneal epithelial cell surfaces utilizing the scanning electron microscope. *Invest. Ophthalmol.* 13:906, 1974.

47. Harnisch, J. P., et al. Ultrastructural identification of type I and II collagen in the cornea of the mouse by means of enzyme labelled antibodies. *Albrecht Von Graefes Arch. Klin. Exp. Ophthalmol.* 208:9, 1978.

48. Hay, E. D., and Revel, J. P. Fine Structure of the Developing Avian Cornea. In A. Wolsky and P. S. Chen (Eds.), *Monographs in Developmental Biology*, Vol. 1. Basel: Karger, 1969.

49. Hirst, L. W., et al. Comparative studies of corneal surface injury in the monkey and rabbit. *Arch. Ophthalmol.* 99:1066, 1981.

50. Hoffman, F., and Schweichel, J. U. The microvilli structure of the corneal epithelium of the rabbit in relation to cell function. *Ophthalmol. Res.* 4:175, 1972.

51. Hogan, M. J., Wood, I., and Fine, M. Fuchs' endothelial dystrophy of the cornea. *Am. J. Ophthalmol.* 78:363, 1974.

52. Hogan, M. J., Alvarado, J. A., and Weddell,

J. E. Histology of the human eye. Philadelphia: Saunders, 1971.

53. Irvine, A. R., and Irvine, A. R. Variations in normal human corneal endothelium. Preliminary report of pathologic human corneal endothelium. *Am. J. Ophthalmol.* 36:1279, 1953.

54. Iwamoto, T., and Smelser, G. K. Electron microscopy of the human corneal endothelium with reference to transport mechanisms. *Invest. Ophthalmol.* 4:270, 1965.

55. Jakus, M. A. The Fine Structure of the Human Cornea. In G. K. Smelser (Ed.), *The Structure of the Eye.* New York: Academic, 1961.

56. Jakus, M. A. Further observations on the fine structure of the cornea. *Invest. Ophthalmol.* 1:202, 1962.

57. Kaufman, H. E. Epithelial erosion syndrome: Metaherpetic keratitis. *Am. J. Ophthalmol.* 57:983, 1964.

58. Kayes, J., and Holmberg, A. The fine structure of Bowman's layer and the basement membrane of the corneal epithelium. *Am. J. Ophthalmol.* 50:1013, 1960.

59. Kenney, C., et al. Analyses of collagens from ultrastructurally pure Descemet's membrane and cultured endothelial cells. *Invest. Ophthalmol. Vis. Sci.* 17(Suppl.):253, 1978.

60. Kenyon, K. R. Ocular Ultrastructure of Inherited Metabolic Diseases. In M. F. Goldberg (Ed.), *Genetic and Metabolic Eye Disease.* Boston: Little, Brown, 1974. P. 139.

61. Kenyon, K. R. Mesenchymal dysgenesis in Peters' anomaly, sclerocornea and congenital endothelial dystrophy. *Exp. Eye Res.* 21:125, 1975.

62. Kenyon, K. R. Recurrent corneal erosion: Pathogenesis and therapy. *Int. Ophthalmol. Clin.* 19(2):169, 1979.

63. Kenyon, K. R. Non-infected corneal ulceration. *Ophthalmology* 89:44, 1982.

64. Kenyon, K. R., and Maumenee, A. E. Further studies of congenital hereditary endothelial dystrophy. *Am. J. Ophthalmol.* 76:419, 1973.

65. Kenyon, K. R., Berman, M. B., and Hanninen, L. A. Tissue adhesive prevents ulceration and inhibits inflammation in the thermal burned rabbit cornea. *Invest. Ophthalmol. Vis. Sci.* 18(Suppl.):1196, 1979.

66. Kenyon, K. R., Stark, W. J., and Stone, D. L. Corneal endothelial degeneration and fibrous proliferation after pars plana vitrectomy. *Am. J. Ophthalmol.* 81:486, 1976.

67. Kenyon, K. R., Van Horn, D. L., and Edelhauser, H. F. Endothelial degeneration and posterior collagenous proliferation in aphakic bullous keratopathy. *Am. J. Ophthalmol.* 85:329, 1978.

68. Kenyon, K. R., et al. Regeneration of corneal epithelial basement membrane following thermal cauterization. *Invest. Ophthalmol. Vis. Sci.* 16:292, 1977.

69. Kenyon, K. R., et al. Prevention of stromal ulceration in the alkali-burned rabbit cornea by glued-on contact lens: Evidence for the role of polymorphonuclear leukocytes in collagen degradation. *Invest. Ophthalmol. Vis. Sci.* 18:570, 1979.

70. Kessler, E., Mondino, B., and Brown, S. I. The corneal response to *Pseudomonas acruginosa*: Histopathological and enzymatic characterization. *Invest. Ophthalmol. Vis. Sci.* 16:116, 1977.

71. Keutner, K. E., et al. Proteinase inhibitors activity in connective tissues. *Experientia* 30:595, 1974.

72. Khodadoust, A. A., et al. Adhesion of regenerating corneal epithelium: The role of basement membrane. *Am. J. Ophthalmol.* 65:339, 1968.

73. Krachmer, J. H., Schnitzer, J., and Fratkin, J. Cornea pseudoguttata: A clinical and histopathologic description of endothelial cell edema. *Arch. Ophthalmol.* 99:1377, 1981.

74. Kuwabara, T., Perkins, D. G., and Cogan, D. Sliding of the epithelium in experimental corneal wounds. *Invest. Ophthalmol.* 15:4, 1976.

75. Leuenberger, P. M. Lanthanum hydroxide tracer studies on rat corneal endothelium. *Exp. Eye Res.* 15:85, 1973.

76. Leuenberger, P. M., and Novikoff, A. B. Localization of transport adenosine triphosphate in rat cornea. *J. Cell Biol.* 60:721, 1974.

77. Matsuda, H., and Smelser, G. K. Electron microscopy of corneal wound healing. *Exp. Eye Res.* 16:427, 1973.

78. Maurice, D. M., Zauberman, H., and Michaelson, I. C. The stimulus to neovascularization in the cornea. *Exp. Eye Res.* 5:168, 1966.

79. Mishima, S. The effects of the denervation and the stimulation of the sympathetic and trigeminal nerve on the mitotic rate of corneal epithelium in the rabbit. *Jpn. J. Ophthalmol.* 1:67, 1957.

80. Mondino, B. J., et al. Autoimmune phenomena in ocular cicatricial pemphigoid. *Am. J. Ophthalmol.* 83:443, 1977.

81. Nakanishi, I., and Brown, S. I. The histopathology and ultrastructure of congenital central corneal opacity (Peters' anomaly). *Am. J. Ophthalmol.* 72:801, 1971.

82. Neufeld, A. H., et al. Influences on the density of beta-adrenergic receptors in the cornea and iris-ciliary body of the rabbit. *Invest. Ophthalmol. Vis. Sci.* 17:1069, 1978.

83. Olsen, J. S., and Neufeld, A. H. The rabbit cornea lacks cholinergic receptors. *Invest. Ophthalmol. Vis. Sci.* 18:1216, 1979.

84. Perlman, M., Baum, J. L., and Kaye, G. I. Fine structure and collagen synthetic activity of monolayer cultures of rabbit corneal endothelium. *J. Cell Biol.* 63:306, 1974.

85. Perry, H. D., et al. Corneal complications after closed vitrectomy through the pars plana. *Arch. Ophthalmol.* 96:401, 1978.

86. Pfister, R. R. The healing of corneal epithelial abrasions in the rabbit: A scanning electron microscopic study. *Invest. Ophthalmol.* 14:468, 1975.

87. Pfister, R. R., and Burstein, N. The normal and abnormal human corneal epithelial surface: A scanning and electron microscope study. *Invest. Ophthalmol. Vis. Sci.* 16:614, 1977.

88. Robb, T. M., and Kuwabara, T. Corneal wound healing: II. An autoradiographic study of the cellular components. *Arch. Ophthalmol.* 72:401, 1964.

89. Rodrigues, M. M., Fine, B. S., and Laibson, P. R. Disorders of the corneal epithelium: A clinicopathologic study of dot, geographic and fingerprint patterns. *Arch. Ophthalmol.* 92:475, 1974.

90. Savage, C. R., and Cohen, S. Proliferations of corneal epithelium induced by epidermal growth factor. *Exp. Eye Res.* 14:135, 1972.

91. Shapiro, M. S., Friend, J., and Thoft, R. A. Corneal reepithelialization from the conjunctiva. *Invest. Ophthalmol. Vis. Sci.* 21:135, 1981.

92. Sholley, M. M., Gimbrone, M. A., and Cotran, R. A. The effects of leukocyte depletion on corneal neovascularization. *Lab. Invest.* 38:32, 1978.

93. Smelser, G. K., and Ozanics, V. Reaction of the cornea to injury and wound healing. *Trans. New Orleans Acad. Ophthalmol.* 1972. P. 239.

94. Sommer, A., Green, W. R., and Kenyon, K. R. Bitot's spots responsive and nonresponsive to vitamin A. Clinicopathologic correlations. *Arch. Ophthalmol.* 99:2014, 1981.

95. Sommer, A., Green, W. R., and Kenyon, K. R. Clinical histopathologic correlations in xerophthalmic ulceration and necrosis. *Arch. Ophthalmol.* 100:953, 1982.

96. Stone, D. L., Kenyon, K. R., and Stark, W. J. Ultrastructure of keratoconus with healed hydrops. *Am. J. Ophthalmol.* 82:450, 1976.

97. Stone, D. L., et al. Congenital central corneal leukoma (Peters' anomaly). *Am. J. Ophthalmol.* 81:173, 1976.

98. Thoft, R. A., and Friend, J. Biochemical transformation of regenerating ocular surface epithelium. *Invest. Ophthalmol. Vis. Sci.* 16:1, 1977.

99. Thoft, R. A., Friend, J., and Murphy, H. Ocular surface epithelium and corneal vascularization in rabbits: I. The role of wounding. *Invest. Ophthalmol. Vis. Sci.* 18:85, 1979.

100. Thoft, R. A., Friend, J., and Kenyon, K. R. Ocular surface response to trauma. *Int. Ophthalmol. Clin.* 19(2):111, 1979.

101. Trobe, J. D., and Laibson, P. R. Dystrophic changes in the anterior cornea. *Arch. Ophthalmol.* 87:378, 1972.

102. Van Horn, D. L., and Hyndiuk, R. A. Endothelial wound repair in primate cornea. *Exp. Eye Res.* 21:113, 1975.

103. Van Horn, D. L., et al. Regenerative capacity of the corneal endothelium in rabbit and cat. *Invest. Ophthalmol. Vis. Sci.* 16:597, 1977.

104. Waring, G. O., Laibson, P. R., and Rodrigues, M. Clinical and pathologic alterations of Descemet's membrane: With emphasis on endothelial metaplasia. *Surv. Ophthalmol.* 18:325, 1974.

105. Wolter, J. R. Reactions of the cellular elements of the corneal stroma. *Arch. Ophthalmol.* 59:873, 1958.

106. Zauberman, H., et al. Stimulation of neovascularization of the cornea by biogenic amines. *Exp. Eye Res.* 8:77, 1969.

3. IMMUNOLOGY

Gilbert Smolin

At the heart of immunology lie cell memory, cell specificity, and the recognition of nonself. These mechanisms increase our chances of survival in this world. In the course of this chapter I shall attempt to define these terms and to describe various interrelated aspects of the immune system.

GENERAL CONSIDERATIONS OF THE IMMUNE REACTION

COMPONENTS

ANTIGENS

An antigen (or immunogen) is any substance that evokes an immune response when it is introduced into an organism. The immune response may be expressed by the production of antibodies, cell-mediated immunity, or immunologic tolerance. These reactions will be discussed in detail below. The vast majority of antigens are proteins and vary widely in their molecular weight. Generally speaking, the larger the protein the more antigenic it is.

Antigens can be mixed with substances that enhance the immune response. These substances, called adjuvants, of which Freund's complete adjuvant is an example, are useful in research. They act by retaining the antigen in the tissue and thus prolonging the immune response [76], or as carriers delivering antigens to the sites where lymphocytes are to be found.

Although some materials are not antigenic in themselves, when linked covalently to carrier molecules, they can function as antigenic groups that direct the specificity of the immune response. These materials are called haptens. The portions of an antigen molecule that induce an immune response, and that react in turn with antibody or sensitized lymphocytes, are referred to as antigenic determinants.

The body's own proteins are called autoantigens and do not normally elicit immune responses. In certain disease states, however, this situation can be altered, and an autoimmune disease, i.e., an attack on "self" proteins, results.

Antigens can be broken down into several groups: (1) those from another member of the same species (allogeneic or homologous), (2) those from another species (xenogeneic or heterologous), (3) those characteristic of a single individual (individual-specific or idiotypic), (4) those that are specific for a given organ in the same or different species (organ-specific), and (5) those common to the members of a given species (species-specific).

The antigens carried on the surfaces of nucleated cells of almost all tissues are called histocompatibility or human-leukocyte (HLA) antigens. The differences in these HLA antigens are the main reason why tissues from unrelated donors cannot be freely exchanged without graft rejection. The HLA antigens are present on the chromosomes in the nucleus. Each chromosome carries genes in the form of DNA. The position of a gene along a chromosome is called the gene locus. Several genes may have the same locus and are then called alleles. The HLA antigens are determined by four genes: one gene allele at each of two gene loci on each number 6 chromosome.

The histocompatibility loci are labeled A, B, C, and D. The HLA antigens located at these loci have been defined by serologic and cellular laboratory methods. The HLA A, B, and C loci code for antigens that are present on almost all cells in the body and are serologically defined. The D locus was originally defined by means of cellular techniques (proliferation in a primary mixed-lymphocyte culture), but recently serologically detected antigens associated with the D locus (DR) have been found with limited tissue distribution. The antigens associated with this DR locus are called Ia (immune-associated) antigens and may be present in ocular tissues, e.g., in Langerhans' cells at the corneal limbus, or in macrophages [91].

To complicate matters, cellularly defined antigens have been found for the A, B, and C loci.

The significance of HLA antigens will be discussed later in the section on graft rejections.

HLA antigens whose identity is still debatable are called workshop (W) antigens.

In humans, certain diseases are associated with an increased frequency of HLA-B8/DRW3. They include recurrent herpes labialis, dermatitis herpetiformis, coeliac disease [154], Addison's disease [151], Sjögren's syndrome [152], sarcoidosis, arthritis, Graves' disease [155], myasthenia gravis [50], and hepatitis. Other associations are Behçet's disease with HLA-B5; pemphigus vulgaris with HLA-A10; rheumatoid arthritis with HLA-DW4 [147]; atopic dermatitis with HLA-A1, HLA-A3, HLA-A9, HLA-B5, HLA-B8, and HLA-B12 [102]; ankylosing spondylitis with HLA-B27; and multiple sclerosis with HLA-DW2 and HLA-DRW2 [86].

B-LYMPHOCYTES

B-lymphocytes arise in the bone marrow of humans and differentiate in the bursa of Fabricius of chickens and in the gastrointestinal tract or fetal liver of other animals. A few antigens—e.g., pneumococcal polysaccharide, dextran—can trigger B-lymphocytes directly to produce antibody. They are called T-independent antigens, and the antibody produced is almost entirely IgM. Tolerance is readily induced, and little memory results. Most antigens are not T-independent and require T cell assistance to trigger B-lymphocytes into producing antibody.

The most likely sequence of events is as follows: A foreign antigen is digested or ingested by a macrophage, resulting in the manufacture of an informational type of RNA that contains antigen fragments. This stimulates a T-lymphocyte (helper cell) to produce nonspecific soluble factors (lymphokines) that send a nonspecific signal to the altered antigen, and these combined signals then trigger the B-lymphocyte to produce antibody. When sensitized, these lymphocytes are transformed into immunoblasts, which eventually develop into plasma cells. The Golgi apparatus is prominently developed, and the rough-surfaced endoplasmic reticulum is increased.

The B-lymphocytes, by way of their plasma cell derivatives, can form an antibody immunoglobulin (Ig) that will combine specifically with the provocative antigen. The antibodies fit closely to a part of the surface of the antigen. The forces that hold the antibody to the antigen are (1) the coulombic force, i.e., the electrostatic attraction between oppositely charged ionic groups on protein side chains (e.g., an ionized amino group $[NH_3^+]$ on one protein can be attracted to an ionized carboxyl group $[COO^-]$ on the other); (2) hydrogen bonding between a proton donor on the antigen and an acceptor on the antibody, or between an acceptor on the antigen and a donor on the antibody; (3) Van der Waals forces, which are due to the interaction between two atoms that are close; and (4) hydrophobic forces owing to the interaction of nonpolar surfaces.

All of the several distinct classes of immunoglobulins have a basically similar structure consisting of two identical long, heavy chains and two identical short, light chains of amino acids that are linked covalently by interchain disulfide bonds.

One-half of the light chain—the half with the carboxyl terminal end—has the same amino acid sequence from one light chain to another; the other

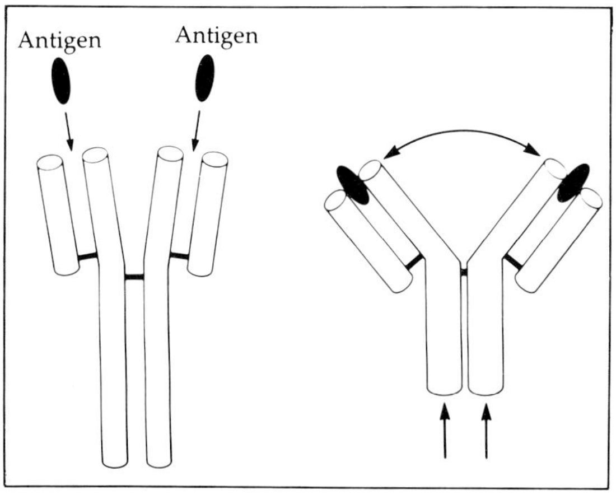

FIGURE 3-1. *The basic structure of an immunoglobulin molecule. The Y configuration and heavy and light chains are obvious. After interaction with antigen, the fragment crystallizable (Fc) section of the molecule may shorten.*

half—the half with the amino terminal end—has many different amino acid sequences from one light chain to another. This arrangement shows the high degree of variability in this half of the light chain, and similar variations are found in the amino terminal half of the heavy chain. These variable regions are the idiotypic regions of the Ig molecule (Fig. 3-1).

In this idiotypic region, there are certain areas of hypervariability that probably form the antigen-binding site. Their heterogeneity ensures diversity in the combining specificities—a diversity that is the result of variations in the shape and nature of the surface of the hypervariability areas.

The specificity of the Ig molecule seems to be determined by the heavy chain [41, 45], but the activation of the molecule requires the light chain. Two pairs of heavy and light chains account for the bivalent antigen-binding activity of the antibody molecules.

Papain can split the Ig molecules into three fragments. Two are identical, can combine with antigen, and are called the fragment antigen-binding [F(ab)$_2$] portions; the third fragment, which does not combine with antigen, is called the fragment crystallizable (Fc) portion [121]. The Fc portion is uniform and permits the Ig molecule to combine with complement, skin, mast cells, macrophages, lymphocytes, staphylococcal antigen, and others.

A single plasma cell can produce more than one type of Ig at a time, and clones of a single precursor cell can produce antibodies of different classes, all of which share the combining sites on the antigen [94, 117]. The B-lymphocytes have readily detectable membrane Ig and receptors for complement, antigen-antibody complexes, and the Fc region of Ig. In humans they account for 5 to 15 percent of all peripheral blood lymphocytes, and T-lymphocytes account for about 75 to 85 percent.

The immunoglobulins can be characterized as follows:

IgG

IgG is about 75 percent of the total serum Ig and has a molecular weight of 150,000. It can fix complement, cross the placenta, and interact with killer (K) cells in the antibody-dependent, cell-mediated cytotoxic (ADCC) type of reaction. IgG predominates in the secondary response to a given antigen. Because of its size, it predominates in the interstitial body fluids and thus carries the major burden of neutralizing bacterial toxins and binding to microorganisms to increase their phagocytosis directly or by binding complement. If red bood cells are coated with IgG, they can adhere to B-lymphocytes to form rosettes. IgG has several subclasses.

IgA

IgA is about 15 percent of the total serum Ig [156] and has a molecular weight of 170,000. IgA may form dimers spontaneously through association with a cystine-rich polypeptide known as the J chain.

A special form of IgA is exocrine or secretory IgA. It is a combination of two IgA molecules with a secretory piece (also called transport piece or T piece). The secretory piece is synthesized by local epithelial cells, e.g., lacrimal gland epithelium [46, 145]. Exocrine IgA is stabilized against proteolysis and so can continue to act as an antibody in an environment rich in proteolytic enzymes—an environment common to the tissues and body fluids susceptible to IgA action, i.e., saliva, tears, lung, gastrointestinal tract, nasal fluids. Specialized tissues in the intestinal tract (gut-associated lymphoid tissue), lung (bronchus-associated lymphoid tissue), and eye (conjunctiva-associated lymphoid tissue) appear to serve as the major sites of antigen sensitization.

In the gut, the lymphoid tissue is located in Peyer's patches. Lymphocytes sensitized to an antigen in these patches migrate to the draining mesenteric lymph nodes, from these to the circulation via the thoracic duct, and back "home" to the lamina propria of the intestinal tract. A similar situation exists in the eye: Antigen-sensitized lymphocytes in the conjunctiva eventually return to the lacrimal gland. "Homing" without antigen sensitization may also occur and is one type of natural antibody defense mechanism. But the homing of antigen-sensitized lymphocytes would certainly be of much greater magnitude and persistence than homing without antigen sensitization [80].

Exciting new work [158] indicates that sensitized lymphocytes can migrate from their original site to new areas where they can eventually produce IgA when again exposed to the original antigen. For example, the ingestion of an antigen can produce sensitized cells that migrate to the lacrimal gland, and when the subject is challenged, the tears can show IgA from cells residing in the lacrimal gland. All of the mucous membranes may be able to interact in this same way.

IgA antibodies are described as an "immunologic paint" on the body's external surfaces and may well be the body's first line of defense against invading microorganisms [74, 135, 157]. IgA antibodies are reduced in many autoimmune diseases and in children with atopic disease, though just why they are reduced or what effect the reduction has on these diseases is still unknown.

Aggregates of IgA can bind complement through the alternative pathway. IgA does not cross the placenta but is present in colostrum.

IgM

IgM is about 5 percent of the total serum Ig and has a molecular weight of about 900,000. The IgM molecules are pentamers with a high antigen-combining capacity. IgM is the first type of antibody formed after the initial encounter with antigen. IgM antibodies are extremely efficient agglutinating and cytolytic agents. They can fix complement [84], are confined largely to the blood stream, and do not cross the placenta. Many natural antibodies are of the IgM type.

As noted above, the initial exposure to an antigen results in the formation of IgM antibody. When IgG is synthesized, it "shuts off" or slows down IgM synthesis [43], and later (after 10–14 days) the IgG predominates in the immune response. Either rechallenge with or subsequent exposure to the same antigen meets with an accelerated and more prolific production of antibody. This second response is characterized by IgG production from the outset.

IgD

IgD is only 0.5 percent of the total serum Ig and has a molecular weight of 150,000. It is probably a primitive Ig that later gives way to IgM and the other immunoglobulins [2, 126]. It does not cross the placenta. Recently, IgD antinuclear antibodies have

been seen in systemic connective tissue disorders, but this may be only an epiphenomenon.

B-lymphocytes have immunoglobulins on their surfaces (a characteristic that differentiates them from T-lymphocytes), and of these, IgD appears to be the principal Ig.

IgE

IgE is only 0.007 percent of the total serum Ig and has a molecular weight of about 200,000. It does not fix complement but can cross the placenta. The so-called skin-sensitizing antibody is IgE [83]. It remains firmly fixed to the injection site of the skin and is responsible for the anaphylactic type of reaction on the skin (flare and wheal) and in such other tissues as the eye, lung, nose, and gastrointestinal tract.

Contact between an antigen (allergen) and an IgE molecule that is fixed by its Fc fragment to mast cells or basophils results in the release of pharmacologic mediators from these cells. (Basophils can be distinguished from mast cells by the small diameter of the basophils, the multilobular nature of their nuclei, the margination of chromatin in the nucleus, and the large, pink granules in the cytoplasm; in contrast, mast cells are elongated, have one nucleus [usually oval], and often have a nucleolus and numerous smaller granules that tend to stain dark purple. Basophils arise in the bone marrow and are circulating cells, but the origin of the fixed mast cell is unknown.) Although these pharmacologic mediators are responsible for the symptoms associated with allergic disease, this can surely not be the main function of IgE. It is thought, indeed, that its main function is to protect the host from parasitic infestation. Contact between a parasitic antigen and the mast cell–bound or basophil-bound IgE antibody in the gut wall results in the release of vasoactive amines, increased vascular permeability, and, finally, increased ability of the body's defenders (principally IgG) to reach and destroy the parasite.

IgG, on the other hand, can rarely affix to mast cells and so does not produce the type of anaphylactic reaction produced by IgE.

T-LYMPHOCYTES

T-lymphocytes are cells that originate in the thymus, whence they are released into the circulation. Morphologically they are almost impossible to differentiate from B-lymphocytes. Under the scanning electron microscope, B-lymphocytes sometimes have a more irregular, villous, turbulent appearance than T-lymphocytes (Fig. 3-2) [3]. In vitro, human T-lymphocytes can form spontaneous rosettes with uncoated sheep red blood cells [37]; B-lymphocytes

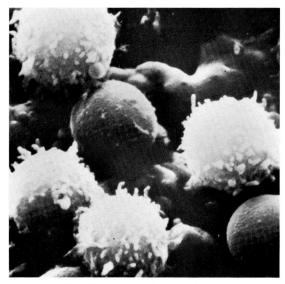

FIGURE 3-2. *Scanning electron microscope demonstrates the villous, turbulent B cell surface.*

can do this only if the sheep red blood cells are coated with IgG.

T-lymphocytes do not have detectable membrane Ig, complement, or Fc receptors for Ig, although new evidence indicates that subsets of T-lymphocytes may have some receptors. In mice, the T cells have receptors for a theta antigen, thymus-leukemia antigen, Ly antigen, and others.

When exposed to certain mitogens—concanavilin A, phytohemagglutinin, and pokeweed mitogen—T cells undergo a lymphoblastic transformation [131]; B cells can do the same thing when exposed to phytohemagglutinin and pokeweed mitogen, and to both purified protein derivative and bacterial lipopolysaccharide. (T cells do not respond to purified protein derivative or bacterial lipopolysaccharide, and B cells do not respond to soluble concanavilin A [131].)

T and B cells can be separated by electrophoresis, by depletion of one or the other by rosette formation, by affinity chromatography, by nylon-wool columns, and by anti-Ig and anti–T cell procedures. They can be differentiated by special staining procedures such as alphanaphthylacetylesterase (ANAE) activity, methyl green-pyronine, and fluorescein staining for Ig light or heavy chains.

Both types of lymphocytes react to the same range of antigens, and the location of the antigen often determines the type of lymphocyte that predominates. For example, antigens in the circulating body fluids stimulate mainly B cells, but fixed antigens in tissue allografts, solid neoplasms, and phagocytized bacteria stimulate mainly T cells.

The B cell is responsible for the humoral antibody–mediated immune response and the T cell for the cell-mediated immune (CMI) response.

As part of the CMI response, the stimulated T-lymphocyte can produce lymphokines, some of which affect macrophages. Migration inhibition factor (MIF) prevents macrophages from leaving the scene of the T cell–antigen interaction. Macrophage aggregation factor brings macrophages to this site, and macrophage arming factor increases the biologic activity of the macrophage. Mitogenic factor increases the blastic transformation of the T cell. Chemotactic factors for neutrophils, basophils, and eosinophils can be produced, and a neutrophil inhibitory factor as well. Other lymphokines are growth inhibitory factor, osteoclast activating factor, cytotoxic factor, skin reactive factor, immune interferon, Ig, interleukin-2, and possibly transfer factor.

There are also subpopulations of T-lymphocytes that can alter B cell antibody response.

The helper T cells have a low density, are radiation- and steroid-sensitive, and have an Fc receptor for IgM. By giving a nonspecific signal, they can play an important role in triggering a B cell response to an antigen. They may also increase the T cell responses, but if too abundant, they may actually inhibit antibody production.

The suppressor T cells can be differentiated from the helper cells by virtue of their high density, their resistance to radiation and steroid, and the fact that they have an Fc receptor for IgG. They act as negative regulators of B cell maturation and have been implicated in virtually every immunologic regulatory mechanism [52, 166], i.e., in the maintenance of tolerance, in antigen competition, in the control of antibody responses to antigens, and in the control of IgE responses.

Depressed levels of suppressor cells may permit an excess of IgE-mediated responses and result in atopy. The suppressor cell population in atopic patients is in fact consistently deficient. Depressed levels of these cells also occur in autoimmune diseases (e.g., lupus erythematosus, Sjögren's syndrome, rheumatoid arthritis) and may partially account for the host's inability to control the body's attack on self, i.e., on its own DNA, lacrimal glands, and joints [164, 165].

KILLER AND NATURAL KILLER LYMPHOCYTES
K cells are lymphocytes that apparently do not carry antigen receptors on their surfaces and may not belong to either the T or B cell series, although recent reports favor the T cell line for both K and natural

killer (NK) cells [88]. K cells, which may also be of macrophage origin, have both complement receptors and Fc receptors for IgG but lack Ig on their surfaces. They arise in response to an antigen and can fuse with the Fc portion of an Ig molecule that has previously entered into combination with cell surface antigen. In this way they can exert a direct cytolytic effect on the cell. Functionally, this mechanism of ADCC would be expected to play a major role in target-cell destruction when the targets— solid tumors, transplants, large parasites—are too large for ingestion by phagocytosis.

NK-lymphocytes are naturally occurring cells that can form without any antigenic stimulus. They contribute to the body's ability to resist or mitigate an attack by a foreign antigen. For example, patients subject to recurrent herpetic vesicles on the lips may have low levels of NK cells [99]. Cortisone can depress NK cell activity [100], and exogenous interferon can elevate it [38, 68]. NK cells may belong to a T cell line, and some of them may have receptors for the Fc portion of IgG [19].

MACROPHAGES (ADHERENT CELLS)
Macrophages possess receptors for the Fc portion of certain classes of IgG molecules and certain complement components (C3). An Ig that fixes to the macrophage membrane is called a cytophilic antibody. Macrophages have no memory of a previously encountered antigen, but a sensitized T cell does have such a memory and can influence the macrophage's activity.

Macrophages process antigen, which then becomes highly immunogenic for T cells, and this complex of antigen, T cells, and macrophages triggers the B-lymphocytes to produce antibody. Macrophages are also scavengers that clear the body of dead or damaged cells, inorganic crystals, and organic debris; active defenders against certain classes of microorganisms, particularly facultative and obligate intracellular parasites; and in vivo regulators of granulopoiesis.

Macrophages have characteristics that suit them for these functions. They are highly phagocytic, can adhere to charged surfaces (which has given them the name *adherent cells*), are motile, possess lysosomal enzymes, and respond to chemotactic stimuli. In culture, activated macrophages seem to secrete plasmin activator, collagenase, elastase, lysozyme, bacteriocidins, endogenous pyrogen, hyaluronidase, prostaglandin E, a stimulatory factor for leukocyte production, and a number of other products [35, 162].

The polymorphonuclear leukocyte (PMN) shares many properties with the macrophage. They are both active phagocytes. In phagocytosis, the following six interdependent steps are taken: (1) random movement, (2) chemotaxis, (3) attachment to the foreign material, (4) ingestion, (5) activation of the macrophage or PMN, and (6) destruction of the foreign material.

Random movement is the nondirectional movement of the phagocytic cell. Chemotaxis is the activation of the phagocyte by a chemotactic factor and then by cell movement [107, 144]. The phagocyte must next attach itself to the foreign material. The attachment is called opsonic adherence or immune adherence. In the immune adherence process, complement participates. The attached phagocytes can then transport particles from the extracellular space to the inside of the phagocyte and its vacuoles (phagosomes). Activation of the phagocyte's intracellular metabolism is required for the destruction of the foreign invader. The metabolic events include an increase of glucose utilization through the hexose monophosphate shunt, an uptake of oxygen, and the production and release of superoxide and hydrogen peroxide [150]. The destruction of the foreign material by the neutrophilic PMN is brought about by the action of peroxidase, the hydroxyl radical, singlet oxygen, superoxide, acid, or lysozyme.

COMPLEMENT
The classical complement system consists of nine individual components, C1 through C9. When activated, these components interact sequentially with one another in a so-called cascade similar to the coagulation sequence. The individual components were numbered in the order of their discovery—not in the order of their activation.

In general, the activation of the components of the complement system requires the enzymatic cleavage of each component into two fragments. The larger of the two fragments joins the preceding activated component, which in turn generates new enzymatic activity that can cleave the next component (Fig. 3-3). The smaller fragments in the earlier steps often have properties of their own. For example, C4C2 fragments resemble kinins, C3b increases phagocytosis, C3a and C5a produce an anaphylatoxin and can cause chemotaxis, and C567 can cause chemotaxis. The anaphylatoxin can result in the release of vasoactive amines (e.g., histamine, platelet-activating factor).

In the classic pathway of complement activation, antibody plays three roles: It selects the target for the complement attack, it serves as a site for the first component of complement to attach to the Fc portion of the Ig molecules, and it triggers the conversion of inactive C1 to enzymatically active C1. C1 has three subunits—C1q, C1r, and C1s. It is the interaction of C1q with the Fc receptor on the Ig molecule that results in the conversion of C1r from a proenzyme to an active enzyme, which in turn converts the C1s proenzyme to an active enzyme [111]. This interaction begins the complement cascade. The last components form a complex that produces functional holes in the cell membrane and leads to cell lysis [63, 149].

The alternative pathway of complement activation, which is also called the properdin system, can be activated by such substances as aggregated immunoglobulins (IgG1, 2, 3, and 4, IgA, and IgE), bacterial endotoxins, bacterial cell walls, and polysaccharides (e.g., inulin). The initiation site of the Ig is the Fab area. This contrasts with the initiation site of the classical pathway, which is the Fc area.

On this alternative pathway, properdin conver-

tase, and then properdin, are activated sequentially. The active properdin then activates a factor D, which in turn activates a factor B. This latter factor can activate C3 with the assistance of C3b, and once C3 is activated, the classical cascade of C3 to C9 proceeds. In this way the alternative pathway bypasses C1, C4, and C2 of the classical pathway.

The system is self-regulatory by virtue first of the instability of some of the components, and then of the production of substances that destroy some of the components.

There are several other enzyme-effector systems—the kinin system, the clotting system, and the plasmin (fibrinolytic) system—that interact with the complement system (Fig. 3-4). Activation of the Hageman factor (clotting factor XII) initiates both the intrinsic coagulation sequence (i.e., the throm-

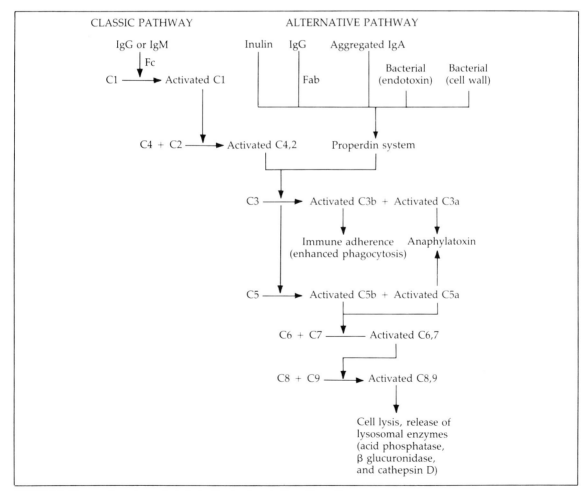

FIGURE 3-3. *The complement cascade includes the classic and alternative pathways.*

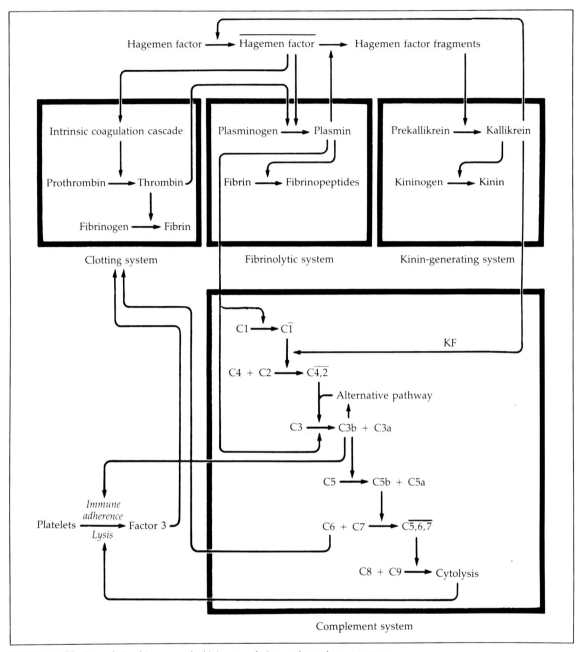

FIGURE 3-4. *The interrelationship among the kinin, coagulation, and complement systems.*

botic occlusion of small vessels) and the plasmin system. Plasmin, in addition to cleaving polymerized fibrin into vasoactive fibrinopeptides, cleaves activated Hageman factor. The cleaved fragments activate the kinin system, which increases vascular permeability, the chemotaxis of neutrophilic PMNs, and the production of a fragment that makes C1 more efficient in the production of C4,2. Plasmin also initiates the complement system by activating C1, and it can increase the release of anaphylatoxin from C3a. The clotting system can be activated by the immune adherence of platelets to C3b.

Defects in the complement system can occur. The best known is the lack of C1 esterase inhibitor, which results in hereditary angioneurotic edema.

ASSOCIATED INFLAMMATION

Inflammation, whether induced by immunologic reactions, tissue damage, or microbial products, plays a vital role in the body's defense system. It is in fact a necessity for the proper functioning of the immune defenses since it attracts all of the circulating substances to the site of foreign invasion. These vital circulating substances are the PMNs, macrophages, lymphocytes, antibodies, complement, C-reactive protein (e.g., a molecule, unrelated to the immunoglobulins, that precipitates with the group-specific C-carbohydrate of pneumococci), and properdin, which can activate the alternative pathway of complement stimulation.

There are neurogenic and nonneurogenic controls of vasomotor activity. The capillaries, precapillaries, and small arterioles are affected by chemicals, and the large vessels near the terminal arterioles are affected by the nervous system. Of the complicated, nonneurogenic controls, the most important are (1) the vasoactive amines, which include histamine, heparin, platelet-activating factor, bradykininlike substances, eosinophil chemotactic factor, and leukotrienes C, D, and E; (2) the serum proteases and polypeptides known as kinins; and (3) the prostaglandins of the E and F series. In specific types of inflammation, some mediators play more prominent roles than others.

The kinins are a family of vasoactive polypeptides that can cause pain, increase vascular permeability, alter vascular tone, contract intestinal smooth muscle, and exert proteolytic activity. As noted above, the kinin system interacts with (1) the clotting system, which can cause platelet release, thrombosis, complement activation, kinin generation, and chemotaxis; (2) the plasmin system, which can cause chemotaxis, an increase in proteolytic activity, kinin generation, thrombolysis, and complement

activation; and (3) the complement system, which was discussed in detail above.

The prostaglandins are potent substances that are liberated locally in the tissues during inflammation. The control of prostaglandin release may depend upon the availability of its precursor; the release or activation of the synthetase enzymes; the cofactor requirements; and changes in the sodium, potassium, and calcium concentrations.

The prostaglandins can cause sustained vasodilatation, can counteract the vasoconstriction caused by substances such as norepinephrine and angiotensin, and can increase vascular permeability, hyperalgesia, granuloma formation, fever, and leukotaxis. The newly arrived leukocytes can release more prostaglandins and continue the inflammatory process. Prostaglandins can suppress human T cell mitogenesis [57] and other functions [115]. Prostaglandin E and prostaglandin F are present in the ocular tissues and tears. Prostaglandins may play an important role in (1) the mediation of anterior and posterior uveitis, (2) the formation of aqueous flare and cells and of miosis after trauma, (3) episcleritis, (4) the elevation of intraocular pressure after alkali burns of the corneal, and (5) the reduction of intraocular pressure after trauma or inflammation [118]. The effects of prostaglandin E on Behçet's disease, on the macular edema associated with aphakia, on corneal graft reactions, and on thermal burns are still uncertain.

CELL ALTERATION

IMMUNOLOGIC TOLERANCE

Under normal circumstances, some potential antigens reach the lymphoid cells during their developing, immunologically immature phase in the prenatal or perinatal period. When the child reaches immunologic maturity, these lymphoid cells or their cell lines suppress any subsequent response to the antigen. In this way, unresponsiveness to one's own bodily components (self) can be established. But any foreign cells introduced into the body during this perinatal period can trick the immune system into treating them as self, and immunologic tolerance to this foreign, nonself material is induced.

Immunologic tolerance can also be induced in adults. There are two levels of antigen dosage at which this can occur: very high doses (high-zone tolerance), and very low doses (low-zone tolerance). In high-dose tolerance, both B- and T-lymphocytes participate. The induction of the tolerance takes a long time, and unless exposure to the antigen persists, the tolerance itself is short-lived at best. Tolerance may be hard to induce because of the B cell with its high concentration of surface receptors. B cell tolerance may also be due to the depletion of specific B cells after their interaction with a plentiful supply of antigen or to the suppression of the B cells by suppressor T cells.

Low-dose tolerance involves T cells [168] and can be achieved in hours. Even in the absence of persistent antigen, it can last for months. T cell tolerance may be due to suppressor cell activity, to the depletion of specific T cells by the antigen (unlikely), or to immune complexes that block the receptor sites of the T cells [169].

Tolerance can be more readily established if immunosuppressive drugs are given, and tolerance to solid tissue can be attained only in this way.

IMMUNOLOGIC ENHANCEMENT
Immunologic enhancement is the achievement of increased survival of foreign antigens by the use of enhancing antibodies. These antibodies, administered or produced under appropriate conditions, combine with the surface antigens of the foreign cells, which are then no longer accessible to the receptors on the sensitized lymphocytes. The combination avoids the activation of complement or K cells.

AUTOIMMUNITY
When there is a breakdown in the mechanism controlling the production of antibodies to self, autoantibodies (i.e., antibodies capable of reacting with self tissues) are produced. Autoantibodies may normally be present in controlled amounts and may routinely dispose of cellular breakdown products [11], but if they are out of control and cause disease, then specific autoimmune disease occurs.

Suppressor T cells are thought to play the major role in controlling autoantibody production. The breakdown in control can occur if there is either a decline of suppressor T cell activity (e.g., in the aged [66], in thymectomized animals [116], or in disease states such as diabetes) or a disturbance in the balance between helper and suppressor cells [153], or if other, as yet unknown, mechanisms occur.

The attack on self can be brought about by a variety of mechanisms. Chemical and physical agents can alter the configuration of protein molecules so that previously hidden antigenic determinants are exposed to the immune system. Isolated antigens may be recognized as nonself after they are in-

troduced to the immune system (e.g., in lens-induced uveitis or Mooren's ulcer). Viruses can form new antigenic determinants on the cell membranes of infected cells, and these new determinants, as well as the intracellular viral protein, can elicit an immune response to the cell in and on which they reside (e.g., disciform keratitis after herpes simplex virus infection of the cornea). Neoplasms can alter body tissues and form new antigens that can elicit immune responses. Haptens can combine with host proteins to render them autoantigenic (e.g., as in hemolytic anemias); exogenous, cross-reacting proteins can produce autoimmune disease (e.g., streptococcal infections); ontogenic tissue that develops late and is not present during uterine life can act as a foreign protein and elicit an autoimmune attack; and abnormal, mutant clones of lymphocytes may be produced that will attack self.

There are organ-specific autoimmune diseases in which the antigens are available only in low doses, tolerance is not firmly established, and the antibodies are organ-specific. In this type of autoimmune disease, the affected tissue is infiltrated by lymphocytes and plasma cells, and there is evidence that the CMI response plays an important role. Examples of these diseases are Hashimoto's thyroiditis, pernicious anemia, pemphigoid, sympathetic ophthalmia, some forms of optic neuritis, and lens-induced uveitis.

There are also non-organ-specific autoimmune diseases in which the antigens are readily accessible, tolerance is usually firmly established, and the antibodies are not organ-specific. The lesions are due to the deposition of antigen-antibody complexes and appear histologically as fibrinoid necrosis [92]. Increased T cell responsiveness has occasionally been noted. Examples of these diseases are systemic lupus erythematosus, rheumatoid arthritis, scleroderma, and dermatomyositis.

Autoimmune diseases exhibit exacerbations and remissions and are not always progressive [125]; increased IgG and IgM levels may be present, and there may be a selective deficiency of IgA [47].

IMMUNOALTERATION BY DRUGS
IMMUNOENHANCEMENT
Potentiation of the reticuloendothelial system in general and of the CMI response in particular has been successful in ameliorating the course of infectious disease and neoplasia. Some of the agents that have been used are transfer factor [130, 148], levamisole hydrochloride [26, 124], various lymphokines [141], *Mycobacterium bovis* (BCG) [142],

muramyldipeptide [104], *Corynebacterium parvum*, vitamin A, thymosin, PG inhibitors, and zinc.

Transfer factor is a dialyzable substance that can convert skin test–negative recipients to positive recipients after inoculation [95]. It has been effective in increasing resistance to disease in many situations [89].

Levamisole hydrochloride, an orally administered anthelmintic agent, can restore CMI in anergic patients, exerting its effect by stimulating macrophage function, T cell function, and the reticuloendothelial system nonspecifically. The data suggest that levamisole hydrochloride acts on cells by altering the intracellular cyclic guanosine 3′,5′-cyclic phosphate (cGMP) to adenosine 3′,5′-cyclic phosphate (cAMP) ratios [123].

BCG and muramyldipeptide can increase the proliferative and cytotoxic T cell response in vitro and the ability of macrophages to kill tumors [104]. *C. parvum* may work by similar mechanisms [42].

Vitamin A greatly increases the number of antibody-forming cells produced by immunization with sheep red blood cells. It also induces nonspecific resistance to infection [29], and it can prevent or lessen the immunosuppressive effect of corticosteroids [87].

Research into both new and established immunoenhancers should yield valuable information that will help us in our efforts to learn how the body can increase its resistance to nonself antigens.

IMMUNOSUPPRESSION

The depletion of unstimulated lymphocytes may depress the immune response effectively. This can be accomplished by such means as neonatal thymectomy, thoracic duct drainage, radiation, and the use of antilymphocyte serum (ALS) or corticosteroids.

ALS is prepared by immunizing one species with the lymphocytes of another species, and then using the serum of the immunized animal to destroy the lymphocytes of the donor [140]. The major effect of ALS is to depress the CMI response [96] by depressing the long-lived, recirculating, small T-lymphocytes. To a lesser degree, the B-lymphocytes are also affected [8]. Unfortunately, ALS evokes many adverse reactions—e.g., serum sickness, antigen-antibody glomerular basement membrane deposits [62]—because ALS is itself a heterogeneous antigen.

Corticosteroids can cause a transient lymphopenia that reaches its maximum in 4 to 6 hours. (T-lymphocytes are more sensitive to the steroids than are B-lymphocytes.) The lymphopenia can be due to lysis or to the redistribution of the lymphocytes from the blood vessels to other tissues, particularly

the bone marrow. Lymphocyte proliferation, function, and circulation are also inhibited, and the proliferative response to mitogenic stimulation by phytohemagglutinin and to antigen can be depressed in vitro. Macrophages are also affected. Steroids reduce the metabolism of the macrophage; reduce its secretion of plasmin activator, collagenase, and elastase [161, 170]; impede its circulation; and interfere with antigen retention on the macrophage surface. Inhibition of macrophage spreading on glass has also been reported [28, 33]. Steroids can also reduce the movement of antigen-antibody complexes across basement membranes [51].

Steroids also affect the inflammatory process directly, and under certain circumstances, as for example, at very low doses, this action may be quite separate from the steroids' direct immunosuppressive action.

Steroids increase the levels of adenyl cyclase at the receptor sites on mast cells, lymphocytes, and other cells; increase the levels of cAMP in human leukocytes; and increase the cAMP response to prostaglandin E. They also potentiate the effects of beta-adrenergic catecholamines on human leukocytes. All of these actions lessen the release of the vasoactive amines from the mast cells and basophils and in this way reduce the symptoms of allergy. The histamine content of the tissues is reduced, and eosinopenia can occur. When applied topically, steroids can constrict the blood vessels in the human eye [60], and this in turn reduces the vascular permeability and postinflammatory neovascularization. There is also a reduction in the number of blood monocytes and of monocytes at inflammatory sites. This reduction and the stabilization of the lysosomal membranes of these cells reduce the inflammation.

Recent work [44] suggests that corticosteroids lessen the accumulation of prostaglandin E by limiting the availability of the substrate for prostaglandin biosynthesis, and that they also decrease the release of prostaglandin from cells.

Immunosuppression by selective destruction of the dividing, differentiating, antigen-stimulated blast cell can be accomplished by alkylating agents, purine and pyrimidine antagonists, folic acid analogues, some antibiotics, and alkaloids. The alkylating agents, e.g., cyclophosphamide, block DNA replication in dividing cells, and mitosis ceases [14]. Purine antagonists, e.g., mercaptopurine and azathioprine, inhibit various steps in the purine synthesis competitively and exert feedback inhibition on the earliest steps of the sequence [23]. The pyrimidine antagonists, e.g., idoxuridine (IDU) and cytarabine, are converted in vivo to metabolites that inhibit thymidine synthesis and competitively exert feedback inhibition at several steps in the chain of pyrimidine synthesis [122].

Folic acid analogues interrupt the supply of tetrahydrofolate, which in turn terminates DNA synthesis. Methotrexate acts by inhibiting the enzyme folic reductase, which converts folic acid to tetrahydrofolate [171]. Some antibiotics, e.g., chloramphenicol, resemble part of the messenger RNA molecule and so compete with it for messenger RNA binding sites on the ribosome [32]. The alkaloids, e.g., colchicine, are potent mitotic inhibitors [20].

Prostaglandin inhibitors can affect the immune response either directly or indirectly by first affecting the inflammation. Experimentally, prostaglandin antagonists (polyphloretin phosphate) and biosynthesis inhibitors (inhibitors of cyclooxygenase such as aspirin, indomethacin, indoxole, flurbiprofen, naproxen, fenoprofen) have been effective in a variety of animal models in altering the effect of prostaglandin as follows: (1) An elevation of intraocular pressure induced by arachidonic acid can be neutralized by many prostaglandin inhibitors [119]. (2) Iridocyclitis after systemic inoculation with a bacterial toxin can be counteracted by aspirin or indomethacin [118]. (3) Inflammation after paracentesis can be counteracted by indoprofen or indomethacin [160]. (4) A rise in intraocular pressure in herpetic keratouveitis can be partially counteracted by aspirin [15]. (5) The corneal immune and inflammatory responses to bovine gamma globulin intracorneal inoculation can be partially counteracted by indomethacin but are unaffected by fenoprofen or indoxole [12, 143].

Nonresponsiveness to a donor idiotype present on the Ig molecule or T cell can result in a type of tolerance to grafted tissue from that donor. This sequence of events will be discussed in the section on graft rejection.

TESTING FOR IMMUNE REACTIONS

Time and space prohibit the listing of all of the available tests one can make when trying to define the immunologic status of a given patient. But in any case, complete laboratory surveys are generally recognized as wasteful, expensive, and of little value to the patient.

On the other hand, wise, carefully selected tests can be of immense value. The selection can only

be accomplished, however, by an understanding of the immunology of the suspected disease, of the immunologic alterations produced by it, and of the tests that would most accurately reflect those alterations and yield the necessary diagnostic information. Assistance can be obtained from general laboratory manuals [127] and from specialists in rheumatology, immunology, or other pertinent fields. In this section, I shall outline briefly a general approach to the solution of an immunologic problem.

The first step is to try to determine whether the causal agent of the disease is infectious or not. Blood tests for complement fixation antibodies, precipitating antibodies, and hemagglutinating antibodies; indirect fluorescent antibody tests; serology testing; and direct agglutination tests can be directed toward a specific infectious antigen, e.g., *Treponema pallidum, Toxoplasma gondii, Leptospira* sp., *Brucella* sp., *Coccidioides immitis, Histoplasma capsulatum, Chlamydia* sp., and herpes simplex virus. Blood tests for noninfectious agents, e.g., an eosinophil count, a test for C-reactive protein, etc., are also available.

The foreign agent may be the patient's self, and the appropriate blood tests would then be one or several of the following: a test for rheumatoid factor (IgM), a test for antinuclear antibodies, a lupus erythematosus preparation, a test for antithyroid antibodies, protein electrophoresis, a serum viscosity determination, a test for heparin-precipitable fibrinogen, or the determination of certain Ig levels.

Lymphocytes can be tested for their responsiveness in general, or to a given antigen in particular, by tests for MIF or other lymphokine levels, by blastogenesis to a given antigen or mitogen, or by mixed-lymphocyte culture reactions.

The total B or T cell population (ANAE stain, E-rosettes) and the suppressor cell levels can also be determined.

Testing for a given antigen (e.g., a circulating immune complex or alpha-fetoprotein) or making nonspecific tests (e.g., white blood cell count and differential count, sedimentation rate determinations) can occasionally be helpful. Determining the patient's HLA type is of limited value in some of the diseases mentioned earlier in the chapter.

Skin testing can indicate specific CMI hypersensitivity to a given antigen or general immune responsiveness. Skin test antigens such as streptokinase-streptodornase, trichophytin, candidin, protein derivative, and mumps can be used to test for anergy, i.e., general immune unresponsiveness.

Special tests such as enzyme-linked immunosorbent assays, which are designed to test for an antibody or a specific antigen; radioimmunosorbent test; or radioallergosorbent test, which is designed to test for IgE, are also helpful in selected cases.

If there is tissue available, routine staining with hematoxylin-eosin may identify the type of immune or nonimmune response by showing the predominant cell type (eosinophils, mast cells, and basophils in allergic states; neutrophilic PMNs in necrosis and toxic states; lymphocytes in viral disease and some immune states). Tissue can also show any alterations in the normal architecture—occlusive vasculitis and fibrinoid necrosis in immune diseases, foreign bodies in granulomas, caseation. Special stains can be used to identify special cell types, e.g., methyl green-pyronine, ANAE, fluorescent antibody.

HYPERSENSITIVITY RESPONSES

TYPE I: ANAPHYLACTIC RESPONSE

Nearly 10 percent of the population suffer in one degree or another from allergies. The participating Ig in this anaphylactic type of response is IgE. On contact with an allergen (which is an antigen that reacts with IgE and evokes an allergic response), the IgE (at least two molecules) attached to the surface of a mast cell or basophil by its Fc portion alters the cell surface so that vasoactive amines are released. The configurational alteration of the cell surface is

believed to interfere with adenyl cyclase activity. Adenyl cyclase is an enzyme that can convert adenosine triphosphate to cAMP, and since cAMP is required to maintain the stability of the mast cell, any reduction in adenyl cyclase leads to a reduction in cAMP and to the release of the pharmacologic mediators (e.g., histamine, heparin) from the granules (Fig. 3-5).

The amount of mediator released depends partially on the amount of IgE on the cell surface and the subsequent stimulus. The number of IgE molecules on the cell surface can range from a few to 90,000. IgE antibody is called homocytotropic because of its adherence to the surfaces of the mast cells or basophils.

The hallmark of allergy is the rapidity of the onset of its symptoms once a sensitized individual is brought into contact with the offending allergen. Sensitivity is normally assessed by the response to intradermal challenge with antigen. The release of histamine and the other mediators rapidly produces a flare and wheal that are maximal within 30 minutes and then subside. The Prausnitz-Küstner test is as follows: The appropriate allergen is injected into the site of the IgE skin attachment 48 hours after the test serum is injected (presumably the test serum contains IgE, which is capable of binding to skin

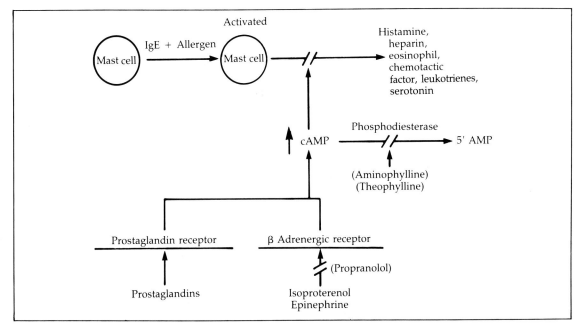

FIGURE 3-5. *The control of adenosine 3',5'-cyclic phosphate in the mast cell. Type I hypersensitivity response.*

tissue and to remain at the site of inoculation); a flare and wheal appear immediately if the reaction is positive.

The level of cAMP can be affected by factors other than the adenyl cyclase level mentioned above. Stimulation of the beta-adrenergic receptor increases the levels of cAMP. Prostaglandin E_1 and E_2 can also act by way of adenyl cyclase to increase the levels of cAMP and thus inhibit mediator release. Phosphodiesterase breaks down cAMP to 5'-AMP, and inhibitors of this action, e.g., aminophylline, theophylline, papaverine, and caffeine, can elevate the levels of cAMP. Stimulation of the alpha-adrenergic receptor by phenylephrine or norepinephrine, plus propranolol, reduces the level of cAMP.

The cholinergic receptor, which can be stimulated by acetylcholine or carbachol, leads to elevated levels of cGMP and mediator release, which is the opposite of elevated levels of cAMP. Atropine can block the stimulation of the cholinergic receptor and thus inhibit mediator release.

Disodium cromoglycate (DSCG), which diminishes the release of the pharmacologic mediators, may work by preventing an influx of calcium into the cell.

The pharmacologic mediators—histamine, platelet activating factor, and leukotrienes C, D, and E —can cause vasodilation and smooth-muscle constriction.

Histamine can interact with specific H_1 receptors and cause allergic manifestations. But it can also interact with H_2 receptors, which cause an increase in intracellular cAMP and in this way turn off the reaction [98].

The eosinophils, which arrive at the target site because of released eosinophil chemotactic factor and histamine, contain eosinophil-derived inhibitor (EDI) of histamine release [78]. The EDI activates adenyl cyclase, which elevates cAMP and inhibits further mediator release. Eosinophils also contain arylsulfatase B and major basic protein, which can inactivate the slow-reacting substance of anaphylaxis; histaminase, which can destroy histamine; and phospholipase D, which can inactivate the platelet-activating factor and thus reduce the serotonin levels [54]. The eosinophils can phagocytize immune complexes, especially allergen-IgE complexes.

T-lymphocytes, especially suppressor cells, may play an important role in terminating mediator release. The concept that elevated IgE levels are secondary to a reduction in the regulatory function of T cells is supported by the observation that elevated serum IgE levels occur in anergic patients with Wiskott-Aldrich syndrome [163] and other entities with impaired cellular immunity [22]. Enhancement of suppressor cell activity can ameliorate the symptoms of allergy and probably accounts in part for the use of transfer factor and levamisole hydrochloride to treat atopic disease.

The more routine forms of therapy are the use of agents that can (1) raise the level of intracellular cAMP (e.g., prostaglandin, epinephrine, caffeine, papaverine, aminophylline, theophylline, DSCG, cortisone), (2) lower the level of cGMP (e.g., atropine), (3) ameliorate the symptoms directly with vasoconstrictors (e.g., cortisone, naphazoline hydrochloride), or (4) compete with histamine for the cellular receptors (e.g., antihistamines). Antihistamines can also reduce capillary permeability directly. They can be given topically or systemically.

Immunotherapy has been used in severe cases. An attempt is made to change the relative IgE/IgG (antiallergen-antibody) ratio in favor of the latter since IgG can bind the allergen without inducing an allergic biologic response [129]. Immunization by the transmucosal route produces a preponderance of IgE antibodies, and parenteral immunization produces a striking increase in IgG antibodies [97]. In an attempt to reduce clinical symptoms, we can therefore produce blocking IgG antibodies by parenteral immunization [31].

The commonest ocular manifestations of the hay fever type of anaphylactic reaction are rapid vascular congestion and conjunctival chemosis. The conjunctiva looks milky or pale pink. The exudative material is clear or whitish if the ocular reaction is acute, and whitish, thick, and stringy if the reaction is chronic. There may be mild papillary hypertrophy. Lid chemosis can occur concomitantly with the conjunctival chemosis or corneal edema. All these signs are the sequelae of the release of the vasoactive amines. The symptoms are itching, tearing, and burning. If the cornea is affected, photophobia and blurred vision may result.

In the vernal or atopic type of keratoconjunctivitis with its giant papillae, a mononuclear cell infiltrate occurs. The presence of lymphocytes and macrophages suggests that this type of reaction has a slightly different pathogenesis from the strictly anaphylactic, hayfever type of reaction that produces the signs and symptoms listed above. It is believed that the CMI response (cutaneous basophilic hypersensitivity reaction) plays a particularly important role in the vernal atopic entities. (This is an example of the nonclassic form of CMI in which mast cells predominate.)

TYPE II: CYTOTOXIC RESPONSE

The cytotoxic response is the one that participates in the immune protection of the host from pyogenic bacteria, transplanted tissue, and tumor cells. The action of the antigen on the foreign cell, combined with antibody (IgG or IgM), causes the death of the affected cell by bringing about its contact with phagocytes or K cells. Phagocytosis is accomplished by a reduction in surface charge; opsonic adherence directly through the Fc portion of the antibody, the phagocytes adhering to antibody without the assistance of complement; or immune adherence through bound C3b, the phagocytes adhering to antibody with the assistance of complement. The activation of complement occasionally occurs and results in cell death (Fig. 3-6).

Killer cells can bind nonspecifically to the Fc fraction of the antibody, and the final result is the death of the cell.

Circulating cytotoxic antibodies can be identified in vivo by the passive transfer of antibody-containing serum into a normal recipient. In vitro, adding the patient's serum to the target cells in a test tube, or adding the patient's serum to normal cells in the presence of antigen, produces agglutination or lysis if complement is present. Sometimes the antibody fails to produce agglutination unless a second antibody is added. Such nonagglutinating antibodies are called incomplete and may be detected by the Coombs' test [9].

Some examples of these cytotoxic reactions are transfusion reaction, rhesus factor incompatibility, organ transplantation reaction (in part), acute nephritis, many drug reactions, Mooren's ulcer, and mucous membrane pemphigoid.

TYPE III: IMMUNE COMPLEX RESPONSE

In the immune complex response, the injured cells or tissue are innocent bystanders and do not possess the antigenic determinants that can combine with the antibody that caused the injury. The antibody reacts with its antigen, and the resulting immune complex binds complement, attracts PMNs,

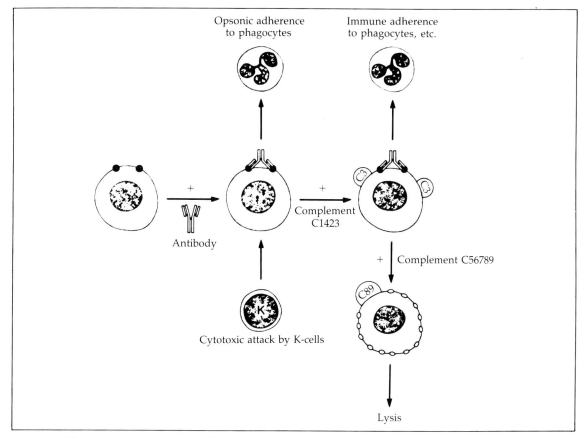

FIGURE 3-6. *The cytotoxic (type II) hypersensitivity response.*

and then directly or indirectly injures tissues that are in the vicinity. The result can be catarrhal ulceration; a Wessely ring in response to antigen injected into the cornea, to antigen on a contact lens over the cornea, or to viral antigen; or peripheral infiltrates in a variety of conditions, e.g., rheumatoid arthritis, polyarteritis nodosa. The distribution of the injury to the tissue is determined by the sites where the immune complexes form or are deposited (Fig. 3-7).

The mechanism of immune complex–induced injury is complicated. The size of the complex is important: Large complexes are easily phagocytized by the reticuloendothelial system and do not localize in tissues; small complexes persist in the circulation but may be too small to localize in tissues. It is the intermediate sizes that localize in tissues, but the vascular permeability must increase before they can localize in the extravascular areas, e.g., the kidney or limbus. The vasoactive amines may play a crucial role in increasing this permeability, and platelets, complement, anaphylatoxins, and mast cells or basophils combined with IgE may also be sources of these vasoactive amines.

Previous damage (nonimmunologic or immunologic) to the blood vessels can also increase their permeability and pave the way for the subsequent deposition of immune complexes in the surrounding tissues (the Auer reaction). This phenomenon may play a significant role in recurrent uveitis.

The damage caused by the complexes can be due to the release of proteolytic enzymes from the PMNs, elevated blood viscosity (associated with the larger complexes [85]), and the activation of Hageman factor.

When there is an excess of antigen, the complexes that form are soluble and can produce lesions in the walls of the blood vessels and in the perivascular spaces. The clinical picture consists of fever, swollen lymph nodes, a generalized urticarial rash, and painful joints (as in serum sickness).

When there is an excess of antibody, insoluble complexes form and produce the Arthus reaction. This reaction causes an intense infiltration of the complex site (usually within venules) with PMNs and occlusion of blood vessels. This severe reaction can reach a peak within hours of the introduction of the antigen into the hyperimmunized recipient.

TYPE IV: CELL-MEDIATED IMMUNE RESPONSE

The CMI response is due entirely to the activity of thymus-dependent lymphocytes and cannot be transferred from sensitive to nonsensitive individuals by way of serum antibodies; lymphoid cells or soluble transfer factor are required [34, 146].

The T-lymphocyte responds primarily to fixed rather than soluble antigens, participating in reactions to many bacteria, viruses, fungi, tissue allografts, and neoplasms. There are two types of this delayed hypersensitivity response (so-called because of the delayed immune response, i.e., it takes 48 hours for maximal skin test response to an antigen injected into a sensitized host). The two types are the classic, tuberculin type in which T cells and macrophages participate; and the cutaneous, basophil type (previously called the Jones-Mote reaction)

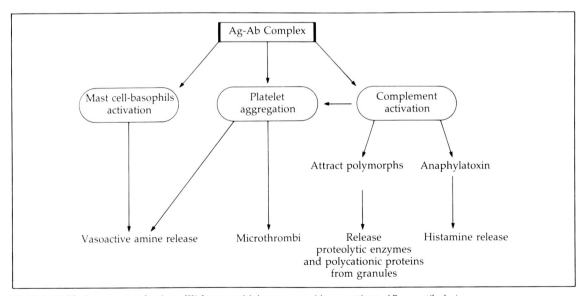

FIGURE 3-7. *The immune complex (type III) hypersensitivity response. (Ag = antigen, AB = antibody.)*

in which T cells, macrophages, mast cells, basophils, and eosinophils participate.

The CMI reaction is probably initiated by the combining of macrophage-processed antigen with the receptors on the surface of an appropriate T cell, one of a clone of memory cells previously exposed to the antigen. The cell membrane becomes activated, and the signal is transmitted to the interior of the cell, which is then transformed into a large immunoblast and undergoes mitosis. As previously noted, plant lectins can induce this change non-specifically. The immunoblast can now release the lymphokines, which will mediate the response [13, 59, 136].

Tissue damage can be caused by the lymphokines as well as by complement. Histologically, the classic CMI response is characterized by perivascular cuffing with lymphocytes, particularly when it is early in the course of the reaction, and by a granulomatous response later. There is usually a core of macrophages (many of them engorged with ingested antigenic material and called epithelioid cells) surrounded by the lymphocytes. The chemotactic mediators account for the presence of other cell types.

Defects in the CMI response are present in a variety of congenital diseases—combined immunodeficiency, Di George's syndrome, ataxia-telangiectasia, Wiskott-Aldrich syndrome, and Nezelof's syndrome—and in certain diseases that develop later—Hodgkin's disease, sarcoidosis, lepromatous leprosy, diabetes mellitus, severe lupus erythematosus, advanced malignancy, uremia, severe burns, xeroderma pigmentosum, viral diseases, chronic mucocutaneous candidiasis, and heroin addiction.

Malnutrition [25], advanced age [16], and immunosuppressive therapy can also depress cell-mediated immunity.

The CMI response plays a role in the following disease states:

INFECTION

Infection is a process that establishes a specific relationship between host and parasite. Its essential steps are the entrance of the parasite into the host, or its adherence to the host, and the multiplication of the parasite within the host.

In the first step, some microorganisms can produce aggressins in order to invade the host; others lack this ability and gain entrance to the host by accident—through a break in the skin, a break in the cornea, or the bite of an insect or other arthropod vector. Once the integrity of the barrier is breached, the organisms can be disseminated by the blood stream, the lymphatic system, or tissue mi-

gration of the organisms themselves or of phagocytic cells containing them [16].

Virulence is the term usually applied to an organism's ability to produce disease. Microorganisms can exercise their virulence in a number of ways. As integral parts of their structure, some possess antiphagocytic properties (e.g., the capsule of the pneumococcus and the M proteins of streptococcal cell walls) that repel the host's phagocytes by negative chemotaxis; others (gram-negative bacteria) possess endotoxins as part of their cell walls; still others produce exotoxins that are toxic to all of the cells of the reticuloendothelial system. Staphylococcal coagulase causes the deposition of fibrin around each coccus, coating it protectively, and around abscesses, the osmotic barrier preventing the entrance of immunoglobulins.

Organisms can be disseminated more readily with the help of hyaluronidase, fibrinolysins, and streptokinase (which is elaborated by most strains of group A streptococci).

The following are a few examples of the adaptations bacteria have made in their struggle for survival:

Bacteria can elaborate collagenases (e.g., *Pseudomonas*), amylases, nucleases, and other enzymes and in this way enhance their pathogenicity. In the presence of an antibiotic, some microorganisms (e.g., *Staphylococcus aureus*) can undergo transition to L forms (viable bacteria minus cell walls), and then reemerge as fully virulent organisms when the antibiotic is withdrawn. Many parasites (e.g., *Mycobacterium tuberculosis*, *Listeria monocytogenes*, *Francisella tularensis*) can resist destruction if phagocytized by macrophages. *Borrelia recurrentis* is a versatile parasite that apparently undergoes an antigenic change of coats in vivo that increases its longevity. *S. aureus* is covered by a substance called protein A. The Fab cannot combine with protein A, only the Fc. This reversed attachment blocks phagocytosis by both macrophages and neutrophils [110]. Plasmids contribute directly to virulence by converting the organism to phagocytosis-resistant forms. This they accomplish by producing toxins and by resisting the bactericidal activity of the serum [93].

The eye is particularly vulnerable to virulent bacteria: Some ocular tissues are avascular and have few mesenchymal cells (e.g., the cornea, lens, and vitreous) and are thus highly susceptible to infection. Many ocular tissues can be easily injured, permitting bacterial entrance. Many chemotherapeutic agents used to treat ocular trauma, and even infection (e.g., corticosteroids, IDU), can also suppress the host's immunologic defense mechanisms.

The host's three main lines of defense against these ingenious bacteria are the barriers provided by the intact conjunctiva, skin, and mucous membranes; the nonspecific immune defenses; and the specific immune defenses. Most bacteria cannot long survive on the skin because of the inhibitory effect of the skin's lactic acid and fatty acids and the low pH that these substances generate. The ciliated epithelium in the respiratory tree prevents the bulk of inhaled organisms from reaching the alveoli, and the expulsive forces of sneezing and coughing protect the host mechanically. By competing for the viral enzyme neuraminidase, the mucous secretions inhibit the penetration of cells by viruses. The specific ocular defenses will be discussed later in this chapter.

In connection with the nonspecific immune defenses, the role of secretory IgA alone or with complement has been discussed. Natural IgM antibodies present in the serum of normal individuals respond to repeated contact with the many bacterial antigens present normally in the gut. Lysozyme is an antibacterial substance that has a minimal inhibitory effect on bacteria on the surface of the eye. Cells can produce interferon (not the lymphokine variety) in response to a viral infection, and the interferon can protect other cells by preventing adherence, penetration, and viral multiplication. Interferon acts on two enzymes that prevent the availability of messenger RNA for viral replication.

Among the specific immune defenses are the humoral [24] and CMI [113] responses to the particular microorganism. Humoral immunity plays a major role in resisting many microorganisms and their toxins (e.g., group A streptocci, *Haemophilus influenzae*, pneumococci, poliovirus, influenza virus). Humoral immunity can neutralize extracellular viral particles.

The CMI response plays a part in the host's defense against the following microorganisms: *Salmonella* sp., *Brucella* sp., *Treponema pallidum*, *Listeria monocytogenes*, *Franciśella tularensis*, herpes simplex virus, herpes zoster virus, cytomegalovirus, vaccinia virus, measles virus, *Candida* sp., *Aspergillus* sp., *Histoplasma capsulatum*, *Coccidioides* sp., *Toxoplasma gondii*, and *Plasmodium* sp.

Contact between T cell and antigen occurs at the site of infection or in the paracortical areas of the draining lymph nodes. Specifically, sensitized T cells function in different ways to protect the host: They may produce lymphokines, they may lyse infected host cells directly, or they may increase antibody production.

In viral infections, when the infected and noninfected cells are destroyed, the virus becomes extracellular and is then destroyed by circulating antibody. The viral antigen incorporated into the cell membrane (e.g., in stromal herpetic keratitis or in the subepithelial opacities of epidemic keratoconjunctivitis) is destroyed by K cells or sensitized T cells. The virus may change the normal HLA antigen on the membranes of infected cells in such a way that it is recognized as foreign by the host's lymphocytes and is ultimately lysed [173]. If this type of reaction continues until unaltered membrane antigens of similar, noninfected cells are destroyed, an autoimmune process may result. (Multiple sclerosis may be an example of this sequence of events.)

Cell death may be beneficial or detrimental, depending on the tissue under attack. In lymphocytic choriomeningitis (LCM), T cells are sensitized by LCM-infected brain cells and are then directly cytotoxic for those cells [40]. This cytotoxicity is detrimental to the infected host because it is directed against such vital tissues as the meninges, ependyma, and choroid plexus. The rationale for the use of steroids in corneal herpetic stromal disease is based partially on this concept, i.e., that the cytotoxic effect on visually important tissues is due to immunologic mechanisms and not to replicating live virus.

In this ocular situation, the theoretical benefit of suppressing the immune response to protect vital tissues must be weighed against the following facts: (1) Cortisone can increase melting and decrease healing. (2) Immunosuppression can increase viral and other microbial growth in the affected area. (3) The unaltered course of herpetic stromal keratitis in uncompromised hosts is self-limited. (4) A healed, untreated eye may ultimately have remarkably good visual acuity.

Immune interferon is produced as a lymphokine by sensitized T cells [105]. It may not only affect viral activity in the cell directly by tying up the messenger RNA [101] but also may enhance the activity of the NK cells, which, in turn, can favorably alter the course of an infection.

TUMORS

The CMI response also plays a major role in tumor control. The immune system polices the body's cells, keeping watch for altered cells. This immunologic surveillance mechanism works because tumor cells have different surface antigens called tumor-specific transplantation antigens (TSTA). The cells that are infected by oncogenic viruses have new transplantation antigens on their surfaces that are characteristic of the infecting virus (viral TSTA) [79]. All tumors induced by the same virus contain the same TSTA [36]. Immunization with material from one tumor confers resistance to subsequent challenge with any other syngeneic tumor induced by the same virus.

The action of chemical carcinogens is largely a random interaction between the chemical and the cell's DNA. The resultant tumors are all antigenically different [114]. Tumors derived from the same type of cell often have a common differentiation antigen that is also present on embryonic cells. Examples of these oncofetal antigens are the alpha-2 fetal protein in hepatic carcinoma [1] and the carcinoembryonic antigen in cancer of the intestine [56]. Testing for these antigens may prove to be a helpful diagnostic tool.

Specific antibodies form in response to malignant tumors [55, 109], but they are not necessarily damaging to the tumor unless it is of lymphoid origin. K and T cells are the principal effective cells needed for an attack on a solid tumor. K cells attack the antibody-coated tumor; lymphokines from T cells play a complex but yet to be defined role [58, 70].

It is believed that we all face the development of numerous tumors during our lifetimes. The body's defense mechanisms recognize the foreign antigen and destroy it. We need, then, to ask why some tumors succeed in growing and eventually destroying the host organism.

Apparently tumor antigenicity can vary. Tumor antigens are in general relatively weak when compared with transplantation antigens, and the less antigenic of these tumors may survive.

If the host's immune responsiveness is unfavorably altered, then the tumor may survive. For example, children with immunologic deficiencies [48], patients whose immune systems have been suppressed by drugs for long periods of time in attempts to prolong the survival of transplanted tissue [39], and the elderly [114] all exhibit a higher than average frequency of malignancies. There are also lapses in a person's immunologic competence during his life owing to infections, surgery, severe stress, general anesthesia, and other reasons, and these periods of relative immunodepression may allow tumors to become established. The more prolonged the suppression, the more likely it is that this may happen.

Blocking factors, which are probably antigen-antibody complexes, can combine with specific receptors on sensitized T cells, thus altering the T cells' ability to destroy the tumor [134]. They can also adsorb to the surfaces of the tumor cells and block the cytotoxic K or T cells, preventing them from gaining access to the antigenic sites on the tumor cell surfaces [10].

In certain cases, the body may become tolerant of the tumor because of prolonged exposure to small amounts of antigen (low-zone tolerance).

If any of these mechanisms allows the tumor to grow appreciably, the host's CMI response may not be able to handle it because of its mass.

Therapy includes surgical extirpation and chemotherapy.

Immunologically speaking, attempts have been made to reduce the blocking factors by removing the bulk of the tumor, plasmapheresis, and the inoculation or production of unblocking antibodies [71]. Attaching an anticancer drug to monoclonal tumor-antigen antibodies may increase the tumor-killing properties of the drug. Liposomal preparations of the anticancer drugs insure their prolonged localized targeting. Increasing the patients' CMI response by thymosin [69], *Corynebacterium parvum* [67], BCG [103], or *Bordetella pertussis* [103] may inhibit tumor growth and increase the likelihood of its rejection.

CORNEAL GRAFT REJECTION

There are a variety of organ- and species-specific corneal antigens that incite the immunologic response to an allograft. HLA antigens are present on the surfaces of the corneal cells and play a major role in the rejection phenomenon. More specifically, it is the immune-associated (Ia) antigen associated with the HLA-DR locus that may play the key role. These Ia antigens are present on the surfaces of B cells, some T cells [73], macrophages, and Langerhans' cells. The Langerhans' cells are a subpopulation of epidermal cells. They have Fc receptors for IgG and C3 receptors, and they are present at the corneal limbus and in the peripheral corneal epithelium [91].

The soluble and particulate corneal allograft antigen can diffuse from the cornea, exit via the corneal blood vessels in neovascularized corneas, and exit via the corneal lymphatic channels in neovascularized corneas. Once the antigen has reached the limbus, it enters the conjunctival lymphatics and proceeds to the lymph nodes.

Antigen present in the anterior chamber may diffuse from it and make the graft recipient tolerant and not sensitive to the antigen because of its unusual method of sensitizing the host. But if the host is sensitized, he can mount an immunologic response that manifests itself by the sensitization of T cells [159] and the production of lymphokines [132], antibody production [17, 112], and subsequent coating of the allograft's surface antigen and K cell attack (ADCC) of the antibody-coated antigen [61]. The host is apparently sensitized within a week to the corneal donor tissue, but it is the ability of the effector cells to reach the target graft that may prevent any clinically observable rejection phenomenon. For this reason, the degree of vascularization of the donor bed is crucial [27, 90].

The first signs of rejection are a mild uveal reaction shown by flare and cells, an accumulation of fine keratic precipitates (KPs) on the endothelium, and circumlimbal injection. In the peripheral type of graft rejection, the KPs are in the lower part of the graft or at its margin near the heaviest vascularization. A line of KPs may form and migrate centripetally. The donor cornea becomes edematous when the endothelium is compromised by the accumulation of lymphocytes. In the less common, diffuse type of rejection, the KPs spread diffusely over the endothelium, and a few days later the cornea becomes edematous. In both types of response, the development of a membrane on the posterior surface of the corneal button may be a late manifestation [27].

In endothelial rejections, the rejection line consists principally of T cells accompanied by fibrin on the endothelial surface (Fig. 3-8). The T cells infiltrate the endothelium, often replacing the endothelial cell cover and in some areas exposing Descemet's membrane to the anterior chamber [81]. Stromal edema overlies the areas of severe damage. The rejected endothelial cells are often rounded or globular and have greatly thickened centers. The endothelial nuclei are irregularly thickened. Tight junctions between adjacent endothelial cells disappear [120]. Precipitates consisting of lymphocytes, other monocytes, and fibrin appear on the endothelium. The lymphocytes are said to reach the endothelium through the unhealed Descemet's membrane from the blood vessels and wandering cells that have entered the corneal stroma. Descemet's membrane heals in several months, and this route of lymphocyte ingress is then closed. When grafts are being rejected, or have been rejected, the healing of Descemet's membrane may be delayed [82].

The reparative process depends on the spreading of the surviving endothelial cells of both host and

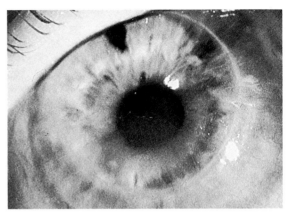

FIGURE 3-8. *An endothelial rejecting line in a corneal graft reaction.*

donor. If the endothelial destruction is severe, a retrocorneal membrane may form. The cells that make up the membrane are fibroblasts that probably come from the edge of the graft through the disrupted Descemet's membrane. Some investigators [106] feel that metaplasia of the endothelial cells leads to the formation of the retrocorneal membrane.

The prevention and treatment of corneal graft rejection will be discussed in terms of their immunologic implications. Several surgical maneuvers can minimize rejection: (1) The removal of the donor epithelium in suitable cases reduces the antigenic load and may in particular eliminate Ia antigens or Langerhans' cells. (2) The use of a small, centrally placed graft reduces the antigenic load and moves the donor tissue away from the blood vessels with their effector cells. (3) The removal of interrupted sutures as soon as possible, or the use of running sutures, minimizes vascularization. (4) The preplacement of a lamellar graft in the heavily vascularized graft bed before penetrating keratoplasty moves blood vessels away from the allograft. (5) The use of keratoprostheses in very selected cases eliminates the foreign antigen.

Soaking the donor graft in the recipient's serum may remove passenger lymphocytes (with their Ia antigens) and reduce the rejection rate. Soaking the donor tissue in antilymphocyte globulin may reduce or eliminate the Ia antigen–bearing cells and coat the endothelium with noncytotoxic antibodies, in this way preventing an ADCC and K cell attack. Hyperbaric oxygen may alter Ia antigens, and donor tissue treated with hyperbaric oxygen may be less antigenic.

Matching the HLA antigens of donor and recipient (especially the D locus) in high-risk cases may be an effective way of preventing graft rejection, and the use of monoclonal antibodies facilitates the procedure.

Sterile T-lymphocytes from a donor of the same species can be mixed with recipient T-lymphocytes in a mixed lymphocyte culture. The blasts that form are the recipients and are given back to the recipient in a regularly scheduled pattern of delivery. After several weeks the recipient may become tolerant of the donor's idiotypic antigen, and although he may still reject grafted tissue from another donor of the same species, he will no longer reject any grafted tissue from the present donor [123]. This idiotype tolerance is strong, lasts a long time, and may play an important role in future grafting procedures.

Reducing inflammation by a corticosteroid remains the mainstay of the prevention of rejection, and reducing inflammation and immunosuppressing the graft recipient by high doses of corticosteroids remains the mainstay in the treatment of rejection.

CONTACT DERMATITIS

The skin is the major interface between the body and its environment. Contact dermatitis serves as a clinical model of the adverse effects of environmental agents. The sensitizing substances, called haptens, are of low molecular weight, can penetrate the skin (i.e., are lipid soluble), and can form strong covalent bonds with proteins of the skin [75].

Some of the commonest sensitizers (listed in decreasing order of frequency) are the following: nickel sulfate, -caine mixtures, thimerosal (present in many ophthalmic solutions, especially contact lens solution), neomycin sulfate, and ammoniated mercury [21, 128]. The conjugates formed in the skin reach the regional lymph nodes by way of the rich lymphatic system. After the T cells have been sensitized, they undergo blastogenic transformation and form clones of committed T cells [53]. And within 12 to 14 hours, T cells and macrophages accumulate in the area of the skin where the sensitizer was applied (Fig. 3-9).

Sensitivity may persist for as short a time as 1 year in patients who are only slightly sensitive to an uncommon sensitizer, or it may last for many years.

OCULAR CONSIDERATIONS AFFECTING THE IMMUNE RESPONSE

BLOOD VESSELS

The lacrimal artery, the superior and inferior medial palpebral arteries, and the muscle branches of the ophthalmic artery (with their anterior ciliary branches) form the rich blood supply of the conjunctiva, eyelids, and lacrimal glands. The uveal tract and retina are also well supplied with blood vessels [172]. (The cornea, lens, and vitreous, on the other hand, are avascular.) This rich blood supply can be thought of as a natural immunologic defense. Ocular inflammation first dilates the blood vessels and then increases their permeability. This permits the leakage of vital elements of the immune response, e.g., Ig, B cells, T cells, macrophages.

Since the cornea is devoid of blood vessels and exposed to the external environment, it is in an especially precarious situation if the surface barrier is broken or penetrated by aggressive microorganisms, e.g., *Corynebacterium diphtheriae* or *Neisseria gonorrhoeae*. The failure of the immune system to recognize foreign antigens in the cornea, and the cornea's inability to attract effector cells to itself, accounts for this situation. This status is altered, however, if the cornea becomes vascularized. In fact, anticorneal antibodies may arise nonspecifically when chronic corneal inflammation and neovascularization develop [72].

Both the cornea and the lens have organ-specific antigens. The organ-specific antigens of the cornea reside in the epithelium [70] and anterior one-fourth of the stroma [65] (Fig. 3-10). Since both the lens and the cornea are devoid of blood vessels, the immune system fails to recognize these antigens. Should lens protein escape from its isolation (as it may at the time of cataract extraction or in hypermature cataracts), the body may consider this antigen (the lens protein) as nonself and produce autoantibodies to it. Lens-induced uveitis may then be the result.

The cornea may behave in the same way. Recognition of its organ-specific antigen or of a slightly modified version thereof (by a microorganism or other agent), may be the pathogenesis of Mooren's ulcer.

LYMPHATICS

There are lymphatics in the conjunctiva. Those in the bulbar conjunctiva begin at the limbus in a series of arcades. There are two plexuses: a superficial plexus composed of small vessels just beneath the vascular capillaries, and a deep plexus consisting of large vessels in the fibrous layer of the conjunctiva. On the lateral side, both plexuses drain into the preauricular and parotid lymph nodes. This can be seen in Parinaud's syndrome and in epidemic keratoconjunctivitis (Fig. 3-11). On the medial side, both plexuses drain into the submandibular lymph nodes.

The normal cornea does not have lymphatic vessels, but if the cornea vascularizes, there is a concomitant ingrowth of cell-lined lymphatic channels

[30, 137]. Corneal and conjunctival immunologic reactions are often associated with immunologic activity in the draining lymph nodes [139].

There are no true lymphatic vessels inside the eye; nevertheless, drainage to regional lymph nodes does occur after an injection of antigen into the vitreous [64]. Antigen is slowly released by the vitreous, and this increases the immune response—an adjuvant effect. The anterior chamber is a privileged site, not only because of the absence of lymphatic channels but also because of an aberrant central processing of an antigen, i.e., the antigen encounters the blood vessels before it encounters the lymph node. This leads to tolerance of antigen introduced into the anterior chamber, not to sensitization to it.

TEAR FILM

The tear film's neutral pH and the blinking process are important natural defense mechanisms. The tears contain several antibacterial substances, e.g., lysozyme, lactoferrin, beta lysin [49], secretory IgA, IgG, and complement. The lysozyme comes from type A cells in the lacrimal gland [7]. The large amounts of secretory IgA, some IgG, and complement [18] are probably supplied by the normally abundant plasma cells lying beneath the conjunctival epithelium and in the stroma of the lacrimal gland. The IgA may trap, coat, and lyse bacteria in addition to neutralizing viruses and toxins. The IgG may neutralize toxins and viruses, lyse bacteria, and form immune complexes. Complement components C1q, C3, C4, C5, properdin, and properdin factor B, are found in the cornea as well [108]. In the conjunctiva, in addition to the large number of inflammatory cells present [6], there also appear to be areas of lymphoid accumulation, similar to Peyer's patches in the intestine, that can function in the same manner. Antigen may enter here and eventually cause sensitization and IgA production in the lacrimal gland. This area may be part of the mucous membrane–associated lymphoid tissue system also present in the gut, lungs, and other areas. During inflammation, the Ig components of the tears may change significantly (IgG increases). IgE and histamine have been found in the lacrimal gland and tears of normal persons, and at higher levels in patients with vernal keratoconjunctivitis.

ANTIBODY PRODUCTION

There is some controversy about the ability of the ocular tissues to produce antibody when challenged with a new antigen. A primary ocular challenge

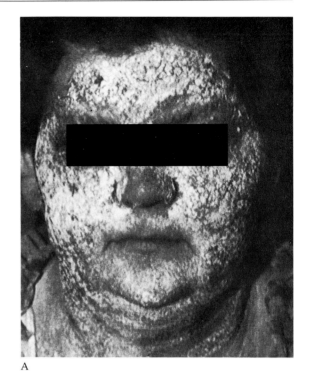

A

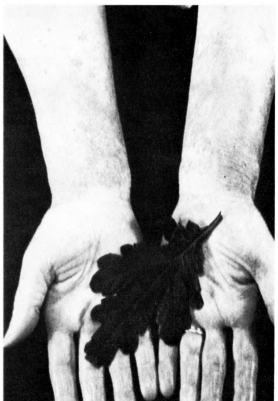

B

FIGURE 3-9. *A and B. Contact dermatitis of the skin.*

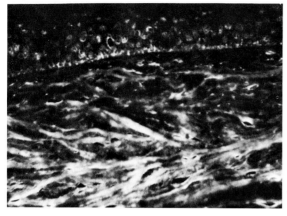

FIGURE 3-10. *Immunofluorescence demonstrating the organ-specific antigen in the anterior stroma of the bovine cornea.*

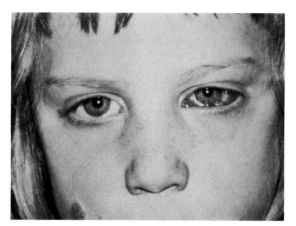

FIGURE 3-11. *Parinaud's syndrome. Enlarged preauricular glands are noted in this disorder.*

probably elicits its initial immune response at a distant site, e.g., from a draining lymph node, the spleen, or the bone marrow. The sensitized effector cells (lymphocytes and plasma cells) then travel back to the ocular source of the antigen and reside there, awaiting the stimulus that would cause them to release the appropriate mediators, e.g., Ig, lymphokines [133, 138].

There is an abundance of Ig in the external ocular tissues. The conjunctiva has a rich supply—IgA, IgG, IgM—that probably comes from the rich vascular supply, the abundant plasma cells, and the lacrimal gland [4]. The levels of IgG and IgA in the central and peripheral cornea are the same, the IgG level being one-half the serum level and the IgA level only one-fifth the serum level. IgM is found less often and has only rarely been detected in the central, avascular cornea [5]. The immunoglobulins are found principally in the stroma.

The iris is usually free of immunoglobulins. The usual double-walled vessels of the iris, with their junctions between the endothelial cells, may explain this lack. The stroma of the ciliary body and choroid, but not the epithelium, contains all five immunoglobulins.

REFERENCES

1. Abelev, G. I. Production of embryonal serum and globulin by hepatomas. *Cancer Res.* 28: 1344, 1968.
2. Abney, E. A., and Parkhouse, R. M. E. Candidate for immunoglobulin D present on murine B lymphocytes. *Nature* 252:600, 1974.
3. Alexander, E. L., and Wetzel, B. Human lymphocytes. *Science* 188:732, 1975.
4. Allansmith, M. R., and O'Connor, G. R. Immunoglobulins. *Surv. Ophthalmol.* 14:367, 1970.
5. Allansmith, M. R., and McClennan, B. Immunoglobulins in the human cornea. *Am. J. Ophthalmol.* 80:123, 1975.
6. Allansmith, M. R., et al. Plasma cell content of main and accessory lacrimal glands and conjunctiva. *Am. J. Ophthalmol.* 82:819, 1976.
7. Allen, M., Wright, P., and Reid, L. The human lacrimal gland. *Arch. Ophthalmol.* 88:493, 1972.
8. Allison, A. C. Effects of antilymphocytic serum on bacterial and viral infections and virus oncogenesis. *Fed. Proc.* 29:167, 1970.
9. Alper, C. A., and Rosen, F. S. Studies of the in vivo behavior of human C3 in normal subjects and patients. *J. Clin. Invest.* 46:2021, 1967.
10. Baldwin, R. W., et al. Immunity in the tumor-bearing host and its modification by serum factors. *Cancer* 34:1452, 1974.
11. Bankhurst, A. D., Torrigiani, G., and Allison, A. C. Lymphocytes binding human thyroglobulin in healthy people and its relevance to tolerance for autoantigens. *Lancet* 1:226, 1973.
12. Belfort, R., Jr., et al. Indomethacin and the corneal immune response. *Am. J. Ophthalmol.* 81:650, 1976.
13. Bennett, B., and Bloom, B. R. Reactions *in vivo* and *in vitro* produced by a soluble substance associated with delayed-type hypersensitivity. *Proc. Natl. Acad. Sci. U.S.A.* 59:756, 1968.
14. Bennett, L. L., Jr., et al. The primary site of inhibition of 6-mercaptopurine on the purine biosynthetic pathway in some tissues in vivo. *Cancer Res.* 23:1574, 1963.
15. Bhattacherjee, P. Prostaglandins and inflammatory reactions in the eye. *Meth. Find. Exp. Clin. Pharmacol.* 2:17, 1980.

16. Bigley, N. J. *Immunologic Fundamentals.* Chicago: Year Book, 1975. Pp. 1–9, 140–147.

17. Binder, P. S., Chandler, J. W., and Kaufman, H. E. *In vitro* demonstration of cytotoxic antibodies and their possible role in corneal graft rejection. *Invest. Ophthalmol.* 15:481, 1976.

18. Bluestone, R., et al. Lacrimal immunoglobulins and complement quantified by counterimmunoelectrophoresis. *Br. J. Ophthalmol.* 59:279, 1975.

19. Bolhuis, R. L. H., et al. Characterization of NK cells and K cells in human blood: Discrimination between NK and K cell activities. *Eur. J. Immunol.* 8:731, 1978.

20. Bruchovsky, N., et al. Effects of vinblastine on the proliferative capacity of L cells and their progress through the division cycle. *Cancer Res.* 25:1232, 1965.

21. Brun, R. Epidemiology of contact dermatitis in Geneva. *Contact Dermatitis* 1:214, 1975.

22. Buckley, R. H., Wray, B. B., and Belmaker, E. Z. Extreme hyperimmunoglobulinemia E and undue susceptibility to infection. *Pediatrics* 49:59, 1972.

23. Caskey, C. T., Ashton, D. M., and Wyngaarden, J. B. The enzymology of feedback inhibition of glutamine phosphoribosylpyrophosphate aminotransferase by purine ribonucleotides. *J. Biol. Chem.* 239:2570, 1964.

24. Centifanto, Y. M., Little, J. M., and Kaufman, H. E. The relationship between virus chemotherapy, secretory antibody formation and recurrent herpetic disease. *Ann. N.Y. Acad. Sci.* 173:649, 1970.

25. Chandra, R. K. Rosette-forming T lymphocytes and cell-mediated immunity in malnutrition. *Br. Med. J.* 545:608, 1974.

26. Churchill, W. H., Jr., and David, J. R. Levamisole and cell-mediated immunity. *N. Engl. J. Med.* 289:375, 1973.

27. Ciba Foundation Symposium. *Corneal Graft Failure.* Amsterdam: Associated Scientific Publishers, 1973.

28. Claman, H. H. How corticosteroids work. *J. Allergy Clin. Immunol.* 55:145, 1975.

29. Cohen, B. E., and Elin, J. R. Vitamin A–induced nonspecific resistance to infection. *J. Infect. Dis.* 129:597, 1974.

30. Collin, H. B. Lymphatic drainage of I^{131}-albumin from the vascularized cornea. *Invest. Ophthalmol.* 9:146, 1970.

31. Connell, J. T., and Sherman, W. B. The effects of treatment with the emulsions of ragweed extract on antibody titers. *J. Immunol.* 91:197, 1963.

32. Coutsogeorgopoulos, C. On the mechanism of action of chloramphenicol in protein synthesis. *Biochim. Biophys. Acta* 129:214, 1966.

33. Dannenberg, A. M., Jr. The antiinflammatory effects of corticosteroids. *Inflammation* 3:329, 1979.

34. David, J. R., et al. Delayed hypersensitivity *in vitro. J. Immunol.* 93:264, 1964.

35. David, J. R. Macrophage activation by lymphocyte mediators. *Fed. Proc.* 34:1730, 1975.

36. Defendi, V. Effect of SV40 virus immunization on growth of transplantable SV40 and polyoma virus tumors in hamsters. *Proc. Soc. Exp. Biol. Med.* 113:12, 1963.

37. Dickler, H. B., Adkinson, N. F., and Terry, W. D. Evidence of individual human peripheral blood lymphocytes bearing both B and T cell markers. *Nature* 247:213, 1974.

38. Djeu, J. Y., et al. Augmentation of mouse NK cell activity by interferon and interferon inducers. *J. Immunol.* 120:175, 1979.

39. Doak, P. B., et al. Reticulum cell sarcoma after renal homotransplantation and azathioprine and prednisone therapy. *Br. Med. J.* 4:746, 1968.

40. Doherty, P. C., and Zinkernagel, R. M. H-2 compatibility is required for T cell mediated lysis of target cells infected with lymphocytic choriomeningitis virus. *J. Exp. Med.* 141:502, 1975.

41. Edelman, G., et al. Reconstitution of immunologic activity by interaction of polypeptide chains of antibodies. *Proc. Natl. Acad. Sci. U.S.A.* 50:753, 1963.

42. Ellouz, F., et al. Minimal structural requirements for adjuvant activity of bacterial peptidoglycan derivative. *Biochem. Biophys. Res. Commun.* 59:1317, 1974.

43. Finklestein, M. S., and Uhr, J. W. Specific inhibition of antibody formation by passively administered 19S and 7S antibody. *Science* 146:67, 1964.

44. Floman, N., and Zor, U. Mechanism of steroid action in ocular inflammation. *Invest. Ophthalmol. Vis. Sci.* 16:69, 1977.

45. Franek, F., and Nezlin, R. Recovery of antibody combining activity by interaction of different peptide chains isolated from purified horse antitoxins. *Folia Microbiol.* (Praha) 8:128, 1963.

46. Franklin, R. M., Kenyon, K. R., and Tomasi, T. B. Immunohistologic studies of human lacrimal gland. *J. Immunol.* 11:984, 1973.

47. Fraser, K. J. IgA immunoglobulins and autoimmunity. *Lancet* 2:804, 1969.

48. Fraumeni, J. F. Constitutional disorders of man leading to leukemia and lymphoma. *Natl. Cancer Inst. Monogr. Hemopoietic Neoplasms* 32:221, 1969.

49. Friedland, B. R., Anderson, D. R., and Forster,

R. K. Non-lysozyme antibacterial factor in human tears. *Am. J. Ophthalmol.* 74:52, 1972.

50. Fritz, D. C., et al. HLA antigens in myasthenia gravis. *Lancet* 1:240, 1974.

51. Germuth, F. G., et al. A unique influence of cortisone on the transit of specific macromolecules across vascular walls in immune complex disease. *Johns Hopkins Med. J.* 122:137, 1968.

52. Gershon, R. K. T Cell Control of Antibody Production. In M. D. Cooper and N. L. Warner (Eds.), *Contemporary Topics in Immunobiology.* New York and London: Plenum, 1974. P. 1.

53. Giminez-Camaraja, J. M., et al. The lymphocyte transformation test in contact nickel dermatitis. *Br. J. Dermatol.* 92:9, 1975.

54. Goetzl, E. J. Modulation of human eosinophil polymorphonuclear leukocyte migration and function. *Am. J. Pathol.* 85:419, 1976.

55. Gold, P., and Freedman, S. Demonstration of tumor-specific antigens in human colonic carcinomata by immunological tolerance and absorption techniques. *J. Exp. Med.* 121:439, 1965.

56. Gold, P., and Freedman, S. Specific carcinoembryonic antigens of the human digestive system. *J. Exp. Med.* 122:467, 1965.

57. Goodwin, J. S., Bankhurst, A. D., and Messner, R. P. Suppression of human T-cell mitogenesis by prostaglandin. *J. Exp. Med.* 146:1719, 1977.

58. Granger, G. A., and Kolb, W. P. Lymphocyte *in vitro* cytotoxicity. *J. Immunol.* 101:111, 1968.

59. Granger, G. A. Mechanisms of lymphocyte-induced cell and tissue destruction *in vitro*. *Am. J. Pathol.* 59:469, 1970.

60. Greeson, T. P., et al. Corticosteroid-induced vasoconstriction studied by xenon-clearance. *J. Invest. Dermatol.* 61:242, 1973.

61. Grunnet, N., et al. Occurrence of lymphocytotoxic lymphocytes and antibodies after corneal transplantation. *Acta Ophthalmol.* 54:167, 1976.

62. Guttman, R. D., et al. Treatment with heterologous antithymus sera. *Transplantation* 5:1115, 1967.

63. Hadding, U., and Müller-Eberhard, H. J. The ninth component of human complement. *Immunology* 16:719, 1969.

64. Hall, J. M. Specificity of antibody formation after intravitreal immunization with bovine gamma globulin and ovalbumin. *Invest. Ophthalmol.* 10:775, 1971.

65. Hall, J. M., Smolin, G., and Wilson, F. M., II. Soluble antigens of the bovine cornea. *Invest. Ophthalmol.* 13:304, 1974.

66. Hallgre, H. M., and Yunis, E. J. Suppressor lymphocytes in young and aged humans. *J. Immunol.* 118:2004, 1977.

67. Halpern, B., et al. The effect of *Corynebacterium parvum* on tumor resistance. *Nature* 212:853, 1966.

68. Hansson, M., et al. Effect of interferon and interferon inducers on the NK sensitivity of normal mouse thymocytes. *J. Immunol.* 125:2225, 1980.

69. Hardy, M. A., et al. The effect of thymosin on human T cells from cancer patients. *Cancer* 37:98, 1976.

70. Heise, E. R., and Weiser, R. S. Factors in delayed hypersensitivity. *J. Immunol.* 103:570, 1969.

71. Hellstrom, K. E., and Hellstrom, I. Lymphocyte-mediated cytotoxicity and blocking serum activity to tumor antigens. *Adv. Immunol.* 18:209, 1974.

72. Henley, W. L., Okas, S., and Leopold, I. H. Clinical experiments in cellular immunity in eye disease. *Invest. Ophthalmol.* 12:520, 1973.

73. Henry, C., et al. Fluorescence visualization of Ia antigens on T cells. *Cell Immunol.* 53:125, 1980.

74. Heremans, J. F. Immunoglobulin formation and function in different tissues. *Curr. Top. Microbiol. Immunol.* 45:131, 1968.

75. Hjorth, N., and Fregert, S. Contact Dermatitis. In A. Rook, J. Ebling, and D. Wilkinson (Eds.), *Textbook of Dermatology.* London: Blackwell, 1972. Pp. 305–424.

76. Holt, L. B. Quantitative studies in diphtheria prophylaxis. *Br. J. Exp. Pathol.* 32:151, 1951.

77. Holt, W. S., and Kinoshita, J. H. The soluble proteins of the bovine cornea. *Invest. Ophthalmol.* 12:114, 1973.

78. Hubscher, T. Role of the eosinophil in the allergic reactions. *J. Immunol.* 114:1379, 1975.

79. Huebner, R. J., et al. Specific adenovirus complement-fixing antigens in virus-free hamster and rat tumors. *Proc. Natl. Acad. Sci. U.S.A.* 50:379, 1963.

80. Husband, H. J., and Gowans, J. G. The origin and antigen-dependent distribution of IgA-containing cells in the intestine. *J. Exp. Med.* 148:1146, 1978.

81. Inomata, H., Smelser, G., and Polack, F. M. The fine structural changes in the corneal endothelium during graft rejection. *Invest. Ophthalmol.* 9:263, 1970.

82. Inomata, H., Smelser, G. K., and Polack, F. M. Fine structure of regenerating endothelium and Descemet's membrane in normal and rejecting corneal grafts. *Am. J. Ophthalmol.* 70:48, 1970.

83. Ishizaka, K., and Ishizaka, T. Human reaginic antibodies and immunoglobulin E. *J. Allergy* 42:330, 1968.

84. Ishizaka, T., et al. C^{1}1 fixation by human isoagglutinins. *J. Immunol.* 97:716, 1966.

85. Jasin, H. E., Lospalluto, J., and Ziff, M. Rheumatoid hyperviscosity syndrome. *Am. J. Med.* 49:484, 1970.

86. Jersild, C. B., et al. Histocompatibility determinants in multiple sclerosis. *Transplant. Rev.* 22:148, 1975.

87. Jurin, M., and Tannock, I. F. Influence of vitamin A on the immunologic response. *Immunology* 23:301, 1972.

88. Kaplan, J., Callewaert, D. M., and Peterson, W. D. Expression of human T lymphocyte antigens by killer cells. *J. Immunol.* 121:1366, 1978.

89. Khan, A., Kirkpatrick, C. H., and Hill, N. O. *Immune Regulators in Transfer Factor.* New York: Academic, 1979.

90. Khodadoust, A. A., and Silverstein, A. M. Studies on the nature of the privilege enjoyed by corneal allografts. *Invest. Ophthalmol.* 11:137, 1972.

91. Klareskog, L., et al. Expression of Ia antigen–like molecules on cells in the corneal epithelium. *Invest. Ophthalmol. Vis. Sci.* 18:310, 1979.

92. Klemperer, P., Pollack, A. D., and Baehr, G. Diffuse collagen disease. *JAMA* 119:331, 1942.

93. Kline, B. C. Pili, plasmids, and microbial virulence. *Mayo Clin. Proc.* 51:3, 1976.

94. Kolb, H., and Bosma, M. J. Clones producing antibodies of more than one class. *Immunology* 33:461, 1977.

95. Lawrence, H. S. The cellular transfer of cutaneous hypersensitivity to tuberculin in man. *Proc. Soc. Exp. Biol. Med.* 71:516, 1949.

96. Levey, R. H., and Medawer, P. B. Nature and mode of action of anti-lymphocytic antiserum. *Proc. Natl. Acad. Sci. U.S.A.* 56:1130, 1966.

97. Lichtenstein, L. M., Holtzman, A., and Burnett, L. S. A quantitative *in vitro* study of the chromatographic distribution and immunoglobulin characteristics of human blocking antibody. *J. Immunol.* 101:317, 1968.

98. Lichtenstein, L. M. Sequential analysis of the allergic response. *Int. Arch. Allergy Appl. Immunol.* 49:143, 1975.

99. Lopez, C., and O'Reilly, R. J. Cell-mediated immune responses in recurrent herpesvirus infections. *J. Immunol.* 118:895, 1977.

100. Lotzova, E., and McCredie, K. B. Natural killer cells in mice and man, and their possible biological significance. *Cancer Immunology Immunotherapy* 4:215, 1978.

101. Marcus, P. I., and Salb, J. M. Molecular basis of interferon action. *Virology* 30:502, 1966.

102. Marsh, D. G., and Bias, W. B. The Genetics of Atopic Disease. In M. Samter (Ed.), *Immunological Disease* (3rd ed.). Boston: Little, Brown, 1978. P. 119.

103. Mathe, G. Attempts at using systemic immunity adjuvants in experimental and human cancer therapy. In *Immunopotentiation* (Ciba Foundation Symposium). Amsterdam: Associated Scientific Publishers, 1973.

104. Matter, A. The effects of muramyldipeptide in cell-mediated immunity. *Cancer Immunol. Immunother.* 6:201, 1979.

105. Merigan, T. C. Host defenses against viral disease. *N. Engl. J. Med.* 290:223, 1974.

106. Michels, R. G., Kenyon, K. R., and Maumenee, A. E. Retrocorneal fibrous membrane. *Invest. Ophthalmol.* 11:822, 1972.

107. Miller, M. E. Leukocyte movement. *J. Pediatr.* 83:1104, 1973.

108. Mondino, B. J., et al. Alternate and classical pathway components of complement in the normal cornea. *Arch. Ophthalmol.* 98:346, 1980.

109. Morton, D. L., et al. Demonstration of antibodies against human melanoma by immunofluorescence. *Surgery* 64:233, 1968.

110. Mudd, S., and Shayegani, M. Delayed-type hypersensitivity to *S. aureus* and its uses. *Ann. N.Y. Acad. Sci.* 236:244, 1974.

111. Naff, G. B., and Ratnoff, O. D. The enzymatic nature of C1r. *J. Exp. Med.* 128:571, 1968.

112. Nelken, E., and Nelken, D. Serological studies in keratoplasty. *Br. J. Ophthalmol.* 49:159, 1965.

113. Ogra, P. L., et al. Implications of secretory immune system in viral infections. *Adv. Exp. Med. Biol.* 45:271, 1973.

114. Old, L. J., et al. Antigenic properties of chemically-induced tumors. *Ann. N.Y. Acad. Sci.* 101:80, 1962.

115. Parker, C. W. Control of lymphocyte function. *N. Engl. J. Med.* 295:1180, 1976.

116. Penhale, W. J., et al. Spontaneous thyroiditis in thymectomized and irradiated Wistar rats. *Clin. Exp. Immunol.* 15:225, 1973.

117. Penn, G. M., Kunkel, H. G., and Grey, H. M. Sharing of individual antigenic determinants between IgG and a IgM protein in the same myeloma serum. *Proc. Soc. Exp. Biol.* 135:660, 1970.

118. Perkins, E. S. Prostaglandins and the eye. *Adv. Ophthalmol.* 29:2, 1975.

119. Podos, S., Becker, B., and Kass, M. A. Indomethacin blocks arachidonic acid–induced elevation of intraocular pressure. *Prostaglandins* 3:7, 1973.

120. Polack, F. M. Scanning electron microscopy of the host-graft endothelial junction in corneal graft reaction. *Am. J. Ophthalmol.* 73:704, 1972.

121. Porter, P. R. Chemical structure of γ globulin and antibodies. *Br. Med. Bull.* 19:197, 1963.

122. Prussoff, W. H. Substitution of DNA with Base Analogs. In P. N. Campbell (Ed.), *Interaction of Drugs and Subcellular Components in Animal Cells.* London: Churchill, 1968.

123. Renoux, G., and Renoux, M. Inhibition par la theophylline de la stimulation immunologique par le phenylimidothiazole. *C. R. Acad. Sci.* 274D:3149, 1972.

124. Renoux, G., et al. Potentiation of T-cell mediated immunity by levamisole. *Clin. Exp. Immunol.* 25:288, 1976.

125. Roitt, I. *Essential Immunology* (2nd ed.). London: Blackwell, 1974.

126. Rome, D. S., et al. IgD on the surface of peripheral blood lymphocytes of the human newborn. *Nature* 242:155, 1973.

127. Rose, N. R., and Friedman, H. *Manual of Clinical Immunology.* Washington, D.C.: American Society of Microbiology, 1976.

128. Rudner, E. J., et al. The frequency of contact sensitivity in North America. *Contact Dermatitis* 1:277, 1975.

129. Salvaggio, J. E., et al. A comparison of the immunologic response of normal and atopic individuals to intranasally administered antigen. *J. Allergy Appl. Immunol.* 35:62, 1964.

130. Schulkind, M. L., et al. Transfer factor in the treatment of a case of chronic mucocutaneous candidiasis. *Cell Immunol.* 3:606, 1972.

131. Sell, S. *Immunology, Immunopathology, and Immunity* (2nd ed.). New York: Harper & Row, 1975. P. 39.

132. Sher, N. A., et al. Macrophage migration inhibition factor activity in the aqueous during experimental corneal xenograft and allograft rejection. *Am. J. Ophthalmol.* 82:858, 1976.

133. Shimada, K., and Silverstein, A. M. Local antibody formation within the eye. *Invest. Ophthalmol.* 14:573, 1975.

134. Sjögren, H. O., et al. Suggestive evidence that blocking antibodies of tumor-bearing individuals may be antigen-antibody complexes. *Proc. Natl. Acad. Sci. U.S.A.* 68:1372, 1971.

135. Smith, C. B., Bellanti, J. A., and Chanock, R. M. Immunoglobulins in serum and nasal secretions following infection with type 1 parainfluenza virus and injection of inactivated vaccines. *J. Immunol.* 99:133, 1967.

136. Smith, R. T., Baucher, J. A. C., and Adler, W. H. Studies of an inhibitor of DNA synthesis and a nonspecific mitogen elaborated by human lymphoblasts. *Am. J. Pathol.* 60:495, 1970.

137. Smolin, G., and Hyndiuk, R. A. Lymphatic drainage from vascularized rabbit cornea. *Am. J. Ophthalmol.* 72:147, 1971.

138. Smolin, G., Hall, J., and Stein, M. Afferent arc of the corneal immunologic reaction. *Can. J. Ophthalmol.* 7:336, 1972.

139. Smolin, G., and Hall, J. M. The afferent arc of the corneal immunologic reaction. *Arch. Ophthalmol.* 90:231, 1973.

140. Smolin, G., and Wilson, F. M., II. Antilymphocyte serum. *Surv. Ophthalmol.* 18:200, 1973.

141. Smolin, G., Tabbara, K., and Okumoto, M. Guinea pig herpes simplex keratitis treated with a lymphocyte extract. *Am. J. Ophthalmol.* 78:921, 1974.

142. Smolin, G., Okumoto, M., and Belfort, R., Jr. The treatment of experimental herpetic keratitis with BCG. *Can. J. Ophthalmol.* 10:385, 1975.

143. Smolin, G., et al. Failure of fenoprofen to affect the corneal immunologic reaction. *Ann. Ophthalmol.* 10:351, 1978.

144. Snyderman, R., and Stahl, C. Defective Immune Effector Function in Patients with Neoplastic and Immune Deficiency Diseases. In J. A. Bellanti and D. H. Dayton (Eds.), *Phagocytic Cell in Host Resistance.* New York: Raven, 1975. Pp. 167–281.

145. South, M. A., et al. The IgA system. *J. Exp. Med.* 123:615, 1966.

146. Spitler, L. E., and Lawrence, H. S. Studies on lymphocyte culture. *J. Immunol.* 103:1072, 1969.

147. Stasny, P. Association of the B cell alloantigen DRW4 with rheumatoid arthritis. *N. Engl. J. Med.* 298:869, 1978.

148. Steele, R. W., Myers, M. G., and Vincent, M. M. Transfer factor for the prevention of varicella-zoster infection in childhood leukemia. *N. Engl. J. Med.* 303:355, 1980.

149. Stolfi, R. L. Immune lytic transformation. *J. Immunol.* 100:46, 1968.

150. Stossel, T. P. Phagocytosis. *Semin. Hematol.* 12:83, 1975.

151. Strober, W. Abnormalities of the HLA system and gastrointestinal disease. In J. Dausset and A. Svejgaard (Eds.), *HLA and Disease.* Copenhagen: Munksgaard, 1977. P. 168.

152. Svejgaard, A., and Ryder, L. P. Association between HLA and Disease. In J. Dausset and A. Svejgaard (Eds.), *HLA and Disease.* Copenhagen: Munksgaard, 1977. P. 46.

153. Talal, N. Disordered immunologic regulation and autoimmunity. *Transplant. Rev.* 31:240, 1976.

154. Thorsby, E. The human major histocompatibility system. *Transplant. Rev.* 18:51, 1974.

155. Thorsby, E. E., et al. The frequency of major histocompatibility antigens (SD and LD) in thyrotoxicosis. *Tissue Antigens* 6:54, 1975.

156. Tomasi, T. B. Jr., et al. Characteristics of an immune system common to certain external secretions. *J. Exp. Med.* 121:101, 1965.

157. Tomasi, T. B. The gamma A globulins. *Hosp. Pract.* 2:25, 1967.

158. Tomasi, T. B., Jr.   Overview of the IgA System and Its Role in Mucosal Defense. In G. R. O'Connor (Ed.), *Immunologic Diseases of the Mucous Membranes.* New York: Masson, 1980. P. 1.

159. Ugrinski, P. S., and Kirkpatrick, C. H.   Corneal cellular immunity in the guinea pig. *Am. J. Pathol.* 74:365, 1974.

160. Unger, W. G., Cole, D. F., and Hammond, B. R.   Disruption of the blood-aqueous barrier following paracentesis in the rabbit. *Exp. Eye Res.* 20:255, 1975.

161. Vassalli, J. D., Hamilton, J., and Reich, E.   Macrophage plasminogen activator. Cell 8:271, 1976.

162. Wahl, S. M., et al.   The role of macrophages in the production of lymphokines by T and B lymphocytes. *J. Immunol.* 114:1295, 1975.

163. Waldmann, T. A., et al.   Immunoglobulin E in immunologic deficiency diseases. *J. Immunol.* 109:304, 1972.

164. Waldmann, T. A., et al.   Role of suppressor T cells in pathogenesis of common variable hypogammaglobulinemia. *Lancet* 2:609, 1974.

165. Waldmann, T. A., et al.   Defect in IgA secretion and in IgA specific suppressor cells in patients with selective IgA deficiency. *Trans. Assoc. Am. Physicians* 89:215, 1976.

166. Waldmann, T. A., and Broder, S.   Suppressor Cells in the Regulation of the Immune Response. In R. Schwartz (Ed.), *Progress in Clinical Immunology.* New York: Grune & Stratton, 1977. Vol. 3, p. 155.

167. Waldorf, D. S., Wilkens, R. F., and Decker, J. L.   Impaired delayed hypersensitivity in an aging population. *JAMA* 203:831, 1968.

168. Weigle, W. O.   Recent observations and concepts in immunologic responsiveness and autoimmunity. *Clin. Exp. Immunol.* 9:437, 1971.

169. Weigle, W. O., Chiller, J. M., and Habicht, G. S.   Effect of immunological unresponsiveness on different cell populations. *Transplant. Rev.* 8:3, 1972.

170. Werb, Z.   Biochemical actions of glucocorticoids on macrophages in culture. *J. Exp. Med.* 147:1695, 1978.

171. Werkheiser, W. C.   The biochemical cellular and pharmacological action and effects of the folic acid antagonists. *Cancer Res.* 23:1277, 1963.

172. Wolff, E.   *Anatomy of the Eye and Orbit.* Philadelphia: Saunders, 1961.

173. Zinkernagel, R. M., and Doherty, P. C.   Immunological surveillance against altered self-components by sensitized T lymphocytes in lymphocytic choriomeningitis. *Nature* 251:547, 1974.

4. MICROBIOLOGY

Infectious Agents: BACTERIA

Masao Okumoto

Bacterial infections of the cornea are one of the major causes of blindness in underdeveloped countries, and in developed countries such infections may lead to serious visual impairment. If the causal agent can be established early in the infectious process, a more effective therapeutic regimen is possible, particularly if the causative bacterium can be isolated to determine its drug sensitivity spectrum. Thus some basic knowledge concerning the organism is important.

A classification of the important species of bacteria is outlined at the beginning of this section. The morphologic, staining, and cultural characteristics of each organism are discussed in detail, as are laboratory tests useful in securing a rapid, reliable diagnosis. Finally, currently available information dealing with pathogenic mechanisms is presented.

Almost any bacteria are capable of establishing a focus of infection in the cornea if the normal barriers or defense mechanisms are compromised [17, 43, 53, 54]. However, certain bacterial groups appear to be particularly predisposed to localizing in the cornea. These include the staphylococci, the streptococci, the pseudomonads, and *Moraxella*. Other groups, such as *Serratia marcescens* [39], *Mycobacterium fortuitum* [40], *Neisseria* sp. [21], *Proteus* sp. [22], *Azotobacter* sp. [41], and *Nocardia* sp. [24], are infrequently associated with infections of the cornea.

CLASSIFICATION
Most microbiologists follow the classification system used in *Bergey's Manual of Determinative Bacteriology*, currently in its eighth edition [8]. With rare exception, the Bergey system is followed throughout this section.

STAPHYLOCOCCUS
Staphylococcus is placed in the family Micrococcaceae, which includes five genera. The only other

genus of ocular importance in this family is the *Micrococcus*. The genus *Staphylococcus* is separated into three species: *S. aureus*, *S. epidermidis*, and *S. saprophyticus*.

STREPTOCOCCUS

The streptococci are placed in the family Streptococcaceae with five genera, but none of the others are of ocular significance. There are many species in the genus *Streptococcus*, but *S. pyogenes* and *S. pneumoniae* are the most important in clinical medicine as a cause of morbidity and mortality. In recent years there has been an increased incidence of corneal infections caused by the alpha-hemolytic variety of streptococci.

The alpha-hemolytic streptococci, also known as viridans streptococci, are a heterogeneous group and include a number of species such as *S. salivarius*, *S. mutans*, *S. sanguis*, *S. mitis*, and *S. pneumoniae*. *S. pneumoniae* is sometimes discussed separately in this section because of a number of distinctive features that set the pneumococci apart from the other members of this group.

PSEUDOMONAS

Pseudomonas is placed in the family Pseudomonadaceae with two other genera, but the other two are of no medical interest. *P. aeruginosa* is the principal species in corneal infections, but *P. maltophilia* and *P. cepacia* are occasionally encountered. *P. acidovorans* and *P. stutzeri* have been reported recently as unusual causes of corneal ulcers [6].

MORAXELLA

Moraxella is now in the family Neisseriaceae. There are five species: *M. lacunata*, *M. bovis*, *M. nonliquefaciens*, *M. phenylpyruvica*, and *M. osloensis*. Only the first three species are of concern in ocular infections, with the second species, *M. bovis*, being encountered only in veterinary medicine. *M. liquefaciens* is now classified as a variant of *M. lacunata*.

MORPHOLOGY AND STAINING CHARACTERISTICS

STAPHYLOCOCCUS

The staphylococci are spherical bacteria that divide in three planes and produce grapelike clusters. The individual coccus is approximately 1 μ in diameter and stains strongly gram-positive (Fig. 4-1). Like most cocci, they are nonmotile and lack flagella or pili. No spores are produced, but they are rather hardy organisms and may remain viable in contaminated material for many weeks. Capsulated strains

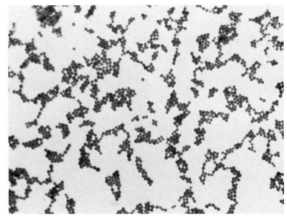

FIGURE 4-1. *Gram stain of a culture showing* Staphylococcus aureus *in typical grapelike clusters.*

are uncommon, but a number of such strains have been reported [62].

STREPTOCOCCUS (*EXCLUDING* S. PNEUMONIAE)

The streptococci divide in a single plane and may produce long chains of cocci when grown in liquid media. On solid media or in scraping specimens, long chains are difficult to demonstrate (Fig. 4-2). The individual coccus is generally oval or elliptic, although spherical forms resembling staphylococci can be encountered. The coccus measures 0.5 to 1.0 μ in diameter, depending on the strain being examined; there is little variation in size in any given specimen. Streptococci are uniformly gram-positive.

Group A streptococci elaborate a hyaluronic acid capsule, but because of the production of hyaluronidase by this organism, the capsule is demonstrable only in very young cultures. Group D streptococci have been reported to possess flagella, but motility is a rare characteristic among the coccoid forms of bacteria. No spores are produced by any of the streptococci.

S. PNEUMONIAE

The pneumococcus is a gram-positive diplococcus; owing to the production of autolytic enzymes, however, gram-negative forms may be seen. The pneumococcus, like all streptococci, divides in a single plane and may occasionally produce chains, but characteristically is seen in pairs. Even in a chain, the elements of the chain can be seen as pairs of cocci. The morphology of the paired cocci is rather distinctive and referred to as lancet-shaped. The individual coccus is elliptic; in a pair, in which the two cocci are attached end to end, the adjoining ends

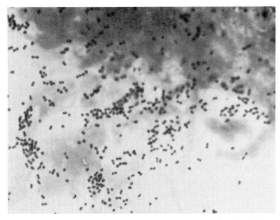

FIGURE 4-2. *Gram-stained corneal scraping showing beta-hemolytic streptococci. Note lack of chaining.*

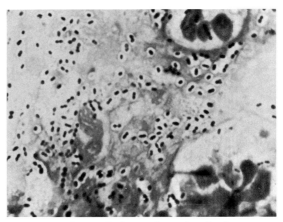

FIGURE 4-3. *Gram-stained corneal scraping showing pneumococci, some with capsulation.*

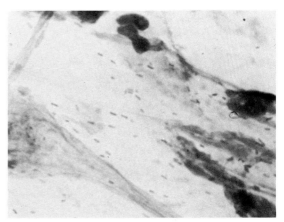

FIGURE 4-4. *Gram-stained corneal scraping showing* Pseudomonas aeruginosa.

appear blunted, and the opposite ends appear pointed (Fig. 4-3). With appropriate staining a polysaccharide capsule may be seen. In culture material, the capsule is best seen in young cultures grown in serum-containing media.

PSEUDOMONAS
The pseudomonads are all gram-negative rods. *P. aeruginosa*, the most important member of this group, can be described as a slender rod with parallel sides, straight or slightly curved, with rounded ends when seen in light microscopic specimens. The width of the rods is rather constant at approximately 0.5 μ. Length is variable, ranging from 1.5 to 3 μ (Fig. 4-4).

The pseudomonads are almost always found as single rods with a distinct absence of any tendency to form pairs, chains, or clusters. The pseudomonads are motile organisms—all produce polar flagella. *P. aeruginosa* has a single flagellum at one end, whereas *P. cepacia* and *P. maltophilia* exhibit a tuft of three or more flagella at one pole [27]. Definite capsules are not produced, but strains of *P. aeruginosa* isolated from patients with cystic fibrosis usually display a mucoid slime layer loosely surrounding the rods. No endospores are produced.

MORAXELLA
The *Moraxella* sp. are among the easiest of the ocular bacteria to identify in smears or scrapings. Their outstanding morphologic feature is the constant occurrence of rods in diplobacillus form with the individual rods joined end to end. These are large bacilli, measuring approximately 1 to 1.5 μ in diameter and 2 to 3 μ in length. Occasional strains may measure 2 to 3 μ in width [46]. The rods are symmetric and uniform in size and shape when seen in tissue scrapings (Fig. 4-5). In culture material, pleomorphism is not uncommon; long filamentous forms may be seen as well as diplococcoid forms. The rods tend to appear thick in relation to their length, so they are described as plump rods. Occasionally chains are seen, but it is apparent that the chains are composed of pairs of rods.

The *Moraxella* sp. are gram-negative. In thick smears or hastily performed Gram-stained smears or scrapings, they often appear as gram-positive rods; however, the distinctive diplobacillus morphology will reveal its true identity. Capsules are not seen in ocular scrapings, but there are several reports of capsulated *Moraxella* [5, 58]. No spores or flagella are produced.

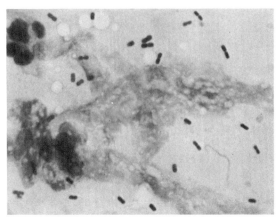

FIGURE 4-5. Moraxella nonliquefaciens *in a Gram-stained corneal scraping.*

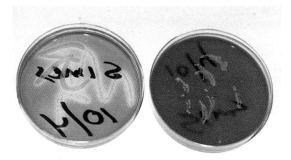

FIGURE 4-6. Staphylococcus aureus *cultured from a corneal ulcer on blood and mannitol agar.*

CULTURAL CHARACTERISTICS

STAPHYLOCOCCUS

Staphylococci are among the easiest bacteria to grow on artificial media. Almost any noninhibitory bacteriologic medium will allow isolation of this bacterium.

For routine use, blood agar is probably the best for several reasons. It is a medium widely used in clinical laboratories everywhere. Fresh blood plates are readily available from many sources. Blood is not necessary for the growth of the staphylococci, but its presence allows the bacteriologist to note the degree of hemolysis surrounding the colonies. The blood also provides lipids that are necessary for the optimum development of pigmentation in the colonies, which aids in the identification of the various staphylococcal species. Tiny colonies can be seen on blood agar after overnight incubation. By 48 hours, the typical colony morphology is apparent. *S. aureus* colonies are usually hemolytic—a clear zone of beta-hemolysis surrounding the colonies is characteristic of this species (Fig. 4-6). Isolated colonies are several millimeters in diameter, round, and flat, with a smooth surface. The majority of *S. aureus* strains are pigmented, varying from light beige to golden yellow. The *S. epidermidis* strains are usually nonhemolytic and nonpigmented. No special odor is associated with the staphylococci.

Thygeson [57] reported a number of years ago that mannitol salt agar is an excellent medium for differentiating staphylococci based on the fermentation of mannitol. With rare exceptions, only pathogenic strains are able to ferment mannitol. The Proctor Foundation microbiology laboratory has been using mannitol salt agar for many years as a supplementary medium to the blood plate, and we have found it to be a very useful medium for differentiating pathogenic staphylococcal strains from harmless saprophytes. This medium also has high sodium chloride content (7.5 percent), which is inhibitory to almost all other bacterial species, so that staphylococci are selectively isolated even when large numbers of other bacterial species are present.

STREPTOCOCCUS

With a few exceptions, the streptococci, including the pneumococci, are fastidious organisms and require a nutritionally more complex medium than do the staphylococci. Fortunately, blood agar is well suited to the growth requirements of the streptococci, and hemolysis of the blood provides important information for identifying and differentiating the streptococci. Sheep blood agar is the medium of choice. Sheep blood is most commonly used in the United States for making blood agar and is recommended for the isolation of the streptococci. Horse blood is used in some laboratories, but atypical hemolysis of horse blood is produced by some of the nonhemolytic streptococci, whereas sheep blood hemolysis is more typical and familiar to most microbiologists. The streptococci are facultatively anaerobic bacteria, utilizing a less efficient fermentative metabolic pathway. They produce tiny colonies.

The characteristic features of the streptococci vary with the species and the age of the culture. The most useful cultural feature in identifying the streptococci is the type of hemolysis on 5% blood agar. The *S. pyogenes* strains are all beta-hemolytic; the relatively wide zone of clear hemolysis surrounding the colony is highly diagnostic. The colonies are only about a millimeter in diameter, and the hemolytic zone is several times the size of the colony. Young colonies may be smooth, but after 24 hours the colonies may appear rough and dry.

Alpha-hemolytic colonies are characterized by incomplete lysis of the red blood cells: A relatively narrow zone of greenish hemolysis is produced around the colony. Intact red cells are always present in this zone of incomplete hemolysis. Beta-hemolysis is accompanied by complete lysis of all red blood cells in the immediate vicinity of the colony. The gamma or nonhemolytic streptococci are the most difficult to identify on gross examination of the blood plate. Fortunately, this variety is rarely encountered in corneal infections.

The pneumococci are all alpha-hemolytic and produce small colonies very similar to those of the alpha-hemolytic streptococci. When first seen at 24 hours, the two kinds of colonies are often identical, but by 48 hours the pneumococcal colonies appear flat with a central depression described as pitting. The alpha-hemolytic streptococci are elevated and appear more opaque, but occasional strains may be flat and translucent and may be confused with the pneumococci.

Human blood is used in a few laboratories, but this is to be discouraged since inhibitory substances such as antibody or antibiotics may be present. There are a number of other media such as chocolate agar, Trypticase soy agar, and liquid media that will allow good growth of the streptococci, but hemolysis cannot be observed. However, there may be special cases in which these media may be useful.

PSEUDOMONAS
As with the staphylococci, the pseudomonads are highly adaptable to growing on almost any bacteriologic medium. A clear agar medium such as Mueller-Hinton, which is widely available in hospital bacteriology laboratories, has a decided advantage in bringing out the water soluble pigments pyoverdin (fluorescein) and pyocyanin that diffuse into the surrounding medium and that can be a very useful aid in the early detection of P. aeruginosa and other pigment-producing pseudomonads.

Blood agar, also an excellent medium, will allow hemolysis to be manifested. Although its appearance is somewhat delayed, pigment can be detected in 48 to 72 hours in the clear hemolyzed zones surrounding the Pseudomonas colonies.

P. aeruginosa colonies are easily identified from a number of distinctive features, such as hemolysis, odor, autoplaquing, and pigmentation. The colonies are moderate in size, raised, mucoid, and somewhat irregular in form (Fig. 4-7). Hemolysis is usually not apparent at 24 hours on primary isolation, but by 48 hours, it is usually quite evident. Altenbern has shown that the hemolytic enzyme is released in small amounts at 24 hours, but an in-

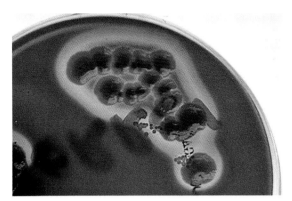

FIGURE 4-7. Pseudomonas aeruginosa *cultured on blood agar. Note pigmentation in hemolyzed area.*

creasingly greater output is noted at 48 to 72 hours [1]. Since most gram-negative bacilli are nonhemolytic, this is a useful identifying feature. The water soluble pigments pyoverdin (fluorescein) and pyocyanin are produced by almost all strains. These pigments diffuse into the agar medium and are easily seen in clear media; on blood agar, they are obscured by the red cells. However, when the erythrocytes hemolyze, the blue-green color in the agar can be detected by holding the plate against a diffuse light source. The odor of P. aeruginosa on culture media is diagnostic. It is sweet and aromatic and associated by many with the smell of grapes. As the culture ages, an underlying putrid odor also develops.

Another interesting phenomenon often seen in P. aeruginosa cultures is autoplaquing. This is the spontaneous occurrence of lytic areas on the surface of the colonies, which produces an iridescent or metallic plaquelike lesion. Pillich and associates [47] investigated the importance of these autoplaques and found that they occur frequently and resemble lytic lesions produced by bacteriophages although they are unrelated to the action of any phage.

MORAXELLA
The medium of choice for *Moraxella* is the Loeffler coagulated serum prepared in a Petri plate. This medium supports good growth of all *Moraxella* sp. and has the advantage of differentiating the *M. lacunata, M. liquefaciens,* and *M. nonliquefaciens* on the basis of their capacity to liquefy the coagulated serum.

None of the *Moraxella* species is hemolytic, but blood agar is also a good choice since it is widely available. *M. lacunata* on blood agar is easily identified owing to its distinctive colony appearance. Even at 48 hours the colonies remain pinpoint size and appear almost transparent. *M. liquefaciens* and *M. nonliquefaciens* produce considerably larger colonies. These two species are difficult to separate on colony morphology alone. Their general appearance is reminiscent of that of gram-negative bacteria with a slightly mucoid look, but the *Moraxella* sp. generally produce smaller colonies than do the enteric bacilli. Isolated *Moraxella* colonies are moderately elevated in the center with a translucent periphery and opaque centers. The *Moraxella* species are all nonhemolytic, nonpigmented, and nonodorous.

The three *Moraxella* species are easily differentiated when grown on Loeffler medium. *M. lacunata* and *M. liquefaciens* digest the surface of this medium, and visible colonies of the conventional type are not formed. *M. lacunata* will produce tiny pits resembling the lacunae of bone on the surface of this medium—hence the species name. *M. liquefaciens* exhibits a much greater digestive capacity and actively liquefies the coagulated serum. *M. nonliquefaciens* lacks the digestive enzymes and so produces colonies on the surface like those of most bacteria grown on conventional medium.

Moraxella are sensitive to acidity, and their growth is inhibited in the presence of *S. aureus*, which produces an acid reaction. I have noted that in cases of angular blepharoconjunctivitis in which scrapings show a mixture of *Moraxella* and staphylococci with both organisms present in large numbers, blood agar plates yield growth of *S. aureus*, but *Moraxella* fail to grow.

TESTS FOR IDENTIFICATION

STAPHYLOCOCCUS

The colony appearance of staphylococci is usually adequate for genus identification, but further tests are required for separation of *S. aureus* from the nonpathogenic variety. A number of biochemical and enzymatic reactions such as acid production from mannitol and the clotting of plasma by coagulase [64], the hydrolysis of DNA by deoxyribonuclease [15] or thermonuclease [45], and the lysis of *Micrococcus lysodeikticus* by lysozyme [26] are tests available for identifying *S. aureus*. The single most reliable test, however, is the production of the enzyme coagulase by all strains of *S. aureus*. The anaerobic mannitol fermentation test is also highly

reliable [16] but results are sometimes not available for 7 days. The more convenient aerobic plate test is used in clinical laboratories. The aerobic method, however, leads to a considerable percentage of staphylococcal strains becoming mannitol-positive and coagulase-negative. Taxonomically these would be categorized *S. epidermidis*, but I feel that such strains are potentially more virulent than the mannitol-negative and coagulase-positive strains.

STREPTOCOCCUS

The hemolytic varieties of streptococci are easily identified, but the nonhemolytic type may present problems. In such cases the catalase test offers a simple and effective means of differentiating streptococci from other gram-positive cocci [20].

Once the organism has been identified as a streptococcus, it may be important to determine its grouping. In ocular specimens, it is rare to encounter groups other than A, D, and the viridans type (including *S. pneumoniae*). Of these, group A (*S. pyogenes*) and the pneumococci are most virulent and produce the most acute and severe infections of the cornea.

Just recently Analytab Products Inc. (Plainview, New York) introduced a testing kit for streptococci that incorporates 20 biochemical reactions that allow grouping of groups A through G and Q as well as speciation of a number of Group D and viridans species. This kit is similar to the API 20E, widely used in testing the enteric bacilli and *Pseudomonas* species.

PSEUDOMONAS

P. aeruginosa identification on culture is relatively easy. For the other *Pseudomonas* sp. it may be necessary to employ one of the commercial biochemical testing systems on the market. Probably one of the most extensively used is the API 20E (Analytab Products Inc.).

All *Pseudomonas* species are oxidase-positive except for *P. maltophilia*. A rapid screening test for *Pseudomonas* may be carried out by using a commercial oxidase disc on any colony under question. A positive reaction is grossly observable by a series of color changes in the colony—from pink to purple to coal black in a matter of minutes.

MORAXELLA

Standard biochemical testing procedures for *Moraxella* are generally not feasible because these organisms are nonfermentative and exceptionally inactive biochemically, being unable to metabolize polysaccharides, disaccharides, polyalcohols, or even glucose (with one exception) [3]. *M. liquefaciens* does have gelatinase activity; inoculation of a gelatin tube will allow identification of this subspecies.

PATHOGENICITY

STAPHYLOCOCCUS

TOXINS

At least 30 different biologically active substances have been identified from *S. aureus* [60]. A number of these are toxins: alpha, beta, gamma, and delta toxins; exfoliative toxin; leukocidin; and enterotoxin. Thygeson [56] showed some years ago that alpha toxin, also known as dermonecrotic factor, was the principal mechanism by which *S. aureus* attacks the eye. One major difficulty in working with alpha toxin has been its extreme instability [9]. There is general agreement that alpha toxin acts on cell membranes to cause increased permeability. The hemolytic and dermonecrotic properties of alpha toxin are well known; it also produces constriction of coronary arteries. Its lethal effect in the rabbit is the result of rapid collapse of brain bioelectric activity [50]. Beta toxin, commonly called beta-hemolysin, is cytotoxic to a variety of cell types and damages the plasma membrane of red cells, leukocytes, and macrophages. Identified as sphingomyelinase C, beta toxin damages sensitive cells by degradation of membrane sphingomyelin [2]. Gamma toxin has been accepted as a distinct entity only recently. Little is known about its cytotoxic effect [5]. Delta toxin is quite different from other bacterial membrane-damaging toxins. It is heat-stable, has a low degree of cellular specificity, and is relatively hydrophobic. It affects cell membranes by way of its detergentlike properties [50]. In 1932, Panton and Valentine described an extracellular staphylococcal product called leukocidin that had an effect on polymorphonuclear leukocytes and macrophages in rabbits and humans [50, 61].

Exfoliative toxin is responsible for the entity variously known as staphylococcal scalded-skin syndrome, toxic epidermal necrolysis, or Ritter's disease. The production of this toxin appears to be under the control of a plasmid [49]. Exfoliative toxin is produced mainly by phage group 2 staphylococci, which comprise approximately 3 to 5 percent of the clinical isolates of *S. aureus*. Occasionally other phage groups produce this toxin, but exfoliative toxin produced by other groups differs somewhat from the typical phage group 2 toxin [37]. The mechanism of action is felt to be the splitting of desmosomes in the granular layer of the epidermis, which results in bullae formation with subsequent separation and peeling of the superficial epidermis, leaving a raw scalded-skin appearance.

ENZYMES

Coagulase is often considered to be an important virulence factor since it is the most reliable indicator for separating the pathogenic *S. aureus* from the less virulent *S. epidermidis*. The production of coagulase is thought to provide a protective barrier around the organism that inhibits phagocytosis.

Lysozyme is produced by almost all strains of *S. aureus* and approximately 8 percent of *S. epidermidis* strains [29]. It may be important in eliminating competing strains of lysozyme-sensitive bacteria.

Hyaluronidase is also produced by most strains of *S. aureus*. It presumably aids in dissemination of the staphylococci.

Other enzymes such as deoxyribonuclease, staphylokinase, and lipase have been identified with staphylococcal organisms, but their relationship to pathogenesis has not been clarified.

STREPTOCOCCUS PYOGENES

TOXINS

S. pyogenes produces three toxins that have been intensively investigated. Two of these are cytolytic toxins: streptolysin O (SLO) and streptolysin S (SLS); the third is erythrogenic toxin. SLO, produced by virtually all strains of *S. pyogenes*, damages susceptible cells by acting on the cell membrane. Only cells containing cholesterol are affected by SLO. Its activity is lost on exposure to oxygen but restored by sulfhydryl compounds [12, 13, 23, 30, 55]. SLS is closely associated with SLO and shares some of the toxic properties of the latter, such as the ability to lyse red blood cells and platelets, damage leukocytes, inhibit phagocytosis, and damage mitochondrial and liposomal elements [14].

Most Group A streptococci produce a toxin known as erythrogenic toxin (ET) that is serologically separable into three distinct types, A, B, and C. Owing to its potent fever-inducing property, ET is also referred to as streptococcal pyrogenic exotoxin. The fever is due to the toxin's ability to cross the blood-brain barrier and directly stimulate the hypothalmic fever response control center [25, 51]. ET also enhances Arthus and delayed hypersensitivity reactions [36, 52].

ENZYMES

A number of enzymes are elaborated by Group A streptococci, but the relationship of most of these enzymes to pathogenicity is not clearly established

[4]. Hyaluronidase presumably allows dissemination of the infecting microorganisms, but there is little evidence that it enhances infection. On the contrary, it may have an opposite effect, as shown by Foley and Wood [18]. Streptokinase, an extracellular enzyme produced by the majority of Group A streptococci, is able to lyse fibrin and other protein substrates. This enzyme is felt to contribute to the pathogenesis of streptococcal infection by lysing the fibrin barrier created by the host and allowing the spread of the organisms or their products [38].

STREPTOCOCCUS PNEUMONIAE

TOXINS

For many years, it was accepted that the pneumococcus does not produce any toxins and that pathogenesis of the pneumococci is a function of its invasiveness. However, several reports have appeared that suggest that a hemolytic agent produced by *S. pneumoniae* has toxic properties for the cornea [31, 32]. Johnson and Allen were able to purify and concentrate a pneumococcal extract (designated as cytolysin or ocular toxin) that when injected into rabbit corneas produced complete opacification in 24 hours. Opacification lasted at least 30 days. The authors felt that the corneal damage was probably the result of this toxic agent's activating host enzymes such as collagenase [30, 31].

ENZYMES

All strains of *S. pneumoniae* studied by Kilian and coworkers [35] and Male [44] produced IgA1 protease. This enzyme appeared rapidly to cleave human IgA1 and some secretory IgA but not IgA2, IgG, or IgM. Since the mucosal surface of the eye is protected by IgA, it is possible that the pneumococcus is able to colonize and invade mucosal tissue by inactivating this part of the normal host defenses.

PSEUDOMONAS AERUGINOSA

TOXINS

Since Liu's [42] pioneering work on *Pseudomonas* exotoxin A, numerous investigators have studied this toxin. Exotoxin A is a unique product of *P. aeruginosa*. Approximately 90 percent of all strains produce this toxin [10]. It is highly toxic, being 10,000 times more lethal for experimental animals than is the endotoxin from the bacterium [63]. Human macrophages are extremely sensitive to exotoxin A: Exposure to as little as 10 ng per milliliter will cause cell death [48]. The mechanism of action is identical to that of diphtheria toxin; the result is the inhibition of protein synthesis.

ENZYMES

For some years the destructive action of the *Pseudomonas* organism on the cornea was attributed to the production of a potent collagenase, but Brown and colleagues have demonstrated that the cornea-destroying enzyme of *P. aeruginosa* is not a collagenase [7]. Kessler and coworkers [34] purified the extracellular protease from a virulent strain of *P. aeruginosa* and, after extensive testing, concluded that the dissolution of the cornea by *Pseudomonas* infection results essentially from the degradation of the protein backbone of corneal proteoglycan. Kessler's group [33] also demonstrated the important contribution of host-derived enzymes in the pathogenesis of *Pseudomonas* corneal infections.

Although not an enzyme or toxin, the glycocalyx of *Pseudomonas* enables the bacteria to adhere to susceptible cells and to each other to produce large aggregates that resist phagocytosis [28].

MORAXELLA

TOXINS

As one would expect from a gram-negative bacterium, *Moraxella* sp. have endotoxic activity [11]. Intradermal injection of a partially purified preparation into rabbits in microgram amounts elicited the characteristic response of edema and erythema within 12 hours, with a peak response in 12 to 48 hours.

ENZYMES

Since the early days of bacteriology, proteases have been associated with the pathogenicity of these organisms [59]. Several factors suggesting the proteolytic nature of the *Moraxella* have been the liquefaction of gelatin and Loeffler coagulated serum, as well as the excoriation and maceration of the angles of the eyelid. The enzymes from human species have not been specifically identified, but Frank and Gerber [19] have biochemically defined a number of enzymes from *M. bovis*.

REFERENCES

1. Altenbern, R. A. Formation of hemolysin by strains of *Pseudomonas aeruginosa*. *Can. J. Microbiol.* 12:231, 1966.
2. Arbuthnott, J. P. Staphylococcal Toxins. In C. Schlessinger (Ed.), *Microbiology*. Washington, D.C.: American Society of Microbiology, 1975. Pp. 267–271.
3. Baumann, P., Doudoroff, M., and Stanier, R. Y. Study of the *Moraxella* group. *J. Bacteriol.* 95:58, 1968.
4. Bernheimer, A. W., Lazarides, P. D., and Wilson, A. T. Diphosphodyridine nucleotidase as an extracellular product of streptococcal growth

and its possible relationship to leucotoxicity. *J. Exp. Med.* 106:27, 1957.

5. Bottone, E., and Allerhand, J. Association of mucoid encapsulated *Moraxella duplex* var. *nonliquefaciens* with chronic bronchitis. *Appl. Microbiol.* 16:315, 1968.

6. Brinser, J. H., and Torczynski, E. Unusual *Pseudomonas* corneal ulcers. *Am. J. Ophthalmol.* 84:462, 1977.

7. Brown, S. I., Bloomfield, S. E., and Tam, W. I. The cornea-destroying enzyme of *Pseudomonas aeruginosa*. *Invest. Ophthalmol.* 13:174, 1974.

8. Buchanan, R. E., and Gibbons, N. E. *Bergey's Manual of Determinative Bacteriology* (8th ed.). Baltimore: Williams & Wilkins, 1974.

9. Coulter, J. R. Production, purification and composition of staphylococcal alpha toxin. *J. Bacteriol.* 92:1655, 1966.

10. Cross, A. S., et al. Evidence for the role of toxin A in the pathogenesis of infection with *Pseudomonas aeruginosa* in humans. *J. Infect. Dis.* 142:538, 1980.

11. Davis, R. H., and Palazzolo, A. M. Evidence for the existence of endotoxic activity in three strains of *Moraxella*. *Can. J. Ophthalmol.* 21:668, 1975.

12. Dourmashkin, R. R., and Rosse, W. F. Morphologic changes in the membranes of red blood cells undergoing hemolysis. *Am. J. Med.* 41:699, 1966.

13. Duncan, J. L. Characteristics of streptolysin O hemolysis: Kinetics of hemoglobin and rubidium release. *Infect. Immun.* 9:1022, 1974.

14. Duncan, J. L., and Mason, L. Characteristics of streptolysin S hemolysis. *Infect. Immun.* 14:77, 1976.

15. Elston, H. R., and Fitch, D. M. Determination of potential pathogenicity of staphylococci. *Am. J. Clin. Pathol.* 42:346, 1964.

16. Evans, J. B., and Page, C. A. Method for determining anaerobic fermentation of mannitol by staphylococci. *Int. J. Systemic Bacteriol.* 30:557, 1980.

17. Feaster, F. T., Nisbet, M., and Barber, J. C. *Aeromonas hydrophila* corneal ulcer. *Am. J. Ophthalmol.* 85:114, 1978.

18. Foley, M. J., and Wood, W. B., Jr. Studies of the pathogenicity of group A streptococci. *J. Exp. Med.* 110:617, 1959.

19. Frank, S. K., and Gerber, J. D. Hydrolytic enzymes of *Moraxella bovis*. *J. Clin. Microbiol.* 13:269, 1981.

20. Fung, D. Y. C., and Petrishko, D. T. Capillary tube catalase test. *Appl. Microbiol.* 26:631, 1973.

21. Grayson, M. *Diseases of the Cornea.* St. Louis: Mosby, 1979. P. 38.

22. Gutierrez, E. H. Bacterial Infections of the Eye. In D. Locatcher-Khorazo and B. C. Seegal (Eds.), *Microbiology of the Eye*. St. Louis: Mosby, 1972. P. 69.

23. Halbert, S. P., Bircher, R., and Dahle, E. The analysis of streptococcal infections: V. Cardiotoxicity of streptolysin O for rabbits *in vivo*. *J. Exp. Med.* 113:759, 1961.

24. Halde, C., and Okumoto, M. Ocular mycoses: A study of 82 cases. *Excerpta Medica Int. Cong. Ser.* 146:705, 1966.

25. Hanna, E. E., and Watson, D. W. Enhanced immune response after immunosuppression by streptococcal pyrogenic exotoxin. *Infect. Immun.* 7:1009, 1973.

26. Holt, R. J. Lysozyme production by staphylococci and micrococci. *J. Med. Microbiol.* 4:375, 1970.

27. Hugh, R., and Gilardi, G. L. Pseudomonas. In E. H. Lennette et al. (Eds.), *Manual of Clinical Microbiology* (3rd ed.). Washington, D.C.: American Society of Microbiology, 1980. Pp. 288–317.

28. Hyndiuk, R. A. Experimental *Pseudomonas* keratitis: I. Sequential electron microscopy. II. Comparative therapy trials. *Trans. Am. Ophthalmol. Soc.* In press, 1982.

29. Jay, J. Production of lysozyme by staphylococci and its correlation with three other extracellular substances. *J. Bacteriol.* 91:1804, 1966.

30. Jelyaszewicz, J., and Wadstrom, T. (Eds.). *Bacterial Toxins and Cell Membranes.* London: Academic, 1978.

31. Johnson, M. K., and Allen, J. H. Ocular toxin of the pneumococcus. *Am. J. Ophthalmol.* 72:175, 1971.

32. Johnson, M. K., and Allen J. H. The role of cytolysin in pneumococcal ocular infection. Pt. II. *Am. J. Ophthalmol.* 80:518, 1975.

33. Kessler, E., Mondino, B., and Brown, S. I. The corneal response to *Pseudomonas aeruginosa*: Histopathological and enzymatic characterization. *Invest. Ophthalmol. Vis. Sci.* 16:116, 1977.

34. Kessler, E., Kennan, H. E., and Brown, S. I. *Pseudomonas* protease, purification, partial characterization, and its effect on collagen proteoglycan and rabbit corneas. *Invest. Ophthalmol. Vis. Sci.* 16:488, 1977.

35. Kilian, M., Mestecky, J., and Schrohenloher, R. E. Pathogenic species of the genus *Haemophilus* and *Streptococcus pneumoniae* producing immunoglobulin A 1 protease. *Infect. Immun.* 26:143, 1979.

36. Kim, Y. B., and Watson, D. W. A purified group A streptococcal pyrogenic exotoxin. *J. Exp. Med.* 131:611, 1970.

37. Kondo, I., Sakurai, S., and Sarai, Y. New type of exfoliatin obtained from staphylococcal strains belonging to phage groups other than group II, isolated from patients with impetigo and Ritter's disease. *Infect. Immun.* 10:851, 1974.

38. Krasner, R. I., and Jannach, J. R. The strep-tokinase-plasminogen system: II. Its effect on development of local streptococcal infections in rabbit skin. *J. Infect. Dis.* 112:134, 1963.

39. Lass, J. H., et al. Visual outcome in eight cases of *Serratia marcescens* keratitis. *Am. J. Ophthalmol.* 92:384, 1981.

40. Lazar, M., et al. *Mycobacterium fortuitum* keratitis. *Am. J. Ophthalmol.* 78:530, 1974.

41. Liesgang, T. J., Jones, D. B., and Robinson, N. M. *Azotobacter* keratitis. *Arch. Ophthalmol.* 99:1587, 1981.

42. Liu, P. V. The roles of various fractions of *Pseudomonas aeruginosa* in its pathogenesis: III. Identity of the lethal toxins produced *in vitro* and *in vivo*. *J. Infect. Dis.* 116:481, 1966.

43. MacDonald, R., Blatt, M., and Edwards, W. C. *Shigella* corneal ulcer. *Am. J. Ophthalmol.* 60:136, 1965.

44. Male, C. J. Immunoglobulin A 1 protease production by *Haemophilus influenzae* and *Streptococcus pneumoniae*. *Infect. Immun.* 26:254, 1979.

45. Menzies, R. E. Comparison of coagulase, deoxyribonuclease, and heat-stable nuclease tests for identification of *Staphylococcus aureus*. *J. Clin. Pathol.* 30:606, 1977.

46. Murray, R. G. E., and Truant, J. P. The morphology, cell structure, and taxonomic affinities of the *Moraxella*. *J. Bacteriol.* 67:13, 1954.

47. Pillich, J., Kazdova, A., and Pulverer, G. Importance and evaluation of autoplaques in clinical strains of *Pseudomonas aeruginosa*. *Pathol. Microbiol.* 40:79, 1974.

48. Pollack, M., and Anderson, S. E., Jr. Toxicity of *Pseudomonas aeruginosa* exotoxin A for human macrophages. *Infect. Immun.* 19:1092, 1978.

49. Rogolsky, M., and Wiley, B. B. Production and properties of a staphylococcal plasmid for exfoliative toxin synthesis. *Infect. Immun.* 15:726, 1977.

50. Rogolsky, M. Nonenteric toxins of *Staphylococcus aureus*. *Microbiol. Rev.* 43:320, 1979.

51. Schlievert, P. M., and Watson, D. M. Group A streptococcal pyrogenic exotoxin: Pyrogenicity, alteration of blood-brain barrier, and separation of sites for pyrogenicity and enhancement of lethal endotoxin shock. *Infect. Immun.* 21:753, 1978.

52. Schlievert, P. M., Bettin, K. M., and Watson, D. W. Reinterpretation of the Dick test: Role of group A streptococcal pyrogenic exotoxin. *Infect. Immun.* 26:467, 1979.

53. Stern, G. A., Hodes, B. L., and Stock, E. L. *Clostridium perfringens* corneal ulcer. *Arch. Ophthalmol.* 97:661, 1979.

54. Tabbara, K. F., and Tarabay, N. *Bacillus licheniformis* corneal ulcer. *Am. J. Ophthalmol.* 87:717, 1979.

55. Thelestam, M., and Mollby, R. Interaction of streptolysin O from *Streptococcus pyogenes* and theta toxin from *Clostridium perfringens* with human fibroblasts. *Infect. Immun.* 29:863, 1980.

56. Thygeson, P. Bacterial factors in chronic catarrhal conjunctivitis. *Arch. Ophthalmol.* 18:373, 1937.

57. Thygeson, P. Mannitol fermentation as an indicator of conjunctival pathogenicity of staphylococci. *Arch. Ophthalmol.* 20:274, 1938.

58. Van Bijsterveld, D. P. New *Moraxella* strains isolated from angular conjunctivitis. *Appl. Microbiol.* 20:405, 1970.

59. Van Bijsterveld, D. P. Bacterial proteases in *Moraxella* angular conjunctivitis. *Am. J. Ophthalmol.* 72:181, 1971.

60. Waldstrom, T. Biological properties of extracellular proteins from staphylococcus. *Ann. N.Y. Acad. Sci.* 236:343, 1974.

61. Ward, P. D., and Turner, W. H. Identification of staphylococcal Panton-Valentine leucocidin as a potent dermonecrotic toxin. *Infect. Immun.* 27:393, 1980.

62. Yoshida, K., and Takeuchi, Y. Comparison of compact and diffuse variants of strains of *Staphylococcus aureus*. *Infect. Immun.* 2:523, 1970.

63. Young, L. S. The role of exotoxins in the pathogenesis of *Pseudomonas aeruginosa* infections. *J. Infect. Dis.* 142:626, 1980.

64. Zarzour, J. Y., and Belle, E. A. Evaluation of three test procedures for identification of *Staphylococcus aureus* from clinical sources. *J. Clin. Microbiol.* 7:133, 1978.

Infectious Agents: VIRUSES

Jang O. Oh

Viruses constitute a unique class of infectious agent. Their name derives from the Latin word *virus*, meaning "poison." They were originally distinguished by their extremely small size and their obligatory intracellular parasitism. These properties are shared by some small bacteria, however; the truly distinctive features of viruses are now known to be their simple organization and composition and their unique way of replicating (Table 4-1). A virus contains only a single species of nucleic acid, which may be either DNA or RNA and either single- or double-stranded. A virus lacks constituents fundamental for growth and multiplication, e.g., ribosomes, which are enzyme systems required for the synthesis of both nucleic acids and protein and for generating ATP. A virus does not multiply by binary fission, and its coat does not contain muramic acid, which is found in most other classes of microorganisms.

STRUCTURE OF VIRUSES
In a complete virus particle (*virion*), viral nucleic acid is surrounded by a protective protein coat (*capsid*) that consists of many identical protein subunits (Fig. 4-8). The proteins on the capsid have a specific affinity for complementary receptors on the surfaces of susceptible cells. They also contain antigenic determinants that are responsible for the production of protective antibodies by the infected animal. The structural units of the capsid, or the group of units, may be visualized by electron microscopy as morphologic units called *capsomers*. The capsid has either *cubic symmetry* if the protein coat is *isometric*, or *helical symmetry* if the protein coat is *tubular*. The combined nucleic acid and capsid are called the *nucleocapsid*.

Three structural classes of animal viruses have been distinguished (Fig. 4-8): isometric nucleocapsids that are "naked" (e.g., the adenoviruses); isometric nucleocapsids enclosed within a lipoprotein envelope (*peplos*), which is released from the host's cells (e.g., herpesviruses); and tubular nucleocapsids, which in animals are always surrounded by an envelope (e.g., measles virus).

CLASSIFICATION OF ANIMAL VIRUSES
The official classification adopted by the International Committee on the Taxonomy of Viruses is presented in Table 4-2. The major bases for viral classification are (1) the chemical nature of the virus's nucleic acid (whether DNA or RNA); (2) the symmetry of the nucleocapsid (whether helical or cubic); (3) the presence or absence of an envelope; and (4) certain measurements, e.g., the size of the virion, the triangulation number, and the number of capsomers. Although latinized names, ending in -*virus* for a genus and -*viridae* for a family, have been widely accepted, there has been no support for latinized specific names, i.e., for a latinized binomial nomenclature. In Table 4-2 and Figure 4-9, only family names are listed. Full information on the classification of animal viruses can be found in the Third Report of the International Committee on the Taxonomy of Viruses [20].

PATHOGENESIS OF VIRAL INFECTION
The development of a viral infection depends on the nature of the infecting virus (including its virulence), the susceptibility of the host's cells, host resistance, and immunologic and other systemic factors.

NATURE OF THE INFECTION
Viral infections can affect host cells in several different ways. The following sections describe various

TABLE 4-1. *Biologic and Chemical Features of Microorganisms*

Feature	Bacteria	Mycoplasmata	Rickettsiae	Chlamydiae	Viruses
Grow in cell-free medium	+	+	−	−	−
Divide by binary fission	+	+	+	+	−
Nucleic acid	D and R	D and R	D and R	D and R	D or R
Contain ribosomes	+	+	+	+	−
Coats contain muramic acid	+	−	+	+	−

D = DNA; R = RNA.

changes that may be observed in host cells infected with viruses.

CYTOPATHIC EFFECTS

Cytopathic effects (CPE) are morphologic alterations of the cells and usually result in cell death. The precise causes of the various CPE are not known, but several factors appear to contribute to their development—for example, the synthesis of cellular macromolecules and alterations of cell membranes. Paramyxoviruses and herpesviruses form multinucleated giant cells (polykaryocytes) (Table 4-3) when infected cells fuse with adjacent uninfected cells to form a common cytoplasm as a result of an alteration of cell membranes.

Cytopathic changes without any replication of the infectious virus (a toxic effect) may be initiated by a high concentration of virions or viral-coat proteins. For example, a high concentration of vaccinia virus can rapidly kill cultures of macrophages and other cells without any viral multiplication. The CPE of the adenoviruses is produced by a purified capsid protein of the virus, the penton antigen. Viral toxic effects occur also in animals. In mice, for example, intravenous injection of highly concentrated preparations of certain viruses (e.g., influenza, mumps, and vaccinia viruses) causes death within hours, with hemorrhage and cellular necrosis in various organs but without much viral multiplication.

INCLUSION BODIES

Some intracellular inclusions arise as a consequence of the accumulation of virions and unassembled viral subunits (nucleic acid and protein) in the nucleus (e.g., adenovirus inclusions), in the cytoplasm (e.g., rabies virus Negri bodies), or in both nucleus and cytoplasm (e.g., measles virus inclusions). These large accumulations of viral materials appear to disrupt the structure and function of the cells and cause their death. Other inclusion bodies develop at the sites of earlier viral synthesis but do not contain detectable virus particles or their components; thus, the eosinophilic intranuclear inclusion bodies in cells infected by herpes simplex virus (HSV) are "scars" left by earlier viral multiplication. The types of inclusions produced by various viruses are listed in Table 4-3.

CHROMOSOMAL ABERRATIONS

Cells of primary cultures infected with a variety of viruses commonly show chromosomal aberrations, such as breaks or constrictions. Aberrations have been reported for measles virus, several herpesviruses, oncogenic adenoviruses, polyomavirus, simian virus 40, and Rous sarcoma virus. Measles virus produces similar chromosomal abnormalities in peripheral leukocytes during natural infections. Herpesvirus induces chromatid breaks in certain specific chromosomes (numbers 1, 9, and 16) [25]. Chromatid breaks may continue to occur during the multiplication of cells that survive infection by HSV or polyomavirus, which suggests persistent infection of the cell clones.

CELL TRANSFORMATION

Tumor-producing viruses may affect cells (1) by stimulating the synthesis of cellular DNA, (2) by causing surface alterations recognizable by the incorporation of new antigenic specificities distinct from those of virion subunits, (3) by causing chromosomal aberrations, and (4) by altering the growth properties of the cells. This conversion of a normal cultured cell to one resembling a malignant cell is called transformation and is indicated by changes in the cellular morphology, for example, a rounding of cells, a piling up of cells that normally grow as a monolayer, and the growth of cells in

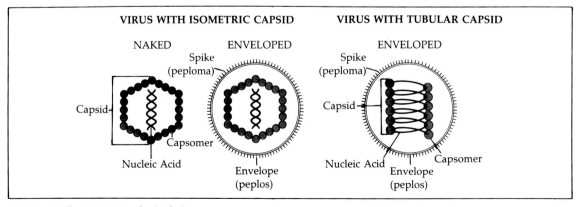

FIGURE 4-8. *The components of animal viruses.*

semisolid medium under conditions in which normal cells do not grow.

4. MICROBIOLOGY

117

SUSCEPTIBILITY OF CELLS TO VIRUSES

Host-cell susceptibility plays a critical role in viral infection. Differences in cell susceptibility usually come into play in early stages in the virus-cell interaction, e.g., the attachment of the virions or the release of their nucleic acid in the cells. The resistance of cells to animal viruses is often caused by adsorption failure. In species in which the susceptibility to viruses varies markedly with age, there is often a parallel variation in the ability of the organs to adsorb the virus. Whether or not there are receptors for viral adsorption on the cell surfaces depends on both physiologic and genetic factors. Cultivation in vitro may markedly alter the susceptibility of cells to viruses. For example, polioviruses do not grow in the kidney of a living monkey but multiply well in kidney cultures, owing to the presence in the cultured cells of receptors that are absent in the intact kidney. Marked changes in susceptibility accompany the maturation of animals. Many viruses (e.g., HSV) are much more virulent for newborn than for adult animals; others (e.g., lymphocytic choriomeningitis virus) are more virulent for adult animals.

HOST RESISTANCE TO VIRAL INFECTION

In both primary infection and reinfection of the eye with viruses, the principal purpose of the host's defenses is to prevent the establishment of infection; if infection has already been established, their purpose is to interfere with virus multiplication, limit

TABLE 4-2. *Classification of Animal Viruses*

Family	Capsid Symmetry	Envelope	Size of Virus (nm)	Number of Capsomers	Typical Member
			DNA Animal	Viruses[a]	
Parvoviridae[b]	Cubic	−	18–26	32	H-1 virus, adeno-associated virus
Papovaviridae[c]	Cubic	−	45–55	72	Human papilloma virus, mouse polyomavirus
Adenoviridae	Cubic	−	70–90	252	Human adenoviruses
Iridoviridae	Cubic	+	130	1500	African swine fever virus
Herpesviridae	Cubic	+	100	162	Herpes simplex virus, varicella-zoster virus, cytomegalovirus, EB virus
Poxviridae	Complex	Complex coat	230 × 300	Unknown	Variola virus, vaccinia virus
			RNA Animal	Viruses	
Picornaviridae[e]	Cubic	−	20–40	32	Poliovirus, Coxsackie virus, ECHO virus, enterovirus 70
Reoviridae[f]	Cubic	−	60–80	32–92	Human rhinovirus
Togaviridae	Cubic	+	40–60	32–42	Group A & B arbovirus, rubella virus, yellow fever virus
Orthomyxoviridae	Helical	+	80–120	Unknown	Influenza viruses A, B, C
Paramyxoviridae	Helical	+	150–300	Unknown	Mumps virus, measles virus, Newcastle disease virus, parainfluenza virus, respiratory syncytial virus
Rhabdoviridae	Helical	+	60 × 180	Unknown	Rabies virus, vesicular stomatitis virus
Retroviridae	Helical	+	100	Unknown	Visna virus, Rous sarcoma virus
Arenaviridae	Helical	+	50–300	Unknown	Lymphocytic choriomeningitis virus, Lassa fever virus
Coronaviridae	Helical	+	80–130	Unknown	Human respiratory coronavirus
Bunyaviridae	Helical	+	100	Unknown	Group C arbovirus

[a]All have double-stranded DNA except members of Parvoviridae, whose DNA is single-stranded.
[b]*Parvo* = small.
[c]*Papova: Pa* = papilloma; *po* = polyoma; *va* = vacuolating agent.
[d]All have single-stranded RNA except members of Reoviridae, whose RNA is double-stranded.
[e]*Picorna: Pico* = small; *rna* = ribonucleic acid.
[f]*Reo: Respiratory enteric orphan.*

SOURCE. Data from R. E. F. Matthews [20].

DNA VIRUSES

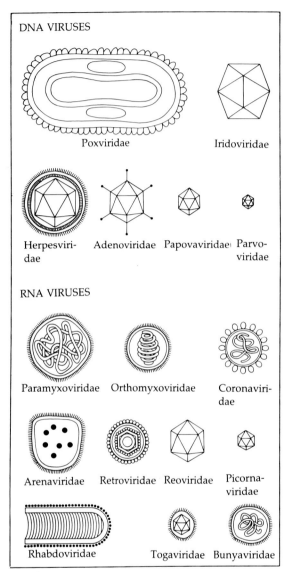

Poxviridae   Iridoviridae

Herpesviri-   Adenoviridae   Papovaviridae Parvo-
dae   viridae

RNA VIRUSES

Paramyxoviridae   Orthomyxoviridae   Coronaviri-
                                     dae

Arenaviridae   Retroviridae   Reoviridae   Picorna-
                                           viridae

Rhabdoviridae   Togaviridae Bunyaviridae

FIGURE 4-9. *Diagram of animal viruses of the major taxonomic groups showing their shapes and relative sizes. (Modified from F. Fenner,* Medical Virology. *New York: Academic Press, 1974.)*

the spread of infection, and finally eliminate the virus. To achieve these feats, a complex host-defense mechanism has to be in operation.

In primary ocular infection, nonspecific host resistance represents the main line of defense during the first few days of infection. It consists of preexisting defense mechanisms, e.g., physical barriers (intact epithelium, mucus) to viral penetration, and phagocytosis that leads to viral destruction. Another series of nonspecific antiviral factors are in-

troduced soon after infection has taken place. Among these are interferon, elevations of temperature, and acid pH at the inflammatory site. By interfering in these ways with the early stage of a viral attack, the nonspecific host defenses may be important in determining the outcome of a viral infection. Final recovery from a fully established infection, however, is brought about by specific immune responses that appear only some days later in the infection.

Specific host immune responses are the main line of host defense against reinfection with the same or antigenically related organisms. These responses are mounted by cells of the lymphoid system and by antibodies produced by B-lymphocytes. Antibodies neutralize extracellular virus, and cellular immunity is mediated by sensitized T-lymphocytes. There is intense interaction between the immune responses of B and T cells to viral infections. Other elements—complement, macrophages, polymorphonuclear leukocytes, and null cells—also participate.

In the following sections, various host factors that may share in the eye's defense against viral infection will be considered on the basis of evidence obtained in studies of both ocular and nonocular tissues.

EPITHELIUM AND MUCUS
The intact corneal and conjunctival epithelial and mucous layers form physical barriers that protect the eye from viral infection [8]. Trauma is thought to break the resistance of the intact conjunctiva and cornea to virus in the following ways: Corneal or conjunctival trauma may break the physical barrier formed by the mucous layer covering the epithelial surface; trauma may expose epithelial cells in the deep ocular layers of the eye, which are more susceptible to the virus; or trauma may generate prostaglandins, which have been shown to increase the susceptibility of cells to HSV [14].

IMMUNOGLOBULINS
IgG, IgM, and IgA can all neutralize viruses. The neutralization of HSV by IgM is greatly increased by complement [12]. When antibody comes into contact with large numbers of viral particles, inactivation is often incomplete because a small fraction of virus is subject to steric hindrance from debris or other antibody molecules and cannot be neutralized. Such an infectious HSV-IgG complex has been detected in vesicular fluid from herpes labialis [6] and in tears from herpetic eyes [3]. The presence of an infectious HSV-IgG complex is thought to be a possible reason for the persistence of HSV in humans with high titers of circulating antibodies.

In addition to neutralizing HSV, antibodies bind

to herpesvirus antigens on the cell surface, and, with the help of complement, can cause lysis of the infected cell. Virus-specific antigens are known to have appeared on the cell surface early enough and in sufficient quantity to bring about cytolysis before the full production of virus, and in this way to have minimized viral dissemination [10]. As described later in this chapter, antibodies also participate in antibody-dependent cell-mediated cytotoxic reactions by macrophages, killer cells, and polymorphonuclear leukocytes.

INTERFERON

The interferon (IFN) system is one of the earliest of the host defenses to develop. IFN whose production is stimulated by viruses (type 1 interferon, IFN-α, IFN-β) can be produced by virtually all nucleated body cells when they become infected with viruses. The process appears to be regulated by genes located on chromosome 9 in humans [27]. Immune IFN (type 2 interferon, IFN-γ) is one of the lymphokines produced by sensitized T-lymphocytes during the immune response.

IFN does not inactivate virus. It reacts instead with the membranes of surrounding cells to depress a gene encoded for intracellular antiviral protein(s). This gene is located on human chromosome 21 [38] and probably codes for IFN receptor molecules. The antiviral protein within the cell does not prevent subsequent viral penetration, but it inhibits the intracellular multiplication of most viruses by inhibiting the synthesis of essential viral protein at the level of translation, probably by affecting ribosomes. It also augments killer cell and natural killer cell activities [13, 26].

T-LYMPHOCYTES

Sensitized T-lymphocytes can react with virus-specific antigens on the surfaces of infected cells and cause cell destruction. The virus-specific antigens appear on the surface of infected cells sufficiently early in the viral growth cycle to permit immune destruction before the full yield of infectious virus has appeared [10].

In addition to the direct cytolytic effect exerted by sensitized T-lymphocytes on virus-infected cells, effector T-lymphocytes, when they react with virus-specific antigen on target cells, may produce a variety of mediators of cellular immunity (lymphokines). The mediators may be chemotactic factor, macrophage migration inhibition factor, lymphotoxin, or IFN.

MACROPHAGES

Although macrophages may act against virus in conjunction with the immune system (i.e., with antibody and sensitized T-lymphocytes), they may also act alone to engulf virus present in the extracellular fluid. The effect of phagocytosis of the virus by macrophages is to reduce the level of virus in the body fluid (as during viremia) and thus to minimize its dissemination. These effects can occur only if the virus is destroyed by the macrophages, as is usually the case in the cells of normal adults. However, if the virus replicates in the macrophages, as is usually the case in the cells of newborns, the infected macrophages may aid in transmitting the virus to other body cells.

TABLE 4-3. *Virus-Induced Inclusions and Polykaryocytes*

Virus	Inclusion Bodies		Polykaryocytes (multinucleated cells)
	Nuclear	Cytoplasmic	
Herpes simplex	+ (E)	−	+
Varicella-zoster	+ (E)	−	+
Cytomegalovirus	+ (E)	+ (B)	+
Adenovirus	+ (E—early) (B—late)	−	−
Measles	+ (E)	+ (E)	+
Vaccinia	−	+ (E)	−
Variola	−	+ (E)	−
Molluscum contagiosum	−	+ (E) ·	−
Newcastle disease	−	+ (E)	+
Rabies	−	+ (E)	−

E = eosinophilic; B = basophilic.

In addition to phagocytosis, when macrophages are directed by specific antibody they may attack and lyse cells containing virus-specific surface antigens. This interaction occurs through the Fc receptors on macrophages [30]. Macrophages can also be activated to attack virus-infected cells, not only by antibody but also by sensitized T-lymphocytes.

POLYMORPHONUCLEAR LEUKOCYTES
A recent study has suggested that polymorphonuclear leukocytes (PMNs) can act as effector cells in the antibody-dependent cell-mediated cytotoxicity system [32]. PMNs are known to have receptors for the Fc fragment of IgG, and human PMNs can damage HSV-infected target cells sensitized with antiviral antibody. PMNs are much less effective as killer cells than are peripheral blood mononuclear cells, but as PMNs are the predominant inflammatory cells within HSV lesions, they may be quantitatively more important than the mononuclear cells in the human host defenses against recurrent HSV infection. The cytotoxic effects of PMNs can be significantly reduced by prostaglandins or hydrocortisone.

KILLER CELLS AND NATURAL KILLER CELLS
Killer cells (K cells), which have been shown to mediate antibody-dependent cell-mediated cytotoxicity in cells actively infected with virus in vitro [35], appear to require IgG binding through Fc receptors on the cell surface. The efficiency of the resulting cell lysis is apparently many times greater than that of antibody plus complement.

Natural killer cells (NK cells), unsensitized lymphocytes from normal humans, can lyse or damage a variety of target tumor cells as well as virus-infected cells [4]. This activity is independent of antibody and complement and does not reflect conventional phagocytic activity.

IMMUNE-MEDIATED DISEASE
The evidence available suggests that the immune responses that serve, in most circumstances, to control viral replication and promote recovery may in some virus-host relationships contribute to the pathogenesis of the infection. The most convincing experimental data supporting this concept have come from studies of experimental animal models (e.g., lymphocytic choriomeningitis of mice).

The primary mechanisms through which immune responses may have deleterious effects on the host are (1) deposition of immune complexes (e.g., in EB virus or hepatitis B virus infection); (2) lysis of virus-infected cells by antibody and complement (e.g., in HSV infection); (3) damage to virus-infected cells by immune effector cells (e.g., in lymphocytic choriomeningitis, measles, mumps, HSV infection); and (4) combined cytotoxicity of effector cells and antibody (e.g., in influenza and HSV infection).

PATTERNS OF VIRAL DISEASE
Viruses cause three basic patterns of infection: localized, disseminated, and inapparent. In herpesvirus infections, latent infection also occurs.

LOCALIZED INFECTION
In localized infection, viral multiplication and cell damage remain localized near the site of entry (e.g., the skin, respiratory or gastrointestinal tract, conjunctiva, or cornea), spreading from the cells infected first to neighboring cells by diffusion in intercellular spaces and by cell contact. The virus then forms a single lesion or group of lesions, e.g., the lesions of HSV infection on corneal epithelium.

In a less strictly localized pattern, the virus is transported by excretions or secretions within connected cavities, causing diffuse infection of an organ. Thence it may in time spread to distant sites, but this is not essential for the production of the characteristic illness.

DISSEMINATED INFECTIONS
Disseminated infections develop by way of the following sequential steps: (1) The virus undergoes primary multiplication at the site of entry and in regional lymph nodes. (2) Viral progeny spread through the blood stream and lymphatics (primary viremia) to additional organs. (3) Further multiplication takes place in these organs. (4) The virus disseminates to the target organs through the blood or lymph vessels (secondary viremia). (5) The virus multiplies in the target organs, where it causes damage, pathologic lesions, and clinical disease. Such a pattern of disseminated infection can be seen in HSV infection in newborn infants.

INAPPARENT INFECTIONS
In addition to the acute infections described above, many transient viral infections occur without producing overt disease. They are very common and epidemiologically important, often representing unrecognized sources of viral dissemination and conferring immunity. Several factors contribute to the production of these inapparent infections: virus attenuation; the host's immunity, including the host's ability to produce a prompt secretory antibody response; and failure of the virus to reach the target organ.

LATENT INFECTIONS

It is a common observation of those afflicted with HSV, and one of the oldest puzzles of virology, that latent herpesvirus infections can persist for many years. HSV infection in the form of herpes labialis or herpes keratitis can be activated from its latency by a wide range of stimuli. Herpesviruses can be recovered from nerve ganglia of infected animals or human cadavers, which suggests that somehow the virus can maintain an association with ganglion cells. No one as yet knows how this relationship is maintained, but two major hypotheses have been proposed—the dynamic-state and the static-state hypotheses.

The dynamic-state hypothesis suggests that virus replication and shedding from affected ganglia occurs continuously but at a slow rate. According to the hypothesis, the virus migrates to skin or mucosa and produces microfoci of infection, but the host's immune responses, if uncompromised, control the degree of virus-induced cytopathologic changes. Thus no clinical disease occurs. Support for this hypothesis comes from the observation that virus shedding occurs intermittently or continuously in the absence of visible lesions. Recently it has been proposed that local environmental conditions may increase the susceptibility of the epithelial cells to infection with the continuously shed virus [14]. The rate of virus replication is then greater, and this leads to clinical lesions.

The static-state hypothesis suggests that the virus is present in the ganglia in some unknown state, either integrated or free, but not replicating, possibly because the specific neurons harboring it lack a functional transcriptase required for replication, or because of some immunologic control of replication. After some reactivation stimulus that alters the biochemical or immunologic balance, the virus migrates centrifugally along the axon to initiate an active site of replication in the epithelial cells. The virus grows if it is uncontrolled by the immune response and if the epithelial cells are susceptible.

Neither of these hypotheses adequately explains why the infected ganglion cells are not killed by a virus that is usually extremely cytocidal. Nor do we know what factors can result in reactivation.

ANTIVIRAL CHEMOTHERAPY

Rational design of antiviral chemotherapeutic agents must be based on exploitable biochemical differences among three factors—the normal host cell, the virus-infected cell, and the virus itself. Since viruses are obligatory cellular parasites, their growth is largely dependent on the cell's structural and enzymatic equipment. Viruses also contain virus-coded, specific, functional molecules that de-

anions tested, heparin has shown promising results. Heparin, a negatively charged polysaccharide, exhibits antiviral activity against herpesviruses in cell cultures [40]. Its addition to virus preparations sharply reduces their infectivity: By forming a noninfectious virus-heparin complex, the heparin molecule prevents attachment of the virus particle to the cell.

AMANTADINE HYDROCHLORIDE

Amantadine hydrochloride has received considerable attention for its ability to prevent virus penetration. A unique, symmetric, primary amine, it exists as an ammonium ion at pH 7.4. Its molecular weight is 15, and it is readily soluble in water. In cell cultures, amantadine hydrochloride prevents the infection of cells by several viruses: myxoviruses, paramyxoviruses, rubella virus, and pseudorabies virus (one of the herpesviruses) [7, 19, 23].

IDOXURIDINE

The first clinically effective antiviral nucleoside, idoxuridine (IDU), was synthesized in 1959 by Prusoff [28] as part of an anticancer program. It was active only against certain oncogenic RNA viruses and certain DNA viruses including herpesvirus [29]. It appears to exert its inhibitory effect on viral DNA synthesis with some degree of specificity. Series of enzyme systems—thymidine kinase, thymidylate kinase, DNA polymerase, and cytidine diphosphoreductase—are affected, but a conclusive molecular biologic reason for the high antiviral activity is still not known. IDU has an antiviral effect when applied topically in herpetic keratitis [16], but it does not prevent recurrences, and it is toxic to corneal and conjunctival cells.

CYTARABINE

Cytarabine (ara-C), a synthetic nucleoside, is active against poxvirus, herpesviruses, and adenovirus. Several studies [18, 39] have also clearly shown that ara-C has antiviral activity in vivo, especially in herpetic keratitis. It interferes with viral DNA synthesis, and DNA replicating polymerase is a major enzyme that is affected by it. When systemically applied, ara-C can cause toxic effects on the host's lymphatic system that might result in immunosuppression.

VIDARABINE

Vidarabine (ara-A) has a rather broad spectrum of antiviral activity against DNA viruses (e.g., herpesviruses and poxviruses). In herpesvirus-infected cells, its main effect is the inhibition of DNA synthesis. Its unique characteristics are the preferential inhibition of viral DNA synthesis relative to cellular DNA synthesis, the differential inhibition of the DNA-dependent DNA polymerase system, and differences in the kinds of linkages of ara-A molecules that have been incorporated into the DNA in host cells and in the virus. The drug is effective when used topically in herpetic keratitis [24] and appears to be effective against some herpesviruses that are resistant to IDU. Ara-A also has an effect on herpetic encephalitis, particularly when patients are treated early [41]. A disadvantage of ara-A, however, is its lack of solubility and rapid conversion in humans to an inactive form as a result of deamination by adenosine deaminase.

TRIFLURIDINE

Trifluridine (F_3T) is a potent and specific inhibitor of the replication of herpesvirus in vitro and herpes simplex and vaccinial keratitis [17]. F_3T is incorporated into viral DNA, which results in the formation of small pieces of DNA and leads to incomplete transcription of late mRNA and to the synthesis of defective proteins.

ACYCLOVIR

One of the most promising new antiherpes compounds is 9-(2-hydroxyethoxymethyl) guanine. Formerly known as acycloguanosine, it is now called acyclovir (trade name Zovirax). It has marked antiviral activity in animal and human herpetic eye infections [9, 15] and very low toxicity by virtue of its specificity for virus-induced enzymes. The compound is apparently phosphorylated to a monophosphate by a herpesvirus-specific thymidine kinase, an event that does not often take place in uninfected cells. The monophosphate is converted to triphosphate to a much greater extent in herpes-infected cells than in uninfected cells. Furthermore, acyclovir is much more active against virus-specific DNA polymerase than against corresponding host-cell enzymes. It causes very little ocular irritation and has an extremely low level of metabolic degradation after systemic administration; these features make it an attractive candidate for both topical and systemic antiviral chemotherapy.

5-(2-BROMOVINYL)-2'-DEOXYURIDINE

5-(2-Bromovinyl)-2'-deoxyuridine (BVDU), with low toxicity, is highly selective in inhibiting the replication of HSV and varicella-zoster virus (VZV). Unlike acyclovir, it is less inhibitory to HSV-2 than to HSV-1. BVDU is readily phosphorylated in HSV- or VZV-infected cells (but not in uninfected cells) by the virus-encoded thymidine kinase to monophosphate and diphosphate forms, which are subsequently converted to BVDU-triphosphate by host cell kinase. The BVDU-triphosphate inhibits virus DNA polymerase more effectively than does cellular DNA polymerase. BVDU has been shown to be effective in the treatment of herpes simplex keratitis in experimental animals [21] and human patients [22]. However, BVDU does not cross the blood-brain barrier well, which could limit its usefulness in systemic therapy for herpetic encephalitis.

PHOSPHONOACETIC ACID
Phosphonoacetic acid has restricted but highly specific antiviral activity, inhibiting HSV and several other herpesviruses selectively [11, 34]. Its main effect is to inhibit DNA synthesis in infected cells through its inhibitory influence on herpesvirus-induced DNA-dependent DNA polymerase.

RIBAVIRIN
A synthetic nucleoside analogue of guanosine, ribavirin (Virazole), appears to be effective against herpesvirus and influenza virus in experimental animals [36] by inhibiting steps leading to the biosynthesis of guanylic acid nucleotides. Since ribavirin is apparently somewhat toxic, it cannot be administered systemically for extended periods.

2-DEOXY-D-GLUCOSE
2-Deoxy-D-glucose can prevent or reduce the severity of herpetic keratitis in rabbits [5, 31]. It is believed to interfere with the synthesis or elongation of the oligosaccharides that are incorporated into the viral-specific glycoproteins. These glycoproteins are essential for the formation of the envelopes of myxoviruses and herpesviruses. Although the protection bestowed by 2-deoxy-D-glucose is not dramatic, it suggests that sugar analogues may be useful antiviral compounds.

RIFAMPIN
Rifampin inhibits the growth of poxviruses and adenoviruses and can prevent the maturation of infectious virus until quite late in the viral growth cycle [37]. It apparently inhibits the cleavage of a protein precursor that would otherwise be cleaved at the time of the protein's assembly into smaller polypeptides. These small polypeptides are required for the assembly of the virus core. To inhibit growth, however, large concentrations of rifampin are needed.

THIOSEMICARBAZONES
Two thiosemicarbazones have been found to exhibit antiviral activity: isatin-β-thiosemicarbazone and 1-methylisatin-3-thiosemicarbazone (Methiazone).

Both are effective prophylactic agents in humans exposed to smallpox [2], both are valuable for the treatment of vaccinia gangrenosa and disseminated vaccinia [1]. In the presence of these drugs, late viral mRNA synthesis is inhibited. As a result, the number of polysomes formed by viral mRNA is greatly reduced, and viral proteins programmed to be translated thereafter are not formed. Thiosemicarbazones also affect the cleavage of a precursor protein molecule of the virus core.

LABORATORY DIAGNOSIS OF VIRAL INFECTIONS OF THE EYE
Many animal viruses can cause eye disease (Table 4-5). The conventional isolation and serologic procedures used for the laboratory diagnosis of viral infections can provide only a retrospective indication of the causal agent. Although such information is very useful in the epidemiologic study of viral diseases, it is of limited value for the immediate clinical management of the patient. Fortunately, various new methods offer considerable promise for more rapid and more specific diagnosis of viral infections.

There are three basic approaches to the identification of viral infections (Table 4-6): the direct examination of clinical materials for virus or viral antigen, the isolation and identification of viruses from clinical specimens, and serologic diagnosis based on the demonstration of a major increase in viral antibody during the patient's illness.

DIRECT EXAMINATION OF CLINICAL MATERIALS
Direct examination of clinical materials permits the most rapid recognition and identification of viral

TABLE 4-5. *Viruses Known to Cause Human Eye Disease*

DNA Viruses	RNA Viruses
Papilloma	Poliovirus
Adenovirus	Coxsackie
Herpes simplex	Enterovirus 70
Varicella-zoster	Rhinovirus
EB	Arbovirus
B	Influenza
Cytomegalovirus	Mumps
Variola	Measles
Vaccinia	Newcastle disease
Orf	Rabies
Molluscum contagiosum	Rubella
	Marburg

ISOLATION AND IDENTIFICATION OF VIRUSES FROM CLINICAL SPECIMENS

agents. In a few viral infections, caused, for example, by herpesviruses or poxviruses, examination of materials from the ocular lesions by light or electron microscopy can be used to detect viruses, and the morphology of their CPE or of the virus particles discloses the major group to which each causal agent belongs. However, direct examination procedures in which the specimen is treated with specific viral antibody (e.g., immunofluorescence microscopy, immune peroxidase) permit both the rapid detection and specific identification of the viral agent.

Although immunologic approaches to the detection of viral antigens in clinical materials offer great advantages in terms of rapidity of diagnosis, they also have certain limitations compared with virus isolation. Diagnostic capability is restricted to those agents for which suitable immune reagents are available. Whenever possible, therefore, the clinical specimens should be inoculated into appropriate host systems for isolation as a backup to direct examination.

Various approaches have been developed in recent years that permit rapid and efficient identification of viral isolates. The first prerequisite for the successful isolation of a viral agent is the collection of material most likely to harbor the agent. The specimen must be taken at optimal times during the early acute phase of the illness—the sooner after onset the better since the opportunity for successful isolation diminishes rapidly with time, the rallying defense mechanisms and antibody formation exerting an increasing influence on the course of the disease. Once collected, the material must be inoculated into susceptible cells. The susceptible cells for a number of viruses known to infect the eye are listed in Table 4-6.

After the CPE or other signs of infection develop in a host system, it is efficient to use selected antisera or conjugates and to proceed directly to the definitive identification of the virus by immunologic methods. Determination of the physical and chemical properties of a virus—e.g., its size, ether sensitivity, and nucleic acid content—can also identify viral isolates, but the necessary procedures require considerable time and effort.

TABLE 4-6. *Laboratory Diagnosis of Viral Infections of the Eye*

Virus	Direct Examination (light microscopy)	Virus Isolation (host systems)	Serodiagnostic Tests
Herpes simplex	Intranuclear inclusions (eosinophilic), multinucleated cells	Various animal cells	NT, CF, IHA, ELISA
Varicella-zoster	Intranuclear inclusions (eosinophilic)	Human embryonic cells	CF, IFA
Cytomegalovirus	Intranuclear inclusions (eosinophilic), cytoplasmic inclusions (basophilic), cytomegalic cells	Human embryonic lung cells	CF, IHA
Adenovirus	Intranuclear inclusions (eosinophilic in early stage; basophilic in late stage)	Human cells	CF, HI
Measles	Intranuclear and cytoplasmic inclusions (both eosinophilic), multinucleated cells	Primary human or simian cells	CF, HI
Rubella	—	African green monkey kidney cells; rabbit kidney cells (RK-13)	HI, CF

NT = neutralization test; CF = complement fixation; IHA = indirect hemagglutination; ELISA = enzyme-linked immunosorbent assay; IFA = indirect fluorescent antibody; HI = hemagglutination inhibition.

SEROLOGIC DIAGNOSIS

Serologic diagnosis is based on the demonstration of a major increase (fourfold or more) in antibody to a given virus over the course of an illness. This requires testing, in parallel and in the same run, an acute-phase serum specimen collected as early as possible after the onset of the illness and a convalescent-phase serum specimen taken at least 2 weeks later. However, in reinfection or recurrent infection with certain viruses (e.g., HSV), antibody titers do not rise; therefore serodiagnosis is not a useful tool for identification of the infection. Also, heterologous serologic responses to HSV have been observed in herpes zoster patients and to herpes zoster virus in HSV patients [33]. The conventional methods used for the serodiagnosis of viral infections are neutralization, hemagglutination inhibition, complement fixation, and indirect fluorescent antibody staining; to a much lesser extent, passive hemagglutination, immunodiffusion, and counterimmunoelectrophoresis are also used. Recently a number of new methods for detecting viral antibodies—immune adherence hemagglutination, radioimmunoassay, and enzyme-linked immunosorbent assay (ELISA)—have been devised. These methods offer the advantages of simplicity, rapidity, and sensitivity over conventional serologic methods.

REFERENCES

1. Bauer, D. J., and Sadler, P. W. The structure-activity relationship of the antiviral chemotherapeutic activity of isatin-β-thiosemicarbazone. *Br. J. Pharmacol. Chemother.* 15:101, 1960.
2. Bauer, D. J., et al. Prophylaxis of smallpox with Methiazone. *Am. J. Epidemiol.* 90:130, 1969.
3. Centifanto, Y. M., Little, J. M., and Kaufman, H. E. The relationship between virus chemotherapy, secretory antibody formation and recurrent herpetic disease. *Ann. N.Y. Acad. Sci.* 173:649, 1970.
4. Ching, C., and Lopez, C. Natural killing of herpes simplex virus type 1-infected target cells: Normal human responses and influence of antiviral antibody. *Infect. Immun.* 26:49, 1979.
5. Courtney, R. J., Steiner, S. M., and Benyesh-Melnick, M. Effects of 2-deoxy-D-glucose on herpes simplex virus replication. *Virology* 52:447, 1973.
6. Daniels, C. A., and LeGoff, S. G. Shedding of infectious virus/antibody complex from vesicular lesions of patients with recurrent herpes labialis. *Lancet* 2:524, 1975.
7. Davies, W. C., et al. Antiviral activity of 1-adamantanamine (amantadine). *Science* 144:862, 1964.
8. Edwards, P. A. W. Is mucus a selective barrier to macromolecules? *Br. Med. Bull.* 34:55, 1978.
9. Elion, G. B., et al. Selectivity of action of an antiherpetic agent 9-(2-hydroxyethoxymethyl) guanine. *Proc. Natl. Acad. Sci. U.S.A.* 74:5716, 1977.
10. Ennis, F. A. Host defense mechanisms against herpes simplex virus: I. Control of infection in vitro by sensitized spleen cells and antibody. *Infect. Immun.* 7:898, 1973.
11. Gerstein, D. D., Dawson, C. R., and Oh, J. O. Phosphonoacetic acid in the treatment of experimental herpes simplex keratitis. *Antimicrob. Agents Chemother.* 7:285, 1975.
12. Hampar, B. A., et al. Heterogeneity in the properties of 7S and 19S rabbit-neutralizing antibodies to herpes simplex virus. *J. Immunol.* 100:586, 1968.
13. Herberman, R. B., Ortaldo, J. R., and Bonnard, G. D. Augmentation by interferon of human natural and antibody-dependent cell-mediated cytotoxicity. *Nature* 277:221, 1979.
14. Hill, T. J., Blyth, W. A., and Harbour, D. A. Trauma to the skin causes recurrence of herpes simplex in the mouse. *J. Gen. Virol.* 39:21, 1978.
15. Jones, B. R., et al. Efficacy of acycloguanosine (Wellcome 248U) against herpes simplex corneal ulcers. *Lancet* 1:243, 1979.
16. Kaufman, H. E. Clinical cure of herpes simplex keratitis by 5-iodo-2′-deoxyuridine. *Proc. Soc. Exp. Biol. Med.* 109:251, 1962.
17. Kaufman, H. E., and Heidelberger, C. Therapeutic antiviral action of 5-trifluoromethyl-2′-deoxyuridine in herpes simplex keratitis. *Science* 145:585, 1964.
18. Kaufman, H. E., and Maloney, E. D. IDU and cytosine arabinoside in experimental herpetic keratitis. *Arch. Ophthalmol.* 69:626, 1963.
19. Maassab, H. F., and Cochran, K. W. Rubella virus: Inhibition in vitro by amantadine hydrochloride. *Science* 145:1443, 1964.
20. Matthews, R. E. F. Classification and nomenclature of viruses: Third Report of the International Committee on Taxonomy of Viruses. *Intervirology* 12:132, 1979.
21. Maudgal, P. C., et al. (E)-5-(2-bromovinyl)-2′-deoxyuridine in the treatment of experimental herpes simplex keratitis. *Antimicrob. Agents Chemother.* 17:8, 1981.
22. Maudgal, P. C., et al. Efficacy of (E)-5-(2-bromovinyl)-2′-deoxyuridine in the topical treatment of herpes simplex keratitis. *Albrecht Von Graefes Arch. Klin. Exp. Ophthalmol.* 216:261, 1981.
23. Neumayer, E. M., Haff, R. F., and Hossmann, C. E. Antiviral activity of amantadine hydro-

chloride in tissue culture and in ovo. *Proc. Soc. Exp. Biol. Med.* 119:393, 1965.

24. Pavan-Langston, D., and Dohlman, C. H.   A double-blind clinical study of adenine arabinoside therapy of viral keratoconjunctivitis. *Am. J. Ophthalmol.* 74:81, 1972.

25. O'Neal, F. J., and Miles, C. P.   Chromosome changes in human cells induced by herpes simplex, types 1 and 2. *Nature* 223:851, 1969.

26. Ortaldo, J. R., et al.   Augmentation of human K-cell activity with interferon. *Scand. J. Immunol.* 12:365, 1980.

27. Owerbach, D., et al.   Leukocyte and fibroblast interferon genes are located on human chromosome 9. *Proc. Natl. Acad. Sci. U.S.A.* 78:3123, 1981.

28. Prusoff, W. H.   Synthesis and biological activities of iododeoxyuridine, an analog of thymidine. *Biochim. Biophys. Acta* 32:295, 1959.

29. Prusoff, W. H., and Goz, B.   Halogenated Pyrimidine and Deoxyribonucleosides. In O. Eicher, A. Farah, H. Herkin, and A. D. Welch (Eds.), *Handbook of Experimental Pharmacology.* Berlin: Springer, Vol. 38, pp. 272–347.

30. Rager-Zisman, B., and Bloom, B. R.   Immunological destruction of herpes simplex virus-infected cells. *Nature* 251:542, 1974.

31. Ray, E. K., et al.   A new approach to viral chemotherapy. Inhibitors of glycoprotein synthesis. *Lancet* 2:680, 1974.

32. Russell, A. S., and Essery, G.   Cellular immunity to herpes simplex virus in man: VII. K-cell activity to HSV-1 infected target cells in disease. *Cancer* 40:42, 1977.

33. Schmidt, N. J., Lennette, E. H., and Magoffin, R. L.   Immunological relationship between herpes simplex and varicella-zoster viruses demonstrated by complement-fixation, neutralization and fluorescent antibody tests. *J. Gen. Virol.* 4:321, 1969.

34. Shipkowitz, N. R., et al.   Suppression of herpes simplex virus infection by phosphonoacetic acid. *Appl. Microbiol.* 26:264, 1973.

35. Shore, S. L., et al.   Detection of cell-dependent cytotoxic antibody to cells infected with herpes simplex virus. *Nature* 251:350, 1974.

36. Sidwell, R. W., et al.   Broad-spectrum antiviral activity of Virazole: 1-β-D-ribofuranosyl-1,2,4-triazole-3-carboxamide. *Science* 177:705, 1972.

37. Subak-Sharpe, J. H., Timbury, M. C., and Williams, J. F.   Rifampicin inhibits the growth of some mammalian viruses. *Nature* 222:341, 1969.

38. Tan, Y. H., and Greene, A. E.   Subregional localization of the gene(s) governing the human interferon induced antiviral state in man. *J. Gen. Virol.* 32:153, 1976.

39. Underwood, G. E.   Activity of l-β-D-arabino-furanosylcytosine hydrochloride against herpes simplex keratitis. *Proc. Soc. Exp. Biol. Med.* 111:660, 1962.

40. Vaheri, A.   Heparin and related polyionic substances as virus inhibitors. *Acta Pathol. Microbiol. Scand.* (Suppl.) 171:1, 1964.

41. Whitley, R. J.   Adenine arabinoside therapy of biopsy-proved herpes simplex encephalitis. *N. Engl. J. Med.* 297:289, 1977.

Infectious Agents: FUNGI

Masao Okumoto

FUNGI IMPORTANT IN CORNEAL INFECTION

Fungi are opportunistic agents of infection. They rarely infect the healthy, intact cornea, but in a compromised or immunosuppressed cornea, almost any fungal species can probably induce infectious keratitis [2, 15, 21, 34, 45, 50, 53–55, 59]. A few genera are encountered much more frequently than others. Although the exact reasons for this are not known, it may be related to a higher degree of virulence for the cornea and a higher population density in the environment.

In the United States, *Fusarium, Candida, Aspergillus,* and *Acremonium (Cephalosporium)* are the most frequent causes of keratomycosis [32]. In cooler areas of the world, *Candida* is the most frequent cause of fungal keratitis [10, 26], whereas in warmer regions *Fusarium* sp. are the most common [11, 39]. There are exceptions: In India, where a hot and humid climate often prevails, *Aspergillus* is the most common fungal species isolated from eyes with keratomycosis and from normal conjunctivae [35, 53, 66].

HABITAT

Fungi are ubiquitous. Their light spores, produced in enormous numbers, are widely disseminated and have a remarkable ability to germinate and subsist on almost any organic substance. The home environment has been examined for the presence of fungi by a number of investigators. In one study done in Tulsa, Oklahoma, more than 44 genera of fungi were identified, with the predominant types being *Alternaria, Hormodendrum, Pullularia, Pencillium,* and *Epicoccum* [38].

Another study investigated the outdoor mold population in Edmonton, Alberta (Canada). In spite of the extremely cold winters, outdoor molds were very common throughout the year, although they were more prevalent in the spring and early summer months [65]. Several fungal genera and species that have been reported in keratomycosis in Tampa, Florida, were isolated from the sandy beaches of that city [8].

Candida sp. are endogenous opportunistic pathogens that normally reside harmlessly on or in mammalian hosts [25]. Approximately 10 percent of seriously ill patients undergoing hyperalimentation develop endophthalmitis, presumably from endogenous *Candida albicans* [29, 58]. In rare cases, endogenous *Candida* endophthalmitis may involve the cornea [46]. A number of cases of *Candida* endophthalmitis among drug abusers have been reported. The source of the *Candida* has not been strictly demonstrated, but the cotton balls and other nonsterile apparatus used by the drug abusers have been suggested [16].

Fusarium sp. are primarily plant pathogens, and keratomycosis caused by these organisms has often been found in agricultural workers [40].

MORPHOLOGY

Morphologically the fungi important in corneal disease can be divided into two broad categories. The yeast type is represented by the *Candida* sp., which are characterized by oval structures with or without buds and in some clinical specimens by the presence of pseudohyphae, which are elongation of the buds resembling hyphae. The filamentous variety produces long branching structures that may or may not be septate.

The cell wall more than any other cellular part defines a fungus and distinguishes it from other living organisms. Eighty to ninety percent of the fungal cell wall is polysaccharide, with most of the remainder consisting of protein and lipid. The polysaccharide is either cellulose or chitin; usually only one type is found in a given fungus [5].

The filamentous fungi can be easily identified if large segments of the hyphae are seen intact, since their long, branching, often septate hyphal structure is very distinctive. The identification of genera and species is usually not possible from morphologic examination of a tissue specimen, since spores and their supporting stucture, which are the principal identifying feature in taxonomy, are absent.

The staining characteristics of these fungi are discussed in Fungal Diseases in Chapter 5.

FUSARIUM

The *Fusarium* sp. are characterized by distinctive spores referred to as macroconidia, and in some species by small coccoid spores known as microconidia. The main identifying morphologic feature of the *Fusarium* is the large canoe- or banana-shaped conidia, which are produced on short lateral hyphae or conidiophores (Fig. 4-10). A small cluster of conidia is produced on the tip of each conidiophore, and the aggregates of macroconidia bear a striking resemblance to a bunch of bananas. Often, the conidia have transverse septation. The microconidia are much less diagnostic since the *Acremonium* sp. produce similar micronidia. Both types of conidia de-

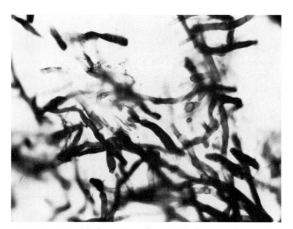

FIGURE 4-10. *Methenamine-silver–stained corneal scraping showing* Fusarium solani.

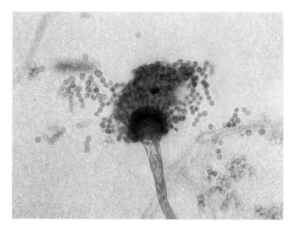

FIGURE 4-11. *Cellophane tape mount of* Aspergillus fumigatus *showing characteristic distribution of conidia in chains on upper portion of vesicle.*

tach readily and are usually found randomly scattered throughout a smear made from sporulating culture.

ACREMONIUM
The *Acremonium* sp. are devoid of macroconidia, producing only microconidia. Like *Fusarium* spores, *Acremonium* spores are produced at the end of lateral hyphae that develop into conidiophores with one or more oval conidia, which has a single central septum. The conidiophore also secretes a sticky mucilaginous substance that holds the conidia together, so that a cluster of microconidia may be seen.

ASPERGILLUS
The *Aspergillus* sp. are among the easiest to recognize from a morphologic standpoint if the spore structures are present. The conidiophore with its swollen terminal end (vesicle) surrounded by flask-shaped sterigma, each of which produces long chains of coccoid conidia that radiate out from the vesicle, is highly diagnostic (Fig. 4-11). The dichotomous branching nature of the hyphae is also diagnostic.

YEAST FORMS
The yeast forms are represented by the *Candida* sp. The presence of budding yeasts in a corneal scraping is almost diagnostic for *Candida*. An inexperienced observer may mistake *Pityrosporum ovale* for *Candida*, but the narrow attachment base of the bud, the lack of symmetry of the yeast, and the off-axis position of the bud in the *Candida* readily sepa-

rates it from *Pityrosporum*. *Candida* also produces pseudohyphae and true hyphae, and both the yeast form and the hyphal form may be seen in a corneal scraping from a *Candida* ulcer (Fig. 4-12). The mycelial form is considered the invasive form. Some investigators have suggested that this is also the most virulent stage, but this remains to be proved [28, 42].

CULTURAL CHARACTERISTICS
The culture media and techniques employed in identifying fungal organisms are described in Fungal Diseases in Chapter 5. The filamentous fungi of ocular importance are all given the general descriptive term *molds*. Their colonies typically appear as a loose cottony growth on the agar surface. The colonies are sometimes white, but a variety of pigmented colonies may also be encountered.

FUSARIUM
There are approximately 40 species of *Fusarium*, but *F. solani* is the principal species that invades the cornea.

The colonies of *Fusarium* sp. are usually white in the early stages of development but often acquire a buff coloration. As the colonies mature, a variety of colored pigments ranging from yellow to red to purple are produced. The pigments are best seen on the undersurface of the colony. This is known as reverse pigmentation (Fig. 4-13).

ASPERGILLUS
Aspergillus is a large genus with many species, but two are particularly prominent: *A. fumigatus* and *A. niger*. *A. fumigatis* colonies are white at first, but as spores are produced the colonies become velvety green owing to the pigmentation of the conidia. An

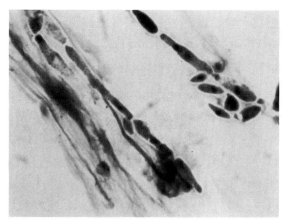

FIGURE 4-12. Candida albicans *from corneal scraping stained with Giemsa.*

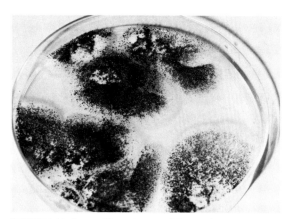

FIGURE 4-14. Aspergillus niger *on Sabouraud agar.*

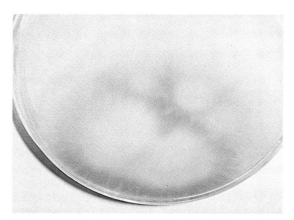

FIGURE 4-13. Fusarium solani *cultured on Sabouraud agar showing reverse pigmentation.*

important avian pathogen, *A. fumigatus* is able to tolerate unusually high temperatures and will grow in vitro at 50°C [17]. *A. niger* colonies are also white during the initial growth phase but turn completely black as they start to sporulate (Fig. 4-14).

ACREMONIUM
Young *Acremonium* colonies are compact and moist but rapidly develop the typical woolly moldlike appearance with an overgrowth of white aerial mycelium. Pigmentations varying from gray to white may be seen. As in *Fusarium* cultures, the pigmentation is seen best by looking at the undersurface of the agar plate.

CANDIDA
Yeast fungi such as the *Candida* exhibit a distinctly different colony appearance from that of the filamentous fungi and may be mistaken for bacterial colonies when seen on blood agar.

The typical *Candida* colony on Sabouraud agar is white and opaque with a smooth, flat, round contour and a pasty, soft consistency (Fig. 4-15). The colonies are a few millimeters in diameter after 48 hours' incubation at 30°C. They will continue to grow for some time, and isolated colonies may reach a diameter of about a centimeter. When grown on blood agar at 35°C, *Candida* colonies may be rather minute and easily mistaken for a micrococcus colony or that of some other bacterial type. They appear as tiny hemispherical colonies without hemolysis and are only about a millimeter or less in diameter at 48 hours. As on Sabouraud agar, colonies grown on blood agar are white to beige, opaque, and smooth with a soft, pasty texture. *Candida* colonies have a distinctly yeasty odor, which is a useful identifying feature.

When *Candida* cultures are kept for several weeks, the colonies appear dull and wrinkled, and pseudohyphae resembling fine rootlike structures that penetrate into the agar depths for a few millimeters may be seen along the periphery or the bottom surface of the colony.

OTHER TESTS FOR IDENTIFICATION
In addition to cultural characteristics, other means of identifying fungi are available. Differentiating *Candida* from other genera of yeasts is fairly simple based on morphologic appearance and characteristics of the culture and stain of the corneal scraping [22]. Other tests that can be used if needed include sugar fermentation, germ tube production [7], immunodiffusion, counterimmunoelectrophoresis (CIE) [33], latex agglutination, crossed electro-

phoresis, enzyme-linked immunosorbent assay, and several commercial systems [9, 37, 51].

The identification of filamentous fungi is based almost entirely on morphologic characteristics. The most widely used method for identification from a culture is the cellophane tape slide mount [18]. The slide culture method can also be used. Antibodies to *Aspergillus fumigatus* can be reliably detected by indirect hemagglutination, indirect immunofluorescence [36], agar gel electrophoresis, and CIE.

PATHOGENICITY

Francois and Rijsselaere have stated that under normal circumstances saprophytic fungi are rapidly destroyed by the humoral and cellular defense reactions of the host [23]. Experimental studies with *Fusarium solani, Aspergillus niger,* and *Aspergillus terreus* showed that intrastromal inoculation of rabbit cornea with large numbers of spores produced only a mild and transient keratitis [23]. Their review of studies by other investigators showed similar findings with *Curvularia, A. terreus, A. flavus, Acremonium,* and *Candida albicans.* The only exception was *Aspergillus fumigatus,* which produced major corneal pathology without concomitant use of corticosteroids. When steroids were used, the previously mentioned fungal species produced considerable corneal pathology, and in the case of *A. fumigatus,* a fulminant keratitis with hypopyon. It appears therefore that fungi (except *A. fumigatus*) are relatively avirulent for the cornea. Indeed, before the introduction of corticosteroids in 1951, corneal infections caused by fungi were mainly limited to *Aspergillus fumigatus* and *Candida* infections [64]. Corticosteroids and other immunosuppressive agents probably increase the virulence of the fungi not by altering their pathogenicity but by weakening the host's tissue defense system [23].

There are a number of publications dealing with the pathogenic mechanisms of the fungi. Wogan's review of mycotoxins lists a class of toxins, the trichothecenes, as being produced by many *Fusarium* and *Acremonium* sp. [70]. At low doses, a single application results in a prolonged inflammatory response; higher doses cause necrosis. A number of trichothecenes have been shown to be cytotoxic or cytostatic to many kinds of aminal cells in culture [70]. Aflatoxin, produced by *Aspergillus,* has been intensively investigated. It is the most potent liver carcinogen yet discovered. Many of the biologic effects caused by this toxin are attributed to pronounced inhibition of DNA and RNA polymerase as well as impairment of protein synthesis.

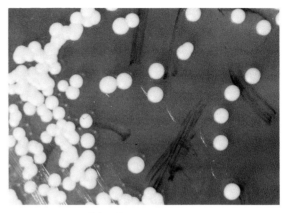

FIGURE 4-15. Candida albicans *on Sabouraud agar.*

However, the relevance of aflatoxin to corneal disease is uncertain because only a few strains of *A. flavus* or *A. parasiticus,* species rarely associated with keratomycoses, seem to produce aflatoxin.

Several reports suggest that the pathogenicity of *C. albicans* is due to the production of proteolytic enzymes that cause lysis of host tissue, which allows the *Candida* to penetrate and invade host tissue [31, 60].

A well-known virulence factor in bacteria is the ability of pathogenic species to adhere to epithelial cells in initiating an infectious process. Sobel and associates have demonstrated that the adherence of *C. albicans* to epithelial cells is aided by a surface protein that binds to epithelial cell receptors [62].

Still another virulence mechanism has been demonstrated by Diamond and associates—a substance liberated by *Candida* that inhibits the contact of human neutrophils with *Candida* pseudohyphae. This inhibitory substance may be a cell wall component or part of a mucus layer secreted by the organism, which would be analogous to the capsule, an important virulence factor among a number of pathogenic bacteria [13].

IMMUNOLOGIC ASPECTS

The cell-mediated immune defense system plays the major role in protecting the host from fungi. The findings of Williams and associates [69] confirm that protection is related not to humoral antibody but to T cell–dependent cellular immunity. Rogers and Balish in their review of immunity to *C. albicans* concluded that resistance to chronic mucocutaneous candidiasis is clearly a function of thymus-dependent cellular immunity, whereas in disseminated candidiasis, resistance is mediated by the innate defense system (such as the elimination of the organism by neutrophils) [56].

Diamond and associates have investigated the ability of neutrophils to damage the pseudohyphae of *C. albicans*, that is, the morphologic form associated with invasiveness. They showed that even in the absence of complement or antibody, neutrophils from normal human subjects were able to attach and spread over the surface of pseudohyphae and cause morphologic changes suggestive of fungal cell death [12]. This fungicidal activity was attributed to the production of myeloperoxidase and hydrogen peroxide in phagocytic granules. Damage to pseudohyphae by neutrophils was inhibited by colchicine, cytochalasin B, and 2-deoxy-D-glucose, all substances known to inhibit neutrophil function [12]. Monocytes from normal patients also damaged *C. albicans* pseudohyphae, and the extent of damage was identical to that observed in the studies in which normal neutrophils were used. The mechanism of fungal damage by monocytes and neutrophils appeared similar in many respects, but important differences were also noted. Monocytes from patients with hereditary disorders of leukocyte function such as chronic granulomatous disease generally did not cause damage to pseudohyphae, but monocytes from one out of four such patients damaged hyphae in the high portion of the range for normal leukocytes. Neutrophils from these patients were inactive or caused minimal damage. Monocytes from patients with myeloperoxidase deficiency caused major hyphae damage, whereas neutrophils from the same patients were uniformly lacking in fungicidal activity. It was suggested that monocytes may have alternative nonoxidative fungicidal activity. Overall, it appeared that oxidative mechanisms were most important in enabling normal monocytes to damage *Candida* hyphae [14].

Many investigators have demonstrated that corticosteroids depress the normal humoral and cellular defense mechanisms and allow opportunistic fungi to invade the cornea [30, 61]. The potentiating effect of antibiotics upon fungal growth has been elucidated to a lesser degree.

MECHANISMS OF ANTIFUNGAL AGENTS
Susceptibility testing of fungi to antifungal agents has not been standardized and utilized to a wide extent. The problem with testing the sensitivity of filamentous fungi to antifungal agents has been lack of agreement among investigators concerning specific methods, inoculum size, incubation conditions, and end-point determination [68]. All of these variables greatly influence the outcome of the results of such tests, so that investigators using one method may report a fungus to be sensitive to a particular drug, whereas those using a different procedure may find it resistant. In spite of these difficulties, many laboratories are performing antifungal susceptibility testing [63].

Although many antifungal agents have been isolated or synthesized, only a few have proved to be of therapeutic value. The most important of these are those that affect the cell membranes: the polyenes and the imidazole compounds. Among the polyenes, the most useful have been amphotericin B and natamycin. For a number of years, amphotericin B has been the most effective antifungal agent against a variety of mycotic infections in humans [3, 6, 24, 27, 41, 63]. The minimum inhibitory concentration of amphotericin B has been particularly good against *Candida* and *Aspergillus* sp. [1]. Early reports indicated that resistance to the polyene antifungal agents did not occur [27], but apparently rare instances of resistance have been noted [1].

Natamycin (pimaricin) has been used for some years as an investigational drug against a variety of keratomycoses and has been demonstrated in extensive clinical usage to be particularly useful in the treatment of *Fusarium* keratitis [24]. Recently natamycin was approved by the Food and Drug Administration for human use, and an ophthalmic preparation (Natacyn) is available from Alcon Laboratories (Fort Worth, Texas).

Clotrimazole, econazole nitrate, ketoconazole, miconazole nitrate, and flucytosine have also been employed in the treatment of keratomycoses [4, 19, 20, 43, 44, 47–49, 52, 57, 60, 67]. A discussion of all of these antifungal drugs is presented in Fungal Diseases in Chapter 5.

REFERENCES
1. Al-Doory, Y. *Laboratory Medical Mycology.* Philadelphia: Lea & Febiger, 1980. P. 150.
2. Azar, P., Aquavella, J. V., and Smith, R. S. Keratomycosis due to an *Alternaria* species. *Am. J. Ophthalmol.* 79:881, 1975.
3. Bannatyne, R. M., and Cheung, R. Comparative susceptibility of *Candida albicans* to amphotericin B and amphotericin B methyl ester. *Antimicrob. Agents Chemother.* 12:449, 1977.
4. Bannatyne, R. M., and Cheung, R. Susceptibility of *Candida albicans* to miconazole. *Antimicrob. Agents Chemother.* 13:1040, 1978.
5. Bartnicki-Garcia, S. Cell wall chemistry, morphogenesis, and taxonomy of fungi. *Ann. Rev. Microb.* 22:87, 1968.
6. Beggs, W. H., Andrews, F. A., and Sarosi, G. A. Synergistic action of amphotericin B and antioxidants against certain opportunistic yeast pathogens. *Antimicrob. Agents Chemother.* 13:266, 1978.

7. Beheshti, F., Smith, A. G., and Krause, G. W. Germ tube and chlamydospore formation by *Candida albicans* on a new medium. *J. Clin. Microbiol.* 2:345, 1975.

8. Bergen, L., and Wagner-Merner, D. T. Comparative survey of fungi and potential pathogenic fungi from selected beaches in the Tampa Bay area. *Mycologia* 69:299, 1977.

9. Bowman, P. I., and Ahearn, D. G. Evaluation of commercial systems for the identification of clinical yeast isolates. *J. Clin. Microbiol.* 4:49, 1976.

10. Chin, G. N., et al. Keratomycosis in Wisconsin. *Am. J. Ophthalmol.* 79:121, 1975.

11. Cuero, R. G. Ecological distribution of *Fusarium solanae* and its opportunistic action related to mycotic keratitis in Cali, Colombia. *J. Clin. Microbiol.* 12:455, 1980.

12. Diamond, R. D., Krzesicki, R., and Jao, W. Damage to pseudohyphal forms of *Candida albicans* by neutrophils in the absence of serum in vitro. *J. Clin. Invest.* 61:349, 1978.

13. Diamond, R. D., et al. Properties of a product of *Candida albicans* hyphae and pseudohyphae that inhibits contact between the fungi and human neutrophils in vitro. *J. Immunol.* 125:2797, 1980.

14. Diamond, R. D., and Haudenschild, C. C. Monoctye-mediated serum-independent damage to hyphal and pseudohyphal forms of *Candida albicans* in vitro. *J. Clin. Invest.* 67:173, 1981.

15. Elliott, I. D., Halde, C., and Shapiro, J. Keratitis and endophthalmitis caused by *Petriellidium boydii*. *Am. J. Ophthalmol.* 83:16, 1977.

16. Elliott, J. H., et al. Mycotic endophthalmitis in drug abusers. *Am. J. Ophthalmol.* 88:66, 1979.

17. Emmons, C. W., et al. *Medical Mycology* (3rd ed.) Philadelphia: Lea & Febiger, 1977. P. 299.

18. Flegel, T. W. Semipermanent microscope slides of microfungi using a sticky tape technique. *Can. J. Microbiol.* 26:551, 1980.

19. Foster, C. S. Miconazole therapy for keratomycosis. *Am. J. Ophthalmol.* 91:622, 1981.

20. Forster, R. K., and Rebell, G. The diagnosis and management of keratomycoses. *Arch. Ophthalmol.* 93:1134, 1975.

21. Forster, R. K., Rebell, G., and Stiles, W. Recurrent keratitis due to *Acremonium potronii*. *Am. J. Ophthalmol.* 79:126, 1975.

22. Forster, R. K., et al. Methenamine silver-stained corneal scrapings in keratomycosis. *Am. J. Ophthalmol.* 82:261, 1976.

23. Francois, J., and Rijsselaere, M. Corticosteroids and ocular mycoses: Experimental study. *Ann. Ophthalmol.* 6:207, 1974.

24. Gadebusch, H. H., et al. Amphotericin B and amphotericin B methyl ester ascorbate: I. Chemotherapeutic activity against *Candida albicans, Cryptococcus. J. Infect. Dis.* 134:423, 1976.

25. Gadebusch, H. H. Candidiasis: An Infectious Disease of Increasing Importance. In D. Schlessinger (Ed.), *Microbiology*. Washington, D.C.: American Society of Microbiology, 1981. P. 199.

26. Halde, C., and Okumoto, M. Ocular mycoses: A study of 82 cases. *Excepta Med. Int. Cong. Ser.* 146:705, 1966.

27. Hamilton-Miller, J. M. T. Chemistry and biology of the polyene macrolide antibiotics. *Bacteriol. Rev.* 37:166, 1973.

28. Hazen, K. C., and Cutler, J. E. Autoregulation of germ tube formation by *Candida albicans. Infect. Immun.* 24:661, 1979.

29. Henderson, D. K., Edwards, J. E., Jr., and Montgomerie, J. Z. Hematogenous Candida endophthalmitis in patients receiving parenteral hyperalimentation fluids. *J. Infect. Dis.* 143:655, 1981.

30. Hogan, M. J., Thygeson, P., and Kimura, S. J. Uses and abuses of adrenal steroids and corticotropin. *Trans. Am. Ophthalmol. Soc.* 52:145, 1954.

31. Howlett, J. A., and Squier, C. A. *Candida albicans* ultrastructure: Colonization and invasion of oral epithelium. *Infect. Immun.* 29:252, 1980.

32. Jones, D. B. Fungal Keratitis. In T. D. Duane (Ed.), *Clinical Ophthalmology*, Vol. 4. Hagerstown, Md.: Harper & Row, 1978.

33. Kaufman, L. Laboratory Diagnosis of Candidiasis. In D. Schlessinger (Ed.), *Microbiology*. Washington, D.C.: American Society of Microbiology, 1981.

34. Krachmer, J. H., et al. Helminthosporium corneal ulcers. *Am. J. Ophthalmol.* 85:666, 1978.

35. Kulshrestha, O. P., Bhargava, S., and Dube, M. K. Keratomycosis: A report of 23 cases. *Indian J. Ophthalmol.* 21:51, 1973.

36. Kurup, V. P., and Fink, J. N. Evaluation of methods to detect antibodies against *Aspergillus fumigatus. Am. J. Clin. Pathol.* 69:414, 1978.

37. Land, G. A., et al. Evaluation of the new API 20C strip for yeast identification against a conventional method. *J. Clin. Microbiol.* 10:357, 1979.

38. Levetin, E., and Hurewitz, D. A one-year survey of the airborne molds of Tulsa, Oklahoma: II. Indoor survey. *Ann. Allergy* 41:25, 1978.

39. Liesgang, T. J., and Forster, R. K. Spectrum of microbial keratitis in south Florida. *Am. J. Ophthalmol.* 90:38, 1980.

40. Lim, G. Distribution of *Fusarium* in some British soils. *Mycopath. Mycologia Appl.* 52:231, 1974.

41. Lou, P., et al. Successful treatment of Candida endophthalmitis with a synergistic combination of amphotericin B and rifampin. *Am. J. Ophthalmol.* 83:12, 1977.

42. Manning, M., and Mitchell, T. G. Morphogenesis of *Candida albicans* and cytoplasmic proteins associated with differences in mor-

phology, strain, or temperature. *J. Bacteriol.* 144:258, 1980.

43. Mark, M. I., and Eichoff, T. C. Application of four methods to the study of the susceptibility of yeast to 5-fluorocytosine. *Antimicrob. Agents Chemother.* 1970. P. 491.

44. McCallan, S. E. A. History of Fungicides. In D. C. Torgeson (Ed.), *Fungicides.* New York: Academic, 1967. Vol. 1, pp. 1–37.

45. McGinnis, M. R. *Laboratory Handbook of Medical Mycology.* New York: Academic, 1980. Pp. 46–55.

46. Michelson, P. E., Rupp, R., and Efthimiadis, B. Endogenous Candida endophthalmitis leading to bilateral corneal performation. *Am. J. Ophthalmol.* 80:800, 1975.

47. Odds, F. C., et al. The activity in vitro and in vivo of a new imidazole antifungal, keto-conazole. *J. Antimicrob. Chemother.* 6:97, 1980.

48. Odds, F. C. Laboratory evaluation of antifungal agents: A comparative study of five imidazole derivatives of clinical importance. *J. Antimicrob. Chemother.* 6:749, 1980.

49. Peterson, E. A., Alling, D. A., and Kirkpatrick, C. H. Treatment of chronic mucocutaneous candidiasis with ketoconazole. *Ann. Intern. Med.* 93:791, 1980.

50. Polack, F. M., Siverio, G., and Bresky, R. H. Corneal chromomycosis: Double infection by *Phialophora verrucosa* (Medlar) and *Cladosporium cladosporoides* (Frescenius). *Ann. Ophthalmol.* 8:139, 1976.

51. Qadri, S. M. H., and Nichols, C. W. Evaluation of a commercial multitest system for identification of yeasts. *Am. J. Med. Technol.* 44:368, 1978.

52. Rabinovich, S., et al. Effect of 5-fluorocytosine and amphotericin B on *Candida albicans* infection in mice. *J. Infect. Dis.* 130:28, 1974.

53. Rao, P. N. S., and Rao, K. N. A. Study of the normal conjunctival flora (bacterial and fungal) and its relations to external ocular infections. *Indian J. Ophthalmol.* 20:164, 1972.

54. Rodrigues, M. M., and Laibson, P. Exogenous mycotic keratitis caused by *Blastomyces dermatitidis. Am. J. Ophthalmol.* 75:782, 1973.

55. Rodrigues, M. M., and Laibson, P. Exogenous corneal ulcer caused by *Tritrachium roseum. Am. J. Ophthalmol.* 80:804, 1975.

56. Rogers, T. J., and Balish, E. Immunity to *Candida albicans. Microbiol. Rev.* 44:660, 1980.

57. Rosenblatt, H. M., et al. Successful treatment of chronic mucocutaneous candidiasis with ketoconazole. *J. Pediatr.* 97:657, 1980.

58. Saltarelli, C. G., Gentile, K. A., and Mancuso, S. C. Lethality of *Candida* strains as influenced by the host. *Can. J. Microbiol.* 21:648, 1975.

59. Schwartz, L. K., Loignon, L. M., and Webster, R. G. Post-traumatic phycomycosis of the anterior segment. *Arch. Ophthalmol.* 96:860, 1978.

60. Shadomy, S. Further in vitro studies with 5-fluorocytosine. *Infect. Immun.* 2:484, 1970.

61. Smolin, G., and Okumoto, M. Antilymphocyte serum potentiation of Candida keratitis. *Am. J. Ophthalmol.* 66:804, 1968.

62. Sobel, J. D., Myers, P. G., and Levison, M. E. Adherence of *Candida albicans* to human vaginal and buccal epithelial cells. *J. Infect. Dis.* 143:76, 1981.

63. Stern, G. A. In vitro antibiotic synergism against ocular fungal isolates. *Am. J. Ophthalmol.* 86:359, 1978.

64. Thygeson, P., and Okumoto, M. Keratomycosis: A preventable disease. *Trans. Am. Acad. Ophthalmol. Otolaryngol.* 78:433, 1974.

65. Tkachyk, S. J., and Khan, R. S. Airborne mold survey—Edmonton. *J. Asthma Res.* 14:103, 1977.

66. Tomar, V. P. S., Sharma, O. P., and Joshi, K. Bacterial and fungal flora of normal conjunctiva. *Ann. Ophthalmol.* 3:669, 1971.

67. Utz, J. P. Chemotherapy for the systemic mycoses: The prelude to ketoconazole. *Rev. Infect. Dis.* 2:625, 1980.

68. Washington, J. A. *Laboratory Procedures in Clinical Microbiology.* New York: Springer, 1981. P. 473.

69. Williams, D. M., Weiner, M. H., and Drutz, D. J. Immunologic studies of disseminated infection with *Aspergillus fumigatus* in the nude mouse. *J. Infect. Dis.* 143:726, 1981.

70. Wogan, G. N. Mycotoxins. *Ann. Rev. Pharmacol.* 15:437, 1975.

Antibiotic Mechanisms

Jules Baum

The practicing ophthalmologist prescribes antibiotics routinely as a prophylactic or treatment for minor external disease. Less commonly, he or she confronts serious bacterial ocular infection, and then judicious selection of antibiotics, with due thought to proper dosage and routes of administration, is often crucial in preventing permanent loss of vision. The busy practitioner, perhaps long out of residency training, often turns to a therapeutic regimen from a standard reference book. However, knowledge of the principles of antibiotic action generates an understanding of the "cookbook" formulas and affords the clinician the opportunity to modify a regimen, if the need occurs, based on a more basic understanding of antibiotic mechanisms and pharmacokinetics. The purpose of this section is to provide a useful background in these areas.

RESISTANCE OF BACTERIA TO ANTIBIOTICS
Resistance or susceptibility to an antibiotic is usually determined in the laboratory by the size of the zone of inhibition of bacterial growth around an antibiotic-impregnated disc, the so-called Kirby-Bauer test. More refined methods, however, are available, such as the broth-dilution test, which can provide information on both the minimal concentration of antibiotic needed to inhibit the bacterial strain (minimal inhibitory concentration, or MIC) and the lowest concentration needed to kill the organisms (minimal bactericidal concentration, or MBC). Nonetheless, the basic information conveyed by the various methods is similar. It must be remembered that the Kirby-Bauer test is designed to reflect susceptibility to levels achievable in the serum. Much higher levels than those in the serum are produced in the tears after local therapy, and much lower ones are achieved in intraocular tissues and fluids.

There are four major mechanisms by which bacteria are resistant to antibiotics. These are bacterial enzymes, permeability barriers, target alteration, and cell wall resistance [28, 34, 45].

BACTERIAL ENZYMES
The bacteria may produce enzymes that inactivate or destroy the antibiotic. This was first discovered with staphylococci that produce penicillinases, enzymes that are liberated into the environment of the bacterium and destroy various penicillins. The "penicillinase-resistant" penicillins such as methicillin, oxacillin, and nafcillin (and later the cephalosporins) were developed because they are relatively resistant to these enzymes and retain activity against staphylococci. The genetic information for production of such enzymes is carried on bacteriophages, small viral-like particles of DNA that can be passed (like a viral infection) throughout the bacteria in a colony of staphylococci, or even from one strain to another. This is called transduction. However, if the bacteria causing an infection lack this information to start with, they will not acquire it in vivo unless a second bacterial strain intrudes.

Gram-negative bacilli produce inactivating enzymes in even wider variety than do gram-positive cocci. Enteric bacilli and *Pseudomonas aeruginosa* may constitutively produce beta-lactamases that destroy a variety of penicillins and cephalosporins. They may also produce aminoglycoside-inactivating enzymes. Other enzymes inactivate chloramphenicol and various other antibiotics. Slight modifications in the antibiotic molecules, however, can confer resistance to these degrading enzymes. Thus, carbenicillin and ticarcillin are active against many strains of *Pseudomonas aeruginosa*, whereas most other penicillins are not. Although the traditional cephalosporins are all without appreciable activity against *Pseudomonas aeruginosa*, the "third generation" congeners such as cefotaxime, moxalactam, ceftriaxone, cefoperazone, and ceftazidime may show activity against this organism, largely because of resistance to the degrading enzymes. Similarly, although gentamicin and tobramycin are active against the large majority (perhaps 95 percent) of gram-negative bacilli in most hospitals, some strains are resistant. Most of the resistant strains (about 80 percent) are still susceptible to amikacin because this agent is less susceptible to the destructive enzymes produced by the organisms.

The genetic information for production of these inactivating enzymes may be carried on the chromosome (constitutively produced) or on bits of extrachromosomal DNA called plasmids. If the organism also possesses the special plasmid segment called resistance transfer factor (RTF), it is capable of producing a pilus, copulating with another bacterium, and passing information on by mating (conjugation). If the RTF becomes linked to an R-determinant and forms an R-factor, (plasmid), there is efficient transfer of the resistance plasmids within species or even among different species of bacteria. Transduction is the major method of passing information among gram-positive bacteria; conjugation is a dominant mechanism for passing genetic information among gram-negative ones.

Recently, species of bacteria that were traditionally highly sensitive to penicillins such as penicillin G and ampicillin have yielded occasional strains that are highly resistant because of production of beta-lactamases. This has been rare with the pneumococcus, but is increasingly commonly encountered with the gonococcus and is now true of 20 to 30 percent of isolates of *Haemophilus influenzae* type b.

Gram-negative bacilli make much better use of the ability to produce antibiotic-inactivating enzymes than do gram-positive cocci. The reasons for this lie in the basic structure of the bacteria. In gram-positive organisms, the peptidoglycan layer or "cell wall," which lies outside the cytoplasmic membrane and is the target of penicillins and cephalosporins, lies exposed to the environment. Although there may be a capsule of some type, there is no important obstacle to prevent antibiotic in the environment from getting to the target. Thus, these organisms must release beta-lactamases in large quantities into the environment in the hope of destroying antibiotic by sheer bulk. In contrast, gram-negative bacilli possess a cell membrane outside the peptidoglycan layer. This membrane serves both as a permeability barrier that reduces antibiotic entry (see below) and as a container that keeps the enzymes in the critical location around the peptidoglycan wall. Thus, small amounts of enzymes, strategically placed where they can readily set upon any drug that passes through the outer membrane, prove highly effective in protecting gram-negative bacteria from beta-lactam antibiotics. This strategic effect also keeps aminoglycoside-inactivating enzymes in the periplasmic space, thereby preventing aminoglycosides from entering the cytoplasm to reach their target, the ribosome.

PERMEABILITY BARRIERS

The bacterium may contain a permeability barrier that prevents antibiotics from reaching the target. The net effect is rather similar to that of inactivating enzymes, but is much less specific, i.e., the barriers that restrict passage of one type of antibiotic often tend to reduce passage of many structurally unrelated drugs. Moreover, the degree of resistance conferred is usually not as great as that produced by enzymatic inactivation, i.e., the MIC may be increased by only severalfold. The frequency of this kind of bacterial resistance is not really known. It appears to be important in the low-level resistance of gonococci to many antibiotics (penicillins, tetracyclines, spectinomycin) and of pneumococci. It probably also contributes to resistance of gram-negative bacilli to aminoglycosides and possibly to other antibiotics.

TARGET ALTERATION

There may be alteration in the target so that the antibiotic no longer has a site to bind to or interfere with. Indeed, humans have virtually no targets with appreciable affinity for beta-lactam antibiotics, which is why they are so nontoxic to the host. In some instances, the species of bacterium has never had an appropriate receptor site and is intrinsically resistant to the antibiotic. In others, resistance is acquired, usually by mutation of the target. However, because the targets of most antibiotics are fundamental to important structural and metabolic functions, extreme mutations are often not compatible with bacterial survival. Thus, this mechanism of acquiring resistance is not a common one clinically. When resistance does occur, it is usually a spontaneous mutation (i.e., it would occur whether or not the antibiotic was present), but the progeny are selected out by the pressure of the antibiotic in the environment. Thus, only the mutants survive. Examples include resistance of tubercle bacilli and gram-negative bacteria to streptomycin and resistance of various bacteria to rifampin. This is one of the reasons we do not generally treat infections with these drugs alone but rather include a second agent that can inhibit or kill the few mutants that may arise. Resistance to sulfonamides typically occurs by virtue of alteration of the target enzymes for folate synthesis. The combination of trimethoprim and sulfamethoxazole is bactericidal in part because the two drugs, acting in sequence on one pathway, rarely induce resistance (which would require a double mutation).

CELL WALL RESISTANCE

There is a special type of methicillin resistance among staphylococci. These organisms are highly resistant to penicillinase-resistant penicillins, not by virtue of the enzymes they produce, but because (apparently) of unusual characteristics of the cell wall. Thus far, such strains are rare in North America.

Recently, interest has focused upon another mode of resistance to cell wall–active drugs. It has become clear that the traditional belief that beta-lactam antibiotics kill bacteria by interfering with cell wall synthesis is an oversimplification. This effect is enough to prevent bacterial multiplication but, for many species, is not enough to cause cell death. Instead, the inhibition of peptidoglycan synthesis is a prelude to the release of autolytic enzymes (housed in the space between peptidoglycan and cytoplasmic membrane) that cause the cell to commit suicide. Some bacteria (primarily gram-positive cocci) are inhibited but not killed by beta-lactam drugs even at high concentrations. They are said to be tolerant to the drugs. The reason appears to be that these organisms are intrinsically deficient in autolytic enzymes. This has been a problem with *Staphylococcus aureus*: As many as 40 percent of strains are tolerant to penicillinase-resistant penicillins in some areas of the country. However, the true frequency of this phenomenon is not known. In summary, staphylococci may be resistant to older penicillins because they produce penicillinases; they may be resistant to penicillinase-resistant penicillins either because they lack autolytic enzymes (methicillin-tolerant strains) or because they have unusual cell wall structure (methicillin-resistant strains). Methicillin-tolerant strains are inhibited but not killed by the drug; methicillin-resistant organisms are not inhibited by the antibiotic.

CATEGORIES OF ANTIBIOTICS ACCORDING TO MECHANISM OF ACTION

INHIBITORS OF CELL WALL SYNTHESIS

Inhibitors of cell wall synthesis act upon the peptidoglycan layer (or cell wall) and interfere with its rigidity, which allows the high osmotic pressure in the bacterial cytoplasm to rupture the cell. The major cell wall–active drugs include the penicillins, cephalosporins, vancomycin and bacitracin. These are generally bactericidal rather than bacteriostatic drugs. (This distinction is explained below.) Alternatively, in a milieu of high osmotic pressure such as the renal interstitium, bacteria may persist as spheroplast or L-forms after antibiotic treatment. Whether such cell wall–defective organisms are the cause of relapse or occult infection is not clear.

INHIBITORS OF PROTEIN SYNTHESIS

Examples of drugs that inhibit protein synthesis include the aminoglycosides such as gentamicin, tobramycin, amikacin, streptomycin, and neomycin, and also chloramphenicol, erythromycin, clindamycin, spectinomycin, and the tetracyclines.

Bacterial protein synthesis takes place in the cytoplasm and occurs in three stages: initiation, elongation, and termination. The antibiotics in this group bind to bacterial ribosomes and "freeze" protein synthesis. The aminoglycosides bind to the 30S subunit of the ribosome; chloramphenicol, erythromycin, clindamycin, spectinomycin, and the tetracyclines bind to the 50S subunit. Each of the

antibiotics seems to bind somewhat differently, and the biochemical processes have been only partially elucidated. Rifampin inhibits RNA synthesis.

ANTIMETABOLITES

Examples of antimetabolites include sulfonamides and trimethoprim.

Mammals depend exclusively on exogenous folate for their metabolic processes. However, bacteria do not appear to incorporate exogenous folate well and must synthesize the vitamin. These differences form the basis for the selective toxicity of sulfonamides against bacteria but not human cells. Trimethoprim acts at a different stage of the same metabolic pathway but, in contrast to the sulfonamides, rapidly inhibits bacterial growth. The combination of these two drugs is synergistic.

ANTIBIOTICS THAT INCREASE CELL PERMEABILITY

Examples of antibiotics that increase cell permeability include the polymyxins, colistin (polymyxin E), and gramicidin. The antibiotics in this group may be thought of as membrane detergents; they kill bacteria by opening up their cell membrane, causing a leak of small essential molecules (phosphate, nucleosides). There is a direct relationship between the extent of the leak and the bactericidal effect of the antibiotic. Why these antibiotics attach to some, but not other, cell membranes has yet to be clarified.

MECHANISMS OF ACTION

BACTERIOSTATIC VERSUS BACTERICIDAL ACTION

Some antibiotics (bactericidal) kill bacteria outright; others (bacteriostatic), which only inhibit bacterial growth, rely more heavily on host defense mechanisms such as phagocytosis, antibodies, and complement to eliminate the infection. Knowledge of these groupings is clinically important. Patients with impaired host defense mechanisms (because of immunosuppression, diabetes, or malnutrition) will fare better with bactericidal (penicillins, cephalosporins, aminoglycosides) than with bacteriostatic (chloramphenicol, tetracyclines, erythromycin) antibiotics. Some "static" antibiotics may become "cidal" at higher concentrations (erythromycin, chloramphenicol) or when exposed to a different environment (sulfonamides within pus). The conjunctiva and cornea are examples of anatomic sites at which high concentrations of antibiotic are developed.

SYNERGISM AND ANTAGONISM

In most instances, simultaneous exposure of a bacterium to two antibiotics produces an additive effect, i.e., the effect is the sum of the effects of the individual agents. In the case of synergy, the total effect is greater than one would expect from the sum of the two independent effects. However, in some instances, the reverse occurs, i.e., the combination is antagonistic—the effect is less than the effect of either drug alone. Although there is a vast literature describing synergy and antagonism of scores of combinations of drugs in vitro, there is little evidence that such interactions are important in vivo. However, occasionally they may be clinically important. Thus, there are data that indicate that the activity of penicillin G may be compromised by the simultaneous administration of tetracycline in pneumococcal meningitis, and that the activity of ampicillin against *Haemophilus influenzae* may be slightly reduced by simultaneous administration of chloramphenicol. Although antibiotics are often given in combination in hopes of a beneficial effect, true synergy is rarely evident. The few situations in which synergy has been well demonstrated include the use of ampicillin (or penicillin G) together with an aminoglycoside for severe enterococcal infection and the use of two drugs to treat tuberculosis (largely because the emergence of resistant organisms is thwarted). It is common practice to give carbenicillin or ticarcillin together with an aminoglycoside for serious *Pseudomonas* infections; however, the evidence that the combination is synergistic is not compelling [40]. It has been suggested, in the case of the enterococcus, that the cell wall–active drug (penicillin) damages the cell wall, permitting the ribosome-active drug to gain access to the cytoplasm. In antagonistic combinations such as those mentioned above, it has been suggested that the use of a bacteriostatic drug inhibits cell division, thereby depriving the cell wall–active drug of the necessary targets for action. Despite this kind of rationale, attempts to derive generalizations that will predict which combinations are synergistic or antagonistic (e.g., combination of bactericidal with bacteriostatic drug) have not been fruitful. Such generalizations are not invariable, and each combination, except perhaps for those mentioned above, must be tested individually. There are other reasons why antibiotic combinations should be avoided if not indicated: the fostering of multiple drug resistance, the clinical confusion that may occur if an adverse reaction occurs that is not clearly attributable to one of the agents, and the enhanced likelihood of bacterial overgrowth because the normal flora is broadly inhibited. However, there are many circumstances in which combination therapy is indicated—mixed infections, infections in which the cause is not known, and instances in which true synergy has been demonstrated.

INACTIVATION

A general rule of drug delivery is to avoid combining drugs in vitro unless it has been demonstrated that one drug does not inactivate the other. In ophthalmic practice, we caution against mixing two antibiotics in the same syringe for a periocular injection, although both drugs soon combine in the sub-Tenon's space. In practical clinical terms, this admonition may be overstated, since even with the worst combination, inactivation of aminoglycoside by carbenicillin, the effectiveness of the aminoglycoside is reduced only 50 percent in 24 hours in vitro and even less in vivo. Since high concentrations of antibiotics in cornea are obtained by topical administration and by periocular injections, inactivation of antibiotics may be a relatively unimportant consideration in the treatment of bacterial corneal infections.

PHARMACOKINETICS

Infectious disease of the cornea is treated, in almost all instances, by topical administration of drops and ointments and by subconjunctival injections. This section discusses and compares the pharmacokinetics of these two routes of administration and evaluates their effectiveness. The pharmacokinetics of parenteral and oral administration are also considered. These comparisons are limited by differences between the rabbit model and the human eye and by variance in experimental protocols among investigators. For instance, Maurice and Ota [39] found that when fluorescein was given as a subconjunctival injection it streamed out the hole made by the injection in the rabbit conjunctiva; however, there was very little reflux seen in humans by slit lamp examination. Moreover, 100 times more fluorescein entered the anterior chamber in humans than in rabbits after comparable subconjunctival injections. A subconjunctival injection raises the serum concentration to a level similar to that following an intramuscular injection. Since the eye-to-body size ratio is much higher in the rabbit than in the human, an equivalent dose administered subconjunctivally produces much higher serum levels in rabbits than in humans. Indeed, the serum levels produced in the rabbit are of a magnitude that would normally be expected using intramuscular or intravenous therapy [2]. They may indirectly contribute to the intraocular levels of drug in a way that would not occur in humans. These differences between rabbit and human suggest caution when extrapolating from one species to the other.

TOPICAL ADMINISTRATION

EYE DROPS

A representative series of studies in rabbits documents that in most instances the concentration of antibiotic was 15 μg per gram or less in the cornea after topical administration of eye drops [2, 13, 14, 24, 25, 29, 30, 31, 37, 47, 49]. The lipophilic antibiotics chloramphenicol and tetracycline produced some of the highest corneal concentrations. Although differences in methods and data reporting prevent direct comparison among all the studies, the following observations can be made: Higher corneal concentrations of drugs were achieved in abraded or inflamed corneas than in normal ones; higher concentrations of administered drug and longer contact times resulted in higher tissue concentrations; and a lipophilic antibiotic such as chloramphenicol, which penetrates corneal epithelium more easily than do nonlipophilic antibiotics, produced higher corneal concentration when administered as an ointment than when given as an eye drop. These data are scanty, and the above are only generalizations. However, there are other data supporting these postulates. Davis and colleagues [21] demonstrated that concentrated eye drops were more effective than less concentrated ones in reducing the bacterial colony count in *Pseudomonas* keratitis in the guinea pig. As an illustration of the effects of longer contact time, Mishima and Nagataki showed that methylcellulose greatly increased peak concentrations of pilocarpine in iris after topical application; the bioavailability was about three times that of the solution without the methylcellulose [42]. They found no advantage in increasing the viscosity of the ophthalmic solution above 10 to 20 cp, which corresponds to hydroxymethylcellulose concentrations of 0.38 to 0.5 percent.

Tear dynamics play a role in determining bioavailability of antibiotic to cornea. The average size of an eye drop from a squeeze bottle is 40 to 50 μl. A recent study showed that increasing drop size of fluorescein from 5 to 20 μl resulted in only a minimal increase in the initial tear concentration of fluorescein [55], which demonstrates a more rapid drainage of the larger eye drop with little time for mixing of fluorescein with tears. In the same study, various volumes of pilocarpine solution (5, 10, 20, and 50 μl) were instilled in the eye, and pupil responses were measured. Increasing the drop size to over 20 μl did little to increase pupil size. Both the fluorescein and pilocarpine studies show that the reflex stimulation of tear flow and poor mixing of drug and tears induced by large drop administration produce a rapid exit of fluid through the lacrimal outflow tract. These data suggest that drop sizes larger than 20 μl are no more effective than smaller ones. Manufacturers should consider reducing drop size for commercial topical medications. Since the maximum volume the eye can hold is 30 μl [41], administration of two successive drops merely increases systemic absorption in some instances without enhancing drug effect. Similar principles apply to the instillation of two different eye drops consecutively. Since it has been demonstrated that reflex stimulation caused by a 1-μl eye drop takes 5 minutes to subside [41], it may be desirable to wait at least 5 minutes before instilling a second eye drop; however, practical considerations frequently require closer spacing of drops.

Instillation of concentrated antibiotic eye drops, made from isotonic tear solutions to which parenteral medications are added, are generally advised for the treatment of a bacterial corneal ulcer. However, such solutions are invariably hypertonic, and the tonicity affects the bioavailability of the drug. The more concentrated the solution, the greater the tonicity. Maurice [38] has shown, after instillation of eye drops containing fluorescein in the human eye, that increasing the tonicity of the drops above that of body fluids leads to their immediate dilution by osmosis, with no increased penetration of fluorescein into the eye. This study suggests that concentrated antibiotic eye drops induce reflex tearing and are therefore further diluted. Hence, corneal tissue concentrations would not be directly proportional to the increased concentration of the eye drop. In contrast, however, as stated above, Davis and coworkers [21] demonstrated increased effectiveness of concentrated antibiotic eye drops in a guinea pig model. This apparent discrepancy may relate less to the model and drug than to the effect of the preservative on drug penetration [17]. More recently, Sidikaro and Jones [50], using human volunteers, measured the kinetics of gentamicin after instillation of solutions with concentrations of 3 and 13.6 mg per milliliter. They detected higher concentrations of gentamicin in the tears over a 1-hour interval after instillation of the more concentrated eye drops. In summary, these data suggest that more concentrated antibiotic eye drops are more effective than those commercially available and should be employed for the treatment of bacterial corneal ulcers. Drug companies should be encouraged, in the public interest, to manufacture such products.

Increased frequency of administration of antibiotic eye drops also helps achieve higher corneal levels of antibiotics. I believe that in treating bacterial corneal ulcers, drops should be given every 30 minutes if possible, to obtain and maintain therapeutic concentrations in the cornea [11, 18, 51].

In de-epithelialized corneas the uptake of antibiotic is greater than in intact corneas [13, 46].

OINTMENTS

I do not use antibiotic ointments to treat bacterial corneal ulcers, because, once applied, they retard subsequent penetration of eye drops [56]. Administration of fortified eye drops every 30 minutes probably results in higher corneal drug levels than ointments do, although there are no studies that substantiate this belief. Ointments do, however, increase corneal and intraocular penetration of pilocarpine [42], fluorescein [57], and tetracycline [54] as compared with eye drops.

SUBCONJUNCTIVAL INJECTIONS
Periocular injections of antibiotics, although called subconjunctival, are in almost all instances anterior sub-Tenon's injections. However, there is probably an insignificant therapeutic difference between the two routes [32, 44, 58]. Antibiotic levels in conjunctiva, cornea, and aqueous are higher after a subconjunctival injection than after a retrobulbar (posterior sub-Tenon's) injection [7].

A representative series of studies in rabbits has shown that the corneal concentrations after subconjunctival injection are all at therapeutic levels and are strikingly high [1, 4, 5, 8–10, 14, 26, 33, 43, 51, 54]. There is no doubt that subconjunctival injections, for almost all antibiotics tested, achieve therapeutic levels soon after injection. However, such injections are routinely administered at 12- to 24-hour intervals, and during this interval corneal concentrations fall off rapidly [4, 8, 10, 11, 14, 43, 49].

A subconjunctival injection leaves a hole, if not a rent, in the conjunctiva through which a drug may exit, decreasing the bolus and increasing drug concentration in the tears. It has been shown that less than 10 percent of a subconjunctival dose is lost to the tears [6]. The rest either enters the ocular tissues directly, is carried away in the systemic circulation, or diffuses posteriorly in the sub-Tenon's space. Large topographic differences in corneal concentrations exist after subconjunctival injections; the highest concentration is nearest the injection site [5, 43]. This unevenness of distribution suggests that most drug enters the cornea by direct diffusion through tissue, rather than through the precorneal tear film. It might be expected that drug concentrations in the cornea would be higher in inflamed than noninflamed eyes; however, no clear trend is seen [5], probably because of a larger flow of drug away from the cornea through the engorged conjunctival vessels in the inflamed eye [6]. A confounding factor lies in the report by Maurice and Ota [39]. Very little reflux of fluorescein was seen coming from the hole after a subconjunctival injection in a human volunteer. In the rabbit, fluorescein poured out of the hole, and there was 100-fold less fluorescein in the rabbit cornea than in the human. Although the authors cast doubt on the clinical relevance of studies of subconjunctival injections in rabbits, their study drew on only three human volunteers. In my opinion, the rabbit has been and will be a valuable, though limited, model.

PROS AND CONS OF TOPICAL VERSUS SUBCONJUNCTIVAL ADMINISTRATION
A bacterial corneal ulcer is a sight-threatening condition that demands prompt sterilization. In the last decade, we have witnessed a dramatic improvement in our ability to sterilize such ulcers, decrease morbidity, and preserve vision, largely owing to the use of new antibiotics and the recognition of the need to achieve higher and more sustained corneal concentration of drug. Augmented corneal drug levels have been achieved by increasing the concentration and frequency of application of topical antibiotic eye drops and by the use of subconjunctival injections.

Although subconjunctival injections are in common use today to treat severe corneal infections, invariably in combination with topical therapy, there are no data to indicate that the subconjunctival route or the combination of routes is more effective than the topical therapy alone. Furthermore, the data that are available concerning the relative efficacy of these two routes generally have been derived either by measuring tissue concentration of the drug after administration or by evaluating the effectiveness of an antibiotic in eradicating an infection, i.e., the number of bacteria killed. The second technique is more direct and gives a more straightforward answer. Curiously, to date, no investigators have employed the two techniques simultaneously.

The data documenting falloff in drug levels hours after a subconjunctival injection suggest that, in the majority of instances, only 0.02 to 0.1 percent of the original amount of drug injected persist 3 to 6 hours after injection (Table 4-7). Such levels are probably therapeutic in most instances. Similarly, a number of studies of experimental bacterial keratitis suggest that subconjunctival injections are effective in killing bacteria [15, 23, 27, 52, 53].

Peak values are not as high after topical administration as after subconjunctival injections. However, drops can be instilled frequently enough (every 15–30 minutes) to maintain high tissue levels of drug. Moreover, in virtually all instances, drug levels are higher in eyes with epithelium absent or deranged over a bacterial corneal ulcer than in normal eyes covered with epithelium.

As stated above, more important than determining tissue concentrations is evaluating the effectiveness of an antibiotic in eradicating bacteria in the infected cornea. Davis and coworkers performed a comprehensive series of experiments, mainly in guinea pigs, in part to determine whether the topical, subconjunctival, or parenteral route was most effective in eradicating organisms from bacterial corneal ulcers. They found the topical route most effective [18–20, 22, 23], especially with more concentrated antibiotic eye drops [21], with more frequent applications [18], when the corneal epithelium was removed [21], and when treatment

was started early [21]. Kupferman and Liebowitz also demonstrated the efficacy of topical therapy in eradicating organisms [35].

That frequent administration of concentrated antibiotic eye drops can eliminate bacteria from infectious experimental corneal ulcers has been adequately demonstrated, as described above. Anecdotal clinical data also attest that such therapy can sterilize bacterial corneal ulcers. That topical therapy in an experimental model is more effective than subconjunctival injections has been demonstrated by Davis and coworkers [22] and recently confirmed by Kupferman and Liebowitz [36]. Yet it is difficult to reconcile these efficacy studies that demonstrate the superiority of topical over subconjunctival administration with studies showing massive concentrations of antibiotic in cornea after subconjunctival injections (Table 4-7).

Clinically, topical and subconjunctival injections are often administered concomitantly in the treatment of bacterial keratitis. If it can be proved that topical therapy is more effective, does it follow that

TABLE 4-7. *Peak Concentration of Antibiotics in Rabbit Cornea After Subconjunctival Administration*

Antibiotic and Dose (mg)	Concentration in Normal Eyes* (μg/g)	Concentration in Inflamed Eyes* (μg/g)	Reference
Pencillin G			
100	3000 (→1500)	—	Bloome et al. [14]
50	300	—	Oakley et al. [43]
Carbenicillin			
100	>300 (→42)	>300 (→25)	Barza et al. [4]
50	15–35	—	Faris and Uwaydah [26]
Methicillin sodium			
100	—	700 (→40)	Kane et al. [33]
Oxacillin			
100	—	2000 (→500)	Kane et al. [33]
Cefazolin			
100	—	600 (→100)	Kane et al. [33]
25	>1000		Abel et al. [1]
12.5	—	150 (→40)	Kane et al. [33]
Cefamandole			
12.5	—	140 (→40)	Barza et al. [8]
Streptomycin			
50	1000	—	Bloome et al. [14]
Gentamicin			
20	—	200 (→25)	Barza et al. [10]
10	—	10	Sloan et al. [51]
5	30	10	Barza et al. [5]
Chloramphenicol			
150	50	—	Sorsby et al. [54]
50	500	—	Oakley et al. [43]
Clindamycin			
34	100	—	Barza et al. [9]

*Parentheses contain concentrations 3 to 6 hr after administration.
SOURCE. Adapted from Barza [2].

subconjunctival injections should be abandoned? The patient would, in fact, be spared the discomfort of the procedure, and the slight possibility of accidental intraocular injection would be eliminated. However, there is the ever-present problem of compliance. How can the physician be assured that eye drops will be administered every 15 to 30 minutes, even in a hospital? Won't an infant or child squeeze or cry out the drops? In the final analysis, the risk-benefit ratio of subconjunctival injections will be determined by the practicing ophthalmologist.

SYSTEMIC ADMINISTRATION

In general, higher serum and, hence, higher corneal tissue levels of antibiotic are achieved after intravenous than after intramuscular or subcutaneous injections [4, 14]. Aminoglycosides (gentamicin, tobramycin), however, may be given by either route. Ocular inflammation enhances the penetration of antibiotics from the systemic circulation into corneal tissues [12, 32]. When corneal concentrations are compared after subconjunctival injections and systemic or oral administration, the latter obviously is an inefficient route of drug delivery to the cornea [3]. In fact, there is no evidence to support the use of oral administration of antibiotic in the treatment of bacterial corneal ulcers, because both topical administration and subconjunctival injections are more effective and because the risk of serious side effects is greater after systemic administration, especially for those antibiotics whose side effects are dose-related (i.e., aminoglycosides). There is no valid reason, in my opinion, to administer systemic antibiotics in the treatment of a nonperforating bacterial corneal ulcer, because of the reasons stated above and because bacteria have never been demonstrated intraocularly before a corneal perforation. Systemic antibiotics are indicated, however, if the cornea perforates, if there is extension to sclera, if *Neisseria gonorrhoeae* is the pathogen, or if *Pseudomonas* [16] or *Haemophilus influenzae* is present in infants, in which instances systemic spread of the infection may ensue.

ACKNOWLEDGMENT

I thank Michael Barza, M.D., for his suggestions and review of this chapter.

REFERENCES

1. Abel, R., Jr., et al. Intraocular penetration of cefazolin sodium in rabbits. *Am. J. Ophthalmol.* 78:779, 1974.
2. Barza, M. Treatment of bacterial infections of the eye. In J. S. Remington and M. N. Swartz (Eds.), *Current Clinical Topics in Infectious Diseases*. New York: McGraw-Hill, 1980. Pp. 159–194.
3. Barza, M., and Baum, J. Penetration of ocular compartments by penicillins. *Surv. Ophthalmol.* 18:71, 1973.
4. Barza, M., et al. Intraocular penetration of carbenicillin in the rabbit. *Am. J. Ophthalmol.* 75:307, 1973.
5. Barza, M., Baum, J. L., and Kane, A. Regional differences in ocular concentration of gentamicin after subconjunctival and retrobulbar injection in the rabbit. *Am. J. Ophthalmol.* 83:407, 1977.
6. Barza, M., Kane, A., and Baum, J. L. The excretion of gentamicin in tears of rabbits after subconjunctival injection. *Am. J. Ophthalmol.* 85:118, 1978.
7. Barza, M., Kane, A., and Baum, J. L. Intraocular penetration of gentamicin after subconjunctival and retrobulbar injection. *Am. J. Ophthalmol.* 85:541, 1978.
8. Barza, M., Kane, A., and Baum, J. L. Intraocular levels of cefamandole compared with cefazolin after subconjunctival injection in rabbits. *Invest. Ophthalmol. Vis. Sci.* 18:250, 1979.
9. Barza, M., Kane, A., and Baum, J. L. Marked differences between pigmented and albino rabbits in the concentration of clindamycin in iris and choroid-retina. *J. Infect. Dis.* 139:203, 1979.
10. Barza, M., Kane, A., and Baum, J. L. The difficulty of determining the route of intraocular penetration of gentamicin after subconjunctival injection in the rabbit. *Invest. Ophthalmol. Vis. Sci.* 20:509, 1981.
11. Baum, J. L., et al. Concentration of gentamicin in experimental corneal ulcers: Topical vs. subconjunctival therapy. *Arch. Ophthalmol.* 92:315, 1974.
12. Baum, J. L., Barza, M., and Weinstein, L. Preferred routes of antibiotic administration on treatment of bacterial ulcers of the cornea. *Int. Ophthalmol. Clin.* 13(4):31, 1973.
13. Benson, H. Permeability of the cornea to topically applied drugs. *Arch. Ophthalmol.* 91:313, 1979.
14. Bloome, M. A., Golden, B., and McKee, A. P. Antibiotic concentration in ocular tissues. Penicillin G and dihydrostreptomycin. *Arch. Ophthalmol.* 83:78, 1970.
15. Bohigian, G., Okumoto, M., and Valenton, M. Experimental *Pseudomonas* keratitis. *Arch. Ophthalmol.* 86:432, 1971.
16. Burns, R. P. *Pseudomonas* eye infection as a cause of death in premature infants. *Arch. Ophthalmol.* 65:517, 1961.
17. Burnstein, N. Preservative alteration of corneal permeability in humans and rabbits. *Invest. Ophthalmol. Vis. Sci.* In press.

18. Davis, S. D., Sarff, L. D., and Hyndiuk, R. A. Antibiotic therapy of experimental *Pseudomonas* keratitis in guinea pigs. *Arch. Ophthalmol.* 95:1638, 1977.

19. Davis, S. D., Sarff, L. D., and Hyndiuk, R. A. Failure of subconjunctival antibiotic in experimental *Pseudomonas* keratitis (abstract). *Invest. Ophthalmol. Vis. Sci.* 17 (Suppl.):228, 1978.

20. Davis, S. D., Sarff, L. D., and Hyndiuk, R. A. Staphylococcal keratitis. Experimental model in guinea pigs. *Arch. Ophthalmol.* 96:2114, 1978.

21. Davis, S. D., Sarff, L. D., and Hyndiuk, R. A. Topical tobramycin therapy of experimental *Pseudomonas* keratitis: An evaluation of some factors that potentially enhance efficacy. *Arch. Ophthalmol.* 96:123, 1978.

22. Davis, S. D., Sarff, L. D., and Hyndiuk, R. A. Comparison of therapeutic routes in experimental *Pseudomonas* keratitis. *Am. J. Ophthalmol.* 87:710, 1979.

23. Davis, S. D., Sarff, L. D., and Hyndiuk, R. A. Experimental *Pseudomonas* keratitis in guinea pigs: Therapy of moderately severe infections. *Br. J. Ophthalmol.* 63:436, 1979.

24. Ellerhorst, B. Ocular penetration of topically applied gentamicin. *Arch. Ophthalmol.* 93:371, 1975.

25. Faigenbaum, S. J., et al. Intraocular penetration of amoxicillin. *Am. J. Ophthalmol.* 82:598, 1976.

26. Faris, B. M., and Uwaydah, M. M. Intraocular penetration of semisynthetic penicillins. *Arch. Ophthalmol.* 92:501, 1974.

27. Furgiuele, F. P., Kiesel, R., and Martyn, L. *Pseudomonas* infection of the rabbit cornea treated with gentamicin: A preliminary report. *Am. J. Ophthalmol.* 60:818, 1965.

28. Gale, E. F., et al. (Eds.) *The Molecular Basis of Antibiotic Action.* London: Wiley, 1972.

29. Golden, B., and Coppel, S. P. Ocular tissue absorption of gentamicin. *Arch. Ophthalmol.* 84:792, 1970.

30. Green, K., and MacKeen, D. L. Chloramphenicol penetration on, and into, the rabbit eye. *Invest. Ophthalmol.* 15:220, 1976.

31. Hardberger, R. E., Hanna, C., and Goodart, R. Effects of drug vehicle on ocular uptake of tetracycline. *Am. J. Ophthalmol.* 80:133, 1975.

32. Hardy, R. G., Jr., and Paterson, C. A. Ocular penetration of ^{14}C-labeled chloramphenicol following subconjunctival or sub-Tenon's injection. *Am. J. Ophthalmol.* 71:1307, 1971.

33. Kane, A., Barza, M., and Baum, J. L. Ocular penetration of subconjunctival oxacillin, methacillin, and cefazolin in rabbits with staphylococcal endophthalmitis. *J. Infect. Dis.* 145:899, 1982.

34. Kucers, A., and Bennett, N. M. *The Use of Antibiotics* (3rd ed.). Philadelphia: Lippincott, 1979.

35. Kupferman, A., and Leibowitz, H. M. Topical antibiotic therapy of *Pseudomonas aeruginosa* keratitis. *Arch. Ophthalmol.* 97:1699, 1979.

36. Kupferman, A., and Leibowitz, H. M. Antibiotic therapy of bacterial keratitis: Topical application or periocular injection (abstract). *Invest. Ophthalmol. Vis. Sci.* 19 (Suppl.):112, 1980.

37. Leopold, I. H., Nichols, A. C., and Bogel, A. W. Penetration of chloramphenicol U.S.P. (Chloromycetin) into the eye. *Arch. Ophthalmol.* 44:22, 1950.

38. Maurice, D. M. The tonicity of an eye drop and its dilution by tears. *Exp. Eye Res.* 11:30, 1971.

39. Maurice, D. M., and Ota, Y. The kinetics of subconjunctival injection. *Jpn. J. Ophthalmol.* 22:95, 1978.

40. Mintz, L., and Drew, W. L. Comparative synergistic activity of cefoperazone, cefoxatime, moxalactam and carbenicillin combined with tobramycin against *Pseudomonas aeruginosa.* *Antimicrob. Agents Chemother.* 19:332, 1981.

41. Mishima, S., et al. Determination of tear volume and tear flow. *Invest. Ophthalmol.* 5:264, 1966.

42. Mishima, S., and Nagataki, S. Conrad Berens Memorial Lecture: Pharmacology of ophthalmic solution. *Contact Lens* 4:21, 1978.

43. Oakley, D. E., Weeks, R. D., and Ellis, P. P. Corneal distribution of subconjunctival antibiotics. *Am. J. Ophthalmol.* 81:307, 1976.

44. Paterson, C. A. Intraocular penetration of ^{14}C-labeled penicillin after sub-Tenon's or subconjunctival injection. *Ann. Ophthalmol.* 5:171, 1973.

45. Pratt, W. B. *Chemotherapy of Infection.* New York: Oxford University Press, 1977.

46. Praus, R., and Krejci, L. Release from hydrophilic gel contact lens and intraocular penetration. *Ophthalmol. Res.* 9:213, 1977.

47. Purnell, W. D., and McPherson, S. D., Jr. The effect of tobramycin on rabbit eyes. *Am. J. Ophthalmol.* 77:578, 1974.

48. Salminen, L. Ampicillin penetration into the rabbit eye. *Acta Ophthalmol.* 56:977, 1978.

49. Salminen, L., Järvinen, H., and Toivanen, P. Distribution of tritiated penicillin in the rabbit eye. *Acta Ophthalmol.* 47:115, 1969.

50. Sidikaro, J., and Jones, D. B. Concentration of gentamicin in preocular tear flow following topical application (abstract). *Invest. Ophthalmol. Vis. Sci.* 20 (Suppl.):109, 1981.

51. Sloan, S. H., Pettit, T. H., and Litwach, K. D. Gentamicin penetration in the aqueous humor of eyes with corneal ulcers. *Am. J. Ophthalmol.* 73:750, 1972.

52. Smolin, G., Okumoto, M., and Wilson, F.

M. The effect of tobramycin on *Pseudomonas* keratitis. *Am. J. Ophthalmol.* 76:555, 1973.

53. Smolin, G., Okumoto, M., and Wilson, F. M. The effect of tobramycin on gentamicin-resistant strains in *Pseudomonas* keratitis. *Am. J. Ophthalmol.* 77:583, 1974.

54. Sorsby, A., Unger, J., and Crick, R. P. Aureomycin, chloramphenicol and Terramycin in ophthalmology. *Br. Med. J.* 2:301, 1953.

55. Sugaya, M., and Nagataki, S. Kinetics of topical pilocarpine in the human eye. *Jpn. J. Ophthalmol.* 22:127, 1978.

56. Waltman, S. R., Buerk, K., and Foster, C. S. Effects of ophthalmic ointment on intraocu-lar penetration of topical fluorescein in rabbits and man. *Am. J. Ophthalmol.* 78:262, 1974.

57. Waltman, S. R., and Kaufman, H. E. Use of hydrophilic contact lenses to increase ocular penetration of topical drugs. *Invest. Ophthalmol.* 9:250, 1970.

58. Wine, N. A., Gornall, A. G., and Basu, P. K. The ocular uptake of subconjunctivally injected C^{14} hydrocortisone: I. Time and major route of penetration in a normal eye. *Am. J. Ophthalmol.* 58:362, 1964.

II. CLINICAL ASPECTS

5. INFECTIOUS DISEASES

Bacterial Diseases

Robert A. Hyndiuk, Kamal F. Nassif, and Eileen M. Burd

The management of infectious corneal ulcers can be one of the most challenging problems in a clinician's practice. Although in some severe, complicated cases, patients must be hospitalized, most patients with infectious corneal ulcers can be well cared for on an outpatient basis by the clinician using equipment available in the office or local hospitals. Current concepts in the pathogenesis, clinical characteristics, microbiologic workup, available antibiotics, and management of bacterial corneal infections are reviewed in this section.

DEFENSE MECHANISMS OF THE EYE

A delicate balance exists between the cornea and its surrounding environment that helps the cornea maintain its integrity in spite of continuous exposure to foreign bodies and pathogens. Corneal ulceration may result when the balance is disrupted and the defense mechanisms are compromised. See Physiology of the Tear Film in Chapter 1 and Chapter 3, Immunology, for more details.

The cornea itself is equipped with a protective lining composed of two layers of mucosubstances. The first, the glycocalyx, is an integral part of the cell membrane. The other is a mucus layer produced by the goblet cells of the conjunctiva. Bacteria have to adhere to epithelium or stroma before they can initiate infection [20, 38, 39]. An intact epithelium acts as a barrier against most organisms except *Neisseria gonorrhoeae*, *Listeria*, *Corynebacterium diphtheriae*, and *Haemophilus aegyptius*, which can probably in-

This work was supported in part by NIH research grants EY-01665 and EY-01463, Ophthalmic Research Center Grant EY-01931, an unrestricted grant from Research to Prevent Blindness, Inc., and the Medical Research Service of the Veterans Administration.

A portion of the research work presented was taken from a thesis (R. A. H.) for membership in the American Ophthalmological Society, accepted by the Committee on Theses, 1981.

vade intact epithelium once they adhere. For all other bacteria, a breach in the integrity of the epithelium is mandatory. The glycocalyx of injured epithelium or the glycocalyx of certain bacteria, especially *Pseudomonas* and gonococcus, play a role in initial adherence. The biologic adhesion allows diffusion of toxins and bacterial products necessary before actual bacterial invasion of stroma [20].

The first line of defense of the host in most nongranulomatous bacterial infections appears to be the polymorphonuclear cell (PMN). The PMN phagocytizes the organism to form a phagosome. This then combines with the intracytoplasmic lysosomes containing cytotoxic and lytic enzymes to form phagolysosomes. These enzymes then act on the organism to destroy it. In systemic infections, humoral immunity plays a role and provides a second line of defense. Cell-mediated immunity plays a questionable role in the cornea except possibly in infections caused by such organisms as mycobacteria and local staphylococcal infections. Although the enzymes elaborated by the PMNs help to combat the invading organisms, they also cause local tissue destruction and in certain tissues such as cornea may cause more harm than benefit [20].

It is easy to envision how certain compromising factors, local or systemic, can affect the balance between the cornea and its surroundings and cause it to break down with the result of corneal infection. Among the local factors, ocular trauma, ocular burns, chronic herpetic keratitis, dry eye states, chronic corneal edema, and contact lens abuse are the most important [17]. In fact, contact lenses, especially soft contact lenses, have become a very common predisposing factor in *Pseudomonas* corneal ulcers (Fig. 5-1). Systemic compromising factors include vitamin deficiency, alcoholism, immunosuppressive therapy, and extensive burns [17].

ROLE OF THE ORGANISM

The lid margins have been found to be normally inhabited with bacteria 100 percent of the time; the conjunctiva is colonized 36 percent of the time [35]. The organisms most frequently recovered from the lid margins are *Staphylococcus* sp., *Corynebacterium* sp., and *Micrococcus* sp. Gram-negative organisms are often found in the flora of patients with dry eyes. The severity of corneal infection usually depends primarily on the organism itself and the enzymes and extracellular toxins it elaborates. Enzymes include, among others, proteases, coagulases, nucleases, fibrinolysins, and lipases. Toxins range from the α, β, δ, and γ toxins of the

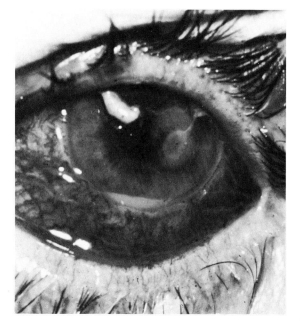

A

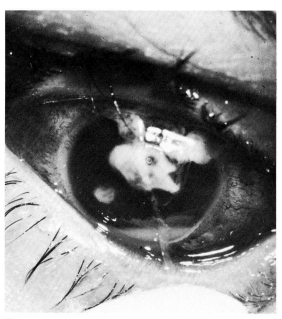

B

FIGURE 5-1. *A.* Pseudomonas *keratitis after overnight wearing of soft contact lens for myopia. B.* Pseudomonas *keratitis precipitated in aphakic patient by soft contact lens.*

staphylococci to the highly potent exotoxins A, B, and C of *Pseudomonas* [2, 20, 23, 24, 32].

Some of these enzymes are antigenic and therefore are involved in the evolution of host defenses against the organism [24]. Others, like the pyocyanase portion of the pyocyanin pigment of

Pseudomonas, have an antibiotic activity, presumably to exclude coexistence of other organisms [32], a phenomenon also noted with staphylococci [19]. Although several of the products of the organisms, such as lipases and proteases, have proven damaging effects on tissues, the pathogenicities of the different organisms have not been attributed to one single component. Among the proteases elaborated by organisms like *Clostridia* sp. are specific collagenases that attack primitive collagen to liberate hydroxyproline. Many strains of *Pseudomonas* elaborate nonspecific collagenases that attack the terminal peptides of native collagen to liberate amino acids. Injected intrastromally, proteases, like proteoglycanases, are capable of breaking down corneal proteoglycan ground substances that normally protect collagen [5]. Proteoglycanase and collagenase activity may either be derived from the organisms themselves or elaborated by the damaged epithelial cells and the invading polymorphonuclear cells (PMNs) [14, 20]. Elastase, another enzyme elaborated by certain bacteria like *Pseudomonas*, breaks down elastin and adds to the damage already produced by these organisms, although its presence is not essential to initiate damage [34]. Hemolysins, such as phospholipase, are elaborated by many organisms such as *Staphylococcus*, pneumococcus, and *Pseudomonas*. Phospholipase breaks down phospholipids that are solubilized by the detergent action of another hemolysin elaborated by these organisms [32].

Toxins produced by some organisms are cytotoxic, acting either on the cell membrane, as in the case of the *Staphylococcus* α toxin, or on cellular protein synthesis, as the *Pseudomonas* exotoxins A, B, and C. While often associated with *Pseudomonas* strains causing severe systemic *Pseudomonas* infection, exotoxin A is not necessary for initiation of corneal damage [34]. Staphylococci elaborate leukocidin, a toxin that acts against neutrophils. They also have surface components that possess antiphagocytic activity [24]. Many strains of *Pseudomonas* possess a glycocalyx that not only helps the bacteria adhere especially to damaged surface epithelium or stroma but also to one another, producing large aggregates or microcolonies that resist phagocytosis [20].

The history is very important. A history of trauma or contact lens wear is often elicited from young patients with ulcers. Atopic disease, previous herpetic infection, and dry eye states in patients with corneal ulcers may direct our attention to opportunistic organisms.

The location of the corneal ulcer may be important in speculating as to the cause of the infection. Corneal ulcers may be conveniently divided into central or peripheral ulcers. Infectious ulcers due to multiplying organisms that start near the limbus tend to spread toward the center of the cornea, away from the vascular limbus, as opposed to noninfectious peripheral ulcers, which remain contiguous to the arc of the limbus (e.g., catarrhal staphylococcal noninfectious ulcers).

The most common cause of peripheral corneal infiltrates and ulcerations are *Staphylococcus*, *Haemophilus* sp., *Moraxella*, *Chlamydia*, and herpes simplex [44]. Other causes include toxins, allergies, and immune phenomena that are discussed elsewhere in this book (see Chapter 3, Immunology; and Ocular Allergies and Ocular Manifestations of the Nonrheumatic Acquired Collagen Diseases, in Chapter 6, Immunologic Diseases).

The most common cause of central infectious corneal ulcers in developed countries is herpes simplex [36]. Bacteria also commonly cause infectious corneal ulceration in both developed and developing countries. Fungal ulcers are on the rise, especially in subtropical and tropical climates. The most common organism involved varies from one geographic area to another, depending on the type of patient seen, the climate, and the condition of the cornea before the infection began (i.e., healthy versus diseased).

Staphylococcus is the most common cause of central bacterial corneal ulcers in Canada and the northern United States (Table 5-1). It is also the most common cause of bacterial ulcers in patients with previous herpetic keratitis, bullous keratopathy, atopic disease, and dry eye syndromes. Pneumococcal ulcers were common in the days of chronic dacryocystitis—before the popularization of dacryocystorhinostomies—but the incidence has declined in most centers. The incidence of gram-negative organisms, especially *Pseudomonas*, is on the rise; these infections are now more common than *Staphylococcus* in some areas in the southern United States such as Georgia and Florida (Table 5-1). *Moraxella* is most common in centers that treat many alcoholics, as these patients are more susceptible to *Moraxella* infections.

The course of the corneal ulcer depends primarily on the virulence of the organism. *Staphylococcus*, *Moraxella*, *Mycobacterium fortuitum*, *Klebsiella*, and *Nocardia* infections usually proceed more slowly than do infections caused by most strains of *Pseudomonas* and *Streptococcus* (including pneumococcus), which are usually more rapidly progressive with more signs of inflammatory response. Clinical characteristics may be atypical in corneal infections that have received some treatment (Fig. 5-2). See Infectious Agents: Bacteria, and Antibiotic Mechanisms in Chapter 4 for more details on the role of the organism in the severity of the disease.

GENERAL CLINICAL FEATURES
The symptoms of corneal ulcers are similar in most patients: decreased visual acuity, photophobia, pain, redness, swelling, and discharge. The severity depends on the organism, the condition of the host, and the duration of symptoms before the patient is examined. The conjunctival reaction is usually not specific and only occasionally helpful in diagnosis. An associated conjunctivitis is often seen in gonococcal, pneumococcal, and *Haemophilus* infections. Chemosis is usually present and may mask the underlying conjunctival reaction. Papillae, which are tufts of capillaries infiltrated by inflammatory cells and separated by septae bound down to the tarsus, usually accompany bacterial infections and are indicative of conjunctival inflammation.

SPECIFIC CLINICAL FEATURES
Ulcers caused by gram-positive cocci tend to remain localized within distinct borders [44]. Gradients of gray, gray-white, or white infiltration are present, with only slight adjacent epithelial and stromal edema, whereas diffuse graying away from the main infiltration is the rule in *Pseudomonas* ulcers.

Ulcers caused by pneumococci usually follow trauma to the cornea. Infiltration starts at the periphery of the site of injury and rapidly spreads toward the center [37]. The anterior chamber reaction is usually severe, with hypopyon formation. Fibrin deposition is usually seen on the endothelial side of the ulcer, and a deep stromal abscess may form, with the intervening stroma relatively spared (Fig. 5-3). If pneumococcal ulcers are left untreated, perforation is imminent. Pneumococcus type 4 is the usual organism recovered. Pneumococcal conjunctivitis does not usually result in corneal ulceration because the organism involved is usually of a different strain that lacks the type 4 virulence [37].

Beta-hemolytic streptococci cause severe corneal infection without typical features. Alpha-hemolytic *Streptococcus* is a cause of indolent ulceration and is

TABLE 5-1. *Causal Agents of Bacterial Keratitis*

City (Dates)	Staph	Pneumo	Strep	*Pseudomonas*	Klebs	Prot	Morax	Neiss	Other GNR
Vancouver (1977–1980)[a]	42	2	4	—	—	—	4	—	—
Montreal (1978–1980)[b]	23	2	2	6	—	—	4	—	1
New York (1935–1968)[c]	1755	1233	4	194	11	30	77	—	—
Boston (1977–1979)[d]	45	11	6	15	2	3	6	1	15
Milwaukee (1973–1980)[e]	53	8	9	12	2	5	5	2	6
Portland, Oreg. (1974–1975)[f]	5	1	—	1	—	—	1	—	—
San Francisco (1948–1975)[g]	27	26	15	18	—	—	13	1	5
Houston (1972–1979)[h]	79	18	16	57	5	6	4	1	30
Athens and Atlanta, Ga. (1968–1975)[i]	6	6	1	22	2	2	6	—	—
Miami (1969–1977)[j]	70	18	17	74	4	18	4	1	12

[a]J. Richards, S. M. Drance, and J. Bowersox, personal communication, 1981.
[b]D. Lorenzetti, B. Jackson, and J. Rosen, personal communication, 1981.
[c]D. Locatcher-Khorazo, *Microbiology of the Eye.* St. Louis: Mosby, 1972.
[d]C. S. Foster, and J. Haaf, personal communication, 1981.
[e]R. A. Hyndiuk, R. O. Schultz, and E. M. Burd, unpublished data, 1981.
[f]R. P. Burns, personal communication, 1976.
[g]H. B. Ostler, M. Okumoto, and C. Wilkey [36].
[h]D. B. Jones [27].
[i]L. Wilson [45].
[j]T. J. Liesegang and R. K. Forster [31].
Staph = staphylococci, pneumo = pneumococci, strep = streptococci, Klebs = *Klebsiella*, Prot = *Proteus*, Morax = *Moraxella*, Neiss = *Neisseria*, GNR = gram-negative rods.

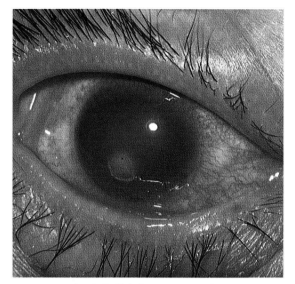

FIGURE 5-2. *Atypical clinical presentation of* Pseudomonas *keratitis with a slowly progressive inflammatory course. The patient was a soft contact lens wearer self-medicating with antibiotics.*

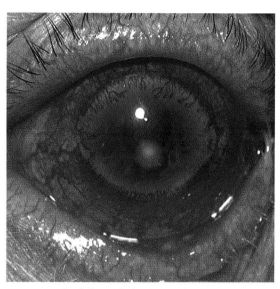

FIGURE 5-4. *Staphylococcal ulcer in an aphakic soft contact lens wearer with atopic keratoconjunctivitis.*

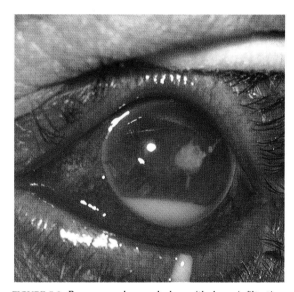

FIGURE 5-3. *Pneumococcal corneal ulcer with dense infiltration and hypopyon.*

often recovered from superinfections of herpetic ulcers.

Staphylococcal ulcers often occur in compromised corneas, i.e., in patients with a history of herpetic keratitis, aphakic bullous keratopathy, dry eyes, rosacea keratitis, or atopic disease. *S. aureus* causes a more severe corneal infiltration with mild to moderate anterior chamber reaction, whereas *S. epider-*

midis causes a more indolent ulceration and infiltration, usually with minimal anterior chamber reaction. Both types of infection tend to remain localized and, early in the course, are usually superficial with surrounding cellular infiltration (Fig. 5-4) [44]. However, long-standing staphylococcal ulcers have a tendency to bore deeply into the cornea and may cause intrastromal abscesses that may lead to perforation (Fig. 5-5). They are occasionally multiple with stromal microinfiltrate satellites that resemble those seen in fungal infections (Fig. 5-6).

Ulcers caused by gram-negative organisms follow one of the following courses. Most common is a rapidly evolving infection leading to perforation and loss of the eye in a relatively short period if left untreated. The less common course is a slowly progressive or even indolent ulceration, probably because of the lack of elaboration of destructive enzymes such as proteases, lipases, and elastases by some strains. The most virulent course is exemplified by the *Pseudomonas* strains, which elaborate proteases, elastases, and exotoxin A. *Pseudomonas* is ubiquitous in our environment, present in ophthalmic solutions, ocular cosmetics such as mascara, and any substance with even a trace of organic carbon [44]. Infection results when a traumatized cornea is exposed to the organism. Signs of infection—superficial edema and microinfiltration of epithelium and stroma on the

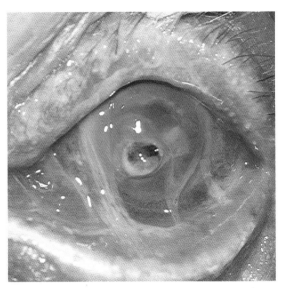

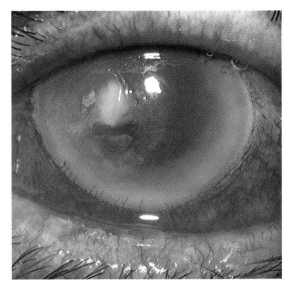

FIGURE 5-7. *Typical* Pseudomonas *corneal ulcer in an aphakic soft contact lens wearer. Note the adherent purulent material and characteristic ground-glass gray appearance over a large area of cornea well away from the actual ulcerative infiltration.*

FIGURE 5-5. *Staphylococcal ulcer with an intrastromal abscess that progressed to a descemetocele. The bacterial infection was superimposed on chronic herpetic keratitis. Such a large descemetocele required an aphakic penetrating keratoplasty, which did well and remains crystal clear despite the patient's severe initial inflammatory reaction.*

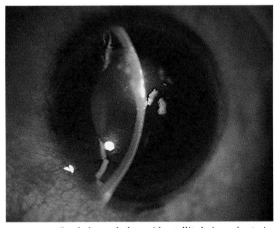

FIGURE 5-6. *Staphylococcal ulcer with satellite lesions of anterior stromal microinfiltration superimposed on keratoconjunctivitis sicca in a diabetic patient. A similar clinical picture may occur in alpha-hemolytic streptococcal ulcers. Both types may simulate fungal keratitis.*

edge of the injury—may be observed biomicroscopically in the area of the epithelial defect as early as 6 to 8 hours after injury. The infiltration extends peripherally and deeply and within 18 to 24 hours is extensive, with severe anterior chamber reaction and hypopyon formation [20]. The ulcer spreads symmetrically and concentrically to involve the whole width and depth of the cornea eventually. Very characteristic of *Pseudomonas* ulcers is the diffuse epithelial graying (inflammatory epithelial edema) that characteristically occurs away from the main site of epithelial and stromal infiltration (Fig. 5-7). A ring ulcer is often seen at 48 to 96 hours in an untreated ulcer. The progressive untreated ulcer is associated with soupy melting of the cornea, with greenish yellow mucopurulent discharge adherent to the ulcer. This leads to a descemetocele and eventual perforation within 2 to 5 days of the onset of infection [20, 44].

Other gram-negative rods such as *Klebsiella, Escherichia coli,* and *Proteus* most commonly cause indolent ulcerations in previously compromised corneas with milder anterior chamber reaction and no other distinguishing features. *Moraxella* is a gram-negative diplobacillus that produces corneal ulcers after trauma in debilitated patients, diabetics, alcoholics, and the chronically malnourished. Its reservoir is the nasopharynx. The ulcer is typically indolent with only mild to moderate anterior chamber reaction. It is usually oval and located in the inferior portion of the cornea. It tends to remain localized, spreading into deep stroma only in its own area [37, 44]. Some *Moraxella* ulcers have prolonged, moderately severe stromal and anterior chamber reactions with endothelial decompensation despite proper treatment [45].

Ulcers caused by anaerobes and high-order bacteria are not very common and usually follow corneal

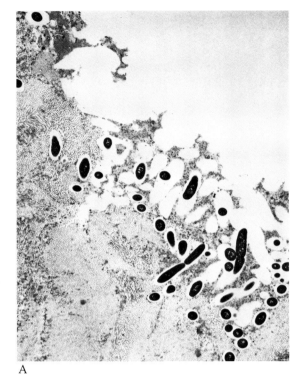

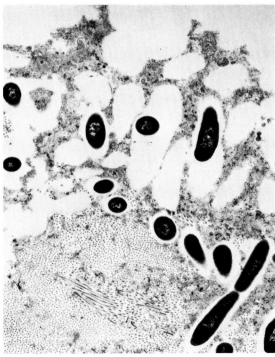

A

B

FIGURE 5-8 A and B. *Transmission EM showing adherence and initial invasion of* Pseudomonas *organisms into the stromal edge of a corneal wound 1 hour after infection. Note the electron-lucent envelope around each bacterium. This envelope may play a role in adherence and invasion.* (A, ×8600; B, ×16,600.)

injuries contaminated with soil [42]. Infections by clostridia should be suggested by the presence of air bubbles in the anterior chamber and corneal stroma and under the epithelium [37]. *Actinomyces*, an anaerobic gram-positive filamentous bacterium, is a common cause of canaliculitis but is only very rarely associated with corneal ulceration [15, 37]. *Nocardia*, a gram-positive branching filamentous bacterium, is a cause of indolent corneal ulceration. *Nocardia* is found in the soil and is introduced into the eye by contamination with soil following trauma to the cornea. *Nocardia* ulcers simulate fungal ulcers in that they are occasionally elevated, have hyphate edges, and often produce satellite lesions. The cornea has been described as having a cracked windshield appearance, which is also occasionally noted with *M. fortuitum* ulcers [29, 37]. *M. fortuitum*, an organism that inhabits the soil, is another cause of indolent corneal ulcer after trauma [43, 46]. The ulcer progresses very slowly over weeks. The bed of the ulcer often appears to have a cracked windshield appearance with minimal surrounding corneal or anterior chamber reaction [29, 45]. Such ulcers are often confused clinically with *Nocardia* or *Moraxella* ulcers [37].

HISTOPATHOLOGY AND STAGES OF CORNEAL ULCERS

The course of corneal ulceration can be divided into three main stages on the basis of histopathologic changes: the progressive stage, the regressive stage, and the healing stage.

PROGRESSIVE STAGE

The progressive stage includes adherence and entry of the organism, invasion of the stroma, host response, multiplication of the organism, diffusion of toxins and enzymes, and resultant tissue destruction.

Within 2 hours of corneal injury, PMNs are seen in the wound. These disappear within 48 hours if no infection ensues, and the epithelium promptly heals. If infection occurs, however, the inflammatory process progresses. Bacteria gain access to the stroma through the injured cornea after they adhere to the injured surface (Fig. 5-8). The adherence is aided in certain bacteria such as *Pseudomonas* and gonococcus by a glycocalyx (slime envelope), which increases bacterial adherence to tissues. Bacteria usually have difficulty adhering to intact epithelium, but they adhere in high numbers to the surface of experimentally wounded corneas (Fig. 5-9). The glycocalyx of injured cells may also promote

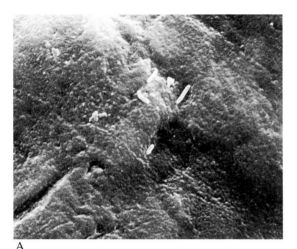

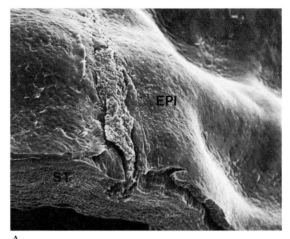

A

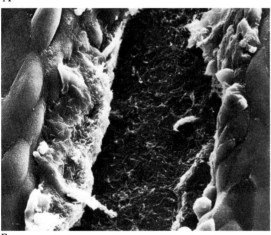

B

FIGURE 5-9A. *Scanning EM of intact superficial corneal epithelium. Only a rare bacterium is found adhering to intact surface. (×500.) B. Scanning EM of injured epithelium and stroma. Multiple bacteria adhere to the injured epithelium and stroma on the sides and base of the injury. (×5000.)*

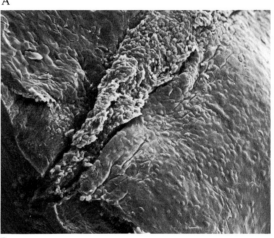

B

FIGURE 5-10 A and B. *Scanning EM of injury site in corneal epithelium (EPI) and stroma (ST) 4 hours after infection. The wound is filled with polymorphonuclear cells, but none is seen on the surface of the intact epithelium. (A, ×100; B, ×200.)*

adhesion, which in turn facilitates corneal stromal invasion. Enzymes released by bacteria and PMNs cause alteration of corneal stroma, which further facilitates stromal invasion of bacteria. Major PMN infiltration is not present until about 4 hours after injury. At that stage, PMNs are found in the wound but rarely on the surface of intact epithelium, the normally "slippery pathway" [20] (Fig. 5-10).

Early in the disease, the tear film is the source of PMNs (Fig. 5-11). These penetrate through the wound and spread deeply and radially toward the limbus. Few PMNs are seen at the limbus in the first 24 hours. Limbal infiltration and limbal vessel contribution to PMN invasion is not important until

approximately 48 hours after infection. Phagocytosis and digestion of bacteria by PMNs are evident in the wound at 4 hours after infection and in anterior stroma at 8 hours (Fig. 5-12). This is the first line of defense against many bacteria. PMN and bacterial infiltration is noted in anterior stroma under intact epithelium adjacent to the wound and probably explains progressive epithelial cell loss around an enlarging ulcer (Fig. 5-13). Stromal keratocytes become necrotic early and are digested by PMNs within 4 to 8 hours after infection. Eight to 16 hours after infection, early collagen degeneration occurs in areas surrounding degranulating PMNs. Major collagen breakdown, however, occurs mainly after 24 hours. During this progression of the ulcer, the bacteria penetrate deeper and are seen either free in the stroma or phagocytized by PMNs. They appear to

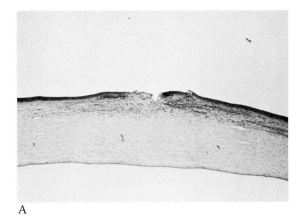

A

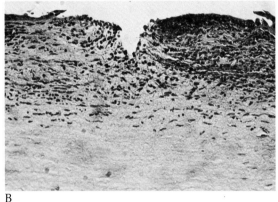

B

FIGURE 5-11 A and B. *Light microscopy of cross-section of cornea 16 hours after infection. Polymorphonuclear cells* (PMNs) *have infiltrated anterior stroma, and adjacent epithelium has broken down. The PMNs adjacent to the wound are arriving from the tear film. The peripheral cornea and limbus show minimal PMN infiltration at this stage. (A, ×16; B, ×63.)*

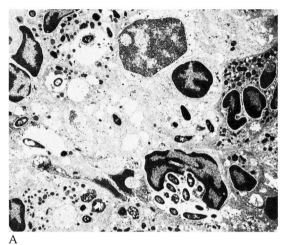

A

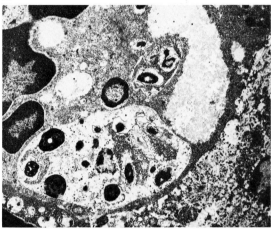

B

FIGURE 5-12 A. *Transmission EM of infected cornea 4 hours after infection. Note aggregate of polymorphonuclear cells* (PMNs) *containing phagocytized bacteria in various stages of digestion. (×6400.) B. Transmission EM of a phagosome containing partially digested bacteria in a PMN 8 hours after infection. Note early collagen degradation associated with electron-dense particles in lower right-hand corner. (×16,600.)*

lose most of their glycocalyx several hours after they penetrate the stroma. Extensive collagen destruction may be noted in certain rapidly progressive ulcers at 48 to 96 hours [20].

REGRESSIVE STAGE
The regressive stage essentially is the regression of the course of events described above. Regression is characterized by decreased pain and other symptoms. The infiltrates decrease in size, the ulcer becomes more demarcated, the collagen destruction is halted, and bacterial multiplication is controlled. Necrotic areas may slough off, mimicking progression even though the inflammation is regressing. The anterior chamber reaction resolves as well.

HEALING STAGE
In the healing stage, the patient's symptoms continue to decrease, and the visual acuity starts to improve. The necrotic stroma is replaced by scar tissue

laid down by fibroblasts, which are transformed histiocytes and keratocytes. Thin areas may be partially replaced by fibrous tissue or may persist as such. Vessels grow in toward the ulcer and bring in fibroblasts with resultant healing. When the healing is completed, the vessels regress into ghost vessels. Bowman's membrane does not regenerate and is therefore replaced by fibrous tissue. Epithelium slowly grows in from all sides to cover the defect. With loss of Bowman's membrane, the epithelium comes in direct contact with bare stroma. The scar never becomes transparent, although its density decreases with time, especially in children and young adults.

TREATMENT OF CORNEAL ULCERS

MICROBIOLOGIC DIAGNOSIS

The definitive diagnosis of ulcers caused by multiplying bacteria can only be arrived at by microbiologic evaluation, despite the suggestive appearance and course of corneal ulcers produced by certain pathogens. Clinical evaluation may be a problem in the inadequately treated bacterial ulcer, the clinical course of which is often atypical. Certain noninfectious corneal ulcers occasionally present a particularly difficult problem in diagnosis when there is considerable concomitant corneal inflammation: some postkeratoplasty corneas with persistent epithelial defects; certain neurotrophic or exposure ulcers; and indolent, postinfectious herpetic ulcers. These entities may sometimes mimic active bacterial corneal infection in appearance. To complicate matters, they often become secondarily infected with bacteria or fungi. When in doubt, a bacterial ulcer workup should be done and the ulcer closely followed. A rapid deterioration of the cornea is probably an indication of a superinfection, and a more aggressive workup and therapeutic approach is indicated.

A microbiologic workup of a suspected infectious ulcer should be done before the start of any antibiotic treatment. After smears and cultures have been taken, the treatment regimen can be started. It can be modified in accordance with the results of the smear, culture, and sensitivity testing. Keep in mind that bacterial yield is markedly decreased if the patient is already taking antibiotics, even if the infection is worsening with inadequate treatment. Cultures are much more sensitive and have a greater yield than smears. The result of either cultures or smears are diagnostic if positive; if negative, infection cannot be ruled out without repeated workups, especially if the patient is taking antibiotics. A corneal biopsy may be necessary to diagnose an infection, especially when a fungal cause is suspected. When culture results are negative but infection is still suspected, as in patients already receiving antibiotic treatment when first seen, cultures should be repeated after discontinuing the antibiotic treatment if the course of the infection permits suspending treatment temporarily. In such patients, the course of the disease and the evaluation of the response to the antibiotic treatment is important.

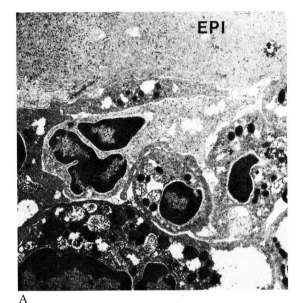

A

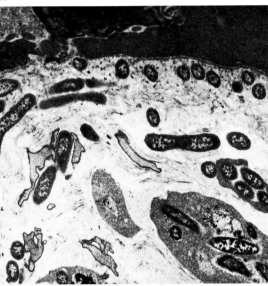

B

FIGURE 5-13A. *Transmission EM of polymorphonuclear cells (PMNs) beneath the corneal epithelium (EPI) near the ulcer 16 hours after infection. Note the interruption of epithelial basement membrane. Early collagen degradation can be seen around PMNs (lower right). (×12,000.) B. Transmission EM showing* Pseudomonas *organisms in anterior corneal stroma lined up beneath intact epithelium adjacent to wound. (×12,000.)*

The first step in the microbiologic workup is to obtain a culture from the lids and conjunctiva of both the infected and the uninfected eye. The patient's own normal flora in the clinically uninvolved eye, which may be important for comparative purposes, is then known. This procedure may also be helpful when no growth is obtained from the ulcer itself, since specimens from the cul-de-sac of the involved eye may grow the causative organism. For culturing lids and conjunctiva, calcium alginate swabs moistened with nutrient broth should be used. Cotton swabs should be avoided because they contain fatty acids that have a proven inhibitory effect on bacterial growth. The yield is also higher when a moistened rather than a dry swab is used. Topical anesthetics should be avoided for this part of the workup, since they are not needed for patient comfort and the preservatives they contain have proven bactericidal properties. The entire cul-de-sac should be wiped and the material streaked on a blood agar plate. The same method is followed for the lid margin.

The corneal ulcer itself should then be cultured. Inoculate directly onto culture media rather than in carrier media, since specimens obtained from the eye usually contain small numbers of organisms or organisms that are often difficult to grow. First anesthetize the eye. Proparacaine hydrochloride (Ophthaine) is recommended since it is the least bactericidal. Use a dry swab to remove superficial debris from the ulcer, and inoculate the same blood agar plate used for lid and conjunctival cultures with this debris. Use a sterile, modified Kimura spatula to scrape the leading edge and center of the ulcer. This spatula has a narrow, tapered, roughened edge that better holds corneal specimens [22]. C-streak this specimen onto a blood agar plate. Any growth on the C-streak may be arbitrarily considered microbiologically meaningful; any off the C-streak is considered probably caused by a contaminant. Inoculate chocolate agar routinely. Include a Sabouraud agar plate without cycloheximide if fungal infection is a possibility. Cycloheximide is toxic to saprophytic fungi capable of causing eye infections. If Sabouraud agar is not available, a blood agar plate may be used and incubated at room temperature. A chopped meat–glucose broth should also be inoculated whenever anaerobic pathogens are a possibility. Thioglycolate medium with hemin and vitamin K may be used as an alternative if it is boiled before being inoculated. Be sure to inoculate below the aerobic indicator (pink) zone. Inoculation of brain-heart infusion medium or other enriched broths may increase the likelihood of recovery of the culprit organism in the face of negative cultures on other media, especially if the patient is already taking antibiotics. Finally, spread multiple specimens on slides for Gram, Giemsa, or Grocott's methenamine silver stains. Gram stain is best for bacteria, and it also shows the yeast phase of dimorphic fungi, which stain gram-positive. Giemsa stain is ideal for cellular detail and cellular response. It shows the outline and septae of fungal hyphae

better than does the Gram stain; however, methenamine silver remains the best stain for fungi. Acid-fast stains are necessary when *M. fortuitum* or *Nocardia* sp. are suspected in cases of indolent corneal ulceration.

The limulus lysate assay, which is very sensitive in detecting gram-negative endotoxin, has recently been recommended and may be a useful adjunct in the initial diagnostic workup of bacterial keratitis caused by gram-negative organisms [31]. As with the smear, however, it may not detect gram-negative organisms in some corneal infections [33].

CHOICE OF ANTIBIOTIC

Until the results of the definitive cultures are available, the Gram stain is a quick and often helpful means of initiating rational antibiotic therapy. However, the ophthalmologist should be cautioned against overreliance on Gram stain results. The frequency of poor correlation between Gram stain and culture results is high. It has been reported to be as high as 30 percent [26]. This is probably due to confusion between normal flora and pathogens, improper staining technique, or decolorization caused by damage to the bacterial cell wall during processing or early antibiotic therapy [3]. This can be minimized and the correlation improved if the staining procedure is meticulously performed. Care should be taken to avoid overly decolorizing the slide with acetone. Fixation in 95% methanol may prove to be better than heat fixation because overheating may damage cell wall integrity. Proper Gram and Giemsa staining techniques have been described in detail elsewhere [22, 27]. If done properly, Gram stain may identify the pathogen in 75 percent of cases caused by a single organism and 37 percent of cases caused by mixed organisms [27]. Caution should be exercised when gram-positive rods or gram-negative cocci are detected or when two or more organisms are observed; these interpretations are misleading in 75 percent of cases [27].

In view of the above-mentioned shortcomings of the available stains, it is not surprising to find controversy regarding the reliance on them for the initial management of corneal ulcers. Some ophthalmologists [3] feel that, in view of the seriousness of corneal infection and the risk of selecting an improper antibiotic based on the stain findings, it is wise to deliver wide-spectrum antibiotic coverage until the final culture results and sensitivities are available. Others [27] argue that wide-spectrum antibiotic coverage increases the risk of antibiotic side effects and antagonism and increases the likelihood of superinfection. The use of such antibiotics may also result in overtreating ulcers that may not be due to a bacterial pathogen.

A method of managing corneal ulcers is clearly outlined by Jones [27] and can be summarized briefly as follows: Initial management should be based mainly on the Gram stain [1, 27, 30] and the clinical impression—severe ulcers warrant more aggressive therapy. If the smear is positive for two organisms, combined therapy is advised, although the high percentage of misinterpretation in such cases should be kept in mind. If only one organism is found, then one antibiotic is recommended, unless the ulcer is severe and the patient is already taking antibiotics, in which case combined therapy is recommended. If the smear results are negative, combined antibiotic therapy is indicated unless the ulcer is not severe and does not clinically appear to be infectious. In that case, treatment should be deferred.

The above method relies heavily on the smear and the technical proficiency of the microbiology lab for diagnosis and on both topical and subconjunctival antibiotic therapy for management. If no organism is observed on the Gram stain, treatment is begun with wide-spectrum antibiotics including topical bacitracin or cephalosporin and an aminoglycoside (gentamicin or tobramycin). In addition to topical therapy, methicillin and gentamicin are injected subconjunctivally every 24 hours for 3 days unless the ulcer is severe or caused by gram-negative rods, in which case the injections are given every 12 hours for 3 days [45]. If gram-positive cocci or rods are seen on the Gram stain, then bacitracin or cephalosporin is given topically and methicillin sodium or gentamicin is injected subconjunctivally. Gram-negative cocci on the smear prompt the use of bacitracin or erythromycin topically and subconjunctivally and intravenous penicillin G, since *Neisseria* is probable. For gram-negative rods, on the other hand, topical and subconjunctival gentamicin and carbenicillin, which have a synergistic effect on gram-negative organisms such as *Pseudomonas,* are recommended. Once an organism is recovered from the cultures and the sensitivities are known, therapy is modified accordingly (Tables 5-2 and 5-3).

Even with a well-equipped ocular microbiology lab in our institution, we prefer initiating treatment with wide-spectrum antibiotic coverage rather than depending heavily on the smear, since the risks of fortified, topically applied, wide-spectrum antibiotics used for brief periods are relatively minor [4].

A wide range of antibiotics is used to treat ocular infections (Table 5-4). The ophthalmologist should familiarize himself with the mechanisms of action of these antibiotics (see Antibiotic Mechanisms in Chapter 4) and their side effects.

The resistance to these antibiotics, as determined by in vitro studies, does not necessarily hold in the treatment of corneal infections, since the antibiotic may be applied topically in very high concentrations without significant systemic or local side effects. Practically, acquired antibiotic resistance in ophthalmology is mainly a problem with nosocomial corneal infections contracted in intensive care or burn units.

Corneal ulcers, except for those caused by *Herpes simplex*, should be considered ocular urgencies. They are best handled in a hospital where the pa-

TABLE 5-2. *Doses of Topical and Subconjunctival Antibiotics for Corneal Ulcers*

Antibiotic	Topical Dose	Subconjunctival Dose	Shelf Life
Erythromycin	5 mg/gm ointment	100 mg/0.5 ml	—
Bacitracin	10,000 units/ml	—	1 week—refrigerate
Vancomycin	25 mg/ml	25 mg/0.25 ml	1 week—refrigerate
Penicillin	—	500,000–1,000,000 units/ml	Decays by 25% in 3 days and by 75% in 7 days
Cephaloridine	50 mg/ml	100 mg/0.5 ml	1 week—refrigerate
Cefamandole	50 mg/ml	100 mg/0.5 ml	1 week—refrigerate
Cefazolin	33 mg/ml	100 mg/0.75 ml	1 week—refrigerate
Methicillin sodium	—	50 mg/0.5 ml	4 days—refrigerate
Amikacin sulfate	10 mg/ml	25 mg/0.5 ml	1 week—refrigerate
Gentamicin	20 mg/ml	20 mg/0.5 ml	30 days at room temperature
Tobramycin	20 mg/ml	20 mg/0.5 ml	30 days at room temperature
Carbenicillin	4 mg/ml	125 mg/0.5 ml	1 week—refrigerate
Polymixin B	1–2 mg/ml	10 mg/0.5 ml	1 week—refrigerate

tient can be closely observed and controlled antibiotic treatment administered.

AMINOGLYCOSIDES
The aminoglycosides are probably the most important antibiotics used in ophthalmology. They are poorly absorbed when given orally and are therefore reserved for parenteral or topical use. Aminoglycoside solutions are very stable at room temperature. Once absorbed, 30 percent of the aminoglycoside is found to be protein-bound and is excreted via the kidneys. The active molecule exerts its bactericidal action through miscoding of genetic information for protein synthesis. The spectrum of aminoglycosides includes *Pseudomonas, Proteus, Klebsiella, E. coli, Salmonella, Shigella, Serratia, Hae-*

mophilus influenzae, and *Staphylococcus.* Enterococci, pneumococci, and *Streptococcus* are usually resistant. Tobramycin is three times as active as gentamicin against *Pseudomonas* on a gram-to-gram basis in vitro. When *Pseudomonas* is resistant to tobramycin and gentamicin, amikacin sulfate may be helpful. The reverse is usually not true. Gentamicin exhibits synergism with ampicillin against *Proteus,* with penicillin against enterococci, and with carbenicillin against *Pseudomonas.*

Aminoglycosides can be highly toxic. They may cause changes leading eventually to nephrotoxicity in proximal tubular cells. Most of these changes,

TABLE 5-3. *Specific Antibiotic Therapy*

| Organism | Antibiotic | | |
	Topical	Subconjunctival	Intravenous
Staphylococcus (penicillin-sensitive)	Penicillin G	Penicillin G	—
Staphylococcus (penicillin-resistant)	Cefazolin Cefamandole	Cefazolin Cefamandole	—
Pneumococcus, streptococcus	Penicillin G Erythromycin Bacitracin Vancomycin	Penicillin G Cephalosporin	—
Anaerobic gram-positive cocci, *Corynebacterium,* anaerobic gram-negative rods	Penicillin G Cefamandole	Penicillin G Cefamandole	—
Acinetobacter	Gentamicin	Gentamicin	—
Mycobacterium fortuitum	Amikacin sulfate Rifampin	Amikacin sulfate	—
Neisseria gonorrhoeae	Penicillin G Bacitracin	Penicillin G	Penicillin G
Enterobacteriaceae	Gentamicin	Gentamicin	—
Pseudomonas	Gentamicin Tobramycin Carbenicillin Amikacin sulfate Polymyxin B	Gentamicin Tobramycin Carbenicillin Amikacin sulfate Polymyxin B	—
Klebsiella	Gentamicin	Gentamicin	—
Nocardia asteroides	Sulfacetamide	Streptomycin	—
Moraxella	Penicillin G Sulfacetamide Gentamicin Colistin Neomycin Zinc sulfate	Gentamicin	—
Haemophilus	Chloramphenicol Cefamandole Tetracycline	Ampicillin	Ampicillin

SOURCE. Modified from D. B. Jones [27].

TABLE 5-4. *Relative Susceptibility of Important Corneal Pathogens to Antibiotics in Vitro*

Pathogen	Ampicillin	Bacitracin	Cefamandole	Chloramphenicol	Erythromycin	Gentamicin	Methicillin	Neomycin	Penicillin	Rifampin	Sulfacetamide	Tetracycline	Tobramycin	Vancomycin
GRAM-POSITIVE COCCI														
Staphylococcus epidermidis	±	+	+	±	±	+	+	±	±	0	−	±	+	+
Staphylococcus aureus	−	+	+	±	±	+	+	±	−	0	−	±	+	+
Streptococcus pneumoniae	+	+	+	+	+	−	+	−	+	+	+	+	−	+
α-Hemolytic *Streptococcus*	+	+	+	+	+	−	+	−	+	−	+	+	−	+
β-Hemolytic *Streptococcus*	+	+	+	+	+	−	+	−	+	+	−	−	−	+
GRAM-POSITIVE BACILLI														
Bacillus sp. (not anthraxis)	0	−	0	+	+	+	0	0	±	0	0	0	+	0
GRAM-NEGATIVE COCCI														
Neisseria sp.	+	+	+	+	+	±	+	0	+	+	+	+	±	−
Haemophilus sp.	+	−	±	+	±	+	−	±	±	0	+	+	+	−
GRAM-NEGATIVE BACILLI														
Pseudomonas aeruginosa	−	−	−	−	−	+	−	±	−	0	−	−	+	−
Proteus mirabilis	+	−	±	±	−	+	−	+	−	+	±	−	+	−
Proteus vulgaris	−	−	±	+	−	+	−	+	−	+	−	±	+	−
Enterobacter sp.	±	−	±	+	−	+	−	+	−	0	±	+	+	−
Serratia sp.	−	−	−	+	−	+	−	+	−	0	−	−	+	−
Klebsiella sp.	−	−	±	+	−	+	−	+	−	+	−	+	+	−
Moraxella sp.	+	0	+	0	+	±	0	+	+	0	0	0	+	0
Mycobacterium fortuitum	0	0	0	0	0	0	0	0	0	+	0	0	0	0
ANAEROBIC BACTERIA														
Gram-positive cocci, streptococci	0	0	±	+	0	−	0	−	+	0	0	±	−	0
Actinomyces sp.	0	0	±	+	+	−	0	−	+	0	0	+	−	0
Bacteroides fragilis	−	0	−	+	0	−	0	−	−	0	0	−	−	0

+ = Susceptible; ± = Variable susceptibility; − = Resistant; 0 = No information.

160

which are observed in 8 percent of patients, are reversible if the drug is discontinued early, but permanent renal damage may persist in 2 to 3 percent of patients. In the presence of renal disease, aminoglycosides may still be used; however, the dosage must be modified according to the creatinine clearance. Ototoxicity occurs in 2 percent of patients receiving systemic aminoglycoside treatment and is reversible in only 50 percent of these cases. Abnormal liver enzymes have been noted. Topical use of aminoglycosides, especially in fortified concentration, is sometimes associated with punctate epithelial keratitis or pseudomembranous conjunctivitis.

PENICILLINS

Penicillins share a common structure consisting of a thiazolidine ring connected to a beta-lactam ring to which a side chain is attached. It is this side chain that determines the characteristics of the individual penicillin. Penicillin G interferes with the cell wall synthesis of bacteria. It is stable in the dry state; however, when in solution, it deteriorates slowly. It is 50 percent protein-bound yet exhibits adequate intraocular penetration, especially when the eye is inflamed. It is acid-labile and therefore is not given orally. Its spectrum includes gram-positive organisms such as pneumococci, *Streptococcus,* and *Staphylococcus,* as well as gonococci and anaerobic bacteria with the exception of *Bacteroides fragilis.* Eighty-five percent of staphylococci produce beta-lactamase, which breaks down penicillin into the inactive penicilloic acid. The renal and ciliary body excretion of penicillin can be partially blocked by 0.5 gm of probenecid given orally every 6 hours. Probenecid should not be given to children under 2 years of age.

The main drawback of the penicillins is the 10 percent rate of allergic reactions, the majority of which are limited to skin rash, contact dermatitis, fever, and eosinophilia. In patients with possible penicillin allergy, a scratch test or intradermal antigen test using penicilloyl-polylysine is indicated before instituting systemic therapy. If test results are negative, the chance that the patient will develop a major allergic reaction is less than 1 percent.

Caution should be exercised when giving large systemic doses of penicillins to patients with renal or cardiac disease because of the danger of potassium overload—every million units of penicillin supplies 1.7 mEq of potassium. Convulsions may also occasionally be triggered in such patients.

SEMISYNTHETIC PENICILLINS

The semisynthetic penicillins include methicillin sodium, oxacillin, cloxacillin, dicloxacillin sodium, and nafcillin. Their main indication is against penicillinase-producing *Staphylococcus.* They are much less active on a gram-to-gram basis than penicillin G; therefore, the latter should be used when the staphylococci do not produce penicillinase. Of the semisynthetic penicillins, methicillin sodium is acid-sensitive and cannot therefore be given orally. However, it is the least protein-bound. The rest of the semisynthetic penicillins are highly protein-bound and therefore less available in the active form although on a gram-to-gram basis are more effective. These opposing properties tend to cancel each other. Therefore all of the semisynthetic penicillins are probably equally effective in clinical situations.

Like penicillin G, the semisynthetic penicillins produce allergic reactions. Interstitial nephritis and agranulocytosis have also been reported as other possible side effects.

EXTENDED-SPECTRUM PENICILLINS

Ampicillin, carbenicillin, and ticarcillin share a broader spectrum that includes gram-positive and several gram-negative organisms. They are, however, ineffective against penicillinase-producing *Staphylococcus.*

Ampicillin is acid-stable and therefore can be taken orally. It is only 20 percent protein-bound. It is as effective as penicillin G against gram-positive bacteria but much more expensive. Its wider spectrum includes *Streptococcus faecalis, H. influenzae, Salmonella* sp., *Shigella* sp., *Proteus* sp., and some strains of *E. coli.* Strains of *H. influenzae* resistant to ampicillin have recently evolved.

Carbenicillin is less effective than penicillin against gram-positive organisms but much more effective against *Pseudomonas,* indole-producing *Proteus,* and anaerobes. It works synergistically with gentamicin against *Pseudomonas.* If given in the same syringe, it decreases the activity of gentamicin by 25 percent. In oral preparation carbenicillin indanyl sodium is available as Geocillin. It is excreted in the urine. Its side effects include allergic reactions, sodium overload, and, when given to patients with renal disease, hemorrhagic manifestations.

Ticarcillin disodium (Ticar) has a similar spectrum to carbenicillin but appears to be slightly more active. It also shares the same side effects.

CEPHALOSPORINS

Like the penicillins, the cephalosporins interfere with cell wall synthesis. They resist beta-lactamase and therefore are effective against penicillin-resistant *Staphylococcus*. Their spectrum also includes pneumococci, *Streptococcus, E. coli, Proteus mirabilis, Klebsiella*, and many anaerobes as well except *B. fragilis*. Cefoxitin, however, is effective against *B. fragilis*. In addition to the above bacteria, cefamandole has been noted to be effective against *Enterobacter*, other *Proteus* sp., *Serratia*, and *H. influenzae*. As a group, in general, the cephalosporins are not effective against enteric streptococci, *B. fragilis*, or *Pseudomonas*. Except for cephalexin (Keflex) which is effective when given orally, cephalosporins are given parenterally. They are given every 6 hours except for cefazolin, which has a longer half-life, achieves higher serum levels, and is therefore given every 8 hours. Many cephalosporins are highly protein-bound. The excretion of cephalosporins through the kidneys may be partially blocked by probenecid. Their side effects include allergic reactions and nephrotoxicity. The incidence of allergic reaction to cephalosporins is about 5 percent. Of those with penicillin allergy, 8 percent are also allergic to cephalosporins. A minor reaction to penicillin, however, is not a contraindication to cephalosporin use. Nephrotoxicity has been shown with cefazolin as well as with cephaloridine, but is more common with the latter, which causes renal tubular damage. Other side effects include hepatic abnormalities, white blood cell and platelet depression, and phlebitis at the site of intravenous injection.

VANCOMYCIN

Vancomycin inhibits cell wall synthesis. Its spectrum includes mainly gram-positive cocci including alpha-hemolytic streptococci and *S. faecalis*. It is nephrotoxic when given systemically. Its use in ophthalmology is restricted to topical application against *Staphylococcus* when the semisynthetic penicillins and cephalosporins are either ineffective or not tolerated. It is sometimes used against enterococci in combination with gentamicin but rarely alone.

TETRACYCLINE

Tetracycline inhibits both mammalian and bacterial protein synthesis. Absorption through the gastrointestinal tract is enhanced by an empty stomach and increased acidity; iron, antacids, chelation, and dairy products interfere with it. It is metabolized by the liver, concentrated in the gallbladder, and excreted in the urine and to a lesser extent in fecal material. The latter route of excretion is the main route for doxycycline, which is therefore given,

when indicated, to renal-failure patients. Tetracycline is available commercially for topical application as a suspension in oil since aqueous solutions are unstable. It is lipid soluble and has good ocular penetration. Its spectrum includes the causal agent of lymphogranuloma venereum, *Chlamydia, Mycoplasma pneumoniae, Treponema pallidum, Rickettsia, Actinomyces*, and *Francisella tularensis*, in addition to gram-positive organisms. It is not used against gram-positive organisms, however, as there are too many resistant strains. It is also a second-line drug against most venereally transmitted infections. Its side effects include gastrointestinal upsets, hepatic dysfunction (especially in pregnant women when given parenterally), toxic granulation, pseudotumor cerebri, phototoxicity, and superinfection with *Candida*, both oral and anogenital. When given to children under 12 years of age or to pregnant mothers, it discolors teeth and arrests bone growth until discontinued.

CHLORAMPHENICOL

Chloramphenicol inhibits protein synthesis. It is available for topical application in ointment form and solution and can be given orally or intravenously. It is well absorbed through the gastrointestinal tract, metabolized by the liver through conjugation with glucuronic acid, and excreted via the kidneys. It is 60 percent protein-bound. Its lipid solubility accounts for its good tissue penetration. The following are included in its spectrum: *E. coli, Klebsiella, Salmonella, Shigella, Proteus*, pneumococci, *Streptococcus, H. influenzae*, and anaerobes including *B. fragilis*. It is also moderately effective against *Staphylococcus*. Ampicillin is still the drug of choice for *H. influenzae;* however, chloramphenicol is invaluable in treating resistant strains.

The most dreaded adverse effect of chloramphenicol is bone marrow depression. This can be either a dose-related, total bone marrow depression, which is reversed 3 weeks after discontinuation of the drug, or an idiosyncratic aplastic anemia related to oral intake of the drug. The latter is unrelated to the dose and is often fatal. Two cases of bone marrow depression following topical use of chloramphenicol ophthalmic solution have been reported. The first case followed prolonged use of massive topical doses [40]; the second was poorly documented [7]. Minor gastrointestinal upsets, optic neuritis, and superinfection with *Candida* sometimes complicate chloramphenicol intake.

ERYTHROMYCIN

Erythromycin shares several characteristics with chloramphenicol and tetracycline. It interferes with protein synthesis, is well absorbed through the gastrointestinal tract, is metabolized by the liver, and is excreted in the urine and bile. It is acid-labile and is therefore given as an enteric-coated tablet. Its spectrum includes *S. aureus, S. epidermidis,* alpha-hemolytic streptococci, *S. faecalis, C. diphtheriae, N. gonorrhoeae, Neisseria meningitidis, H. influenzae,* and *Actinomyces* sp. It is the least toxic of the topically applied antibiotics but penetrates the cornea poorly. Its side effects include gastrointestinal upsets and cholestatic hepatitis when given systemically.

CLINDAMYCIN

Clindamycin, which is derived from lincomycin, exerts its effect by interfering with bacterial protein synthesis. Clindamycin is well absorbed through the gastrointestinal tract. It is 25 percent protein-bound yet produces good tissue levels. It is metabolized by the liver and excreted in the urine. It is effective against anaerobes, especially *B. fragilis* and *Actinomyces* sp.; *H. influenzae;* some gram-positive cocci; and *Toxoplasma.* It has a high rate of side effects. It causes diarrhea in 20 percent of patients—10 percent because of the change in the intestinal flora; 10 percent because of pseudomembranous colitis.

RIFAMPIN

Rifampin interferes with RNA synthesis. It can be given either orally or topically and is excreted in bile and urine. Its main use is in tuberculosis. It has been reported to be useful when applied topically in the treatment of *M. fortuitum* ulcers. It has also been noted to exert some effect against gram-positive and some gram-negative organisms such as *E. coli, Proteus, Pseudomonas,* and *Klebsiella.* Its main side effects are intestinal upsets and bone marrow depression.

PEPTIDE ANTIBIOTICS

The peptide antibiotics include gramicidin, bacitracin, and the polymixins. These share a common structure consisting of peptide-linked amino acids. They are bactericidal but highly toxic.

Bacitracin inhibits protein synthesis and incorporation of protein into the cell wall. It is effective against gram-positive cocci, *H. influenzae, Neisseria, Actinomyces, Clostridium,* and *Bacillus anthracis.* It is restricted to topical use because of its high systemic toxicity. It can cause local epithelial keratitis. Gramicidin is useful topically against gram-positive organisms. It is too toxic for systemic use. Polymixins B and E are bactericidal. They alter cell membrane permeability. They are active against gram-negative organisms including *Pseudomonas* but not against *Proteus* or *Neisseria.*

SPECTINOMYCIN

Spectinomycin is related structurally to the aminoglycosides. It inhibits protein synthesis and has a wide spectrum of activity against both gram-positive and gram-negative organisms. Its clinical use is restricted to the second line of defense against penicillin-resistant gonococci. It is given as a single intramuscular injection and is excreted in the urine. It produces minimal side effects.

SULFONAMIDES

Sulfonamides exert their action by preventing uptake of para-aminobenzoic acid essential for folic acid synthesis. They are bacteriostatic and are used in combination with pyrimethamine against ocular toxoplasmosis. They are useful for treatment of conjunctivitis caused by *H. influenzae* or gram-positive organisms and are recommended in the treatment of corneal ulcers caused by *Nocardia.* Their spectrum also includes *Chlamydia.* They are well absorbed when given orally and are excreted in the urine. Serious side effects occasionally result; sensitization, erythema multiforme (Stevens-Johnson syndrome), and anemia secondary to folate deficiency are the most important.

CHOICE OF ROUTE

Antibiotic solutions are the mainstay in the treatment of corneal infections. Although ointment may stay in contact with the ulcerated cornea longer, it is not known how much of the antibiotic in the ointment is readily released and able to penetrate the cornea. Another drawback is the inability in most places to provide fortified antibiotic concentrations in an ointment vehicle.

Recent investigations have clarified many important factors in the use of topical and subconjunctival antibiotic therapy. Fortified topical antibiotic solutions are more effective than the commercially available ones. The highest safe concentration of antibiotic is the most effective [9]. The epithelial barrier is disrupted when the cornea is ulcerated, which allows for better antibiotic absorption into the cornea. Absorption is less of a problem with the more highly fortified antibiotic solutions [9]. When applied in fortified concentration every 30 minutes topical antibiotics appear to be much more effective than when the same fortified concentration was given every 60 minutes [8]. Giving topical fortified antibiotics every 15 minutes is no more effective than giving the antibiotics every 30 minutes.

What is the best way to achieve high, effective

concentrations of antibiotic in the cornea in ulceration? Fortified antibiotics applied topically appear to be highly efficacious in treating corneal infections [9]. Intensive half-hourly topical therapy with tobramycin for experimental *Pseudomonas* ulcers eradicated 99.9 percent of all organisms within 24 hours of initiation of therapy. The number of *Pseudomonas* organisms continued to decline, and *Pseudomonas* could not be cultured after 6 days of continuous therapy [11]. Davis and associates [12] and Hyndiuk [20] have also shown that more microbial killing can be achieved in the cornea using 2 drops of aminoglycoside (tobramycin) solution (20 mg/ml) applied topically every 30 minutes than using 20 mg injected subconjunctivally. They questioned the value of adjunctive subconjunctival therapy, as Sloan and colleagues had in a previous report [41]. Since then, other reports have supported the concept that frequent topical applications of fortified antibiotics are highly effective [9, 11, 13, 16].

In a recent study using multiple antibiotic treatment trials, one of us (R. A. H.) showed that a short course of either topical fortified solutions or subconjunctival injections were usually almost equally effective when actual microbial killing was assayed [20]. Subconjunctival injections in the same system did not enhance the clinical efficacy of topical application unless only the weaker commercially available aminoglycoside solution (0.3% gentamicin) was used. Also, Baum and Barza have recently completed unpublished studies simultaneously comparing antimicrobial efficacy and tissue concentrations of topical and subconjunctival antibiotics. They utilized gentamicin in *Pseudomonas* and *Staphylococcus* corneal infections and cefazolin in *Staphylococcus* corneal infections. The topical route, using hourly instillation of the antibiotic solutions, and the subconjunctival route were equally effective in sterilizing the experimentally produced ulcers. They concluded that either route of administration may be used effectively, and therefore subconjunctival injections may best be reserved for cases in which compliance is a problem (Baum, J., and Barza, M. Personal communication, 1981). Subconjunctival injections, we feel, are probably worth using in certain ulcers with deep infiltration, when fortified antibiotics are not available for topical application, or when frequent applications are not logistically feasible. Subconjunctivally injected antibiotics reach the cornea through tissue diffusion and leakage through both the conjunctival injection site and intact conjunctiva [20].

We have been treating mild, moderate, and even severe bacterial corneal ulcers mainly with fortified topical antibiotics given every half hour with good results [20]. We resort at times to subconjunctival antibiotic injections for deep infiltrative ulcers and stromal abscesses. Our initial therapy consists of wide-spectrum antibiotic coverage modified by the Gram stain results only when the organism seen on the smear, e.g., *Neisseria*, is known to respond better to a different antibiotic regimen. A cephalosporin and an aminoglycoside are used. Cephalosporins are highly effective against *Staphylococcus* and other gram-positive cocci as well as some gram-negative rods including *Proteus*. Aminoglycosides assure coverage against the possibility of *Pseudomonas* infection. They are also effective against a wide range of gram-negative and gram-positive organisms (including penicillinase-producing staphylococcus). We use cefamandole in 50 mg per milliliter concentration in addition to gentamicin or tobramycin in 20 mg per milliliter concentration, both applied topically every half hour. The therapy is then modified depending on the results of the cultures and sensitivities. If the organism is sensitive to both antibiotics, one of them is discontinued because there does not seem to be any advantage to using both simultaneously [8]. The frequency of the antibiotic application is then decreased gradually, depending on the clinical response and repeat negative cultures. Clinical response is indicated by a decrease in the area and density of the cellular infiltrates, a decrease in corneal edema, epithelial healing over the ulcer bed, a decrease in anterior chamber reaction, and ease of pupillary dilatation. When the defect is epithelialized, an antibiotic ointment may be used instead of the fortified anitbiotic solution. The ointment will provide some antibiotic coverage as well as an emollient effect. During the early stages, repeated gentle debridement is helpful because the debris in the ulcer bed may bind the antibiotic and may also act as a barrier to antibiotic penetration.

If the ulcer responds within 48 hours, we usually do not modify the therapy regardless of the results of cultures and sensitivities. Resistance determined in the lab does not necessarily correlate with the clinical response, because the lab sensitivities are based on the response in systemic infections. Fortified antibiotics can be placed directly in contact with the infected cornea, which provides very high concentrations not achievable in treating many other infections. If cultures remain negative despite the clinical impression, we continue combined topical therapy if the ulcer is responding to treatment. If the ulcer progresses despite continuing treatment, atypical bacteria, herpes, fungus, or other factors such as dry eyes or unnoticed exposure may be playing a role. Sometimes, if cultures are nega-

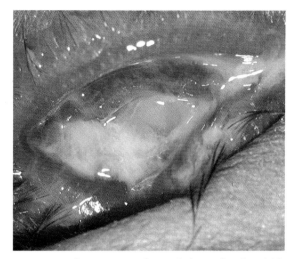

FIGURE 5-14. *Severe gonococcal corneal ulcer and conjunctivitis in an adult male. The eye was saved after intensive topical and systemic antibiotic therapy.*

tive and the ulcer is very slowly progressive, it is best to discontinue antibiotic therapy for 1 or 2 days and reculture and reevaluate diagnostically and therapeutically.

Parenteral antibiotics achieve only relatively low levels in corneal tissue and do not kill intracorneal bacteria. They do not appear to augment the intracorneal antimicrobial effect of topical or subconjunctival antibiotics [20]. Their use is restricted mainly to perforated ulcers, post–perforating injury ulcers, and infections caused by *Neisseria* or *Haemophilus* (Fig. 5-14).

ADJUNCTIVE THERAPY
Cycloplegics should be used as adjunctive therapy to relieve ciliary spasm and to prevent synechiae. Topical 0.25% scopolamine used 2 or 3 times per day is usually adequate.

Collagenase inhibitors have been used as adjunctive therapy, especially in *Pseudomonas* ulcers. The injured epithelium, the PMNs, and the *Pseudomonas* organisms elaborate many enzymes such as specific and nonspecific collagenases that contribute to corneal tissue destruction and melting. Theoretically, collagenase inhibitors should prevent tissue destruction in corneal ulcers. However, to date, no clear evidence is available clinically [45], and they are seldom used by most clinicians even in documented *Pseudomonas* ulcers. Disodium ethylenediaminetetraacetate (EDTA) 0.05% and acetylcysteine (Mucomist) 20% are such inhibitors. Disodium EDTA binds calcium necessary for collagenase activity; acetylcysteine binds to enzyme and inhibits enzyme activity directly [44].

Hyperimmune globulins have been used only in burn patients with *Pseudomonas* ulcers to prevent septicemia and probably have no other application.

Continuous lavage may be helpful in providing constant high concentration of antibiotics in contact with the ulcer. However, this is costly, impractical, and requires patient immobilization. It may cause epithelial injury, and there is some clinical evidence that aminoglycosides given by continuous lavage may cause or play a role in the induction of cataracts (Hyndiuk, R. A. Unpublished observation).

Bandage lenses are usually contraindicated in infected corneal ulcers since they interfere with the penetration of topical drugs and normal wound toileting. They may be helpful if the ulcer becomes indolent with tissue loss but is sterile as documented by cultures and clinical impression. The bandage lens bridges the gap and may help the epithelium grow over the defect.

The most controversial adjunctive therapy in corneal ulcers is the use of corticosteroids. The rationale behind the application of topical steroids to ulcerated corneas is to decrease tissue scarring that may eventually affect visual acuity [30]. Most ophthalmologists would not use corticosteroids for fear of bacterial enhancement or recurrence of the ulcer; this has been shown to occur in *Pseudomonas* ulcers [6, 18]. When the cornea is thin or infiltration is deep, corticosteroids may predispose the cornea to perforation as well. Davis and associates demonstrated, in experimentally induced *Pseudomonas* keratitis, that with optimum topical fortified aminoglycoside therapy, simultaneous administration of intensive topical prednisolone acetate did not adversely alter the microbiologic titer [10]. However, we encourage the ophthalmologist not to use corticosteroids in the treatment of bacterial ulcers. Some recommend use after 4 to 5 days of intensive specific antimicrobial therapy after repeat negative cultures [45]. Corticosteroids, if used in a postinfectious ulcer, should not be used without antibiotic coverage and should be discontinued before the antibiotics themselves are terminated [25, 44].

Cholinergics, especially carbachol and echothiophate iodide (Phospholine Iodide), have been reported possibly to have a role in stimulating epithelial growth if the ulcer becomes indolent. This stimulation may be through the inhibition of adenosine 3′,5′-cyclic phosphate, which is believed by some to be responsible for persistence of epithelial defects [14].

Tissue glue (isobutyl cyanoacrylate or other monomer analogues) may play an important role in the treatment of certain infected, very thin, or perforated corneal ulcers (Fig. 5-15). It is critical in

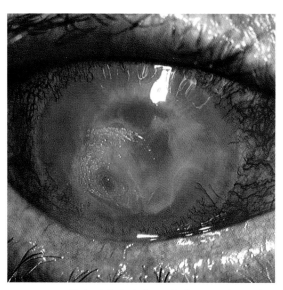

FIGURE 5-15. *Perforated staphylococcal ulcer superimposed on chronic herpetic keratitis after application of tissue adhesive (isobutyl cyanoacrylate). It is important to restore the integrity of the anterior chamber as rapidly as possible in a severely inflamed eye.*

acutely inflamed perforated corneas to restore the integrity of the anterior chamber as quickly and as atraumatically as possible. Often tissue glue is safer than surgical intervention in an inflamed eye. When the ulcer is debrided well and epithelium is removed from its edge, the glue adheres well. The breakdown products of the cyanoacrylate adhesive also have a bacteria-inhibitory effect. The glue is toxic, however, to the endothelium and the lens if it comes in contact with them. It is therefore used for perforations 1 mm or smaller. Larger perforations may be sealed off with a small patch graft and then glued. The patch serves to plug the perforation and keep the glue out of the anterior chamber [21, 28]. Application of a lamellar patch graft while the ulcer is still grossly infected is not advised. A penetrating keratoplasty may be indicated instead, although it carries more risk in an acutely inflamed eye.

Later in the course, after the ulcer has been sterilized, and in the face of a persistent epithelial defect and major stromal loss, a partial conjunctival bridge flap may be indicated if the ulcer is peripheral. Such a flap promotes healing. However, total conjunctival flaps should be avoided in central ulcers and are rarely indicated in bacterial ulcers except in those with associated factors (e.g., keratitis sicca, severe necrotizing herpes) creating healing problems.

ACKNOWLEDGMENTS
We gratefully acknowledge the help of our colleagues Starkey Davis, M.D., Diane Hatchell, Ph.D., Mrs. Kathleen Divine, Larrie Sarff, M.D., and Harlan Pederson. We thank Teresa Auer and Kathy Wichman for typing the manuscript. Ivory Parks and Linda Mader gave excellent technical help in the electron microscopy studies.

REFERENCES
1. Allen, H. F. Current status of prevention, diagnosis and management of bacterial corneal ulcers. *Ann. Ophthalmol.* 3:235, 1971.
2. Arbuthnott, J. P. Staphylococcal Toxins. In D. Schlessinger (Ed.), *Microbiology 1975.* Washington, D.C.: American Society for Microbiology, 1975. Pp. 267–271.
3. Baum, J. L. Initial therapy of suspected microbial corneal ulcers: I. Broad antibiotic therapy based on prevalence of organisms. *Surv. Ophthalmol.* 24:97, 1979.
4. Baum, J. L. Antibiotic Use in Ophthalmology. In T. D. Duane (Ed.), *Clinical Ophthalmology.* Hagerstown, Md.: Harper & Row, 1978. Vol. 4, chap. 26.
5. Brown, S. I., Bloomfield, S. E., and Tam, W. F. The cornea-destroying enzyme of *Pseudomonas aeruginosa. Invest. Ophthalmol.* 13:174, 1975.
6. Burns, R. P. *Pseudomonas aeruginosa* keratitis: Mixed infections of the eye. *Am. J. Ophthalmol.* 67:257, 1969.
7. Carpenter, G. Chloramphenicol eye-drops and marrow aplasia (letter). *Lancet* 2:326, 1975.
8. Davis, S. D., Sarff, L. D., and Hyndiuk, R. A. Antibiotic therapy of experimental *Pseudomonas* keratitis in guinea pigs. *Arch. Ophthalmol.* 95:1638, 1977.
9. Davis, S. D., Sarff, L. D., and Hyndiuk, R. A. Topical tobramycin therapy of experimental *Pseudomonas* keratitis. An evaluation of some factors that potentially enhance efficacy. *Arch. Ophthalmol.* 96:123, 1978.
10. Davis, S. D., Sarff, L. D., and Hyndiuk, R. A. Corticosteroid in experimentally induced *Pseudomonas* keratitis. *Arch. Ophthalmol.* 96:126, 1978.
11. Davis, S. D., Sarff, L. D., and Hyndiuk, R. A. Bacteriologic cure of experimental *Pseudomonas* keratitis. *Invest. Ophthalmol. Vis. Sci.* 17:916, 1978.
12. Davis, S. D., Sarff, L. D., and Hyndiuk, R. A. Comparison of therapeutic routes in experimental *Pseudomonas* keratitis. *Am. J. Ophthalmol.* 87:710, 1979.
13. Davis, S. D., Sarff, L. D., and Hyndiuk, R. A. Relative efficacy of the topical use of amikacin, gentamicin and tobramycin in experimental *Pseudomonas* keratitis. *Can. J. Ophthalmol.* 15:28, 1980.

14. Doughman, D. J. Treatment of corneal thinnings and perforation. *JCE Ophthalmol.* January 1978, pp. 15–23.

15. Duke-Elder, S. S., and Leigh, A. G. Diseases of the Outer Eye, Part 2. In S. S. Duke-Elder (Ed.), *System of Ophthalmology.* St. Louis: Mosby, 1965. Vol. 8, p. 789.

16. Furgiuele, F. P., Kiesel, R., and Martyn, L. *Pseudomonas* infection of the rabbit cornea treated with gentamicin: A preliminary report. *Am. J. Ophthalmol.* 60:818, 1965.

17. Grayson, M. *Diseases of the Cornea.* St. Louis: Mosby, 1979. Chap. 4.

18. Harbin, T. Recurrence of a corneal *Pseudomonas* infection after topical steroid therapy: Report of a case. *Am. J. Ophthalmol.* 58:670, 1964.

19. Hsu, C., and Wiseman, G. M. Antibacterial substances from staphylococci. *Can. J. Microbiol.* 13:947, 1967.

20. Hyndiuk, R. A. Experimental *Pseudomonas* keratitis (Thesis). *Trans. Am. Ophthalmol. Soc.* 79:541, 1982.

21. Hyndiuk, R. A., Hull, D. S., and Kinyoun, J. L. Free tissue patch and cyanoacrylate in corneal perforations. *Ophthalmic Surg.* 5:50, 1974.

22. Hyndiuk, R. A., and Seideman, S. Clinical and Laboratory Techniques in External Ocular Disease and Endophthalmitis. In H. B. Fedukowicz (Ed.), *External Infections of the Eye* (2nd ed.). New York: Appleton-Century-Crofts, 1978. Chap. 5.

23. Johnson, M. K., and Allen, J. H. Ocular toxin of the pneumococcus. *Am. J. Ophthalmol.* 72:175, 1971.

24. Joklik, W. K., and Willett, H. P. The Staphylococci. In D. B. Amos (Ed.), *Zinsser Microbiology* (17th ed.). New York: Appleton-Century-Crofts, 1980. Chap. 26.

25. Jones, D. B. Early diagnosis and therapy of bacterial corneal ulcers. *Int. Ophthalmol. Clin.* 13(4):1, 1973.

26. Jones, D. B. A plan for antimicrobial therapy in bacterial keratitis. *Trans. Am. Acad. Ophthalmol. Otolaryngol.* 79:95, 1975.

27. Jones, D. B. Initial therapy of suspected microbial corneal ulcers: II. Specific antibiotic therapy based on corneal scrapings. *Surv. Ophthalmol.* 24:97, 1979.

28. Kinyoun, J. L., Hyndiuk, R. A., and Hull, D. S. Treatment of corneal perforations with cyanoacrylate. *Wis. Med. J.* 73(Suppl.):117, 1974.

29. Lazar, M., et al. *Mycobacterium fortuitum* keratitis. *Am. J. Ophthalmol.* 78:530, 1974.

30. Lemp, M. A., Blackman, H. J., Koffler, B. H. Therapy for bacterial and fungal infections. *Int. Ophthalmol. Clin.* 20(3):135, 1980.

31. Liesegang, T. J., Forster, R. K. Spectrum of microbial keratitis in South Florida. *Am. J. Ophthalmol.* 90:38, 1980.

32. Liu, P. V. Extracellular toxins of *Pseudomonas aeruginosa. J. Infect. Dis.* 130 (Suppl.):94, 1974.

33. McBeath, J., Forster, R. K., and Rebell, G. Diagnostic limulus lysate assay for endophthalmitis and keratitis. *Arch. Ophthalmol.* 96:1265, 1978.

34. Ohman, D. E., Burns, R. P., and Iglewski, B. H. Corneal infections in mice with toxin A and elastase mutants of *Pseudomonas aeruginosa. J. Infect. Dis.* 142:547, 1980.

35. Okumoto, M. Normal Flora in the Defense of the Conjunctiva Against Infection. In G. R. O'Connor (Ed.), *Immunologic Diseases of the Mucous Membranes: Pathology, Diagnosis and Treatment.* New York: Masson, 1980. Chap. 5.

36. Ostler, H. B., Okumoto, M., and Wilkey, C. The changing pattern of the etiology of central bacterial corneal (hypopyon) ulcer. *Trans. Pacific Coast. Oto-Ophthalmol. Soc.* 57:235, 1976.

37. Ostler, H. B., Thygeson, P., and Okumoto, M. Infectious diseases of the eye: III. Infections of the cornea. *JCE Ophthalmol.* September, 1978, pp. 13–26.

38. Ramphal, R., McNiece, M. T., and Polack, F. M. Adherence of *Pseudomonas aeruginosa* to the injured cornea: A step in the pathogenesis of corneal infections. *Ann. Ophthalmol.* 13:421, 1981.

39. Reed, W. P., and Williams, R. C. Bacterial adherence: First step in pathogenesis of certain infections. *J. Chronic Dis.* 31:67, 1978.

40. Rosenthal, R. L., and Blackman, A. Bone marrow hypoplasia following use of chloramphenicol eye drops. *JAMA* 191:136, 1965.

41. Sloan, S. H., Pettit, T. H., and Litwack, K. D. Gentamicin penetration in the aqueous humor of eyes with corneal ulcers. *Am. J. Ophthalmol.* 73:750, 1972.

42. Tsutsui, J. Tetanus infection of the cornea. *Am. J. Ophthalmol.* 43:772, 1957.

43. Turner, L., and Stinson, I. *Mycobacterium fortuitum* as a cause of corneal ulcer. *Am. J. Ophthalmol.* 60:329, 1965.

44. Vastine, D. Infections of the Ocular Adnexa and Cornea. In G. A. Peyman, D. R. Sanders, and M. F. Goldberg (Eds.), *Principles and Practice of Ophthalmology.* Philadelphia: Saunders, 1980. Chap. 5.

45. Wilson, L. A. Bacterial Corneal Ulcers. In T. D. Duane (Ed.), *Clinical Ophthalmology.* Hagerstown, Md.: Harper & Row, 1978. Vol. 4, chap. 18.

46. Zimmerman, L. E., Turner, L., and McTigue, J. W. *Mycobacterium fortuitum* infection of the cornea. A report of two cases. *Arch. Ophthalmol.* 82:596, 1969.

Fungal Diseases

Richard K. Forster

During the past decade there has been an increase in awareness and recognition of the clinical signs of fungal keratitis, particularly in geographic areas where these infections tend to be more commonly seen (e.g., rural areas and warm climates). This has led to better and more frequent diagnosis and to improved management. Fungal keratitis remains a diagnostic and therapeutic challenge to the ophthalmologist, however, because of its tendency to mimic other types of corneal stromal inflammation, because it may be inadvertently enhanced if corticosteroids are used, and because its management is restricted by the availability of effective antifungal agents and the extent to which they can penetrate into corneal tissue. It is important, therefore, to understand the clinical picture presented by mycotic keratitis and, as an aid in interpreting culture results, to know the fungi that most commonly cause it. Above all, it is important to have a rational and informed approach to the use of both diagnostic laboratory techniques and antifungal compounds and therapeutic alternatives. In this section, the current status of mycotic keratitis is summarized. Now well documented are the importance of prompt and adequate laboratory diagnosis by scraping and culture, the use and value of the polyene antimycotic natamycin in the medical treatment of most cases of mycotic keratitis, and the appropriate place of surgical intervention. Less well documented and still much in need of research are the reasons for occasional natamycin treatment failures; the effectiveness of other antimycotic agents, such as the imidazole compounds; and the whole question of the pathogenesis of mycotic keratitis and the role of immunity and other host resistance factors in susceptibility, cure, and complications.

INCIDENCE

Increased awareness of the occurrence and the frequency of fungal keratitis, better recognition of the clinical features of these infections, and improved laboratory diagnostic techniques of direct examination of stained smears and culture of the causative fungi have all led to an increase in the frequency of correct diagnosis. The growing population in south-

Supported in part by Public Health Service grant EY00674 from the National Eye Institute and the Florida Lions Eye Bank.

ern climates, as in the case of South Florida, for example, has probably also contributed to greater interest in diagnosing mycotic infections [8].

At the Bascom Palmer Eye Institute in Miami, fungal keratitis now accounts for approximately 15 percent of all stromal microbial keratitis for which laboratory studies are performed. During a 9-year period ending in 1977, Liesegang and I reported the culture and staining characteristics of 663 corneal ulcers [14]. Of these, 238 were bacterial, 133 were fungal, and the remaining 292 (44 percent) were culture negative. Fungal keratitis, as a group, was second only to *Pseudomonas* keratitis in frequency [14]. In general, fungal keratitis is more common in the southernmost parts of the United States and in the tropics than it is in the temperate regions.

ETIOLOGY

Although at least 35 genera of fungi have been reported to be associated with corneal infections, several genera and species seem to predominate. The experience in Miami appears to be representative. Infections caused by the same or related species may present a generally similar picture and respond similarly to antifungal agents in vitro and clinically. Over the last several years in Miami we have been able to recognize and catalog certain fungi as frequent or repeated causes of mycotic keratitis. Between 1969 and 1977, of 134 isolates in fungal keratitis, 76 (57 percent) were due to the single species *Fusarium solani,* 28 (21 percent) to other nonpigmented filamentous fungi, 20 (15 percent) to dematiaceous or brown-pigmented fungi, and 10 (7 percent) to yeasts, mainly *Candida albicans* [14] (Table 5-5). A list of the more frequent causes of fungal keratitis would include, in addition to *F. solani,* other species of *Fusarium, Aspergillus fumigatus* and *A. flavus, Paecilomyces lilacinus, Petriellidium boydii,* and, among the pigmented fungi [4], species of *Curvularia, Drechslera, Alternaria,* and *Phialophora,* as well as such tropical fungi as *Lasiodiplodia* and *Colletotrichum,* which are associated with lesions in plants. Any of these species isolated from ulcerative stromal inflammation would be highly suspect as being the causative agent, as are other fungi when they are isolated from carefully made cultures, as described below under Laboratory Methods. Although *F. solani* may be especially common as a cause of keratitis in South Florida, it is also by far the most common isolate received from other parts of the United States, other Western Hemisphere nations, and in fact all parts of the world. Before 1974, nearly 50 percent of reported cases of keratomycosis were attributed to *Aspergillus,* nearly 25 percent to *Candida albicans,* and the remaining 25 percent to diverse fungi among which *F. solani* was increasingly commonly identified after 1970 [7]. This change probably resulted from improved mycologic identification rather than a real change in prevalence.

Most of the fungi implicated in keratitis may be called opportunistic organisms and are ubiquitous as plant pathogens or in the soil. How they become established in the corneal stroma after minor trauma presumably involving implantation of the organism from some outdoor plant material is not adequately understood. There are a number of cases in which the association between infection (after trauma or

injury to the cornea) and plant material is well documented.

An early report of fungal ulcers from South Florida showed an absence of keratitis during the hot, humid, rainy months of June to September [11]. In recent years, however, fungal keratitis, most frequently caused by filamentous fungi other than *F. solani* and yeasts, has also been seen during the summer months. November and March, usually dry, cool, and windy months in South Florida, remain the peak months for the occurrence of fungal keratitis [14]. There is possibly an association of keratitis with dry, windy weather following a wet period suitable for fungus growth. It is of interest, however, that November is also the peak month for bacterial keratitis in South Florida.

Zygomycetes (Phycomycetes) and dermatophytes (ringworm fungi) are rarely reported as causes of fungal keratitis. Many or perhaps most fungi may have the potential to cause keratitis, given the right combination of organism, trauma leading to implantation, and host factors. However, the most common causes appear to be those most frequently encountered after apparently negligible trauma.

CLINICAL FEATURES

Kaufman and Wood described the salient clinical features of mycotic keratitis in 1965 [12]. Some of these features, such as satellite lesions, presumed immune rings, and endothelial plaques, are probably not unique to fungal keratitis but are general features of the stromal inflammatory response in the cornea. However, there are two features that should lead one to suspect a fungal cause: first, stromal infiltrates with feathery, hyphate edges (Fig. 5-16) and second, infiltrates that tend to be dry, gray, and somewhat elevated above the level of the corneal surface (Figs. 5-17 and 5-18). In contrast to this typical picture in mycotic keratitis caused by filamentous fungi (Hyphomycetes), stromal keratitis caused by yeasts such as *C. albicans* may be more localized and have a "collar button" configuration, often with a small ulceration and an expanding although discrete stromal infiltrate (Fig. 5-19). However, it is most important to be aware that although certain features might lead one to suspect a fungal cause, any stromal infiltrate with an overlying ulceration, and rarely also one with an intact epithelium, should in general be considered microbial and probably caused by either bacteria or fungi. A complete microbiologic diagnostic workup, including provisions for the isolation of both bacteria and fungi [9], should, therefore, be done in the

TABLE 5-5. *Fungi Isolated from Eyes with Keratitis (Miami, 1969–1977)*

Organism	No. of Patients
MONILIACEOUS FILAMENTOUS FUNGI	
Fusarium solani	76
Other *Fusarium* species	6
F. episphaeria (dimerum)	3
F. moniliforme	1
F. nivale	1
F. oxysporum	1
Aspergillus	6
A. fumigatus	3
A. flavus	3
Acremonium (Cephalosporium)	4
Penicillium	4
Paecilomyces	2
Petriellidium boydii	2
(Allescheria boydii)	
Geotrichum candidum	1
Myrathecum	1
Volutella	1
Cylindrocarpon	1
DEMATIACEOUS (BROWN-PIGMENTED) FILAMENTOUS FUNGI	
Curvularia	8
C. senegalensis	3
C. verruculosa	1
C. pallescens	1
Unidentified species	3
Sphaeropsidales	5
(Lasiodiplodia theobromae)	
Melanconiales	3
(Colletotrichum atramentum)	
Alternaria	2
Drechslera (Helminthosporium)	1
Cladosporium	1
YEASTS	
Candida albicans	10
Total	134*

*In 133 patients (more than one organism in one patient).
SOURCE. Modified from T. J. Liesegang and R. K. Forster [14].

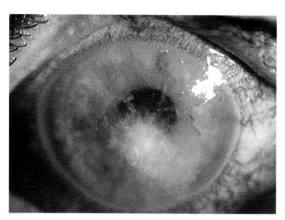

FIGURE 5-16. *Stromal infiltrate with feathery, hyphate edges.* Fusarium episphaeria (dimerum).

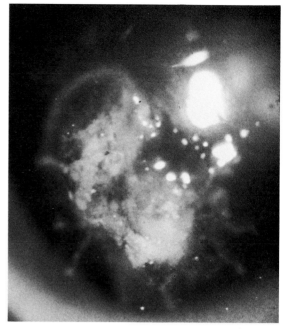

FIGURE 5-18. *Stromal infiltrate with pseudopods, satellites, and immune ring.* Fusarium solani.

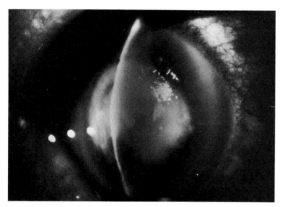

FIGURE 5-17. *Slit lamp biomicroscopic view of fungal keratitis* (Fusarium solani) *with dry infiltrate elevated above level of corneal surface.*

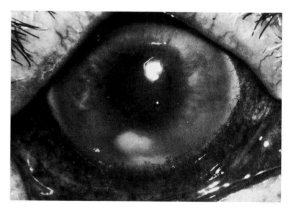

FIGURE 5-19. *Stromal keratitis caused by* Candida albicans. *Localized, discrete infiltrate underlying small ulceration.*

case of all such infiltrates. The unrecognized and undiagnosed fungal keratitis inadvertently treated with corticosteroids may show enhancement in severity and delay in healing. As the consequence of educational efforts and increased awareness of the problem, referring physicians are now more frequently and correctly diagnosing fungal keratitis. In a series of 28 consecutive private referrals, mycotic keratitis was diagnosed correctly in 17 cases, with herpes simplex keratitis being probably the most common condition simulating fungal keratitis [1].

Although fungal keratitis may be an indolent infection, it is usually manifested first as a fairly rapidly developing process, with the onset often resembling that of bacterial keratitis. In my experience, *Pseudomonas* ulceration presents a more

fulminating course, with a shorter delay before referral, than does fungal keratitis. A comparison of fungal keratitis and keratitis caused by *Pseudomonas* (the most common bacterial cause of corneal ulcer in southern regions of the United States) can be summarized as follows [14]: The average age at presentation in fungal keratitis was 44 years compared with 54 years in *Pseudomonas* keratitis. Initiating trauma was seen in 60 percent of the fungal cases, compared with 22 percent of *Pseudomonas* cases. Contrary to expectations and prior teaching, patients developing fungal keratitis tended to be younger and healthier than those with *Pseudomonas* ulcers and often had associated trauma, but rarely had concomitant ocular disease or had used steroids or antibiotic medications before the onset of keratitis. Only 2 percent of patients with fungal keratitis were contact lens wearers, compared with 33 percent of those with *Pseudomonas* keratitis. Prior ocular inflammation had been detected in 6 percent of fungal keratitis eyes, compared with 20 percent of *Pseudomonas* keratitis eyes. Initiating trauma and absence of prior ocular problems or treatment, therefore, distinguished fungal keratitis. In only three of 133 cases of fungal keratitis were steroids known to have been used before the onset of keratitis. However, in 25 percent of cases, steroids were added to the management regimen after the keratitis had developed but before a fungal cause was diagnosed. Antiviral agents were used in 10 percent of fungal ulcers before laboratory diagnosis, which supports the impression that herpes simplex is a common misdiagnosis in cases of fungal keratitis. Major medical disease was seen in 10 percent of patients with fungal keratitis, in contrast to 37 percent of patients with *Pseudomonas* keratitis [14].

LABORATORY DIAGNOSIS

After obtaining a careful clinical history and documenting the clinical features of ulcerative stromal keratitis, the next essential step is to obtain prompt laboratory studies [18, 22]. Laboratory studies consist of obtaining inflamed corneal material by means of a Kimura-like platinum spatula and plating the scraped material onto appropriate culture media and slides for microscopic examination. It is important to obtain multiple samples from the corneal lesion, scraping especially the base and the leading edges of the infiltrate, using slit lamp biomicroscopy, and being certain that corneal stromal material has been obtained before plating it on the culture media or applying it to slides. Occasionally in the case of deep keratitis it will be necessary to obtain corneal material via keratectomy or by loosening deeper corneal material with the aid of a disposable needle. Such scrapings should be performed with the aim of performing ideal laboratory studies, while at the same time in a practical manner, recognizing that there are limitations of available culture media and appropriate stains and that a small infiltrate limits the amount of scraped material available, which therefore must be distributed optimally between slides for staining and culture media. Since bacterial and fungal keratitis can be clinically similar, the scraped material should be plated onto media that will support the growth of either fungi or

bacteria. We therefore routinely inoculate two blood agar plates: one to be maintained at room temperature for fungus growth; the other, at body temperature (35–37°C) for bacterial growth. A Sabouraud agar plate containing gentamicin (50 μg/ml) but without cycloheximide (which tends to inhibit saprophytic fungi) should also be inoculated and incubated at room temperature. A chocolate agar plate is incubated at 37°C in a candle jar. Thioglycolate broth is also routinely inoculated and incubated for possible anaerobic growth at 35 to 37°C. Until recently, a liquid brain-heart infusion (BHI) broth maintained on a rotary shaker at room temperature was also used, mainly as a backup fungus isolate medium. By convention, in order to indicate the site of inoculation on solid medium, material is inoculated in the form of a C-streak, with each row of C-streaks on each medium being made from a separate scraping (Fig. 5-20). Therefore, it is apparent that in order to produce two or three rows of C-streaks, 10 to 15 individual scrapings of the corneal inflammatory material will be required. In addition to the cultures, scraped material is placed on three or four slides for Gram and Giemsa stains as well as on a gelatin- or albumin-coated slide to be used for Grocott's methenamine silver (GMS) stain. If adequate corneal material is available, it is appropriate to smear an additional slide that can be held in reserve for special or repeat stains. Since it is rare for keratitis to progress to endophthalmitis or for the hypopyon associated with keratitis to be infected (even in fungal disease), I do not recommend that anterior chamber paracentesis be performed as an initial diagnostic step in any routine stromal keratitis. The risk of transferring organisms for the cornea or external ocular surface into the eye by paracentesis probably outweighs its questionable diagnostic benefits.

Review of our laboratory results in cases of culture-proven keratitis indicate that Gram stains of corneal scrapings were positive for hyphal elements in 55 percent of the cases, Giemsa stains in 66 percent, and the KOH preparations in 33 percent [14] (Fig. 5-21). In many cases, the KOH preparations were negative in the presence of either positive Gram or Giemsa stains; therefore, we have discontinued making KOH mounts in evaluating ulcerative keratitis. My colleagues and I have, however, described a shortened 1-hour modification of the GMS stain for fungi that has proved highly reliable in confirming the diagnosis of fungal keratitis from scrapings [5] (Fig. 5-22). These stains have been positive in 18 of 21 consecutive cases of fungal

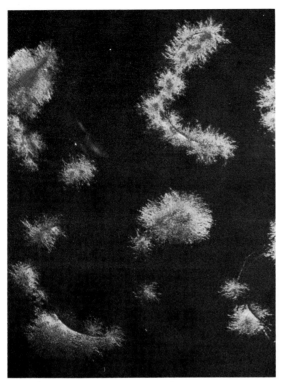

FIGURE 5-20. C-*streaks with early growth of* Fusarium solani *48 hours after inoculation.*

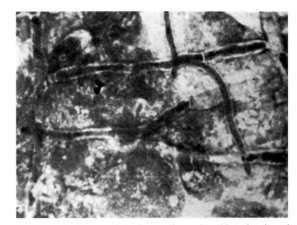

FIGURE 5-21. *Giemsa-stained corneal scraping. Note that fungal cell walls and septa do not stain.*

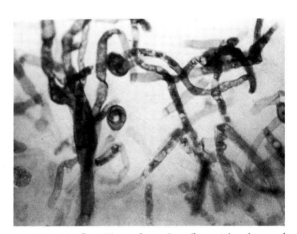

FIGURE 5-22. *Grocott's methenamine silver stain of corneal scraping. Note staining of cell walls and septa.*

keratitis. The GMS stain can also be used for restaining Gram- and Giemsa-stained slides and will often reveal hyphae not clearly shown by the nonspecific staining procedures. In our series of 133 culture-proven cases of fungal keratitis [14], Gram and Giemsa stains were performed in 94 cases. Fungal hyphae were present on two or more slides in 60 percent of these and on only one slide in 21 percent. No hyphae were seen in 19 percent. Although Sabouraud agar with gentamicin and without cycloheximide incubated at room temperature is still the most sensitive medium for isolating fungi, sheep or rabbit blood agar incubated at room temperature is nearly as successful. Blood agar at 37°C was positive for fungi in about 35 percent of the cases, and liquid BHI medium maintained on a rotary shaker at room temperature was positive for fungi in about 50 percent of isolates. Fungal isolates were detected on one or more media in 84 of 105 consecutive cases and on only one medium in 21 cases. In each instance of growth limited to a single medium, the presence of fungus was confirmed by microscopic examination of the scraping.

Contrary to the teaching concerning systemic fungal disease—that cultures for fungi should be incubated for 2 weeks—in my experience almost all ocular fungal isolates grow out and become evident in 48 to 72 hours. Most, in fact, are visible with the dissecting microscope or naked eye within less than 36 hours. One should wait a week before declaring a culture negative for fungi. Some reports indicate slower growth of fungi from eye cultures and a lower incidence of detection by solid media or stained scrapings [16]. These reports are, however, in sharp contrast to the results obtained in a series of 134 isolations from 133 ocular fungus infections [14].

Secondary fungal keratitis was documented in two patients of 133 fungal cases. One case followed an initial *Streptococcus pneumoniae* infection; the other, herpes simplex keratitis. In two proven fungal ulcers, streptococcal superinfections developed subsequently. In my experience, mixed bacterial growth and fungal keratitis is uncommon, and it is rare in cases of fungal keratitis to see growth of bacteria on blood agar at either room temperature or 37°C. There is little evidence that topical antibiotics aggravate fungal keratitis. Likewise, fungi do not seem to alter in a major way the normal ocular flora of the conjunctival surface and the cul-de-sac.

See Infectious Agents: Fungi in Chapter 4 for the culture characteristics of the fungi.

HISTOPATHOLOGY

The classic histopathologic findings in fungal keratitis include two features that are considered to be suggestive of progressive pathogenicity: fungal hyphal elements oriented perpendicular to the normal corneal lamellae, and a tendency for hyphal elements apparently to penetrate Descemet's membrane [15]. We examined approximately 40 ocular specimens histopathologically (Fig. 5-23). Some were whole eyes, but most were from therapeutic penetrating keratoplasty after medical treatment failures in which the infection had progressed to frank or impending perforation. We noted the presence of limbal infiltrates (Fig. 5-24) and a tendency toward progressive keratitis in cases of impending perforation and abscess formation. We also recognized the following syndrome: After initial laboratory proof of fungal keratitis and treatment with topical antifungal agents, there was initial improvement, followed, after approximately 2 weeks of therapy, by progressive ulceration that necessitated penetrating keratoplasty or keratectomy with a conjunctival flap. In these cases, abnormal degenerated hyphal forms were seen histopathologically, sometimes associated with negative cultures obtained at the time of surgery [3]. This finding suggests the need to evaluate factors that contribute to progressive keratitis even in the presence of antifungal treatment that leaves nonviable fungal elements in the corneal stroma. In certain of these histopathologic specimens, a localized inflammatory reaction at the limbus characterized by a collection of round cells and plasma cells was also observed. This suggests that perhaps immune mechanisms contribute in certain instances to progressive ulceration and the apparent failure of medical management.

Progressive keratitis in laboratory animals is difficult to establish without corticosteroids, and fungal keratitis has to date been reported infrequently in animals such as the dog and horse.

TREATMENT

ANTIFUNGAL AGENTS

Before 1969, most cases of fungal keratitis were treated with topical amphotericin B. In Miami, this treatment was effective in only seven of 21 *Fusarium*

ulcers treated [11]. Subsequently, the related polyene natamycin was used investigationally to treat 53 cases of mycotic keratitis. Healing occurred in 46 of these, with a final vision of 20/40 or better in 25 cases [2, 10]. In our experience, a 5% suspension of natamycin used as the initial therapy in fungal keratitis has been successful in approximately 85 percent of *F. solani* infections, 60 percent of those caused by other moniliaceous (nonpigmented) fungi, 90 percent of those caused by dematiaceous (brown-pigmented) fungi, and 75 percent of yeast infections [2]. Failure of infections to heal when treated with natamycin has not necessarily been due to in vitro resistance, but rather to as yet unidentified factors contributing to progressive keratitis, as discussed above. In some of the keratoplasty specimens from cases of failed medical treatment, hyphal fragments were seen by GMS staining but were nonviable by culture.

In 1979, the Food and Drug Administration approved natamycin for topical ocular use, and Alcon Laboratories (Fort Worth, Tex.) made the 5% suspension (Natacyn) commercially available on a case-by-case basis (it can be obtained by calling 817-293-0450). Although amphotericin B is highly effective in vitro against most fungal isolates from keratitis, its record in the treatment of clinical fungal keratitis has in general not been as good as that of natamycin [10]. Although natamycin has been highly successful in the treatment of *F. solani* infections, the results in keratitis caused by other fungi have been more variable. Therefore interest has turned to alternative antifungal agents such as miconazole, clotrimazole, and ketoconazole. With the exception of flucytosine, compounds used against mycotic infections are in general rather insoluble in water. This low solubility limits blood levels in vivo and the range of concentration that can be tested for antifungal effects in vitro. Current medical interest in ketoconazole is high because the agent can be taken orally.

With the exception of that of pencillin, the mechanisms of action of few antibiotics have been studied as extensively as that of the antifungal polyenes. These agents exert their effect by binding to sterols present in the cell membrane of eukaryotic cells [13]. They have no effect on cell membranes in which sterols are absent. They tend to have a greater affinity for ergosterol (fungus membrane sterol) than for cholesterol (animal membrane sterol). This apparently accounts for their in vivo selective antifungal effect in the treatment of mycotic disease in animals. However, their affinity for cholesterol is considerable, which tends to make them toxic. Of the three principal polyene antimycotics used in medicine (amphotericin B, nystatin, and natamycin) only amphotericin B can be administered systemically, although its use and effectiveness is compromised by its toxicity. Local ocular toxicity, although clinically apparent with amphotericin B solubilized by bile salts (unless it is used as a dilute solution), does not seem to be a problem with the other polyene agents, perhaps because of their poor absorption. Amphotericin B, however, is probably also poor in penetrating into the cornea or other intraocular tissues when administered via either systemic or periocular routes.

Functionally, the polyene antibiotics are divided into two classes: large polyenes, with 35 or more carbon atoms, such as amphotericin B and nystatin, and smaller polyenes, with 30 or less carbon atoms, such as natamycin. Although both large and small polyenes bind to sterols, they differ in their subsequent effect on the cell membranes as a consequence of their size difference. As shown in Figure 5-25, the larger polyenes approximate the length of the cell membrane phospholipids and, therefore, by grouping together, can form narrow circular channels for the passage of potassium, chloride, and other small ions. This free passage for small ions apparently leads to electrolyte imbalance and subsequent death of the cell. The lethal effect of the large polyenes therefore may be blocked or reversed by osmotic and electrolyte control of the surrounding medium, since except for these channels the cell membrane, although leaky, remains intact. The molecular length of the small polyenes such as natamycin, however, is less than that of the phospholipids; hence these polyenes do not span the width of the membrane to form channels. Instead, they accumulate in the membrane and form "blisters" that disrupt it and cause the sterol-phospholipid film to break down. This phenomenon is not reversed by osmotic or electrolye control of the external media. Consistent with this interpretation, we have observed that an increase of sodium in the external medium markedly increases the antifungal effect of the large polyenes but does not alter that of small polyenes. The fungicidal end point of natamycin observed in vitro also tends to be more absolute and independent of time of incubation. Whether or not this difference between natamycin and the larger polyenes is clinically important is not known. The polyene antibiotics can be relied upon to be effective in vitro against almost all fungi.

According to current research, the imidazole compounds such as clotrimazole, miconazole, and

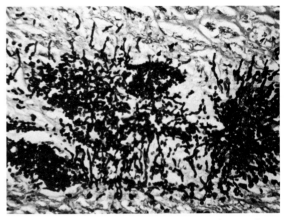

FIGURE 5-23. *Penetrating keratoplasty specimen showing abscess formation and arrangement of hyphal elements perpendicular to corneal lamellae.*

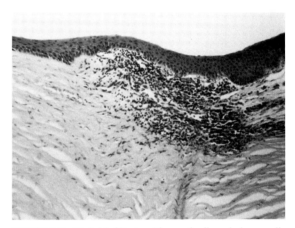

FIGURE 5-24. *Limbal infiltrate with round cells and plasma cells associated with progressive stromal ulceration.*

ketoconazole owe their antifungal effects to two mechanisms affecting the cell membrane [20]. One is an interference with the synthesis of ergosterol, the fungus membrane sterol. The second mechanism is a direct action on cell membranes causing them to become leaky—according to one interpretation by the binding of the imidazole to fatty acids. Free fatty acids are present in the membrane of eukaryotic cells but appear to vary in quantity depending on the organism and other factors. Fungal cells seem to have more fatty acids in their membranes than do animal cells, which may account for the selective antifungal effect of the imidazole compounds in the treatment of mycotic disease. Clotrimazole has a greater tendency to bind to fatty acids, including phospholipid moieties, than does miconazole or ketoconazole. It is also more toxic and is not administered systemically. Unlike the

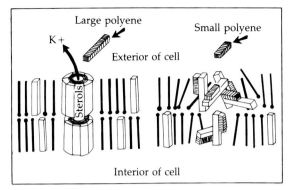

FIGURE 5-25. *Comparison of mechanism of action of large and small polyenes.*

polyenes, the imidazoles also have some antibacterial effect, especially against gram-positive bacteria, as well as a clinical effect against a variety of protozoa and helminths.

Unlike the polyenes and the imidazoles, which act on the cell membrane, flucytosine is incorporated into the fungal RNA and interferes with protein synthesis. Wagner and Shadomy have reviewed the literature and carried out detailed studies of their own on the mechanism of action of flucytosine [21]. The sequence of events in *Candida* begins with the entry of the drug into the yeast cell by a permease. Once in the cell, the flucytosine is rapidly deaminated to fluorouracil. This fluorinated analogue of uracil is incorporated into the fungal RNA, particularly transfer RNA, which leads to the production of nonfunctional protein and ultimately cessation of growth.

Performing careful tube dilution sensitivity studies on a variety of human fungal isolates allows one to tabulate the likely sensitivity pattern for a large number of isolates from ocular mycoses. The other approach is to send fungal isolates to a regional reference laboratory where sensitivity testing can be performed, but this tends to take several days and does not provide the necessary information for the practicing ophthalmologist as quickly as a summarized table of sensitivities, listing the principal known causes of ocular mycotic infections.

We have found, for example, that *F. solani* is not uniquely more sensitive to natamycin but rather is quite uniformly sensitive, and less sensitive to nystatin and amphotericin B, as compared with other fungi. It is, however, considerably less sensitive in vitro to the imidazole compounds than to natamycin. Most other *Fusarium* species seem to share this property of relative resistance to imidazole compounds in vitro. Sensitivity to imidazole compounds appears on the basis of assays performed in tissue culture medium in our recent studies to be quite uniform in the case of most fungi from keratitis, *Fusarium* species excepted. All isolates of filamentous fungi tested with the imidazoles seem to fall into two groups, those that are sensitive, such as *Curvularia* and *Aspergillus,* and those that are relatively insensitive, predominantly *Fusarium* species. In vitro, clotrimazole seems to be the most effective imidazole, but, as I have noted, it is also the most toxic, owing perhaps to its binding to phospholipid fatty acid moieties as well as to free fatty acids.

Synergism between the polyenes, such as amphotericin B, and the imidazole compounds does not occur. The in vitro results show that each drug acts independently and that the combined effect is perhaps slightly less than that obtained with the most effective of the two compounds alone. Combined treatment with flucytosine and amphotericin B, of proven efficacy in yeast infections, is probably not warranted unless the fungus is specifically sensitive to flucytosine alone. Synergism occurs close to the effective flucytosine concentration, but we have also found evidence of antagonism between the two compounds at lower concentrations of flucytosine.

It has often been assumed that failure to respond successfully to antifungal therapy indicates in vitro resistance [7]. In my experience, there is little to support in vitro resistance per se as a cause of treatment failure. Rather, progressive keratitis is probably related to undetermined factors such as poor penetration of the fungal agent and inflammatory and immunologic effects that may persist even after the fungus has been rendered nonviable.

SURGICAL MANAGEMENT
Before 1969, 15 keratoplasties were performed at the Bascom Palmer Eye Institute after medical therapy failure in fungal keratitis. In 13 of these cases, active fungal disease was eliminated. However, useful vision was retained in only three eyes [19]. In contrast, of 61 cases of mycotic keratitis since 1969, including 53 treated with natamycin, 13 were considered medical treatment failures and 11 required therapeutic surgery. A final visual acuity of 20/70 or better was achieved in six of the 11 cases, including five of nine with therapeutic penetrating keratoplasties [3]. In four of the eyes that required surgery, ulceration had progressed in spite of natamycin treatment, but fungal cultures were negative at the time of surgery. Although therapeutic surgery is at times required in the management of fungal keratitis (to remove infectious or antigenic elements or both), it is probably reasonable to try first to treat the patient with natamycin or other

agents for a considerable period in order to render the fungus nonviable before resorting to surgery [17]. This in turn probably improves the general prognosis. Although a rationale is lacking for the use of conjunctival flaps if there is active fungal disease, primarily because of viable fungi deep in the cornea, there are scattered reports from parts of the world where antifungal medical therapy is unavailable that show that debridement alone, presumably resulting in removal of fungal agents, and conjunctival flaps are in some cases successful in controlling fungal keratitis.

The two groups of patients that seem to respond most poorly to medical antimycotic therapy are those with deep corneal infection, presumably because of the penetration limitations of antifungal agents, and those who have been treated with corticosteroids before the diagnosis of fungal keratitis. Like herpesvirus, whose replication is enhanced by corticosteroids, fungi are aided in their growth in tissue by corticosteroids. There is, therefore, little if any rationale for using corticosteroids in presumed or confirmed fungal keratitis; nor is there evidence that a combined steroid-antifungal treatment is either safe or efficacious. However, if the observations that suggest that an immune response contributes to progressive keratitis are correct and can be confirmed, then there may be a place for corticosteroid modification of the inflammatory response to nonviable fungal elements after effective antimycotic treatment.

MANAGEMENT REGIMEN

Prompt, appropriate, rational therapy for fungal keratitis, rests on clinical evaluation and laboratory investigation. Since about 75 to 80 percent of stromal keratitis confirmed by culture to have a fungal cause can be detected by microscopic examination of the scraped material after appropriate staining, it is reasonable to restrict initial antifungal therapy to those cases with a fungus-positive scraping. If by 24 hours after scraping, the culture growth is consistent with a bacterial infection, then in spite of the clinical history and appearance, therapy should not include an antifungal agent. On the other hand, a scraping positive for fungal elements or the appearance of fungal growth by 36 to 48 hours after culture should prompt the initiation of antifungal therapy.

At this time therapy should be started with 5% natamycin suspension (50 mg/ml), usually hourly during the day and every 2 hours at night. The therapy should also include cycloplegic agents and careful monitoring of the intraocular pressure with use of appropriate antiglaucoma medications when indicated. As with other forms of keratitis, in fungal keratitis immediate or prompt improvement in the clinical picture is unusual; one must be patient and allow time for stabilization, lack of progression, and finally improvement in the corneal stromal infiltrate and ulceration. If the infection appears to be progressing in the presence of a confirmed fungal cause, particularly when there is a deep stromal infiltrate, then consideration should be given to adding or substituting another antifungal agent such as miconazole [6]. Miconazole, available as a 1% solution (10 mg/ml) (Monistat), can be used hourly or more frequently topically and can be injected periocularly or subconjunctivally in a dosage of 10 mg. In my experience, injectable miconazole appears much less locally toxic than amphotericin B. It must be emphasized, however, that a body of data similar to that for natamycin testifying to the efficacy of imidazole compounds does not exist, and the presumption of better penetration into the corneal stroma is also not fully proved.

The management of yeast keratitis (C. albicans) can be more difficult than that of infections with filamentous fungi because in cases of yeast infection there are often underlying local ocular abnormalities and sometimes general defects in host resistance. Since yeast infections tend to occur in either immunosuppressed or locally compromised eyes, there appears to be a greater disparity in antifungal sensitivities among cases of Candida infection than among infections with filamentous fungi. One must, therefore, attempt to stabilize the ocular surface and consider using antifungal agents more specifically directed against yeast infections such as flucytosine. Yeasts grow quickly and usually become evident on culture by 24 to 36 hours, and they can perhaps be best treated by combined therapy using natamycin, nystatin, miconazole, and flucytosine. Sensitivity studies should be performed with the particular yeast since there is a high incidence of both acquired resistance and de novo resistance to flucytosine. Clinically, nystatin was the first antifungal polyene to be used. Although not commercially available as an ocular medication, it can be prepared as an eye drop in a concentration of 50,000 units per milliliter. The dermatologic cream preparation can also be utilized for ocular infections. Its use in yeast infections is traditional, although it does not appear to be as effective against yeast infections as natamycin is against filamentous fungi.

ACKNOWLEDGMENT

I acknowledge the invaluable contribution and expertise of Gerbert Rebell in our studies on fungal keratitis and in the preparation of this text.

REFERENCES

1. Forster, R. K., and Rebell, G. The diagnosis and management of keratomycoses. I. Cause and diagnosis. *Arch. Ophthalmol.* 93:975, 1975.

2. Forster, R. K., and Rebell, G. The diagnosis and management of keratomycoses: II. Medical and surgical management. *Arch. Ophthalmol.* 93:1134, 1975.

3. Forster, R. K., and Rebell, G. Therapeutic surgery in failures of medical treatment for fungal keratitis. *Br. J. Ophthalmol.* 59:366, 1975.

4. Forster, R. K., Rebell, G., and Wilson, L. A. Dematiaceous fungal keratitis: Clinical isolates and management. *Br. J. Ophthalmol.* 59:372, 1975.

5. Forster, R. K., et al. Methenamine-silver–stained corneal scrapings in keratomycoses. *Am. J. Ophthalmol.* 82:261, 1976.

6. Foster, C. S. Miconazole therapy for keratomycosis. *Am. J. Ophthalmol.* 91:622, 1981.

7. Jones, B. R. Principles in the management of oculomycosis. *Trans. Am. Acad. Ophthalmol. Otolaryngol.* 79:15, 1975.

8. Jones, D. B. Fungal Keratitis. In L. A. Wilson (Ed.), *External Diseases of the Eye.* Hagerstown, Md.: Harper & Row, 1979.

9. Jones, D. B. Decision-making in the management of microbial keratitis. *Ophthalmology* (Rochester) 88:814, 1981.

10. Jones, D. B., Forster, R. K., and Rebell, G. *Fusarium solanae* keratitis treated with natamycin (pimaricin). *Arch. Ophthalmol.* 88:147, 1972.

11. Jones, D. B., Sexton, R. R., and Rebell, G. Mycotic keratitis in South Florida: A review of 39 cases. *Trans. Ophthalmol. Soc. U.K.* 89:781, 1969.

12. Kaufman, H. E., and Wood, R. M. Mycotic keratitis. *Am. J. Ophthalmol.* 59:993, 1965.

13. Kotler-Brajtburg, J., et al. Classification of polyene antibiotics according to chemical structure and biological effects. *Antimicrob. Agents Chemother.* 15:716, 1979.

14. Liesegang, T. J., and Forster, R. K. Spectrum of microbial keratitis in South Florida. *Am. J. Ophthalmol.* 90:38, 1980.

15. Naumann, G., Green, W. R., and Zimmerman, L. E. Mycotic keratitis. A histopathologic study of 73 cases. *Am. J. Ophthalmol.* 64:668, 1967.

16. O'Day, D. M., et al. Laboratory isolation techniques in human and experimental fungal infections. *Am. J. Ophthalmol.* 87:688, 1979.

17. Polack, F. M., Kaufman, H. E., and Newmark, E. Keratomycosis: Medical and surgical treatment. *Arch. Ophthalmol.* 85:410, 1971.

18. Rebell, G., and Forster, R. K. Fungi of Keratomycosis. In E. H. Lennette (Ed.), *Manual of Clinical Microbiology* (3rd ed.). Washington, D.C.: American Society for Microbiology, 1980.

19. Sanders, N. Penetrating keratoplasty in treatment of fungus keratitis. *Am. J. Ophthalmol.* 70:24, 1970.

20. Sud, I. J., and Feingold, D. S. Heterogeneity of action mechanisms among antimycotic imidazoles. *Antimicrob. Agents Chemother.* 20:71, 1981.

21. Wagner, G. E., and Shadomy, S. Studies on the mode of action of 5-fluorocytosine in *Aspergillus* species. *Chemotherapy* 25:61, 1979.

22. Wilson, L. A., and Sexton, R. R. Laboratory diagnosis in fungal keratitis. *Am. J. Ophthalmol.* 66:646, 1968.

Viral Diseases: HERPETIC DISEASES

Deborah Pavan-Langston

HERPES SIMPLEX OCULAR DISEASE

Herpes simplex virus (HSV), the most ubiquitous communicable infectious virus in man, is the causal agent of a wide variety of chronically recurring diseases. Ocular herpes simplex, caused primarily by type 1 (oral), but occasionally type 2 (genital), HSV, is the leading infectious cause of corneal blindness in the United States, with approximately 500,000 cases reported annually [16, 89]. Recurrent herpes labialis and dermatitis, also usually caused by type 1 HSV (HSV-1), afflicts approximately one-third of the world population; one-half of these people suffer more than one attack annually. Herpes genitalis, caused primarily by type 2 HSV (HSV-2), is the second most common venereal disease in this country, with approximately 100,000 cases reported annually [41, 89]. In neonates and children, the primary attack of HSV can be devastating. It may be associated with herpetic encephalitis and dissemination of infection, which has a very high degree of morbidity and mortality [51]. Immunologically compromised patients such as leukemics or organ transplant recipients are also at high risk of severe systemic and ocular herpetic infections [88]. Certain human malignancies have been strongly linked to members of the herpes family. HSV-2 and HSV-1 in particular have been associated with uterine cervical carcinoma [71, 73].

EPIDEMIOLOGY

In contrast to the extensive data available on the epidemiology of extraocular HSV, little is known about the epidemiology of ocular infections. Nonetheless, information derived from nonocular herpetic studies is of use in understanding many aspects of the often blinding ocular involvement.

The only natural reservoir of HSV is man, with sources of infection being children with primary disease, adults with recurrent disease, and children and adults as healthy asymptomatic carriers. There is a very high incidence of herpetic neutralizing antibodies in children under 6 months of age, presumably owing to passive transfer via the placenta. This incidence then falls to about 20 percent in children from 6 months to 1 year of age and then rises slowly to about 70 percent by age 15 to 25 years. After this time, there is yet a further increase to about 97 percent by the age of 60 years [6, 78].

Transmission of the virus appears to be primarily by direct contact. In the head area, this would be salivary droplets or direct oral contact leading to a primary infection, usually around the mouth. Although the primary illness is manifested clinically in only about 1 to 6 percent of cases infected with virus, the virus still has access to the trigeminal ganglia, the ganglion that innervates the eye [37, 76, 79]. The incubation period between contact and disease is from 3 to 9 days.

In an attempt to determine some of the basic epidemiologic characteristics of ocular herpes, Bell, Holman, and I recently reviewed the medical records of 141 patients (aged 2–81 years) with infectious epithelial HSV keratitis [2]. We found an overall predominance of male patients resulting entirely from an increased male-to-female ratio in the 80 patients over 40 years of age (1.67 : 1.0; p < 0.03). Of the 65 patients who had more than one episode and for whom the dates of all episodes were known, 34 percent had a mean recurrence ratio of one or more episodes per year. Sixty-eight percent had a mean recurrence rate of one or more episodes every 2 years. There was a median time interval between episodes of 1.5 years (range 1.7 months to 20.8 years). Although we found no patient risk factors for frequent recurrence or for severe disease (age of entry into study, age of first ocular episode, sex, or source of primary eye care) we found that 46 percent of 57 recurrences in 27 patients occurred during the four-month period November through February (p < 0.04). The dates were consistent with a possible role of estrogenic hormones and viral respiratory infections in the pathogenesis of infectious ocular herpes.

In a similar but prospective study by Shuster and coworkers of 119 ocular herpes patients, the recurrence rates were somewhat lower, with 24 percent of patients having recurrences within 1 year and 33 percent within 2 years [77]. This may reflect a difference in recurrence rates in the northeastern United States as opposed to the South and West. Shuster and colleagues also found no correlation between rate of recurrence and either sex or age of the patient but did note a general correlation between short intervals between past attacks and short intervals between future recurrences.

In a sociologic study, Smith and coworkers demonstrated a decrease in the incidence of herpetic antibodies in a large population in England [78]. They attributed this to a general improvement in the social environment, improved housing conditions, and better general hygiene.

LATENCY AND TRIGGER MECHANISMS FOR REACTIVATION

Much of the scarring caused by herpes virus is the result of its pattern of recurring. With each new attack, more permanent damage may be left. One of the most important recent advances in herpetic research is the finding that latent herpetic reservoirs in the neuronal tissues are the source of recurrent viral infection [80]. Data on the character of different viral strains have also indicated that some herpes strains are more likely to cause repeated and severe disease, whereas other strains rarely, if ever, cause recurrences and, consequently, cause little disease after the primary infection [32, 85]. Latent HSV infection is apparently established 2 or 3 weeks after the onset of the primary infection [80]. Neuronal tissue cocultivation studies have shown that latent virus is harbored in the neuronal sensory, trigeminal, or autonomic ganglia and the mesencephalic nucleus in the brain stem beyond the reach of topical medications and travels to the affected surface tissues during reactivation [54, 55, 80, 87]. Latent virus in the ganglionic cells has been hypothesized to exist in one of two states: dynamic or static [73].

The dynamic state is one in which latently infected cells contain slowly replicating virus unable to induce recurrent disease unless host defenses fail. Yamamoto and colleagues have demonstrated the presence of HSV-coded thymidine kinase in latently infected dorsal root ganglia of mice up to 8 weeks after inoculation [90]. This suggests that at least a portion of the viral genome is being continuously or intermittently expressed during the latent phase of the HSV infection and that at least a portion of the viral reservoir would be susceptible to systemically administered antiviral drugs activated by these enzymes. This has already been demonstrated with acyclovir [67].

In the static state, HSV is harbored in cells in which replication of viral genome is totally but reversibly interrupted. Puga and coworkers have reported that HSV-specific mRNA is present in the trigeminal ganglia of mice during the acute but not the latent stage; thus, the viral genome may also be capable of existing as a nonreplicating, truly latent entity and, therefore, not susceptible to systemic antivirals during true latency [70].

The wide variety of factors able to induce recurrent herpetic eruptions in humans (sunlight, local trauma, heat, fever, menstruation, immunologic manipulation, infectious disease, surgery, and emotional stress) have been superbly reviewed in the last two decades [36, 73]. Spontaneous reactivation of virus is not common in laboratory animals but can be provoked by stimuli such as anaphylactic shock, epinephrine, prostaglandins, ultraviolet light, electrical stimulation of the trigeminal ganglion, and epilation [5, 38, 54]. Attempts to reactivate HSV by immunosuppressive agents alone have been generally unsuccessful. However, Openshaw and colleagues have demonstrated reactivation of latent HSV in up to 70 percent of the animals treated with the immunosuppressive drug cyclophosphamide, x-rays, or both [55]. The wide variety of factors capable of affecting recurrence rates in humans and animals are all obviously forms of physical or emotional stress or alterations in the immune status of the host. Such factors should be taken into account, and, if possible, ameliorated, when evaluating the best overall management of patients with ocular herpes.

IMMUNE DEFENSE MECHANISMS
Herpesvirus itself does not directly stimulate an inflammatory response, but the by-products of viral replication and immune alteration of the cornea and iris play an important role in many destructive corneal conditions including necrotizing keratitis, immune rings, limbal vasculitis, and disciform edema [31]. The pathogenesis of these manifestations of herpetic disease has yet to be fully elucidated, but much has been established recently through animal models and histopathologic study of human corneal transplant specimens. Intact HSV is found only occasionally in such transplant specimens. Nevertheless, it seems likely that the persistence of incomplete viral antigens and the viral immune alteration of cell membranes in the corneal stroma incite inflammatory reactions that involve programmed host lymphocytes, antiviral antibodies, serum complement, PMNs, and macrophages [17, 48, 50]. The extent to which the host inflammatory response may be beneficial to the eye in terms of ridding the cornea of viral antigens, as opposed to being detrimental in causing matrix destruction, is not yet understood. It is likely that inflammation may be involved in both of these roles simultaneously. It would be highly useful to be able to separate these two functions and to know when and if there is an appropriate time to use antiinflammatory agents before irreversible damage to the cornea ensures.

Host factors, including hereditary characteristics (HLA type), systemic immune diseases (atopy), and other forms of immune incompetence and hyperimmunity have long been felt to play a role in the nature and severity of reaction to herpetic antigen. Recent studies of HLA type, particularly HLA-DR, HLA-A2, and HLA-A3, have been of interest, but results are at variance with each other, with some investigators reporting a positive correlation and others a negative one [26, 49]. The ability to predict the high-risk patient and his prognosis would greatly enhance our management not only of ocular disease but also of herpetic infections elsewhere in the body.

DIAGNOSTIC TESTS

Diagnosis of either primary or recurrent ocular HSV may be assisted by Giemsa staining epithelial scrapings taken from the skin or corneal ulcers. Microscopic examination of the smear may, but does not invariably, reveal typical eosinophilic viral inclusion bodies of Lipshütz in the nuclei. The epithelial cells themselves show ballooning degeneration, and a monocytic white cell infiltrate characteristic of viral infection is always present.

A more definitive diagnosis can be made if a viral culture can be performed within several days of onset of the disease. Swabbing the ulcerated areas and immediately inoculating into tissue culture results in a viral isolation rate of about 70 percent if antivirals have not been used recently. The virus isolate may then be typed as HSV-1 or HSV-2.

Primary herpes can be differentiated from first ocular occurrence of recurrent disease by drawing paired sera. The initial clotted blood sample should be drawn when the patient is first seen during the acute phase; the second sample, 4 to 6 weeks later. These may be sent to the state laboratory for titers against both type 1 and type 2 HSV. Negligible titers in the first blood sample but appreciable titers in the second indicate a primary infection in a previously nonimmune patient with subsequent appearance of anti-HSV antibodies.

CLINICAL FEATURES

Because nearly 500,000 cases of ocular herpes are diagnosed each year in the United States, ophthalmologists must be concerned about the appropriate therapy for this often baffling disease. To understand the advantages and disadvantages of the many modes of therapy used in managing this disease, it is necessary to understand not only the effects of the drugs themselves but the various presentations and pathogenesis of this multifaceted phenomenon.

Ocular herpes may be classified into three general groups: congenital and neonatal, primary, and recurrent.

CONGENITAL AND NEONATAL OCULAR HERPES

Congenital ocular herpes infections are extremely rare. Hutchison and coworkers recovered type 1 (oral) HSV from the eye of an infant, one of dizygotic twins, born with active herpetic keratitis [30]. The mother had no evidence of cervical herpes by culture or serial immune titers, delivery was by cesarean section, and there had been no premature rupture of the membranes. It was hypothesized (but it could not be proved) that the infection was acquired in utero via the transplacental, not the ascending, route. The second twin also developed periocular HSV a few days after birth. Both infants were treated with topical idoxuridine (IDU) and, because of the chance of disseminated disease, systemic vidarabine (ara-A), and both made a full recovery.

Although the vast majority of all ocular herpes infections are caused by type 1 HSV, because of the usual nature of acquisition 80 percent of neonatal cases are caused by type 2 HSV [51]. Despite the unusual case reported by Hutchison and colleagues [30], neonatal disease is almost invariably secondary to direct exposure to an HSV-2–infected birth canal during the late prenatal period or during passage through the canal at birth itself.

Ocular herpes in the newborn may include one or all of the following: conjunctivitis, epithelial keratitis, stromal immune reaction, cataracts, and necrotizing chorioretinitis [9, 28]. Infants' "protective" transplacental antibodies do not seem sufficient to protect them completely from major ocular disease, although they may escape life-threatening visceral involvement [28]. In almost all reported cases, there has been an associated vesicular eruption of the skin, which is a most useful finding when the physician is faced with the need for a very rapid diagnosis. The clinical course of the ocular disease is similar to that encountered with primary or recurrent infections, depending on whether the infant has passively acquired transplacental antibody from the mother. Epithelial ulcers ultimately respond to antiviral therapy, but stromal involvement may clear or leave a nebulous scar. In the absence of superinfection, the skin lesions heal without scarring.

PRIMARY OCULAR HERPES

As noted above, most newborns are protected, in part, by maternal antiherpetic antibodies transferred passively across the placenta in utero. This partial protection lasts for about 6 months, at which time the passively received antibodies have dwindled to negligible titers and the child becomes nonimmune and susceptible to a primary attack of HSV. Fortunately, more than 94 percent of children do not suffer overt disease when they finally do contract the virus; those who do have overt disease usually manifest it about the mouth and not the eye. All those who are infected (70 percent by age 5) then become viral carriers with the agent resting in latent state in the sensory (trigeminal ganglion) and autonomic nervous system [6, 54, 78].

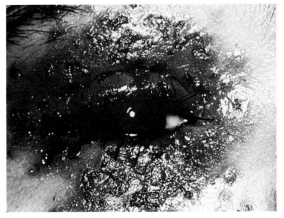

FIGURE 5-26. *Primary herpes simplex periocular vesiculation.*

Primary ocular involvement may present as an acute follicular conjunctivitis or keratoconjunctivitis with nonsuppurative preauricular adenopathy and often with notable vesiculating periocular skin involvement (Fig. 5-26). Pseudomembranes may be present in the fornices. In the absence of skin vesiculation, differentiation from adenoviral infection is aided by a careful search of the lid margins for signs of herpetic blistering.

Primary HSV keratitis is often atypical. Initially, there may be just a nonspecific diffuse punctate keratitis that evolves into multiple scattered microdendritic figures. There may be wandering linear serpiginous ulcers across the entire corneal surface. The diffuse nature of this primary epithelial involvement is probably a function of the host's nonimmune state, which allows more widespread ulceration. Primary disease is, as a rule, confined to the epithelium in terms of clinical findings. Stromal involvement is not seen in this phase of the disease, again because the host is not immunologically programmed against the virus.

RECURRENT OCULAR HERPES
I have found it useful to categorize subsequent herpetic disease as either an infectious or immunologic process. Patients with recurrent herpes have both cellular and humoral immunity against the virus. The disease may present as any one or a combination of the following [58]:

Epithelial infectious ulceration
Epithelial trophic (metaherpetic) ulceration
Stromal disease
  Viral interstitial keratitis, immune rings, limbal vasculitis
  Disciform keratitis
Iridocyclitis and trabeculitis

The incidence of recurrent ocular infections as determined in two recent studies has been discussed above under Epidemiology; it ranges between 24 percent within 1 year to 68 percent within 2 years of a known previous ocular HSV infection [2, 77]. Recurrent disease may occur in the eye even if the primary involvement was clinically manifested elsewhere in the body. The incidence of first ocular occurrence in such cases is not known.

The mechanisms of recurrence are not fully understood. Reservoirs of latent virus residing in the trigeminal and possibly other ganglia are felt to be the source of the infectious component of the disease. Reactivation of the latent organism allows intact virus to travel back down the nerve axons to cause vesicular eruption on the innervated surface. When one considers how much of the population carries HSV in the trigeminal ganglion as a result of oral infection, it is amazing, indeed, that the virus is not directed down the first division of the fifth nerve more often, thus making ocular herpetic infection as common as the oral cold sore.

EPITHELIAL INFECTIOUS ULCERATION
Herpes simplex–induced eruptions of the corneal epithelium are characteristically thin, branching dendritic ulcers; wider, branching dendrogeographic ulcers; or map-shaped geographic lesions. All are caused by live virus. Little inflammatory cell reaction—PMNs but no lymphocytes—is seen in this form of ocular herpes, but many free viruses lie in intracellular and extracellular locations, particularly in the basal epithelium [84].

Signs and symptoms include tearing, irritation, photophobia, and often blurring of vision. As the only presenting clinical findings may be a watery conjunctivitis, the patient should be asked about any trauma; previous corneal ulcers; inflammation inside the eye (iritis); nasal or oral cold sores; genital sores; recent use of topical or systemic steroid or immunosuppressive drugs; and immunologic deficiency states such as malignancy, organ transplants, or chronic eczema.

If corneal examination reveals dendritic or even geographic ulceration, it is HSV until proved otherwise. In herpes, sensation is at least temporarily reduced or absent in the affected cornea. Marked stromal scarring as seen in more chronic forms of herpes results in permanent decrease in sensitivity. Initially, the corneal lesions begin as a fine, transient, punctate keratitis that coalesces to form dendritic, dendrogeographic, or geographic ulcers (Fig. 5-27). In an eye that has had many recurrences, the more subtle stages may be bypassed and the cornea may simply break down in rapidly forming geographic ulceration.

The pathogenesis of the branching ulceration has never been worked out. The popular concept that it is related to neuronal distribution has been disproved [1]. The pattern may simply be a function of viral linear spread by contiguous cell-to-cell movement. Lesions occasionally occur within 2 mm of the limbus. These tend to be much more resistant to antiviral therapy than are central herpetic infections.

Stromal reaction is usually absent or mild and confined to the anterior layers in milder epithelial infections. On occasion, however, even mild epithelial infection may be associated with severe stromal edema and iritis. These eyes are more likely to go on to chronic recurrent immune disease and scarring resulting in visual loss. Concurrent or future stromal disease may be prevented by gentle debridement of the infected epithelium with a sterile cotton-tip applicator before instituting antiviral chemotherapy. Such debridement removes much of the inciting antigen that could penetrate to deep stromal layers.

EPITHELIAL TROPHIC (METAHERPETIC) ULCERATION
Occasionally, despite adequate antiviral therapy, epithelial ulcers do not completely heal or, having healed, break down again in an ovoid or dendriform pattern. This is trophic, or "metaherpetic," keratopathy. This chronic sterile ulceration is secondary to interacting adverse factors including impaired corneal innervation, abnormal tear film stability, and damaged basement membrane [24]. Corneal epithelial cells normally lie on top of their basement membrane attached by hemidesmosomes, rather than interdigitating with the membrane. If the basement membrane is damaged during the infection or the tear film lubricates poorly, the basement membrane takes at least 8 weeks to repair itself and thus slows adequate healing of the overlying epithelium [33]. Gundersen's classic study on the occurrence of trophic ulcers in several hundred patients with herpes revealed that 17 percent of patients receiving no therapy at all developed trophic ulcers. Twenty-six percent treated with partial 10% iodine scrubs of the affected epithelium and 38 percent of those undergoing total epithelial removal with iodine scrubs developed this condition [27].

Clinically, a trophic ulcer may be distinguished from an actively infected ulcer by the appearance of its edge. Trophic ulcers have gray, thickened bor-

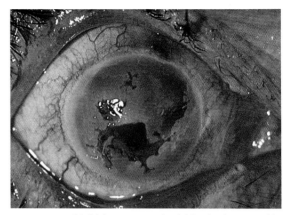

FIGURE 5-27. *Multiple recurrent dendritic, dendrogeographic, and geographic herpes simplex ulcers in cornea with diffuse immune stromal edema.*

ders formed by heaped-up epithelium unable to move across or adhere to the damaged ulcer base (Fig. 5-28). In contrast, actively infected ulcers have discrete flat edges that may change their configuration as the ulcer erodes away newly infected epithelium.

Persistence of trophic ulceration over several weeks or months poses a threat to the integrity of globe. The longer the ulcer is present, the greater the chance of collagenolytic activity with subsequent stromal melting and perforation. This is particularly true in male patients and if the ulcer is located in the central cornea away from peripheral vascularization, which scars but heals [8, 40].

STROMAL DISEASE
Stromal disease may be divided into two categories according to currently presumed pathogenesis: antigen-antibody-complement–mediated (AAC-mediated) disease characterized by viral interstitial keratitis, immune rings, or limbal vasculitis; and delayed hypersensitivity reaction characterized by disciform edema [31, 58].

VIRAL INTERSTITIAL KERATITIS, IMMUNE RINGS, AND LIMBAL VASCULITIS. All three forms of herpetic AAC-mediated disease are thought to be due to immune complex hypersensitivity. The interstitial keratitis presents clinically as single or multiple patches of dense white necrotic infiltration. After several weeks of smouldering, deep, dense leashes of vessels often move in as if in pursuit of the infiltrate(s) (Fig. 5-29). These lesions may remain small and focal or become so severe as to give the cornea a red (vessels) and white (interstitial keratitis) mottled pattern on unaided view. They resemble bacterial or fungal infiltrates but are far more indolent and usually run a course of many months.

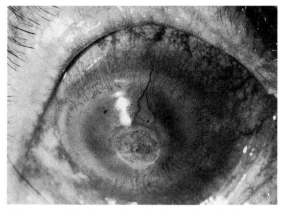

FIGURE 5-28. *Trophic metaherpetic ulcer under thin therapeutic soft contact lens.*

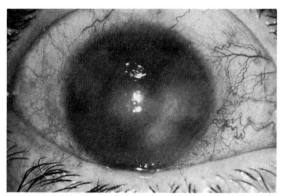

FIGURE 5-29. *Severe herpetic interstitial keratitis with dense blotchy white infiltrates and extensive deep neovascularization.*

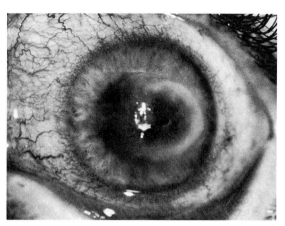

FIGURE 5-30. *Stromal immune (Wessely) ring of ocular herpes simplex.*

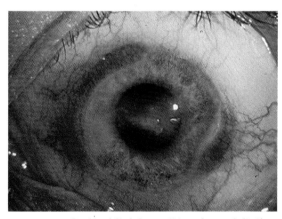

FIGURE 5-31. *Combined limbal vasculitis and central disciform stromal edema.*

Immune (Wessely) rings in the anterior stroma and limbal vasculitis are felt to be two other clinical manifestations of AAC-mediated disease [31, 50, 58]. The immune ring does not seem to incite major neovascularization, but not uncommonly patches of interstitial keratitis may be associated with the ring and stimulate the growth of vessels (Fig. 5-30). Limbal vasculitis is usually focal, although one or more quadrants may be involved in an edematous, hyperemic reaction sufficiently severe to cause dellen formation. There is little to no tendency for these vessels to invade the cornea in the absence of associated interstitial keratitis (Fig. 5-31).

DISCIFORM KERATITIS. Disciform edema of the cornea is a well-known adverse consequence of ocular herpes. It is currently felt that the pathogenesis is a delayed hypersensitivity reaction to HSV-antigenic change of the surface membranes of stromal cells and to the antigenically provocative residue of the viral invasion. The reaction itself is characterized

histopathologically by a mixture of sensitized lymphocytes, plasma cells, and, ultimately, macrophages and PMNs [17, 40, 48].

Clinically, the milder forms of disciform disease present as focal, often disc-shaped stromal edema. There is no necrosis or neovascularization but there may be fine keratitic precipitates (KPs) attacking the endothelium just in the involved area. In some cases there is no anterior chamber reaction, yet KPs are present, which suggests that these programmed lymphocytes are particularly attracted to the focal corneal antigen.

In more severe cases of disciform disease, the stromal edema is more diffuse, Descemet folds are present, and deep and superficial neovascularization is invading. Focal bullous keratopathy may develop, which indicates that the endothelium is severely compromised by the inflammatory attack and that an abnormal amount of fluid is being driven into the cornea by hydrostatic pressure. In the most severe cases, the bullae rupture, and the cornea may become widely ulcerated with subsequent necrosis and melting. In moderate to severe cases of disciform disease, marked iritis is almost invariably present.

Patches of viral interstitial keratitis, immune rings, or limbal vasculitis may be found in eyes with active disciform edema. This combined AAC-mediated disease and delayed hypersensitivity reaction may be mild and readily amenable to therapy or more severe and poorly responsive to the most assiduous treatment.

IRIDOCYCLITIS AND TRABECULITIS

Recurrent nongranulomatous HSV iridocyclitis and trabeculitis may occur without known prior keratitis or without concomitant keratitis. In the presence of active keratitis, however, there is almost invariably some uveal inflammation caused either by reaction to viral antigen in the iris or by the irritative effects of the keratitis (Fig. 5-32). If trabeculitis is present, there is usually a secondary glaucoma unless aqueous production has been markedly reduced by inflammation in the ciliary body.

The pathogenesis of this uveitis is not well understood. Complete viral organisms have been found in the aqueous in several cases and, in one instance, in a retrocorneal membrane [11, 59, 82]. The immune inflammatory component is characterized by diffuse lymphocytic infiltration of the iris stroma.

ANTIVIRAL DRUGS

There are now several antiviral agents with proven efficacy in the treatment of human herpetic keratitis. These drugs are antimetabolites and include IDU (Stoxil, Dendrid, Herplex), ara-A (Vira-A), trifluridine (F$_3$T, Viroptic), acyclovir (Zovirax), and bromovinyldeoxyuridine (BVDU). IDU and F$_3$T work by a mechanism of antiviral action related to the adverse biologic consequences of incorporating these thymidine analogs into viral DNA and by viral enzyme inhibition [69]. Unfortunately, these antimetabolites are also incorporated into the DNA of normal host cells; this may account for the toxicity that may be found during topical or systemic therapy.

Ara-A has been reported to inhibit DNA polymerase and to be incorporated to a small extent into viral and host DNA [56, 60, 69]. Although this drug

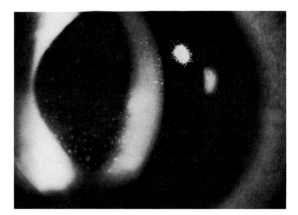

FIGURE 5-32. *Herpetic keratouveitis with fine keratitic precipitates and overlying stromal edema.*

shares some of the toxicity seen with IDU and F$_3$T, it is much less toxic systemically and is, therefore, used not only as a topical agent in the eye but for intravenous therapy of herpetic encephalitis.

Results of controlled clinical studies on these three commercially available ocular antiviral drugs have shown variable therapeutic efficacy. Their recommended frequency of use and concentration in actively infected corneas are shown in Table 5-6. IDU has an average overall cure rate of 76 percent; ara-A and F$_3$T each have overall levels of efficacy approximating 90 to 95 percent [12, 13, 56, 60–62]. F$_3$T, however, appears to be superior to ara-A when steroids are in use. Although all three drugs are effective clinically, their toxicity limits their use in long-term management in many cases. Adverse side effects include superficial punctate keratitis, lacrimal punctal occlusion, follicular conjunctivitis, and contact dermatitis.

Because of this nonspecific toxicity to virus and host systems alike, more benign, highly specific, and therapeutically effective agents have been sought. Two such drugs currently under clinical investigation, both topically and systemically, are acyclovir and BVDU [18, 22, 29, 63, 67]. Both of these drugs are specifically activated by herpesvirus-induced thymidine kinase, thereby effectively bypassing all noninfected normal cells. Viral thymidine kinase initiates the phosphorylation steps that lead ultimately to the production of the therapeutically active triphosphate form of the drugs. These compounds are more inhibitory to herpetic DNA polymerase than to cellular polymerase, thereby preferentially inhibiting the synthesis of viral DNA.

Several clinical studies done in England on 3% acyclovir ointment therapy of ocular herpes have shown that this drug is either equal to or superior to

0.5 and 1.0% IDU ointment and is not toxic to the eye in short-term study [12, 14]. Recent studies in this country have found 3% acyclovir to be therapeutically equal to 3% ara-A [64, 91]. In our own study, we found that ara-A healed 90 percent and acyclovir 95 percent of infected dendritic and geographic ulcers. In addition, acyclovir appeared to be therapeutically superior when steroids were in use, but patient numbers were not sufficient to prove this statistically [64].

Clinical studies on 0.5% BVDU drops in therapy of ocular herpes in Belgium have been equally encouraging. Sixty-nine of 70 patients studied by Maudgal and coworkers healed within a few days of the initiation of therapy with no adverse side effects [45]. In addition, BVDU may have some therapeutic efficacy in stromal disease (E. DeClercq, personal communication, 1981).

PROS AND CONS OF ADJUNCT
CORTICOSTEROID THERAPY

Corticosteroids affect immunologically competent lymphoid tissue by inducing lymphocytolysis of small, nondividing lymphocytes, and arresting or inhibiting RNA, DNA, and protein synthesis in medium and large lymphocytes [43, 44]. These drugs also inhibit white cell amoeboid migration and the release of cellular digestive enzymes through physiologic stabilization of the lysosomal membranes. Ocular studies on the effect of topical steroids in herpes indicate that there is local inhibition of antibody-forming cells (B-lymphocytes) in the cornea and uveal tract. As there is only transient effect on the number of B-lymphocytes in the draining lymph nodes and more on circulating antibody response, the host is still capable of immune reaction once the inflammation-inhibiting steroids are removed [47].

Steroids have also been found to inhibit the formation of both mucopolysaccharides and collagen, two substances critical to the integrity of the corneal matrix and structure. The role of steroids in enhancing the release of collagenolytic enzymes is also of concern in cases of corneal thinning and melts. It

has recently been shown, however, that medroxyprogesterone acetate (Provera) treatment of herpetic keratitis in animals resulted in the suppression of both latent and active collagenase [40]. This was correlated clinically and histologically with a marked reduction in the PMN infiltrate and stromal neovascularization, compared with results in control animals. Epithelial infectious disease was enhanced but could be eliminated by concomitant antiviral therapy. It was felt that medroxyprogesterone acetate, which has an antiinflammatory efficacy roughly equivalent to 0.2% prednisolone, might be a safer steroid to use in herpetic cases threatened by corneal melting.

Although it is known that both topical and systemic corticosteroids may predispose to severe herpetic infection, it has been reported that these drugs do not increase the incidence of recurrence but only its severity if infectious disease does not recur "spontaneously" [35].

The pros for use of steroids in ocular herpes then are a significant inhibition of (1) cellular infiltration, (2) release of toxic hydrolytic enzymes, (3) scar tissue formation, and (4) neovascularization. On the negative side are (1) the suppression of the normal inflammatory responses, which may allow deeper spread of a potentially superficial viral infection; (2) possible "corneal addiction" to steroids by allowing buildup of leukocyte-attracting antigen, the reaction to which must be constantly suppressed; (3) opening the cornea to opportunistic bacterial or fungal infection through suppression of the immune defense system; (4) enhancement of collagenolytic enzyme production by most steroids; and (5) the well-known side effects of steroid glaucoma and cataract.

Having once committed a patient to topical steroid therapy it is sometimes difficult to withdraw treatment. If the steroids are stopped too abruptly, recrudescence of the immune disease may occur and the drugs will have to be reinstituted. Some patients are unable to stop taking these drugs with-

TABLE 5-6. *Usual Concentration and Frequency of Use of Commercially Available Antiviral Drugs*

Drug	Concentration (%)	Frequency
Idoxuridine ointment (Stoxil)	0.5	Five times daily for 14 days
Idoxuridine drops (Stoxil, Herplex, Dendrid)	0.1	Every hour by day, every 2 hours at night for 14 days
Vidarabine ointment (Vira-A)	3	Five times daily for 14 days
Trifluridine drops (Viroptic)	1	Every 1–2 hours by day for total of 9 doses daily for 14 days

out an inflammatory flare-up and may have to continue using "homeopathic" steroid drops once or twice weekly.

A useful rule of thumb to follow in tapering steroids is the 50 percent reduction technique, i.e., each dosage reduction is never more than half of the current level of therapy. An example of this would be to have a patient on 1% prednisolone every 3 hours for 2 to 3 days, then every 6 hours for a week, followed by 1 to 3 weeks at levels of tid, with succeeding 1- to 3-week periods at bid, and qd. At this point, the patient would be switched to $\frac{1}{8}$% prednisolone qid and a similar taper carried out over a several-week period. If a patient is unable to go below 1% prednisolone 2 or 3 times daily, the prognosis for the long run is not good and the chance of steroid and infectious or immune complications greatly increases. It should be noted that less severe disease would warrant starting steroid therapy at levels well below 1% every 3 hours, e.g., $\frac{1}{8}$% 2 or 3 times daily.

TREATMENT

PRIMARY OCULAR AND PERIOCULAR HSV INFECTIONS

In the immunologically competent host, herpetic skin lesions remain fairly localized and are a self-limited disease that resolves without scarring and often without specific therapy. Specific therapy is recommended, however, and may be outlined as follows (see Table 5-6):

1. In the absence of corneal ulceration, prophylactic antiviral ointment to the eyes until skin lesions resolve.
2. In the presence of corneal ulceration, simple debridement of the ulcers with a sterile cotton-tip applicator after topical anesthetic drops followed by antiviral ointment or drops for 14 to 21 days. This may be then stopped or tapered over a several-day period.
3. Eye shields or hand restraints with young children.
4. Topical povidone-iodine (Betadine) gel to badly ulcerated skin, avoiding the eyes; otherwise, no therapy for skin lesions except warm saline soaks and general good hygiene.
5. Topical antibiotics if the cornea is ulcerated.
6. Cycloplegics if iritis is present (rare).

Primary corneal disease responds slowly but well to therapy, and the eye, like the skin, heals without scarring.

RECURRENT INFECTIOUS EPITHELIAL HERPES

Therapy for recurrent infectious herpes is in many ways similar to that for primary disease and may be outlined as follows:

1. Gentle debridement of involved epithelium with a sterile cotton-tip applicator.
2. Antiviral ointment or drops at full recommended dosage for 14 to 21 days. After that time, the therapy is discontinued or rapidly tapered, even if healing is not complete. If viral resistance is suspected, a different class of antivirals at full dosage can again be given.
3. Topical antibiotics should be used while ulcers are present.
4. Cycloplegics should be given, if needed, for iritis.

With antiviral chemotherapy arresting virus replication until the infected cells slough from the eye or with debridement, the infectious epithelial disease heals 90 percent of the time without complication and without need for an antiinflammatory drug. If the ulcer has not healed within 21 days, clinical resistance of the virus, necessitating change to another antiviral, or trophic sterile ulceration should be considered. Limbal ulcers are more resistant to healing but will eventually close over with or without scarring.

There is no place for the use of steroids in infectious epithelial disease uncomplicated by major stromal immune reaction.

TROPHIC POSTINFECTIOUS ULCERS

Therapy for trophic ulcers is aimed at protecting the damaged basement membrane by patching or soft contact lens. Rarely is conjunctival flap used today. In the absence of underlying stromal inflammatory disease that may interfere with basement membrane healing, there is usually no call for topical steroids.

Multiplying virus does not cause the trophic form of disease; there is, therefore, no need for antiviral therapy, which may interfere with healing when used at full dose. Similarly, cauterization may aggravate the condition by further damaging the basement membrane. Scraping off all corneal epithelium results in regrowth of the epithelium up to the borders of the metaherpetic ulcer, but the cells are still unable to adhere to the damaged ulcer base.

Treatment of trophic ulcers may be outlined as follows:

1. A soft contact lens worn continuously around the clock, with twice-daily administration of antibiotic drops; or antibiotic ointment with intermittent 48-hour pressure patching.

3. Antiviral ointment or drops if topical steroids are used during acute ulcerative phase.
4. Topical antibiotic for ulcerative keratitis.
5. Cycloplegics as needed for iritis.
6. Soft contact lens and artificial tears if corneal melting ensues (see Trophic Postinfectious Ulcers).
7. Nonnarcotic or narcotic analgesics for neuralgia days 1 through 10. If the pain is not diminishing, systemic steroids may be used in immunologically competent patients: prednisone 20 mg PO 3 times daily for 1 week, then prednisone 15 mg PO twice daily for 1 week, then prednisone 15 mg PO once daily for 1 week, and continue mydriatics and topical steroids. Monitor frequently for disseminated infection with an internist or dermatologist.

KERATOPLASTY

If a cornea has been sufficiently damaged by herpes zoster ophthalmicus that visual loss is major, it is highly likely that the cornea is sufficiently anesthetic to do very badly if transplantation is attempted. The postoperative eye is very frequently compromised by persistent trophic epithelial defects, melting, superinfection, iritis, and secondary glaucoma, any of which may cause graft failure if not loss of the eye. It is preferable to allow these eyes to heal over a neovascular pannus (autoflap). After 1 or 2 years, these vascular membranes thin out very nicely and there is a notable improvement in vision. In situations in which melting threatens the integrity of the globe, cyanoacrylate glue (see Trophic Postinfectious Ulcers) or a conjunctival flap are the procedures of choice.

REFERENCES

1. Baum, J. Morphogenesis of the dendritic figure in herpes simplex keratitis. *Am. J. Ophthalmol.* 70:222, 1970.
2. Bell, D., Holman, R., and Pavan-Langston, D. Epidemiologic aspects of herpes simplex keratitis. *Ann. Ophth.* 14:421, 1982.
3. Berghaust, G., and Westerby, R. Zoster ophthalmicus—Local treatment with cortisone. *Acta Ophthalmol.* 45:787, 1967.
4. Berman, M. Collagenase inhibitors: Rationale for their use in treating corneal ulceration. *Int. Ophthalmol. Clin.* 15:49, 1975.
5. Blyth, W., et al. Reactivation of herpes simplex virus infection by ultraviolet light and possible involvement of prostaglandins. *J. Gen. Virol.* 33:547, 1976.
6. Buddingh, G., et al. Studies on the natural history of herpes simplex infection. *Pediatrics* 11:595, 1953.
7. Carter, A., and Royds, J. Systemic steroids in herpes zoster. *Br. Med. J.* 2:746, 1957.

8. Cavanagh, H. D. Persistent epithelial defects and anti-inflammatory disease in herpetic ocular disease. *Int. Ophthalmol. Clin.* 15:67, 1975.
9. Cibis, A., and Bunde, R. Herpes simplex virus–induced congenital cataracts. *Arch. Ophthalmol.* 85:220, 1971.
10. Cobo, L. M., et al. Prognosis and management of corneal transplantation for herpetic keratitis. *Arch. Ophthalmol.* 98:1755, 1980.
11. Collin, B., and Abelson, M. Herpes simplex virus in human cornea, retrocorneal fibrous membrane and vitreous. *Arch. Ophthalmol.* 94:1726, 1976.
12. Collum, L., Benedict-Smith, A., and Hillary, I. Randomized double-blind trial of acyclovir and idoxuridine in dendritic corneal ulceration. *Br. J. Ophthalmol.* 64:766, 1980.
13. Coster, D., et al. Clinical evaluation of adenine, arabinoside and trifluorothymidine in the treatment of corneal ulcers caused by herpes simplex virus. *J. Infect. Dis.* 133(Suppl.)A173, 1976.
14. Coster, D., et al. A comparison of acyclovir and idoxuridine as treatment for ulcerative herpetic keratitis. *Br. J. Ophthalmol.* 64:763, 1980.
15. Dauber, R. Idoxuridine in herpes zoster topical therapy. *Br. Med. J.* 2:526, 1974.
16. Dawson, C., and Togni, B. Herpes simplex eye infections. *Surv. Ophthalmol.* 21:121, 1976.
17. Dawson, C., Togni, B., and Moore, R. Structural changes in chronic herpetic keratitis. *Arch. Ophthalmol.* 79:740, 1968.
18. DeClercq, E., et al. (E)-5-(2-Bromovinyl)-2'-deoxyuridine: A potent and selective antiherpes agent. *Proc. Natl. Acad. Sci. U.S.A.* 76:2947, 1979.
19. DeClercq, E., et al. Oral (E)-5-(2-bromovinyl)-2'-deoxyuridine in severe herpes zoster. *Br. Med. J.* 281:1, 1980.
20. Edgerton, A. E. Herpes zoster ophthalmicus. Report of cases and review of the literature. *Arch. Ophthalmol.* 34:40, 114, 1945.
21. Edwards. T. Ophthalmic complications from varicella. *J. Pediatr. Ophthalmol.* 2:37, 1965.
22. Elion, G., et al. Selectivity of action of an antiherpetic agent, 9-(2-hydroxyethoxymethyl)-guanine. *Proc. Natl. Acad. Sci. U.S.A.* 74:5716, 1977.
23. Elliott, R. A. Treatment of herpes zoster with high doses of prednisone. *Lancet* 2:610, 1964.
24. Falcon, M., et al. Management of herpetic eye disease. *Trans. Ophthalmol. Soc. U.K.* 97:345, 1977.
25. Forrest, W. M., and Kaufman, H. E. Zosteriform herpes simplex. *Am. J. Ophthalmol.* 81:86, 1976.

26. Foster, C. S., et al. HLA Phenotypic Expression in Patients with Recurrent and Nonrecurrent Herpes Simplex Keratitis. In R. Sundmacher and J. F. Bergman (Eds.), *Herpetic Eye Diseases*. Munich: Verlag, 1981.

27. Gundersen, T. Herpes corneas: Treatment with strong solution of iodine. *Arch. Ophthalmol.* 12:225, 1936.

28. Hagler, W., Walters, P., and Nahmias, A. Ocular involvement in neonatal herpes simplex virus infection. *Arch. Ophthalmol.* 82:169, 1969.

29. Hettinger, M., et al. Ac₂IDU, BVDU and thymine arabinoside therapy in experimental herpes keratitis. *Arch. Ophthalmol.* 99:1419, 1981.

30. Hutchison, D., Smith, R., and Haughton, P. Conjunctival herpetic keratitis. *Arch. Ophthalmol.* 93:70, 1975.

31. Jones, B., et al. Symposium on herpes simplex eye disease: Objectives of therapy of herpetic eye disease. *Trans. Ophthalmol. Soc. U.K.* 97:305, 1977.

32. Kaufman, H. E. Antimetabolite drug therapy in herpes simplex. *Ophthalmology* (Rochester) 87:135, 1980.

33. Kaufman, H. E. Epithelial erosion syndrome: Metaherpetic keratitis. *Am. J. Ophthalmol.* 57:984, 1964.

34. Keczkes, K., and Basheer, A. Do corticosteroids prevent post-herpetic neuralgia? *Br. J. Dermatol.* 102:551, 1980.

35. Kibrick, S., et al. Local corticosteroid therapy and reactivation of herpetic keratitis. *Arch. Ophthalmol.* 86:694, 1971.

36. Klein, R. Pathogenic mechanisms of recurrent herpes simplex virus infections. *Arch. Virol.* 51:1, 1976.

37. Knox. J. Trench mouth in children. *J. R. Coll. Gen. Pract.* 16:23, 1968.

38. Laibson, P., and Kibric, S. Reactivation of herpetic keratitis by epinephrine in the rabbit. *Arch. Ophthalmol.* 75:254, 1966.

39. Langston, R., Pavan-Langston, D., and Dohlman, C. H. Penetrating keratoplasty for herpetic keratitis. *Trans. Am. Acad. Ophthalmol. Otolaryngol.* 79:577, 1975.

40. Lass, J., et al. Treatment of experimental herpetic interstitial keratitis with medroxyprogesterone. *Arch. Ophthalmol.* 98:520, 1980.

41. Lehner, T., Wilton, J., and Shillitoe, E. Immunological basis for latency, recurrences, and putative oncogenicity of herpes simplex virus. *Lancet* 2:60, 1975.

42. Luby, J., et al. Adenine Arabinoside Therapy of Varicella-Zoster Virus Infection. In D. Pavan-Langston, R. Buchanan, and C. Alford (Eds.), *Adenine Arabinoside: An Antiviral Agent*. New York: Raven, 1975. P. 237.

43. Lundin, R., and Schelin, U. The effect of steroids on the histology and ultrastructure of lymphoid tissue. *Pathology* 1:15, 1966.

44. Makman, M., Nakagawa, S., and White, A. Studies on the mode of action of adrenal steroids on lymphocytes. *Recent Prog. Horm. Res.* 23:195, 1967.

45. Maudgal, P., et al. Efficacy of E-5-(2-bromovinyl)-2'-deoxyuridine in the Topical Treatment of Herpetic Keratitis in Rabbits and Man. In R. Sundmacher and J. F. Bergman (Eds.), *Herpetic Eye Diseases*. Munich: Verlag, 1981. P. 339.

46. Merselis, J., Kaye, D., and Hook, E. Disseminated herpes zoster. *Arch. Intern. Med.* 113:679, 1961.

47. Meyer, R., et al. Effect of local corticosteroids on antibody-forming cells in the eye and draining lymph nodes. *Invest. Ophthalmol.* 14:138, 1975.

48. Meyers, R., and Chitjian, P. Immunology of herpesvirus infections: Immunity to herpes simplex virus in eye infections. *Surv. Ophthalmol.* 21:194, 1976.

49. Meyers-Elliott, R., et al. HLA antigens in herpes stromal keratitis. *Am. J. Ophthalmol.* 89:54, 1980.

50. Meyers-Elliott, R., Pettit, T., and Maxwell, W. Viral antigens in the immune rings of herpes simplex stromal keratitis. *Arch. Ophthalmol.* 98:897, 1980.

51. Nahmias, A., Alford, C., and Korones, S. Infection of the newborn with Herpesvirus hominis. *Adv. Pediatr.* 17:185, 1970.

52. Naumann, G., Gass, D., and Font, R. Histopathology of herpes zoster. *Am. J. Ophthalmol.* 65:533, 1968.

53. Nesburn, A. B., et al. Varicella dendritic keratitis. *Invest. Ophthalmol.* 13:764, 1974.

54. Nesburn, A. B., et al. Reliable in vitro model for latent herpes simplex virus reactivation with peripheral virus shedding. *Infect. Immun.* 15:772, 1977.

55. Openshaw, H., et al. Acute and latent infection of sensory ganglia with herpes simplex virus: Immune control and virus reactivation. *J. Gen. Virol.* 44:205, 1979.

56. Pavan-Langston, D. Clinical evaluation of adenine arabinoside and idoxuridine in treatment of ocular herpes simplex. *Am. J. Ophthalmol.* 80:495, 1975.

57. Pavan-Langston, D. Varicella zoster ophthalmicus. *Int. Ophthalmol. Clin.* 15:171, 1975.

58. Pavan-Langston, D. Ocular Viral Diseases. In G. J. Galasso, T. C. Merigan, and R. Buchanan (Eds.), *Antiviral Agents and Viral Diseases of Man*. New York: Raven, 1979. P. 253.

59. Pavan-Langston, D., and Brockhurst, R. Herpes simplex panuveitis. *Arch. Ophthalmol.* 81:783, 1969.

60. Pavan-Langston, D., and Buchanan, R. Vidarabine therapy of simple and IDU-complicated herpetic keratitis. *Trans. Am. Acad. Ophthalmol. Otolaryngol.* 74:81, 1976.

61. Pavan-Langston, D., Buchanan, R., and Alford, C. *Adenine Arabinoside: A New Antiviral.* New York: Raven, 1975.

62. Pavan-Langston, D., and Foster, C. S. Trifluorothymidine and idoxuridine therapy of ocular herpes. *Am. J. Ophthalmol.* 84:818, 1977.

63. Pavan-Langston, D., Lass, J., and Campbell, R. Acyclic antimetabolite therapy of experimental herpes simplex keratitis. *Am. J. Ophthalmol.* 86:618, 1978.

64. Pavan-Langston, D., et al. Acyclovir and vidarabine in therapy of ulcerative herpes simplex keratitis: A comparative masked clinical trial. *Am. J. Ophthalmol.* 92:829, 1981.

65. Pavan-Langston, D., and McCulley, J. Herpes zoster dendritic keratitis. *Arch. Ophthalmol.* 89:25, 1973.

66. Pavan-Langston, D., and Nelson, D. Intraocular penetration of trifluorothymidine in humans. *Am. J. Ophthalmol.* 87:814, 1979.

67. Pavan-Langston, D., Park, N. H., and Hettinger, M. Ganglionic herpes simplex and systemic acyclovir. *Arch. Ophthalmol.* 99:1417, 1981.

68. Piebenga, L., and Laibson, P. Dendritic lesions in herpes zoster ophthalmicus. *Arch. Ophthalmol.* 90:268, 1973.

69. Prusoff, W., and Ward, D. Nucleoside analogs with antiviral activity. *Biochem. Pharmacol.* 25:1233, 1976.

70. Puga, A., et al. Herpes simplex virus DNA and mRNA sequences in acutely and chronically infected trigeminal ganglia of mice. *Virology* 89:102, 1978.

71. Rapp, F., and Reed, C. Experimental evidence for the oncogenic potential of herpes simplex virus. *Cancer Res.* 36:800, 1976.

72. Refojo, M., Dohlman, C., and Kiliopoulos, J. Adhesive in ophthalmology: A review. *Surv. Ophthalmol.* 15:217, 1971.

73. Roizman, B. An inquiry into the mechanism of recurrent herpes infections of man. *Perspect. Virol.* 4:283, 1965.

74. Rose, C., Breet, E., and Burston, J. Zoster encephalomyelitis. *Arch. Neurol.* 11:155, 1964.

75. Scheie, H. G. Herpes zoster ophthalmicus. *Trans. Ophthalmol. Soc. U.K.* 90:899, 1970.

76. Scott, T. Epidemiology of herpetic infection. *Am. J. Ophthalmol.* 43:134, 1957.

77. Shuster, J., Kaufman, H. E., and Nesburn, A. B. Statistical analysis of the rate of recurrence of herpesvirus ocular epithelial disease. *Am. J. Ophthalmol.* 91:328, 1981.

78. Smith, J., Pentherer, J., and MacCallum, F. The incidence of Herpesvirus hominis antibody in the population. *J. Hyg. Cambr.* 65:395, 1967.

79. Spence, J., Miller, F., and Court, D. *Thousand Family Survey: Newcastle, England.* London: Oxford University Press, 1954.

80. Stevens, J., and Cook, M. Latent herpes simplex virus in sensory ganglia. *Perspect. Virol.* 8:171, 1971.

81. Strachman, J. Uveitis associated with chickenpox. *J. Pediatr.* 46:327, 1955.

82. Sundmacher, R., and Neumann-Haefelin, D. Herpes simplex virus isolations from the aqueous of patients suffering from focal iritis, endothelitis, and prolonged disciform keratitis with glaucoma. *Surv. Ophthalmol.* 27:342, 1981.

83. Thomas, M., and Robertson, W. Dermal transmission of a virus as a cause of shingles. *Lancet* 11:1349, 1968.

84. Van Horn, D., Edelhauser, H., and Schultz, R. Experimental herpes simplex keratitis. *Arch. Ophthalmol.* 84:67, 1970.

85. Varnell, E., Centifanto-Fitzgerald, Y., and Kaufman, H. E. Herpesvirus infection and its effect on virulent superinfection, ganglionic colonization and shedding. *Invest. Ophthal. Vis. Sci.* 20(Suppl.):137, 1981.

86. Waltuch, G., and Sachs, F. Herpes zoster in a patient with Hodgkin's disease. *Arch. Intern. Med.* 121:458, 1971.

87. Walz, M., Price, R., and Notkins, A. Latent ganglionic infection with herpes simplex virus types 1 and 2: Viral reactivation after neurectomy. *Science* 184:1185, 1974.

88. Whitley, R., et al. Adenine arabinoside therapy of herpes zoster in the immunosuppressed. *N. Engl. J. Med.* 294:1193, 1976.

89. Workshop on the Treatment and Prevention of Herpes Simplex Virus Infection. *J. Infect. Dis.* 127:117, 1973.

90. Yamamoto, H., Walz, M., and Notkins, A. Viral-specific thymidine kinase in sensory ganglia of mice infected with herpes simplex virus. *Virology* 76:866, 1977.

91. Yeakley, W., et al. Clinical efficacy and safety of acyclovir versus vidarabine in epithelial herpetic keratitis. *Invest. Ophthal. Vis. Sci.* 20 (Suppl.):135, 1981.

Viral Diseases: ADENOVIRUS AND MISCELLANEOUS VIRAL INFECTIONS

David W. Vastine

The adenovirus and other virus-related diseases discussed here must be differentiated clinically from other causes of acute follicular conjunctivitis (Table 5-7). The infectious agents most frequently causing acute follicular conjunctivitis are adenovirus, herpes simplex, and *Chlamydia trachomatis*. The last two agents and their associated clinical presentations are discussed in other sections of this chapter. Adenovirus and each of the other virus diseases will be considered here according to viral agent, overall incidence, method of transmission, clinical appearance, and management. The viral diseases that affect the external eye and their characteristics are listed in Table 5-8. Clinical manifestations of infections caused by adenovirus, Epstein-Barr virus, poxviruses, RNA-containing viruses including measles and mumps, and enterovirus (hemorrhagic conjunctivitis) will be discussed in detail.

ADENOVIRUS OCULAR INFECTIONS

Adenoviruses are probably the most common cause of acute viral infections of the ocular adnexa and cornea. Because of the self-limited nature of the acute disease, mild cases are not often seen by the ophthalmologist. The adenoviral eye syndromes have three basic clinical presentations: epidemic keratoconjunctivitis (EKC), pharyngoconjunctival fever (PCF), and acute nonspecific follicular conjunctivitis. These ocular syndromes are caused by a variety of adenovirus serotypes. The infections are usually acute and self-limited, but chronic infections have been reported. One case of chronic keratitis has been reported with the isolation of adenovirus type 2 [6]. Darougar and associates [14] have reported a case of recurrent papillary conjunctivitis that lasted 16 months. Adenovirus type 19 was isolated 12 months after onset. Pettit and Holland [55] have described 3 cases of chronic keratoconjunctivitis associated with adenovirus types 3, 4, and 5. In 2 of the 3 cases, active epithelial keratitis was noted; the third patient had recurrent conjunctivitis with pronounced subepithelial opacities. All 3 of these cases had been treated with topical steroids early in the course of infection. Use of steroids may play a role in the chronic form of this disease, although the cases reported by Boniuk and colleagues [6] and Darougar and coworkers [14] were not associated with topical steroid treatment. Other than one report of posterior multifocal placoid pigment epitheliopathy associated with adenovirus type 5 [2], no distinct clinical syndromes have been associated with posterior segment ocular infection.

EPIDEMIC KERATOCONJUNCTIVITIS

The EKC syndrome was first described by Fuchs in 1889 in Vienna as an acute superficial punctate keratitis [23]. Since that time, the disease has been reported worldwide in its epidemic form. The first caused agent (adenovirus type 8) was isolated by Jawetz and associates in 1955 [32, 33]. Since then, multiple types (2–4, 7–11, 14, 16, 19, and 29) have been isolated and shown to be associated with the EKC syndrome [8]. The most common adenovirus types currently associated with outbreaks of this disease are 8 and 19. Adenovirus type 19 appears to have had a recent introduction into the United States, as evidenced by its rapid spread throughout the country in small and large outbreaks [7, 8, 26, 67]. The most recent occurrences of this syndrome exhibit a more hemorrhagic appearance associated with adenovirus type 11.

EPIDEMIOLOGY AND PATHOGENESIS
EKC is the adenoviral ocular infection of most concern to the ophthalmologist. Transmission commonly occurs through direct contact in a hospital or physician's office, but infection throughout a community does occur and has been well established in recent epidemics [17, 26, 39, 67]. The community epidemic pattern in families is associated with transmission by close personal contact. Frequently, transmission occurs in sexually active young adults [58]. A recent report of a mixed adenovirus 13-30/10-19 in Holland has been associated with cervicitis in women as well

TABLE 5-7. *Differential Diagnosis of Acute Follicular Conjunctivitis*

Adenovirus ocular infections
    Epidemic keratoconjunctivitis
    Pharyngoconjunctival fever
    Nonspecific follicular conjunctivitis
Primary herpes simplex
Inclusion conjunctivitis
Acute exacerbations of trachoma
Acute hemorrhagic conjunctivitis
Newcastle disease
Influenza type A
Herpes zoster (rare)
Other viral diseases (rare)
Cat-scratch fever and occasionally other causes of
    Parinaud's syndrome

Table 5-8. *Ocular Viral Infections in Humans*

Virus Group	Distinctive Ocular Characteristics	Associated Systemic Disease	Laboratory Diagnosis with Clinical Specimens
DNA-containing viruses Adenoviruses	Epidemic keratoconjunctivitis (EKC): Follicular conjunctivitis with typical keratitis progressing from superficial punctate to focal with late onset of subepithelial corneal infiltrates.	Minimal systemic symptoms: preauricular adenopathy, occasional pharyngitis.	Virus isolation in HEK cells usually after 7 days with typical cytopathic effect; seroconversion by hemagglutination inhibition or complement fixation. Acute infection may be detected by immunofluorescent staining or conjunctival smear.
	Pharyngoconjunctival fever: Follicular conjunctivitis, frequently with subconjunctival hemorrhage. Corneal lesions like those found in EKC occur in up to 25% of cases with some serotypes such as adenovirus type 4.	Fever, severe pharyngitis, regional adenopathy.	Same as for EKC.
	Nonspecific follicular conjunctivitis: Follicular conjunctivitis with minimal or no keratitis.	May produce fever and pharyngitis.	Same as for EKC.
Herpesviruses Zoster (varicella) virus In children	Mild follicular conjunctivitis; isolated localized corneal lesions rare. Limbal vesicle may be present.	Chickenpox with fever, malaise, and vesicular exanthem. Rarely complicated by pneumonia and encephalitis. Malaise and myalgia may be acute. Microcephaly, deafness, heart disease, and other congenital varicella sequelae may develop.	Virus isolation or antibody seroconversion. Multinucleated giant cells may be found, as with herpes simplex virus types 1 and 2.
In adults	Trigeminal nerve distribution with blepharitis, cutaneous shingles, mild conjunctivitis, mild to severe keratitis, scleritis, iridocyclitis, optic neuritis, and pupillary and oculomotor paralysis. Small elevated dendritic keratitis may be present.	Some patients develop severe postherpetic neuralgia; CNS spread causes myelitis and encephalitis (rare).	Some as for zoster in children.

Table 5-8. *Continued*

Virus Group	Distinctive Ocular Characteristics	Associated Systemic Disease	Laboratory Diagnosis with Clinical Specimens
Cytomegalovirus	Mild follicular conjunctivitis, chorioretinitis.	Infectious mononucleosis-like systemic illness affects immunocompromised hosts. Congenital and venereally transferred infection in perinatal period.	Virus isolation and rise in antibody titer.
Epstein-Barr virus (EBV, infectious mononucleosis)	Secondary keratitis, usually self-limited. Generally mild conjunctivitis, but oculomotor paralysis, optic nerve edema may develop.	Mild to severe infection including lymphadenopathy, fever, lymphocytosis, hepatitis, pericarditis, myositis, and pharyngitis. The mononucleosis syndrome can cause death in leukemic and immunosuppressed hosts.	Presence of atypical lymphocytes in blood smears and positive heterophile antibody response. Also, rise in EBV-specific antibody titer.
Poxvirus			
Smallpox variola virus	Follicular reaction of conjunctiva with hyperemia. May include isolated pocks on lids or conjunctiva, or on cornea with secondary infection.	Small vesicular exanthem associated with fever and death (2–40% mortality), depending on location and virus strain.	Virus isolation, antibody seroconversion, or finding of acidophilic intracytoplasmic inclusion (Guarnieri's bodies) on smear.
Vaccinia virus	Typical severe blepharoconjunctivitis with "kissing" lesions of the lids. May be associated with keratitis in 4% of patients. Secondary sequelae include loss of cilia and minimal corneal opacity.	Generalized vaccinia or just severe local reaction with satellite lesions in area of vaccination may occur.	Virus isolation, antibody seroconversion; scraping from lids may reveal intracytoplasmic acidophilic inclusion (Guarnieri's) bodies on smears stained with H&E, Giemsa, or Papanicolaou's.
Molluscum contagiosum virus	Lesions or lids have umbilicated centers and discharge viral particles into conjunctiva, causing follicular conjunctivitis and keratitis.	May involve skin of face and can be spread by shaving. May be sexually transmitted in some patients.	Virus isolation; smear of exudate from eyelid lesion shows intracytoplasmic acidophilic inclusion (molluscum or Metterson-Patterson's) bodies with Lugol's solution or brilliant cresyl blue stain.
Papovavirus			
Papilloma virus	Papilliform warts of the eyelid with warts on opposing lid margins. May progress to conjunctivitis with mild keratitis.	None.	Electron microscopy of thin tissue sections.

Table 5-8. *Continued*

Virus Group	Distinctive Ocular Characteristics	Associated Systemic Disease	Laboratory Diagnosis with Clinical Specimens
RNA-containing viruses Paramyxoviruses Measles virus	Follicular conjunctivitis, Koplik's spots on conjunctiva or mild diffuse superficial punctate keratitis. In malnourished children, severely ulcerative keratitis with corneal perforation may occur.	Fever, rash, malaise, Koplik's spots on oral mucosa. Severe sequelae with death from pneumonia or encephalitis may occur.	Smear from nasomucosal aspirate stained with H&E, Giemsa, or Papanicolaou's stain may reveal multinucleated giant cells (Warthin-Finkeldey cells); otherwise, rely on viral isolation and seroconversion by humoral antibody.
Mumps virus	Dacryodenitis with follicular conjunctival reaction, rarely with superficial or disciform keratitis, usually without sequelae.	Parotitis, fever, and malaise may be associated with other inflammatory foci such as lacrimal glands and testicles. Encephalitis, aseptic meningitis. CNS paralysis and cerebral nerve palsy are rare.	Viral isolation and seroconversion by humoral antibody.
Newcastle disease virus Picornaviruses	Follicular conjunctival response.	None.	Same as for mumps.
Enterovirus	Follicular conjunctivitis with marked subconjunctival hemorrhage. Short incubation; rapid onset and resolution.	Possible association with CNS symptoms (neurotropic virus).	Virus isolation. Virus is heat-sensitive and grows best at 30–34°C from conjunctival exudate.
Togaviruses Rubella virus Congenital	Microphthalmia, iris hypoplasia, cataract, keratoconus.	Neonatal syndrome with multiple congenital defects.	Virus isolation and humoral antibody seroconversion.
Acquired	Follicular conjunctival response with mild superficial punctate keratitis without sequelae.	Fever, malaise, and cutaneous exanthem; adults may develop synovitis.	Same as for congenital rubella.
Group B arboviruses Orthomyxoviruses	Nonspecific reactions.	Yellow fever, dengue, sandfly fever.	Same as for congenital rubella.
Influenza virus	Follicular conjunctivitis.	Influenza syndrome with bronchopneumonia causing death in elderly people.	No distinctive characteristics. Rely on virus isolation and seroconversion of humoral antibody.

as both EKC and PCF syndromes [58]. These data suggest a possible venereal or sexually transmitted infectious pattern in young adults. It is likely that a continued community reservoir of the endemic syndrome exists with intermittent spread into hospital clinics, industrial infirmaries, and private optometrists' or ophthalmologists' offices. The most common modes of transmission within the hospital or clinic are contaminated fingers [9, 16, 67], solutions [62], and instruments [8, 9]. In most epidemics associated with hospitals or private offices, the transmitting agent is most probably the fingers of physicians or paramedical personnel or contaminated Schiøtz' tonometers. A recent outbreak has been described in which adenovirus type 4 was transferred to medical personnel in an intensive care unit from a patient with fatal type 4 pneumonia. All affected hospital personnel developed the ocular disease. The onset in all patients occurred after discontinuing isolation procedures [44]. Although type 4 adenovirus usually causes respiratory infections, it has also caused an outbreak of conjunctivitis with the typical EKC syndrome in England with minimal respiratory symptoms and very few isolates from sites other than the eye [65]. It is, therefore, extremely important to perform adequate hand washing and cleansing and sterilization of ophthalmic instruments, especially tonometers, between patient examinations to prevent the transmission of EKC in clinical facilities.

Community epidemics of adenovirus conjunctivitis have been frequently reported to be associated with transmission in or about swimming pools. This is a major mode of transmission in Japan. Recently, D'Angelo and coworkers have isolated the virus from swimming pool water, giving credence to the belief that water is the chief source of transmission in these epidemics [12].

CLINICAL FEATURES
EKC is characterized by the sudden onset of an acute watery discharge from the eyes with associated foreign body sensation, enlargement and tenderness of the preauricular lymph nodes, a follicular and papillary conjunctival response (Figs. 5-36 and 5-37) with or without hemorrhage, and mild photophobia with diffuse superficial punctate keratitis. The disease may be unilateral or bilateral; if bilateral, the infection is commonly more severe in one eye than the other. The first eye involved is usually the more severely affected. Infection of the contralateral eye may be delayed 4 to 5 days or more, or the infection may be so mild that the patient fails to

recognize it. During the acute stages, the conjunctival reaction is occasionally so severe that a pseudomembrane forms with eventual conjunctival scarring; small symblepharon may also result (Fig. 5-38). In these patients, a serous or hemorrhagic discharge may develop in the acute phase. In the acute phase, it is characteristic to find a tender preauricular lymph node. Early in the second week of infection, the diffuse superficial punctate keratitis coalesces to form areas of focal keratitis (Fig. 5-39). At this stage, a mild anterior uveitis is occasionally seen [2].

The acute phase gradually resolves, but, during the third week, subepithelial corneal infiltrates characteristic of EKC develop (Fig. 5-40). Centrally located subepithelial infiltrates decrease vision, which may alarm patients and cause them to seek the care of an ophthalmologist after the acute conjunctivitis has resolved. Infiltrates can form anywhere in the cornea. The infiltrates are usually diffusely spread throughout the cornea, and their number, location, and density vary greatly from patient to patient. These infiltrates, which grow to maximum density in the third and fourth weeks of the infection, number from 1 to 50 or more, and may cause a marked decrease in vision for months to years. The more time before onset of infection in the second eye, the less severe the corneal involvement and the fewer the infiltrates in the second eye, possibly because the infection is less intense and less severe.

DIAGNOSIS AND IDENTIFICATION
EKC should be suspected in the presence of follicular conjunctivitis when Giemsa-stained smears of conjunctival exudates show lymphocytes and degenerated epithelial cells with a few PMNs. In patients with pseudomembrane, a predominant PMN response is typical. Isolation of adenovirus from conjunctival swabs or scrapings in human embryonic kidney or WI-38 cell culture is a definitive laboratory test but may take 2 to 28 days or longer. The virus is readily isolated during the first week of the disease, is somewhat less easily isolated in the second, and is isolated from less than 25 percent of patients during the third week of the disease. A fourfold or greater increase in humoral antibody response also suggests recent infection. Newer methods—direct and indirect immunofluorescent staining of conjunctival scrapings from infected patients—have proved to be reliable, rapid, and sensitive in diagnosing the adenoviral syndromes (Fig. 5-41) [59, 66]. The relationship between length of infection and positive immunofluorescent identification by smear has not been established. The virus can also be demonstrated in the epithelial cells from

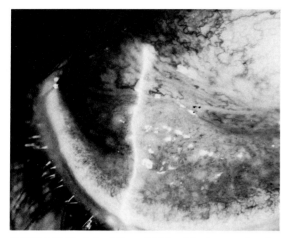

FIGURE 5-36. *Typical gelatinous follicles of the lower conjunctiva in a mild case of epidemic keratoconjunctivitis caused by type 19 adenovirus.*

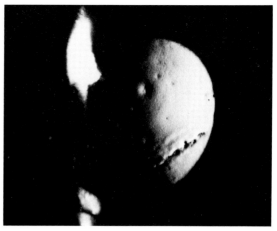

FIGURE 5-39. *Areas of focal keratitis highlighted by the fundus reflex in adenovirus type 8 epidemic keratoconjunctivitis. The typical infiltrates usually form later beneath these focal epithelial lesions.*

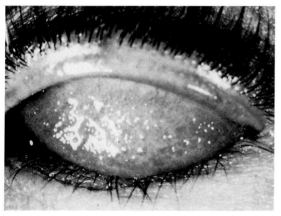

FIGURE 5-37. *Everted upper tarsus of a patient with adenovirus type 19 epidemic keratoconjunctivitis showing follicles buried by intense chemosis and papillary reaction. The follicles are highlighted by the light reflex.*

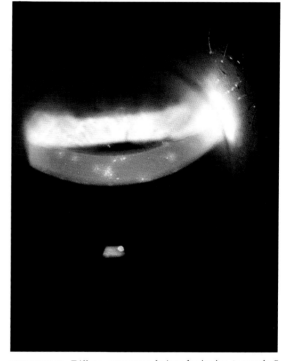

FIGURE 5-40. *Diffuse, numerous lesions beginning to recede 5 months after onset of adenovirus type 8 keratoconjunctivitis in a 65-year-old woman. These lesions appeared to have ironlike pigmentary deposits.*

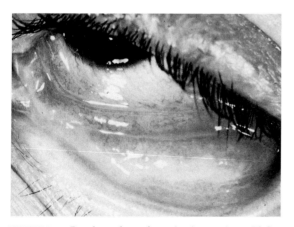

FIGURE 5-38. *Pseudomembrane formation in a patient with hyperacute adenovirus type 19 keratoconjunctivitis. Frequently the membrane may be more extensive, especially on the upper tarsus.*

conjunctival scrapings examined by electron microscopy.

The superficial punctate keratitis seen in the acute stage of EKC should not be confused with the chronic relapsing course of epithelial keratitis described by Thygeson as superficial punctate keratitis [64]. Thygeson's disease is not associated with an acute viral syndrome or with follicular conjunctivitis. The fine punctate superficial keratitis found in EKC is also common to other acute viral infections of the conjunctiva and to toxic reactions from drugs and other agents and is by itself a nonspecific finding.

MANAGEMENT

As soon as the disease is recognized, precautions should be taken to prevent its spread to other family members, fellow patients, or the examining physician, either by the patient himself or by medical personnel. Infected persons should be advised to stay home, use separate linens, and avoid direct oral contact with others. If physicians or other medical personnel are infected, their duties should be suspended immediately until the third week after onset of their disease, when virus transmission is unlikely. Several reports have implicated the contamination of tonometers, usually Schiøtz' tonometers, in the spread of the disease because of the difficulty in cleaning the plunger adequately [72]. Goldmann's tonometers are more easily cleaned by mechanical means with moistened tissue paper [11]. After adequate precautionary measures have been taken, the infected patients should receive follow-up care at least once a week.

The treatment of EKC is controversial. Antibiotics are of no value unless secondary bacterial infections occur. However, no cases of bacterial superinfection were noted in a recent Chicago epidemic [67]. The value of topical steroid use in the acute phase is debatable. Topical steroid therapy in patients with severe conjunctival reactions, pseudomembrane formation, and early symblepharon does provide dramatic relief and appears to result in a decreased number of corneal infiltrates during convalescence [18]. Confirmation of the latter effect is difficult, however, because the disease is so variable from patient to patient.

The natural course and clinical appearance of the corneal lesions have been well documented by Dawson and associates [18] and Laibson and colleagues [38]. The acute punctate keratitis resolves spontaneously, and no specific treatment is recommended. The subepithelial infiltrates develop spon-

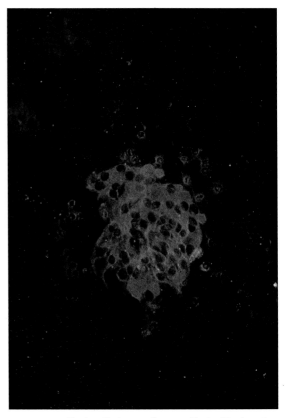

FIGURE 5-41. *Conjunctival smear from a patient with adenovirus keratoconjunctivitis stained by indirect immunofluorescent technique with adenovirus type 2 antiserum. Note the cluster of conjunctival epithelial cells with lengthy fluorescent cytoplasm. Some of the cells have brightly staining nuclei. (× 80.)*

taneously in the second to third week of the disease, as already noted. The number of corneal subepithelial lesions appears to be independent of the severity of the conjunctivitis but relates directly to the extent of the acute focal keratitis (Fig. 5-42).

Without treatment, the corneal infiltrates characteristically recede gradually over a period of months to years and vision improves. The corneal infiltrates are produced by sensitized T-lymphocytes attracted to either viral protein in the cornea or to virions that have been neutralized and rendered inactive by the host defense mechanisms. Similar infiltrates have been identified after primary herpes simplex blepharokeratoconjunctivitis. Suppression of the adenovirus-sensitized lymphocytes by steroids results in complete resolution of the infiltrates. However, since the inciting antigen takes months to years to disappear from the cornea, the infiltrates will reappear when the lymphocyte suppression is released.

The major objection to topical steroid treatment in

acute follicular conjunctivitis is the possibility of misdiagnosis. If the blepharoconjunctivitis or keratitis are the result of herpes simplex virus infection rather than adenovirus, long-term sequelae may be induced by the corticosteroid treatment. Similarly, in acute adult inclusion conjunctivitis, the severity of the infection may be enhanced by topical steroids. Patients receiving antibiotic-steroid combinations without specific activity against *Chlamydia* can develop prolonged infection with extensive pannus. It is this diagnostic dilemma that has increased the need for a rapid and specific diagnostic test that can differentiate these diseases from one another, thus permitting initiation of prompt, appropriate, and specific therapeutic treatment to decrease ocular morbidity. Immunofluorescent and immunoperoxidase staining of conjunctival exudates and smears may serve this purpose.

To date, treatment of EKC with IDU and ara-A has been unsuccessful; the disease progresses in spite of treatment with these agents [20, 29, 53, 68]. The ineffectiveness of these antiviral agents may be due in part to delays in the initiation of treatment.

Early diagnosis by the immunoenzyme technique may provide specific causal verification during the early acute phase of the disease, as already noted, thus permitting prompt antiviral treatment and a resultant decrease in the severity of the infection and in the amount of keratitis and infiltrates.

Laboratory studies in cell culture have demonstrated the effectiveness of F_3T in decreasing production of adenovirus types 8, 19, and 13 [43]. Clinical confirmation of this in vitro effect has yet to be accomplished, however. Because the subepithelial opacities are probably immunologic in origin and the conjunctival disease is self-limited, at present no antiviral therapy is recommended for treatment of adenovirus EKC.

PHARYNGOCONJUNCTIVAL FEVER
PCF is usually caused by adenovirus type 3 and less frequently by types 4 and 7, among others. PCF was first described by Beal in 1907 [3]. The disease is

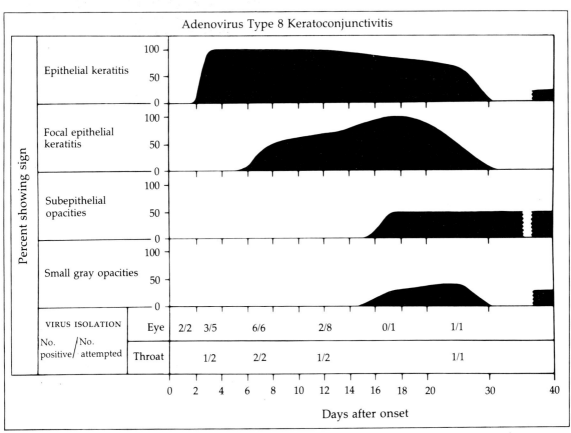

FIGURE 5-42. *The evolution of the epithelial keratitis and subepithelial opacities in epidemic keratoconjunctivitis. (Published with permission from The American Journal of Ophthalmology 69:473, 1970. Copyright by The Ophthalmic Publishing Company.)*

characterized by acute follicular conjunctivitis, which may be hemorrhagic; upper respiratory involvement (pharyngitis); regional lymphoid hyperplasia; tender, enlarged lymph nodes; and fever. The disease is usually unilateral, or less severe on one side, and is spread by upper respiratory contact or droplets. It is most commonly seen in children and is a self-limited disease lasting 7 to 14 days without sequelae [37]. No specific treatment is necessary or effective for the ocular disease. Antihistamines and mild analgesics may decrease upper respiratory symptoms. Patients with PCF do not, as a rule, develop the corneal infiltrates typical of the EKC syndrome. On the other hand, the EKC syndrome described above may also result from infection with adenovirus types 3, 4, and 7 [8, 32, 50, 67]. The keratitis in these patients is usually mild and diffuse; only a small percentage develop focal keratitis and infiltrates. The infiltrates are usually smaller and less intense than those seen in the typical EKC syndrome produced by adenovirus types 8 and 19.

Diagnosis of PCF is confirmed by viral isolation and by a rise in serum antibody levels. The immunofluorescence test on conjunctival smears will be positive for adenovirus, and Giemsa-stained preparations will show a predominant lymphocytic response.

NONSPECIFIC FOLLICULAR CONJUNCTIVITIS

Nonspecific follicular conjunctivitis in children or adults may be caused by many serotypes of adenovirus. The syndrome is so mild that it is usually not seen by the ophthalmologist except in epidemics, when mild cases of conjunctivitis are investigated and adenovirus is isolated. It is this mild form of adenoviral disease in children that probably serves as a reservoir of the adenovirus serotypes that are most frequently associated with EKC.

HERPESVIRUS OCULAR INFECTION

Herpesvirus infections are the most ubiquitous viral diseases in humans. Four herpesviruses produce infections in humans: herpes simplex virus, herpes zoster (varicella) virus, cytomegalovirus (CMV), and Epstein-Barr virus (EBV). Accidental infection with simian B virus may also occur in humans, resulting in serious infections and death. Characteristics of zoster, CMV, and EBV are listed in Table 5-8.

The ocular and systemic diseases caused by herpes simplex and zoster are detailed in the previous section. Ocular involvement with acquired CMV infection is common in compromised hosts

such as renal transplant patients and cancer patients undergoing chemotherapeutic treatment. However, a case of follicular conjunctivitis in an otherwise healthy host suffering from CMV mononucleosis syndrome has been reported [24]. Transmission from contact with another infected person with conjunctivitis was suspected. A case of chorioretinitis in a normal host with CMV infection has also been reported [10]. The shedding of CMV in tears may be a means of transmission of the disease in some patients [24, 69]. The most characteristic intraocular involvement in immunosuppressed hosts is retinitis and uveitis. The conjunctiva is sometimes involved in the CMV mononucleosis syndrome. Corneal involvement has not been recently reported.

CMV may also be spread by blood transfusion. The most common mode of transmission is venereal and the associated congenital CMV syndrome with resultant mental retardation is a major cause of birth defects in humans [51].

EBV is the cause of infectious mononucleosis, which is characterized by extensive lymphadenopathy, fever, lymphocytosis, hepatitis, pericarditis, polyarthritis, myositis, pharyngitis, and occasional follicular conjunctivitis [46]. The disease is transmitted by upper respiratory droplet contamination. In immunosuppressed leukemic patients, the infection can be extremely severe and result in death. Laboratory confirmation of the diagnosis is based on a positive heterophile antibody test and a rise in titer of the indirect fluorescent antibody serologic test.

The ocular manifestations of EBV infection include direct involvement of the eye and adnexa and indirect effects on the central nervous system (CNS) that affect the eye [51, 56, 63]. The virus may affect the lids, conjunctiva, or cornea in the acute phase, producing a follicular or membranous conjunctivitis with or without subconjunctival hemorrhage [4, 45]. Nodular episcleritis and uveitis with secondary involvement of the optic nerve in a patient with CNS infection have been described [4, 56]. Recently, two cases of keratitis associated with severe infectious mononucleosis were reported. In one case, the disease was found late in the course of infection after the use of systemic steroids. It was characterized by bilateral nummular interstitial keratitis, without epithelial involvement, sparing the visual axis and the paralimbal cornea. The lesions were easily suppressed with topical steroids [56]. In the second case, examined earlier in the course of the infection, microdendrites were noted with an ocular viral isolate confirming the presence of EBV. The disease responded to acyclovir ointment with resolution within 2 days of treatment [71]. The late lesions described by Pinnolis and colleagues did not occur [56].

POXVIRUS OCULAR INFECTIONS

The poxviruses are dermatotropic DNA viruses that cause lesions of the eyelids, conjunctiva, and (rarely) the cornea. Diagnosis is made by isolation of the virus from skin lesions, upper respiratory tract, or blood; by demonstration of a fourfold or greater rise in complement-fixing or neutralizing antibody titer; or by immunofluorescent staining of smears taken from pustules. Poxvirus particles may also be recognized by electron microscopy of pustule smears.

VARIOLA

Variola (smallpox) is a severe systemic exanthem that can lead to death in 2 to 40 percent of affected individuals, depending on nutritional status, strain of virus, and geographic location [19]. Fortunately, the disease has been eradicated, with the last known pocket of infection being in the Sudan. Variola may continue to be an extinct viral disease except in the laboratory or in biologic warfare.

After an 8- to 12-day incubation period, the systemic disease is characterized by a febrile course and a diffuse macular eruption, including pustules, sometimes associated with hemorrhage, that resolve during the next 2 to 3 weeks. The scabs flake off, leaving depigmented scars. Direct corneal involvement has been documented, and lesions of the eyelid and conjunctiva can be severe. These severe infections may lead to central corneal scars. The corneal lesions may also become superinfected with bacteria, causing severe corneal ulceration and secondary bacterial endophthalmitis and blindness. The majority of the corneal lesions heal spontaneously with variable, but frequently minimal, visual defects. Adequate antiviral therapy is not available. Some success has been achieved treating smallpox systemically with the antiviral isothiazole thiosemicarbazone shortly after documented exposure [60]. The treatment may prevent death but not the disfiguring effects of the smallpox itself. The most effective treatment is prevention by vaccination.

VACCINIA

The use of vaccinia virus for mass inoculation to prevent smallpox caused more morbidity and mortality than expected from any future unexpected smallpox epidemic [40]. In the United States, withdrawal of compulsory smallpox vaccination resulted from reports by Lane and colleagues [41, 42] and Ruben and Lane [57] detailing the generalized and ocular complications of vaccination. Because smallpox vaccination may be continued on an interim basis for travelers to recently endemic areas, military personnel, and hospital personnel, ophthalmologists may still see patients with accidental

ocular inoculation following vaccination. Overall incidence of accidental vaccinal infections, the majority of which affect the eye, is 18.8 per 1 million vaccinations in all age groups [41]. However, permanent visual sequelae are unusual. Fortunately, generalized vaccinia and the isolated cutaneous inoculations are self-limited and regress spontaneously with adequate production of antibody by the host. Infection of the eyelids is caused by accidental autoinoculation with the fingers or by fomite transmission of virus from the vaccination site to the eye. Rubbing the eye leads to infection of the conjunctiva and eyelid margins with the typical "kissing lesions." These lesions often lead to minor loss of eyelashes.

Accidental corneal involvement with vaccinia virus does occur. It is fortunately rare, but it can cause severe keratitis and subsequent corneal scarring [35, 54, 57]. Severe generalized vaccinia, progressive vaccinia necrosis, and death may occur in immunosuppressed patients, in patients with undiagnosed lymphoproliferative disorders such as Hodgkin's disease and chronic lymphocytic leukemia, and in children with eczema. Death owing to accidental inoculation from siblings in patients with leukemia, eczema, and cutaneous and immune deficiency diseases was an additional incentive to stop vaccination in the United States.

TREATMENT

Topical and systemic vaccinia immune globulin may accelerate the resolution of the disease [22] but may also provide an antigen-antibody complex in the cornea that may lead to larger infiltrates and scarring in patients who develop disciform keratitis [21]. This has been suggested by results from animal studies [22], but because the disease is so rare, no further studies have been done. Nonetheless, in cases of accidental ocular infection, it is generally accepted that vaccinia immune globulin should be used [54].

In addition to specific immune globulin, topical IDU may offer some benefit [25, 34, 36, 54], but its therapeutic effect in humans has never been confirmed. Antiviral activity of this agent has been demonstrated in cell culture experiments [47]. Interferon can also reduce the severity of the keratitis [35].

MOLLUSCUM CONTAGIOSUM

Molluscum contagiosum is a poxvirus infection of the eyelid margins. The viruses form small pearly-pink umbilicated tumors on the eyelid margins. In some cases, conjunctival lesions and subsequent scarring may occur [25]. These lesions secrete large quantities of virus, which causes punctal occlusion, follicular reaction of the conjunctiva, superior keratitis, and vascular pannus of the cornea. The superficial keratitis may be a toxic reaction. The disease is rare but should be considered when an eyelid lesion is associated with a superior pannus and follicular conjunctivitis [15]. The disease is spread by close personal contact and, in the case of both ocular and extraocular lesions, may be transmitted sexually. Molluscum contagiosum is treated by surgical excision of the lesion. Histopathologic examination shows basal epithelial cells with cytoplasmic inclusion bodies. The virus can be seen on electron microscopic evaluation as oval or brick-shaped virions.

PARAMYXOVIRUS OCULAR INFECTIONS
The paramyxoviruses include the causal agents of measles, mumps, and Newcastle disease, all of which may involve the eye. Characteristics of these small RNA viruses are listed in Table 5-8. The RNA-containing viruses (paramyxoviruses, picornaviruses, togaviruses, and orthomyxoviruses), which affect the eyes in several distinct clinical syndromes caused by distinct virus groups, are also listed in Table 5-7.

MEASLES (RUBEOLA)
Infection of the eye with measles results in acute catarrhal conjunctivitis, mild epithelial keratitis, and, occasionally, Koplik's spots on the conjunctiva or semilunar fold. This keratitis is rarely seen in the United States, but when it does occur, it is usually a fine superficial punctate keratitis associated with severe photophobia that is self-limited with little or no permanent visual defect. Interstitial keratitis may occur, but only rarely. Other infrequent ocular manifestations may also develop with the infection; these include chorioretinitis, central vein occlusion, optic atrophy, and isolated extraocular muscle paralysis. Fatal measles encephalopathy and acute retinitis have been described in an immunosuppressed patient [27], which again indicates that patients' incompetent immune systems [30, 31] may be fatally affected by opportunistic viral infections. These infections may be associated with unusual ocular complications.

In developing countries, measles keratitis is severe. Where malnutrition is prevalent, measles infection may become a critically debilitating disease that often results in severe keratitis, keratomalacia,

pneumonia, myocarditis, encephalitis, and, not infrequently, death. Measles virus has been shown to cause an anergy to tuberculin. Children with latent or mild tuberculosis may show renewed activity of this disease following measles.

Diagnosis of measles is made by isolation of the virus from the throat, blood, and mucous membranes, and by determination of the humoral antibody response. There is no effective cure. Adequate prophylaxis may be achieved by vaccination with attenuated measles vaccine.

MUMPS
Mumps occasionally involves the ocular adnexa by causing severe dacryoadenitis, sudden orbital pain, and swelling, with a lacrimal fossa mass. Frequently catarrhal conjunctivitis is noted [48]. The cornea may have fine punctate epithelial keratitis or severe stromal keratitis causing a decrease in vision associated with photophobia and lacrimation but little pain. The disciform keratitis is usually unilateral and may begin 5 to 7 days after onset of the punctate keratitis. In spite of the profound acute changes, including intense stromal haze and folds in Descemet's membrane, the disease resolves spontaneously [13, 15, 49]. Diagnosis is made by the presence of the systemic manifestations, by isolation of the virus, and by humor antibody response. No specific therapy is recommended; however, cycloplegic agents may be helpful in the acute disciform keratitis. Other reported ocular manifestations include episcleritis, scleritis, uveitis, optic neuritis, glaucoma, retinitis, and extraocular muscle paresias [48]. Severe bilateral uveitis associated with mumps in an immunosuppressed leukemia patient has been reported [1]. This is probably related to the abnormalities of the delayed immune system with failure of lymphocytic transformation associated with leukemia and chemotherapy [30, 31].

NEWCASTLE DISEASE
Newcastle disease is an infection limited almost exclusively to poultry workers and laboratory technicians. Infection is manifested by a unilateral follicular conjunctivitis with scanty watery discharge and preauricular adenopathy. The cornea may be rarely affected with fine punctate epithelial keratitis and occasional infiltrates. The disease is diagnosed by history of contact, virus isolation, and humoral antibody response. It is self-limiting, without sequelae, and requires no therapy [25].

PICORNAVIRUS OCULAR INFECTION
A newly recognized acute follicular conjunctivitis, associated with a prominent hemorrhagic conjunctival reaction, has recently been described. The dis-

ease was first reported in Africa as Apollo conjunctivitis [52] and has now been diagnosed in Africa and Asia. It is caused by enterovirus 70 [70], a member of the picornavirus group and is important in the differential diagnosis of acute follicular conjunctivitis. The virus is spread by upper respiratory tract as droplets. The disease has a rapid onset, with an incubation period as short as 24 hours in some patients. Isolation of the infecting virus is made difficult by the very short period of virus shedding from the infected conjunctiva and by the fact that the virus grows best at 30°C.

The disease is characterized by a mild follicular conjunctivitis that usually affects one eye and rapidly spreads to the other. The patient develops a foreign-body sensation, periorbital pain, and mild photophobia that is probably a result of the mild superficial keratitis noted in most patients. Sixty percent of patients develop preauricular adenopathy, and all patients develop a hemorrhagic bulbar conjunctival reaction, more marked temporally, which takes 1 to 2 weeks to resolve. Small petechiae are also observed. These findings are not themselves diagnostic, because infection with other viruses and bacteria may cause a hemorrhagic conjunctival reaction. Fortunately, the ocular disease is self-limited, terminating within a few days, and treatment is symptomatic [70]. Neurologic sequelae have been reported following this infection.

TOGAVIRUSES
Members of this virus group include the causal agents of rubella and the associated congenital rubella syndrome and of the arbovirus group B infections of yellow fever, dengue, and sandfly fever (Table 5-7). All viruses in this group cause hyperemia of the conjunctiva, lid swelling, photophobia, and lacrimation.

RUBELLA
The congenital rubella syndrome includes development of cataracts, glaucoma, purpura, retinopathy, cardiac anomalies, microcornea, microphthalmia, iris hypoplasia, and subretinal neovascularization. Keratoconus and secondary hydrops have been described in the second decade of life in children severely affected with the congenital rubella syndrome. The incidence of keratoconus appears much higher than in the general population [5]. Details of this syndrome will not be covered in this chapter. Seventy percent of children and adults who have the acute viral exanthem may develop a mild catarrhal or follicular conjunctivitis, with fine epithelial keratitis associated with photophobia and tearing in approximately 2 percent of cases. The corneal lesions are confined to the epithelium, are usually

central, and develop about 1 week after the onset of the rash [28, 61]. The delayed development of such epithelial and anterior stromal opacities has not been reported. The disease is self-limited and requires no treatment.

REFERENCES
1. Al-Rashid, R. A., and Cress, C. Mumps uveitis complicating the course of acute leukemia. *J. Pediatr. Ophthalmol.* 14:100, 1977.
2. Azar, P., Jr., et al. Acute posterior multifocal placoid pigment epitheliopathy associated with an adenovirus type 5 infection. *Am. J. Ophthalmol.* 80:1003, 1975.
3. Beal, R. Sur une forme particulière de conjunctivité aigue avec follicules. *Ann. Oculist* 87:1, 1907.
4. Bernstein, A. Infectious mononucleosis. *Medicine* 19:85, 1940.
5. Boger, W. P., III, Petersen, R. A., and Robb, R. M. Keratoconus and acute hydrops in mentally retarded patients with congenital rubella syndrome. *Am. J. Ophthalmol.* 91:231, 1981.
6. Boniuk, M., Phillips, C. A., and Friedman, J. B. Chronic adenovirus type 2 keratitis in man. *N. Engl. J. Med.* 273:924, 1965.
7. Burns, R. P., and Potter, M. H. Epidemic keratoconjunctivitis due to adenovirus type 19. *Am. J. Ophthalmol.* 81:27, 1976.
8. Center for Disease Control. Keratoconjunctivitis due to adenovirus type 19—Canada. *Morbid. Mortal. Weekly Rep.* 23:185, 1974.
9. Charles, S. K. R., Deanmart, J. C., and Barnard, D. L. The disinfection of instruments and hands during outbreaks of epidemic keratoconjunctivitis. *Trans. Ophthalmol. Soc. U.K.* 92:613, 1972.
10. Chawla, M. B., et al. Ocular involvement of cytomegalovirus infection in a previously healthy adult. *Br. Med. J.* 2:281, 1976.
11. Corboy, J. M., Goucher, C. R., and Pornes, C. A. Mechanical sterilization of the applanation tonometer: II. Viral study. *Am. J. Ophthalmol.* 71:891, 1971.
12. D'Angelo, L. J., et al. Pharyngoconjunctival fever caused by adenovirus type 4: Report of a swimming pool–related outbreak with recovery of virus from pool water. *J. Infect. Dis.* 140:42, 1979.
13. Danielson, R. W., and Long, J. C. Keratitis due to mumps. *Arch. Ophthalmol.* 24:655, 1941.
14. Darougar, S., et al. Epidemic keratoconjunctivitis and chronic papillary conjunctivitis in London due to adenovirus type 19. *Br. J. Ophthalmol.* 61:76, 1977.

15. Darrell, R. W. Ocular Infections Caused by the Poxvirus, Togavirus, Myxovirus, Paramyxovirus, and Picornavirus Groups. In D. Locatcher-Khorazo and B. C. Seegal (Eds.), *Microbiology of the Eye*. St. Louis: Mosby, 1972. P. 313.

16. Dawson, C. R., and Darrell, D. Infections due to adenovirus type 8 in the United States: I. An outbreak of epidemic keratoconjunctivitis originating in physician's office. *N. Engl. J. Med.* 268:1031, 1963.

17. Dawson, C. R., et al. Infections due to adenovirus type 8 in the United States: II. Community-wide infection with adenovirus type 8. *N. Engl. J. Med.* 268:1034, 1963.

18. Dawson, C. R., et al. Adenovirus type 8 keratoconjunctivitis in the United States: III. Epidemiologic, clinical, and microbiologic features. *Am. J. Ophthalmol.* 69:473, 1970.

19. Dixon, C. W. Principles of Smallpox Control. In *Smallpox*. London: Churchill, 1962. Pp. 296–360.

20. Dudgeon, J., Bhargava, S. K., and Ross, C. A. Treatment of adenovirus infection of the eye with 5-iodo-2-deoxyuridine: A double-blind trial. *Br. J. Ophthalmol.* 53:530, 1969.

21. Ellis, P. P., et al. Therapy of experimental vaccinal keratitis: Effects of idoxuridine and VIG. *Arch. Ophthalmol.* 74:539, 1965.

22. Ellis, P., and Winograd, L. A. Ocular vaccinia: A specific treatment. *Arch. Ophthalmol.* 68:600, 1962.

23. Fuchs, E. Keratitis punctata superficialis. *Wien. Klin. Wochenschr.* 2:837, 1889.

24. Garau, J., et al. Spontaneous cytomegalovirus mononucleosis with conjunctivitis. *Arch. Intern. Med.* 137:1631, 1977.

25. Grayson, M. Acute and Chronic Follicular Conjunctivitis. In M. Grayson (Ed.), *Diseases of the Cornea*. St. Louis: Mosby, 1979.

26. Guyer, G., et al. Epidemic keratoconjunctivitis: A community outbreak of mixed adenovirus type 8 and type 19 infection. *J. Infect. Dis.* 132:142, 1975.

27. Haltia, M., et al. Measles retinopathy during immunosuppression. *Br. J. Ophthalmol.* 62:356, 1978.

28. Hara, J., et al. Ocular manifestations of the 1976 rubella epidemic in Japan. *Am. J. Ophthalmol.* 87:642, 1979.

29. Hecht, S. D., et al. Treatment of epidemic keratoconjunctivitis with idoxuridine (IDU). *Arch. Ophthalmol.* 73:49, 1965.

30. Hersh, E. M., and Oppenheim, J. J. Inhibition of in vitro lymphocyte transformation during chemotherapy in man. *Cancer Res.* 27:98, 1967.

31. Humphrey, G. B., et al. Impaired lymphocyte transformation in leukemic patients after intensive therapy. *Cancer* 29:402, 1972.

32. Jawetz, E., et al. Studies on the etiology of epidemic keratoconjunctivitis. *Am. J. Ophthalmol.* 40:200, 1955.

33. Jawetz, E., et al. New type of APC virus from epidemic keratoconjunctivitis. *Science* 122:1190, 1955.

34. Jones, B. R., and Al-Hussaine, M. K. Therapeutic considerations in ocular vaccinia. *Trans. Ophthalmol. Soc. U.K.* 83:613, 1963.

35. Jones, B. R., Galbraith, J. E. K., and Al-Hussaine, M. K. Vaccinal keratitis treated with interferon. *Lancet* 1:875, 1962.

36. Kaufman, H., Nesburn, A. B., and Maloney, E. D. Cure of vaccinia infection by 5-iodo-2-deoxyuridine. *Virology* 18:567, 1962.

37. Kimura, S. J., et al. Sporadic cases of pharyngoconjunctival fever in northern California, 1955–1956. *Am. J. Ophthalmol.* 43:14, 1957.

38. Laibson, P. R., et al. Corneal infiltrates in epidemic keratoconjunctivitis: Response to double-blind corticosteroid therapy. *Arch. Ophthalmol.* 84:36, 1970.

39. Laibson, P. R., Ortolan, G., and Dupre-Strachan, S. Community and hospital outbreak of epidemic keratoconjunctivitis. *Arch. Ophthalmol.* 80:467, 1968.

40. Lane, J. M., and Millar, J. D. Routine childhood vaccination against smallpox reconsidered. *N. Engl. J. Med.* 281:1220, 1969.

41. Lane, J. M., et al. Complications of smallpox vaccination, 1968: National surveillance in the United States. *N. Engl. J. Med.* 281:1201, 1969.

42. Lane, J. M., et al. Complications of smallpox vaccination, 1968: Results of ten statewide surveys. *J. Infect. Dis.* 122:303, 1970.

43. Lennette, D. A., and Eiferman, R. A. Inhibition of adenovirus replication in vitro by trifluridine. *Arch. Ophthalmol.* 96:1662, 1978.

44. Levandowski, R. A., and Rubenis, M. Nosocomial conjunctivitis caused by adenovirus type 4. *J. Infect. Dis.* 143:28, 1981.

45. Librach, I. M. Ocular symptoms in glandular fever. *Br. J. Ophthalmol.* 40:619, 1956.

46. McCallum, R. W. Infectious mononucleosis and the Epstein-Barr virus. *J. Infect. Dis.* 121:347, 1970.

47. Meyer, R. F., and Kaufman, H. E. Antiviral agents. In H. E. Kaufman and T. J. Zimmerman (Eds.), *Current Concepts in Ophthalmology*. St. Louis: Mosby, 1976.

48. Meyer, R. F., Sullivan, J. H., and Oh, J. O. Mumps conjunctivitis. *Am. J. Ophthalmol.* 78:1022, 1974.

49. Mickatavage, R., and Amadur, J. A case report of mumps keratitis. *Arch. Ophthalmol.* 69:758, 1963.

50. O'Day, D. M., et al. Clinical and laboratory evaluations of epidemic keratoconjunctivitis due to adenovirus types 8 and 19. *Am. J. Ophthalmol.* 81:207, 1976.

51. Ostler, H. B., and Thygeson, P. The ocular manifestations of herpes zoster, varicella, infectious mononucleosis and cytomegalovirus disease. *Surv. Ophthalmol.* 21:148, 1976.

52. Parrott, W. F. An epidemic called Apollo. *Practitioner* 206:253, 1971.

53. Pavan-Langston, D., and Dohlman, C. H. A double-blind clinical study of adenine arabinoside therapy of viral keratoconjunctivitis. *Am. J. Ophthalmol.* 74:81, 1972.

54. Pettit, T. H. The poxviruses: Vaccinia and variola. *Int. Ophthalmol. Clin.* 15(4):203, 1975.

55. Pettit, T. H., and Holland, G. M. Chronic keratoconjunctivitis associated with ocular adenovirus infection. *Am. J. Ophthalmol.* 88:748, 1979.

56. Pinnolis, M., McCulley, J. P., and Urman, J. D. Nummular keratitis associated with infectious mononucleosis. *Am. J. Ophthalmol.* 89:791, 1980.

57. Ruben, F. L., and Lane, J. M. Ocular vaccinia: An epidemiologic analysis of 348 cases. *Arch. Ophthalmol.* 84:45, 1970.

58. Schaap, G. J. P., et al. A new intermediate adenovirus type causing conjunctivitis. *Arch. Ophthalmol.* 97:2336, 1979.

59. Schwartz, H. S., et al. Immunofluorescent detection of adenovirus antigen in epidemic keratoconjunctivitis. *Invest. Ophthalmol.* 15:199, 1976.

60. Sharma, R. Clinical assessment of an isothiazole thiosemicarbazone against smallpox. *J. Indian Med. Assoc.* 51:610, 1968.

61. Smolin, G. Report of a case of rubella keratitis. *Am. J. Ophthalmol.* 74:436, 1972.

62. Sprague, J. B., et al. Epidemic keratoconjunctivitis: A severe industrial outbreak due to adenovirus type 8. *N. Engl. J. Med.* 289:1341, 1973.

63. Tanner, O. R. Ocular manifestations of infectious mononucleosis. *Arch. Ophthalmol.* 51:229, 1954.

64. Thygeson, P. Further observations on superficial punctate keratitis. *Arch. Ophthalmol.* 66:158, 1962.

65. Tullo, A. B., and Higgins, P. G. An outbreak of adenovirus type 4 conjunctivitis. *Br. J. Ophthalmol.* 64:489, 1980.

66. Vastine, D. W., et al. Cytologic diagnosis of adenoviral epidemic keratoconjunctivitis by direct immunofluorescence. *Invest. Ophthalmol. Vis. Sci.* 16:195, 1977.

67. Vastine, D. W., et al. Simultaneous nosocomial and community outbreak of epidemic keratoconjunctivitis with types 8 and 19 adenovirus.

Trans. Am. Acad. Ophthalmol. Otolaryngol. 81:826, 1976.

68. Waring, G. O., III, et al. Use of vidarabine in epidemic keratoconjunctivitis due to adenovirus types 2, 7, 8, and 19. *Am. J. Ophthalmol.* 82:781, 1976.

69. Weller, T. H. The cytomegaloviruses: Ubiquitous agents with protean clinical manifestations. *N. Engl. J. Med.* 285:203, 1971.

70. Whitcher, J. P., et al. Acute hemorrhagic conjunctivitis in Tunisia. *Arch. Ophthalmol.* 94:51, 1976.

71. Wilhelmus, K. R. Ocular involvement in infectious mononucleosis (letter). *Am. J. Ophthalmol.* 91:117, 1981.

72. Wood, R. M. Prevention of infection during tonometry. *Arch. Ophthalmol.* 68:202, 1962.

Chlamydial Diseases

John P. Whitcher

HISTORIC BACKGROUND

Chlamydial infections of the eye characteristically produce chronic follicular conjunctivitis with associated corneal changes. The chlamydial or psittacosis-lymphogranuloma-trachoma agents responsible for these infections have been producing disease in humans for thousands of years. Trachoma was one of the first diseases in history to be recognized and described as a distinct clinical entity, and as early as the twenty-seventh century B.C. a Chinese medical treatise contained a detailed description of the treatment of trichiasis. Trachoma was epidemic in ancient Egypt; the Ebers papyrus (from 1500 B.C.) describes its exudative and cicatricial features and its treatment with copper salts [29].

It was not until 1907 that the inclusions of trachoma were finally discovered in conjunctival scrapings by Halberstaedter and von Prowazek [13]. They named them chlamydazoa or mantle bodies, because when stained with Giemsa the small reddish elementary bodies appeared to be embedded in a blue matrix or mantle. Halberstaedter and von Prowazek believed that these elementary bodies were the agent of trachoma, and their assumption was verified in the 1930s when Thygeson and others established the developmental cycle of the inclusions [28].

The relationship between trachoma and inclusion conjunctivitis of the newborn was established as early as 1909 when Heyman and Lindner found cytoplasmic inclusions similar to those described by Halberstaedter and von Prowazek in conjunctival scrapings from neonates with conjunctivitis [31]. Lindner described all the essential features of the disease, which he called inclusion blennorrhea [15]. Inclusion conjunctivitis in adults was also described in the early part of the twentieth century. The inclusions were identified, and in 1933 Morax described the clinical characteristics of the disease that differentiated it from acute trachoma [17]. Finally, in 1957 the first isolation of a chlamydial agent was successfully performed when T'ang and coworkers in Peking were able to grow the agent of trachoma in the yolk sac of a developing chick embryo [27].

PREVALENCE OF CHLAMYDIAL DISEASE

Chlamydial ocular infection is one of the most widespread diseases affecting the human species. At present, trachoma affects from 400 to 500 million people, or about one-seventh of the world's population. It is the greatest single cause of preventable blindness and impaired vision in the world today [36]. Although pockets of endemic trachoma have been reported from virtually every area of the globe, the disease remains epidemic in North Africa, the Middle East, other parts of Africa, and South Asia [1]. The Mediterranean basin has throughout history suffered the ravages of epidemic trachoma, but the disease has consistently remained most severe in the countries bordering on the northern Sahara. This pattern continues today; blindness or visual disability from trachoma still remains a number one public health problem in the area [9]. Transmission of the chlamydial agent causing trachoma is by eye-to-eye or hand-to-eye contact. The disease is usually acquired in early childhood and runs its course in adult years when the blinding complications occur. Prevalence and severity of the disease are enhanced by a number of epidemiologic factors including overcrowding, low standards of living, poor hygiene, and a number of other environmental factors.

In contrast, the most common form of chlamydial infection seen in industrialized countries is inclusion conjunctivitis of the newborn. The disease is contracted by the fetus as it passes through an infected birth canal. As a result, 2 to 6 percent of newborn infants born today in the United States are at risk of acquiring a chlamydial infection at birth [26]. The reservoir of the chlamydial agent responsible for inclusion conjunctivitis is the human genital tract. The agent causes urethritis in men and cervicitis in women [25]. The infrequent case of inclusion conjunctivitis in an adult is usually the result of exposure to infective genital tract discharges. The recent increase in venereal disease in general has been paralleled in most industrialized countries by a dramatic rise in the incidence of adult inclusion conjunctivitis. Although the disease does not produce the blinding sequelae of trachoma, it does, however, represent an important public health problem in industrialized countries today [24].

PROPERTIES OF CHLAMYDIAL ORGANISMS

MORPHOLOGY AND LIFE CYCLE

Chlamydial agents are members of the psittacosis-lymphogranuloma-trachoma group. They are obligate intracellular parasites that morphologically resemble gram-negative bacteria in many respects but differ primarily in their lack of energy-yielding metabolic pathways. Therefore, like the viruses, they require a host cell for replication. In clinical disease, the conjunctival epithelial cell provides the medium for growth. The tiny reddish blue elementary bodies (0.25 μ when stained with Giemsa), which are the infectious units, leave behind their protein coats and enter the cytoplasm of the cell where they develop into initial bodies. The initial body, which is bluish (1 μ when stained with Giemsa) and morphologically similar to a bacterium, undergoes division again to produce a mass of elementary bodies. The particles cluster together forming an inclusion body imbedded in a glycogen matrix that hugs the cell nucleus like a cap. The elementary bodies further multiply, rupturing the cell and liberating themselves to invade other epithelial cells. The whole process requires about 48 hours [12].

Although once considered to be large viruses, chlamydiae appear to be more closely related to true bacteria since they possess both DNA and RNA, are sensitive to the action of antibiotics, and have muramic acid in their cell walls. The chlamydiae have a common group antigen (detected by the complement fixation test) but have been divided into two species: *Chlamydia trachomatis*, which includes the agents of trachoma, inclusion conjunctivitis, and lymphogranuloma venereum; and *Chlamydia psittaci*, which includes the agents of psittacosis, feline pneumonitis, guinea pig inclusion conjunctivitis, and others. The *C. trachomatis* agents are distinguished by their sensitivity to sulfonamides and cycloserine and by the presence of glycogen in the cytoplasmic inclusion [6].

GROWTH CHARACTERISTICS
Chlamydial agents are fastidious in their growth requirements. Since the initial isolation of the agent of trachoma by T'ang in the yolk sac of embryonated hens' eggs [27], this medium has become the standard against which all other isolation media are measured. Material from the conjunctiva collected with a sterile spatula or swab is placed in a holding medium containing antibiotics that do not inhibit the growth of the chlamydial agent. When this material is inoculated into the yolk sac of 6- to 8-day-old embryonated hens' eggs and incubated at 35°C, the chlamydial elementary bodies can be observed growing in the yolk sac in 5 to 7 days. Up to five blind passages may be performed successively before a specimen is considered to be negative. The following features are required to identify the agent: (1) elementary bodies in yolk sac smears, (2) chlamydial antigen, (3) serial transmission of the agent to other eggs, (4) no bacterial contamination, and (5) the isolate should not be lethal for mice [22].

More recently, irradiated tissue culture cells have been used for isolation of chlamydial agents. A simplified one-passage technique of culture in irradiated McCoy cells has proven invaluable as a

rapid and sensitive method for the primary isolation of *C. trachomatis*. Conjunctival swabbing and transport of clinical specimens frozen in a cryoprotective medium in liquid nitrogen has increased the sensitivity of the procedure so that chlamydial isolates have been obtained in up to 90 percent of cases of chlamydial ocular infections. The growth characteristics are similar to those seen in yolk sac isolation, but the sensitivity and practicability of irradiated McCoy cells as an isolation medium provide a useful laboratory index, especially for use in epidemiologic and therapeutic studies of trachoma [3].

IDENTIFICATION OF ORGANISMS
SCRAPINGS
GIEMSA
Since the cytoplasmic inclusion of trachoma was first identified in 1907 by Halberstaedter and von Prowazek [13], Giemsa-stained conjunctival scrapings have remained the principal method of diagnosing chylamydial ocular infections. Scrapings from the conjunctival surface are smeared on a glass slide, stained with Giemsa, and examined for cytoplasmic inclusions. An overwhelming PMN cellular response is usually noted in chlamydial infections, although in some chronic cases of inclusion conjunctivitis a mononuclear cellular reaction may predominate. The chlamydial inclusions appear in the cytoplasm of the epithelial cells as a mass of fine reddish blue granules. Occasionally a darker blue initial body may be seen. Inclusions may be single or multiple, but in all cases they appear next to the cell nucleus, hugging it like a cap. In smears in which the epithelial cells have ruptured, free elementary bodies may be seen. Plasma cells and Leber cells (giant debris-laden macrophages) may be noted. Especially in long-standing cases of trachoma or inclusion conjunctivitis, typical cytoplasmic inclusion may not be demonstrable. In cases such as these, positive laboratory diagnosis may depend on the cytologic characteristics of the smear, including the presence of PMNs, plasma cells, Leber cells, and "follicle cells" (aggregates of lymphocytes). Giemsa is an ideal stain to use in appreciating the subtle morphologic characteristics of both the cells and the inclusions themselves. However, since the cytoplasmic inclusions of trachoma and inclusion conjunctivitis are morphologically identical, microscopic examination of Giemsa-stained conjunctival scrapings does not differentiate between the two diseases (Fig. 5-43). Other laboratory methods of identification are necessary.

FLUORESCENT ANTIBODY

Since the early 1960s, the fluorescent antibody (FA) technique has been considered the most sensitive laboratory indicator of chlamydial infection [20]. The FA method depends on the binding of antibodies against the chlamydia inclusion. By fluorescence microscopy, the chlamydia inclusions appear as bright green fluorescing bodies in the cytoplasm of the epithelial cells. The antichlamydial antibodies used in the test may be tagged directly with fluorescein (the direct FA test), or they may be tagged with fluorescein-labeled antibody that is directed against the globulins of the species of the antichlamydial-antibody–containing sera (the indirect FA test) [6]. FA testing requires an adequate conjunctival scraping that is spread on a glass slide and then fixed in chilled ($-20°C$) methanol or acetone, depending on the method of staining to be used. Because of the necessity for freshly cultivated chlamydial agent for producing and testing specific antisera, the FA test has remained mainly a laboratory technique. There is no doubt that it is the most sensitive test for detecting chlamydial agent, however. Schachter and colleagues have found that, in cases of inclusion conjunctivitis in adult men, FA methods are markedly superior (81 percent positive) to Giemsa staining (48 percent positive) as well as to isolation methods (30 percent positive) [23]. In cases of neonatal inclusion conjunctivitis, however, in which maximal levels of agent are being produced, isolation rates are high (67 percent positive) and FA and Giemsa are both positive in 95 percent of the cases [23]. FA staining is also more sensitive than Giemsa in evaluating trachoma, yielding up to 40 percent positive.

IODINE

Iodine staining has also been used to detect chlamydial inclusions, especially in screening large numbers of conjunctival smears in trachoma control programs. Since the inclusions have a glycogen matrix, iodine is rapidly taken up and may easily be seen through the microscope under low power. Iodine is much less sensitive, however, than either Giemsa or FA as a diagnostic stain.

CULTURES

EGG ISOLATION

As a diagnostic tool, isolation of the chlamydial agent is unfortunately cumbersome. Since the trachoma agent was isolated by T'ang and associates [27], egg isolation has continued to be the

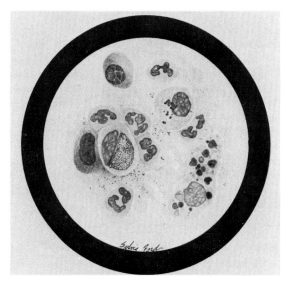

FIGURE 5-43. *Giemsa-stained scraping from chlamydia-infected conjunctiva. Polymorphonuclear leukocytes predominate. Note cytoplasmic inclusions in epithelial cells.*

most successful and readily available method. Swabs or scrapings of the conjunctiva are usually placed in a sterile broth containing streptomycin (2.5 mg/ml), neomycin (0.5 mg/ml), and nystatin (100 units/ml). A portion of the solution (0.25 ml) is inoculated into the yolk sac of 6- to 8-day-old embryonated hens' eggs and incubated at 35°C. The criteria for identification are as previously described.

Eggs are difficult to transport and to store. They are also susceptible to other pathogens. Egg isolation, therefore, is restricted in its clinical usefulness and is primarily a research technique.

TISSUE CULTURE ISOLATION

The availability of irradiated tissue culture cells (usually McCoy cells) for isolation and serial cultivation of chlamydial agents has greatly simplified clinical investigation of chlamydial infections. Specimens are collected from conjunctiva in the same manner as for egg isolation. The irradiated cells are then inoculated and allowed to incubate for 3 days. At that time, the inclusions are stained with iodine or Giemsa and identified, and further serial passages are performed. The enhanced sensitivity and practicability of this method make it ideal for studies in the field as well as for diagnostic clinical testing.

C. trachomatis may also be isolated from the tears of patients with hyperendemic trachoma. Tears collected with cellulose sponges, placed in transport medium, and then inoculated into irradiated McCoy cells yield a high percentage of positive isolations in patients with previously documented disease [4].

epithelial tissues with PMNs and lymphocytes. Because of the neonate's immature immune system, however, follicles cannot develop until the infection has persisted for 6 to 8 weeks. Unlike adults with inclusion conjunctivitis, neonates do develop scarring of the conjunctiva and cornea. A trachomalike corneal pannus at the superior limbus may occur, as well as focal corneal vascularization. Broad scarring of the lower conjunctival fornix may also occur. These cicatricial changes do not occur if the child is treated early in the course of the disease [19].

CLINICAL ASPECTS

TRACHOMA

EPIDEMIOLOGY

In highly endemic areas, trachoma may affect virtually the entire population, producing blindness in a great percentage [7]. One of the outstanding characteristics of trachoma, however, is its extreme variability. A high incidence in an area, for example, may not necessarily be correlated with a high degree of visual impairment; even areas in close proximity may have strikingly different incidences. Preschool children usually serve as the reservoir of acute infection. By the age of 2, all children in hyperendemic areas have been infected, and acute disease declines thereafter, active infectious cases being seen only infrequently in adult life.

The infection is usually acquired by direct inoculation by fingers or fomites into the eye of the affected individual, and mother-to-child transfer is the basic pattern. Cultural and social customs play an important role. In many developing countries where trachoma is endemic, a mixture of lamp black and castor oil called kohl is applied around the eyes of all young children to ward off eye infections. This undoubtedly serves as an excellent method of transferring chlamydial agent between daughters and mother because the same applicator is used on all the female family members. This results also in a higher incidence of acute disease and blindness in women. The conjunctiva is therefore repeatedly inoculated with chlamydial agent from an early age. In addition, there is transfer between siblings in close contact.

Flies also play an important role in the transmission of agent from conjunctiva to conjunctiva. Probably a more important role of flies, however, is in the spread of seasonal epidemics of severe bacterial conjunctivitis. In many developing countries where trachoma is prevalent, seasonal epidemics of bacterial conjunctivitis occur in the spring and fall. The predominant pathogen in these epidemics is *Haemophilus aegyptius*, followed by *Streptococcus*

pneumoniae and *Moraxella* sp. (Fig. 5-44). Bacterial conjunctivitis can produce disastrous complications in eyes already infected with trachoma, and, indeed, bacterial infection may play a greater role than trachoma in producing blinding complications [35]. This phenomenon has been noted for decades: Much of the blindness from trachoma in Egypt is a result of "Egyptian ophthalmia," a combination of trachoma, *Haemophilus aegyptius*, and *Neisseria gonorrhoeae*.

Many other factors affect the prevalence and severity of the disease. There is a definite racial susceptibility, with whites being at greater risk than other racial types. The climate affects prevalence and severity of the disease dramatically. Persons living in hot, dry, dusty climates are at greater risk than those in cool, wet areas with an abundance of water. Poverty, filth, overcrowding, and poor nutritional status all encourage the spread of trachoma and increase the blinding complications of the disease.

CLINICAL PICTURE

Clinically, trachoma is a chronic follicular conjunctivitis that leads to conjunctival and corneal scarring. Because of its unique epidemiologic setting, an acute case of trachoma is rarely observed at onset. In isolated cases, however, it has been observed that the incubation time is approximately 5 days from inoculation until onset of the acute follicular conjunctivitis. In 1908, MacCallan divided the clinical course of trachoma into four stages, based on developmental changes in the follicles, papillary hypertrophy, and scar formation [16]. This classification, which has been used as a guide in all subsequent epidemiologic studies of the disease, provides a useful framework for categorizing the stages of the disease even though there is no provision for grading the intensity of the inflammatory process.

Initially the eye becomes red and inflamed. A purulent discharge and possibly a tender preauricular node may be present. There is usually tearing and discomfort as would be seen in any acute conjunctivitis. This is followed at about the third week by the appearance of follicles on the upper tarsal conjunctiva.

STAGE 1: INCIPIENT TRACHOMA

The first stage of MacCallan's classification is characterized by immature follicles on the upper tarsus, minimal papillary hypertrophy, and faint sub-

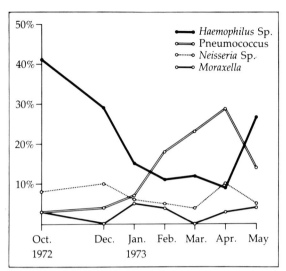

FIGURE 5-44. *Pattern of seasonal bacterial conjunctivitis in an area of severe endemic trachoma. Monthly variations in positive conjunctival cultures in school children in a sub-Saharan oasis village, Tunisia, 1972–1973.*

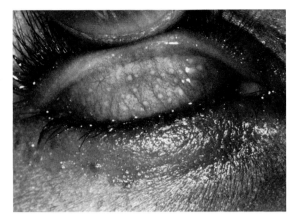

FIGURE 5-45. *Stage 1 trachoma. Note immature follicles on the upper tarsal conjunctiva.*

epithelial opacities with diffuse punctate keratitis (Fig. 5-45). Early pannus formation may be seen.

STAGE 2: ESTABLISHED TRACHOMA

2A: FOLLICULAR HYPERTROPHY PREDOMINANT. Mature, well-developed sagograinlike follicles are present on the upper tarsal conjunctiva (Fig. 5-46). The keratitis is more advanced, and limbal follicles may be present, producing a characteristic serrated edge. The pannus advances and may be associated with subepithelial infiltrates and corneal haze.

2B: PAPILLARY HYPERTROPHY PREDOMINANT. In stage 2b, inflammation is acute. This stage is characterized by papillary hypertrophy obliterating the follicles, intense cellular infiltration, pannus and infiltrates extending from the upper limbus, and necrosis of follicles at the limbus and on the tarsal conjunctiva (Fig. 5-47).

STAGE 3: CICATRIZING TRACHOMA

By stage 3, the follicles have undergone necrosis and scarring, and islands of cellular infiltration and papillary hypertrophy are present between the scars. Trichiasis and entropion may begin to develop, and pannus is grossly visible (Fig. 5-48). An acute attack of trachoma in this stage caused by reinfection may produce disastrous complications as a result of superinfection with bacteria.

STAGE 4: HEALED TRACHOMA

The tarsal conjunctiva is completely cicatrized and smooth or may have a mosaic pattern of scarring. No islands of follicles or papillary hypertrophy remain, and no further inflammatory activity is evident. The cornea is free from subepithelial infiltrates and superficial staining. Variable complications of trichiasis, entropion, corneal opacities, and visual impairment are becoming manifest (Fig. 5-49).

The individual stages of trachoma may last for months or years, with blinding complications occurring frequently during stage 4. The complete corneal picture seen in trachoma, which is of great value in establishing a clinical diagnosis at any time during the disease, includes a micropannus located superiorly, epithelial keratitis, subepithelial infiltrates, limbal follicles, and Herbert's pits [30].

From the standpoint of epidemiologic evaluation, it is also essential to assess the severity of the inflammatory reaction in patients with acute trachoma infections. A method for doing this has been elegantly demonstrated by Dawson and associates, using the standardized World Health Organization criteria for evaluating follicular reaction, papillary hypertrophy, scarring of the conjunctiva and cornea, trichiasis, and entropion formation [8]. The intensity of active inflammatory trachoma may be graded as severe, moderate, or mild, depending mainly on the intensity of the papillary reaction combined with the follicular reaction. This is of value in predicting which patients will ultimately be at risk for blinding complications of the disease. Combinations of severe follicular involvement and papillary hypertrophy associated with cicatrization tend to progress to trichiasis, pannus, and corneal scarring. Other corneal opacities are due to scarring and perforation produced by associated bacterial infections.

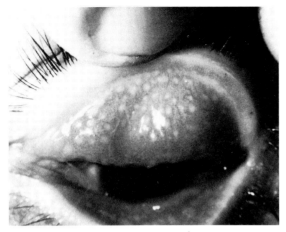

FIGURE 5-46. *Stage 2a trachoma. Note mature follicles on upper tarsus.*

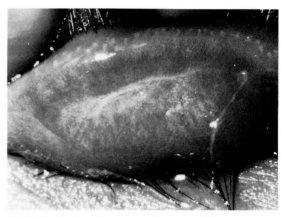

FIGURE 5-48. *Stage 3 trachoma. Note severe inflammatory conjunctival reaction with conjunctival scarring, Herbert's pits, prominent pannus, and corneal infiltrates.*

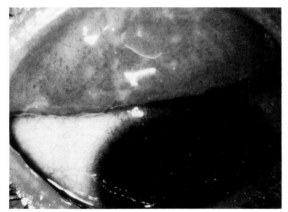

FIGURE 5-47. *Stage 2b trachoma: Hyperacute trachoma with mature follicles partially obscured by papillary hypertrophy. Note early pannus.*

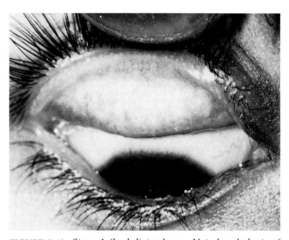

FIGURE 5-49. *Stage 4 (healed) trachoma. Note broad sheets of scarring, corneal scars, and trichiasis.*

TREATMENT

The treatment of individual cases of trachoma has been revolutionized with the advent of antibiotics. Until the development of sulfonamides in the 1930s, the treatment still consisted of the application of copper salts as suggested in the Ebers papyrus (1500 B.C.). Individual and sporadically occurring cases respond well to oral tetracycline 1 to 1.5 gm daily for 3 weeks. Oral triple sulfa (sulfadiazine, sulfamethazine, and sulfamerazine) may also be given in therapeutic doses for 3 weeks in cases that are resistant to tetracycline. Because of the high incidence of allergic reactions to sulfa drugs, their use has been avoided in recent years. Only systemic treatment provides blood levels high enough over a prolonged period of time to eradicate the organisms. Topical tetracycline, sulfisoxazole (Gantrisin),

or erythromycin has a pronounced but short-lived effect on the disease process. It is not necessary to give topical therapy in conjunction with systemic treatment [10].

Areas in which trachoma is hyperendemic and there are associated epidemics of seasonal bacterial conjunctivitis represent a much more difficult public health problem. Combined infection with trachoma and bacterial pathogens leads to severe inflammation, producing potentially blinding complications owing to scarring of the conjunctiva and distortion of the lids. Systemic therapy of all affected persons is virtually impossible because of the potentially hazardous side effects of oral antibiotics given on a large scale. The primary aim then is to prevent blinding complications rather than to attempt to eradicate the disease. Several topical antibiotic regimens have been recommended; the most effective appears to be topical tetracycline or erythromycin applied twice daily for 6 weeks. Results are similar when the medication is applied to the conjunctiva twice daily for 5 days and repeated monthly for 6 months. It is obvious that topical antibiotics are inadequate as a treatment for trachoma itself. Blinding complications are reduced or prevented by topical antibiotics, however, probably by preventing hyperacute bacterial ocular infections that occur during epidemics of seasonal bacterial conjunctivitis [11].

ADULT INCLUSION CONJUNCTIVITIS

EPIDEMIOLOGY

Inclusion conjunctivitis is an oculogenital disease, and as such its epidemiology differs sharply from that of trachoma. The disease was originally reported as being transmitted from genital secretions to the eyes of bathers in swimming pools in Europe. The inclusions were identified in scrapings, and the disease was initially called swimming pool conjunctivitis. Chlorination has now eliminated the chlamydial agent from the water of swimming pools, and the disease in adults is now transmitted by autoinoculation from the genital tract to the eye by the fingers or by genital-to-eye inoculation by an infected sexual partner. The ocular disease is found more frequently in populations with a high venereal disease rate and so is reported more frequently in industrialized societies. The "sexual revolution" has led to an alarming increase of sexually transmitted diseases, with genital chlamydial infections being recognized more and more frequently. In a number of studies, chlamydial strains have been isolated from a high percentage (30–60 percent) of men with symptomatic nongonococcal urethritis. Positive cervical and rectal cultures have also been reported in a large percentage of sexually active women [24]. In contrast to trachoma, eye-to-eye transmission of inclusion conjunctivitis is extremely rare. The main reservoir of the agent remains the genital tract of sexually active men and women. As the incidence of chlamydial genital infection reaches epidemic proportions, there is a parallel increase in the incidence of inclusion conjunctivitis.

CLINICAL PICTURE

Adult inclusion conjunctivitis begins as acute follicular conjunctivitis approximately 5 days after ex-

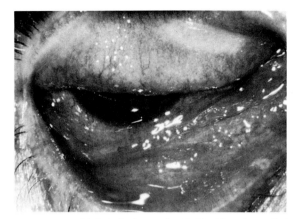

FIGURE 5-50. *Adult inclusion conjunctivitis. Note the marked follicular reaction in the inferior fornix.*

posure, although incubation can range from 2 to 19 days [5]. The patient complains of a unilateral purulent discharge with sticking of the lids on waking. There is an associated nontender preauricular node on the involved side. The initial reaction is usually subacute or acute without the hemorrhages or membrane formation seen in more hyperacute conjunctival infections. If the disease is untreated it usually heals spontaneously but may on occasion persist for longer than a year.

On examination, a marked follicular conjunctival reaction is noted associated with papillary hypertrophy and affecting both the upper and lower conjunctiva (Fig. 5-50). The lower tarsal conjunctiva is involved to the greatest extent, however. During the active stage of the disease, there is usually superficial epithelial keratitis, and micropannus is sometimes recognized. Marginal and central corneal subepithelial infiltrates may also occur, as well as typical "EKC-like" subepithelial opacities. All of these corneal changes rapidly disappear with treatment, and marked pannus or conjunctival scarring does not occur. In marked contrast to trachoma, adult inclusion conjunctivitis subsides without complications. Mild cases of uveitis have been reported in some patients, and otitis media may occur on the same side as the eye involvement in as many as 14 percent of cases [5].

TREATMENT

As in trachoma, topical treatment does not cure inclusion conjunctivitis but only temporarily suppresses the symptoms. The keratitis improves slightly when topical sulfisoxazole is given, but the follicular conjunctivitis persists and continues to remain symptomatic when the drops are discontinued. Patients with a diagnosis of inclusion conjunctivitis confirmed by laboratory studies should

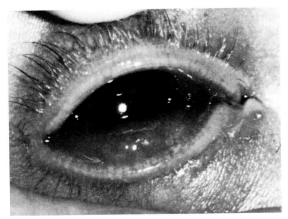

FIGURE 5-51. *Nonspecific conjunctival reaction in neonatal inclusion blennorrhea.*

be given oral tetracycline 1 to 1.5 gm daily for 3 weeks. Oral triple sulfa may also be given in corresponding dosages for 3 weeks in those patients in whom the chlamydial agent is resistant to tetracycline. Patients improve symptomatically in the first week or 2, but follicles may remain visible for a month or more. The patient's sexual partner should also be treated to prevent reinfection.

NEONATAL INCLUSION BLENNORRHEA

EPIDEMIOLOGY

Neonatal inclusion blennorrhea or inclusion conjunctivitis of the newborn is being seen with increasing frequency in industrialized countries and is the most common form of chlamydial eye disease. At present, 2 to 6 percent of newborns acquire chlamydial disease at birth. The eyes become infected as the fetus passes through the infected birth canal of the mother. Cervical carriage of chlamydiae in normal, sexually active women in the United States has been found to be as high as 11 percent in some clinics [24]. The risk of transmission to the newborn is not known, but it is estimated to be in excess of 20 percent. The potential for the newborn to develop systemic chlamydial disease has also been recently documented [26]. A distinctive chlamydial pneumonia syndrome is now recognized, and positive cultures have been obtained from the newborn nasopharynx, throat, lungs, and vagina. The agent has also been found in the feces, which raises the important question of possible chlamydial gastrointestinal infections. In developing countries where the nutritional status of the infant is often precarious, chlamydial infections may contribute to the severity of the diarrhea so common among infants [26].

CLINICAL PICTURE

Neonatal inclusion blennorrhea usually appears on the fifth day after birth, although incubation may vary from 3 to 12 days depending on whether the membranes were prematurely ruptured. Frequently both eyes demonstrate the typical nonspecific signs of neonatal conjunctivitis: lid edema, conjunctival hyperemia, papillary hypertrophy, and mucopurulent discharge (Fig. 5-51). Since the newborn cannot produce follicles for the first 6 to 8 weeks of life, the conjunctival reaction does not contribute to the diagnosis. Large numbers of cytoplasmic inclusions can be seen on conjunctival scrapings stained with Giemsa, however. It is essential to perform scrapings and cultures to rule out gonorrheal conjunctivitis. Untreated, neonatal inclusion blennorrhea may pursue a prolonged course with systemic involvement. Keratitis, corneal pannus, focal vascularization, and conjunctival scarring have been described frequently in the disease. Corneal scarring with visual disability has also been described [18].

TREATMENT

Until recently, it was felt that topical sulfacetamide, tetracycline, or erythromycin applied 4 times daily to the conjunctiva for 3 weeks was adequate for eliminating chlamydial agent from the eyes of newborns and preventing the ocular complications of corneal and conjunctival scarring. The recognition of generalized chlamydial infections in newborns, however, has made evident the necessity for systemic treatment. The treatment now consists of antibiotics (usually erythromycin) by mouth or injection rather than topically.

OTHER OCULAR CHLAMYDIAL INFECTIONS

FELINE PNEUMONITIS

Feline pneumonitis has been reported to cause mild mucopurulent conjunctivitis in humans that persists for more than 3 months. There is follicular conjunctivitis associated with fine epithelial keratitis and subepithelial infiltrates. The disease responds to treatment with oral tetracycline and heals without scars [21].

PSITTACOSIS

Psittacosis, an avian strain, can cause acute follicular conjunctivitis in humans with fine punctate epithelial keratitis. It responds rapidly to a full course of systemic tetracycline [21].

REFERENCES

1. Bietti, G., and Werner, C. *Trachoma: Prevention and Treatment.* Springfield, Ill.: Thomas, 1967. Pp. 1–227.

2. Darougar, S., et al. Rapid serological test for diagnosis of chlamydial ocular infections. *Br. J. Ophthalmol.* 62:503, 1978.

3. Darougar, S., et al. Isolation of *Chlamydia trachomatis* from different areas of conjunctiva in relation to intensity of hyperendemic trachoma in school children in southern Tunisia. *Br. J. Ophthalmol.* 63:110, 1979.

4. Darougar, S., et al. Isolation of *Chlamydia trachomatis* from eye secretion (tears). *Br. J. Ophthalmol.* 63:256, 1979.

5. Dawson, C., et al. Experimental inclusion conjunctivitis in man: III. Keratitis and other complications. *Arch. Ophthalmol.* 78:341, 1967.

6. Dawson, C. Lids, conjunctiva and lacrimal apparatus (annual review): Eye infections with chlamydia. *Arch. Ophthalmol.* 93:854, 1975.

7. Dawson, C., et al. Severe endemic trachoma in Tunisia. *Br. J. Ophthalmol.* 60:245, 1975.

8. Dawson, C., Jones, B., and Darougar, S. Blinding and non-blinding trachoma: Assessment of intensity of upper tarsal inflammatory disease and disabling lesions. *Bull. W.H.O.* 52:279, 1975.

9. Dawson, C., et al. Severe endemic trachoma in Tunisia. *Br. J. Ophthalmol.* 60:245, 1976.

10. Dawson, C., et al. Response to treatment in ocular chlamydial infections (trachoma and inclusion conjunctivitis): Analogies with non-gonococcal urethritis. *Nongonococcal Urethritis and Related Infections.* Washington, D.C.: American Society for Microbiology, 1977. Pp. 135–139.

11. Dawson, C., et al. Chlamydial infections of the eye: Trachoma and inclusion conjunctivitis. *Contact Intraoc. Lens Med. J.* 6:217, 1980.

12. Duke-Elder, S. *System of Ophthalmology,* Vol. 8, Pt. 1. London: Kimpton, 1965.

13. Halberstaedter, L., and von Prowazek, S. Zur Aetiologie das Trachome. *Dtsch. Med. Wochenschr.* 33:1285, 1907.

14. Hogan, M., and Zimmerman, L. *Ophthalmic Pathology: An Atlas and Textbook* (2nd ed.). Philadelphia: Saunders, 1962.

15. Lindner, K. Gonoblenorrhoe, Einschlussblenonorrhoe and Trachoma. *Albrecht Von Graefes Arch. Klin. Exp. Ophthalmol.* 78:345, 1911.

16. MacCallan, A. The epidemiology of trachoma. *Br. J. Ophthalmol.* 15:369, 1931.

17. Morax, V. *Les Conjunctivitis Follicularies.* Paris: Masson, 1933.

18. Mordhorst, C. Studies on oculogenital TRIC agents isolated in Denmark. *Am. J. Ophthalmol.* 63(Suppl.):1282, 1967.

19. Mordhorst, C., and Dawson, C. Sequelae of neonatal inclusion conjunctivitis and associated disease in parents. *Am. J. Ophthalmol.* 71:867, 1971.

20. Nichols, R., et al. Studies on trachoma: II. Comparison of fluorescent antibody, Giemsa, and egg isolation methods for detection of trachoma in human conjunctival scrapings. *Am. J. Trop. Med. Hyg.* 12:223, 1962.

21. Ostler, B., and Schachter, J., and Dawson, C. Acute follicular conjunctivitis of epizootic origin. *Arch. Ophthalmol.* 82:587, 1969.

22. Schachter, J. Recommended criteria for the identification of trachoma and inclusion conjunctivitis agents. *J. Infect. Dis.* 122:105, 1970.

23. Schachter, J., et al. Evaluation of laboratory methods for detecting acute TRIC agent infection. *Am. J. Ophthalmol.* 70:375, 1970.

24. Schachter, J., Causse, G., and Tarizzo, M. Chlamydiae as agents of sexually transmitted diseases. *Bull. W.H.O.* 54:245, 1976.

25. Schachter, J., and Dawson, C. *Human Chlamydial Infection.* Littleton, Mass.: PSG Publishing, 1978.

26. Schachter, J., and Dawson, C. Is trachoma an ocular component of a more generalized chlamydial infection? *Lancet* 1:702, 1979.

27. T'ang, F., et al. Studies of the etiology of trachoma with special reference to isolation of the virus in chick embryo. *Chin. Med. J.* 75:429, 1957.

28. Thygeson, P., and Mengert, W. The virus of inclusion conjunctivitis: Further observations. *Arch. Ophthalmol.* 15:377, 1936.

29. Thygeson, P. Trachoma virus: Historical background and review of isolates. *Ann. N.Y. Acad. Sci.* 98:6, 1962.

30. Thygeson, P. Corneal changes in TRIC agent infections. *Am. J. Ophthalmol.* 63:252, 1967.

31. Thygeson, P. Historical review of oculogenital diseases. *Am. J. Ophthalmol.* 71:975, 1971.

32. Treharne, J., et al. Antichlamydial antibody in tears and sera and serotypes of *Chlamydia trachomatis* isolated from school children in southern Tunisia. *Br. J. Ophthalmol.* 62:509, 1978.

33. Wang, S., and Grayston, J. Immunologic relationship between genital TRIC, lymphogranuloma venereum, and related organisms in a new microtiter indirect immunofluorescence test. *Am. J. Ophthalmol.* 70:367, 1970.

34. Wang, S., and Grayston, J. Human serology in *Chlamydia trachomatis* infection with microimmunofluorescence. *J. Infect. Dis.* 130:397, 1974.

35. Whitcher, J., et al. Severe endemic trachoma in Tunisia: Changes in ocular bacterial patho-

gens in children treated by the intermittent antibiotic regimen. *Rev. Int. Trachome* 4:49, 1974.
36. World Health Organization Methodology for Trachoma Control. W.H.O. Tech. Rep. Ser. No. 703, 1970.

Suspected Infectious Etiology

H. Bruce Ostler

SUPERIOR LIMBIC KERATOCONJUNCTIVITIS

Superior limbic keratoconjunctivitis was described by Thygeson and Kimura [21] under the heading of chronic conjunctivitis with filaments and was given the name superior limbic keratoconjunctivitis by Theodore [15, 16]. The condition is characterized by inflammation of the superior bulbar conjunctiva with marked involvement of the superior limbus, superior epithelial keratitis, and papillary hypertrophy of the upper tarsal conjunctiva. Filaments, though not always present, tend to aggravate the symptoms when they occur.

ETIOLOGY

The cause of superior limbic keratoconjunctivitis is unknown. Thygeson and Kimura [21] suggested that the condition might be caused by a virus. Their studies and subsequent studies at the Proctor Foundation have failed to demonstrate a virus, and there has been no histologic evidence of a virus on biopsy of the conjunctiva [6].

Tenzel [14] and Corwin [4], in 1968, reported an association of superior limbic keratoconjunctivitis with thyroid abnormalities. Since that time as association with an endocrine element (usually hypothyroidism or the use of thyroid or its congeners) has been noted in 26 to 50 percent of patients [2, 3, 26]. In one of my patients, I was impressed by the fact that at onset her disease was bilateral and associated with endocrine exophthalmos. After ablation of the thyroid with radioactive iodine and later replacement therapy with thyroid, the exophthalmos decreased in one eye, and the superior limbic keratoconjunctivitis in that eye also disappeared. The fellow eye continued to manifest severe signs and symptoms. It was only several years later, when the exophthalmos in the fellow eye also disappeared, that the patient was free of symptoms of superior limbic keratoconjunctivitis.

Other suggested causes of superior limbic keratoconjunctivitis include keratoconjunctivitis sicca and an autoimmune process [2]. Several patients have been found to have keratoconjunctivitis sicca, but such findings are uncommon. Most patients have normal Schirmer tear test scores and tear lysosome levels. Although autoimmunity was suggested as a possible cause, there is no convincing argument that this is the case. In fact, in most instances, corticosteroids seem to have no beneficial effect on the course of the disease, and in several cases in which I have obtained laboratory studies for autoimmune processes, the results have been negative.

PATHOGENESIS

Wright's suggestion that the initial pathologic process of superior limbic keratoconjunctivitis resides in the upper tarsal conjunctiva is an attractive one [26]. His explanation of the pathogenic mechanisms—that a chronically inflamed upper tarsal conjunctiva acts to disturb the normal maturation of the bulbar conjunctiva—may be correct, but it is difficult to identify whether the bulbar conjunctiva or the tarsal conjunctiva is the initial site of inflammation.

The following hypothesis is made only as an attempt to explain the findings in superior limbic keratoconjunctivitis, namely, (1) its association with thyroid abnormalities in many but not all patients, (2) the insidious nature of its onset, (3) the laxness of the upper bulbar conjunctiva, (4) the papillary hypertrophy of the upper tarsal conjunctiva, (5) the thickened bulbar conjunctiva with biopsy evidence of abnormal maturation of the bulbar conjunctiva, (6) the superiorly located epithelial keratitis, (7) the presence of filaments in many patients, (8) the temporary relief of symptoms obtained by the application of silver nitrate to the upper tarsal conjunctiva or the mechanical removal of the surface cells of the conjunctiva, and (9) the prolonged relief of symptoms by the removal of the superior bulbar conjunctiva and underlying Tenon's capsule.

The upper eyelid is tensely applied against the upper bulbar conjunctiva and the cornea because of a thyroid abnormality, endocrine exophthalmos, or specific or nonspecific chronic inflammation. The laxness of the bulbar conjunctiva may be of congenital origin or arise from aging, but it constantly subjects the bulbar conjunctiva to movement as the tense upper eyelid opens and closes. The abnormal movement results in a chronic irritation of the bulbar conjunctiva owing to mechanical factors. The papillary hypertrophy and cellular infiltration of the upper tarsal conjunctiva also arise because of the mechanical factors.

The insidious onset of superior limbic keratoconjunctivitis results from the gradual thickening of the bulbar conjunctiva and the gradual development of papillary hypertrophy of the upper tarsal conjunctiva. Once these factors develop, a vicious circle results.

Filaments frequently occur when mucus production is abnormal. The abnormal mucus production arises from the mechanical irritation of the bulbar conjunctiva.

The temporary relief of symptoms with the application of silver nitrate to the conjunctiva or the mechanical removal of the surface conjunctival cells is caused by the sloughing of the surface cells and the loss of the abnormal conjunctiva that has arisen from improper maturation. Once the conjunctival epithelium regenerates, the abnormal maturation begins anew and symptoms recur. The permanent or prolonged relief of symptoms and signs of superior limbic keratoconjunctivitis after the above treatment, on the other hand, results from the development of adhesions between the regenerated conjunctiva and the subconjunctival tissues preventing the abnormal movement of the bulbar conjunctiva.

PATHOLOGY

Bacterial cultures of the conjunctiva in superior limbic keratoconjunctivitis reflect normal conjunctival flora and include primarily *Staphylococcus epidermidis* and diphtheroids. Giemsa-stained scrapings of the tarsal conjunctiva reveal a predominant PMN reaction with some keratinization of the tarsal conjunctival epithelium. Giemsa-stained scrapings of the involved bulbar conjunctiva reveal keratinization of the epithelial cells in almost all cases and a moderate number of PMNs in some cases. Papanicolaou-stained scrapings of the superior bulbar conjunctiva have been reported to show condensed chromatin arranged in the shape of an S or in the form of a coil or bar [24].

Biopsy sections of the bulbar conjunctiva disclose keratinization of the epithelium, acanthosis, degeneration of the nuclei, and intracellular accumulation of glycogen [6]. The conjunctival epithelial cells moreover show an abnormal distribution and aggregation of the nuclear chromatin with filament forms within the nucleus and cytoplasmic filaments surrounding it that cause strangulation of the nucleus and the formation of multilobed nuclei or multinucleated epithelial cells [3]. Biopsy sections of the palpebral conjunctiva reveal inflammatory cellular infiltration consisting of PMNs, lymphocytes, and plasma cells. The conjunctival epithelium appears normal [18].

CLINICAL FEATURES

Patients with superior limbic keratoconjunctivitis generally complain of irritation and redness associated with minimal or no discharge from the eye. In some instances, the irritation is more marked when the patient looks up. Less common symptoms include a burning sensation, a foreign-body sensa-

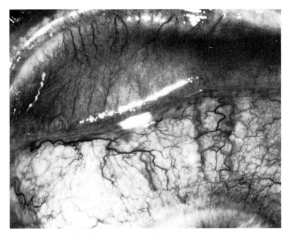

FIGURE 5-52. *Papillary hypertrophy of the superior tarsal conjunctiva with hyperemia and thickening of the upper bulbar conjunctiva in superior limbic keratoconjunctivitis.*

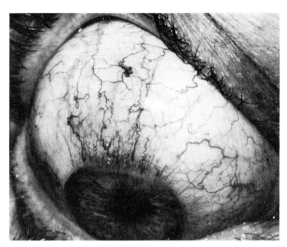

FIGURE 5-53. *Hyperemia of the upper bulbar conjunctiva in superior limbic keratoconjunctivitis.*

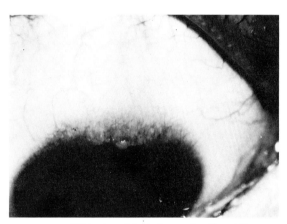

FIGURE 5-54. *Thickening of the bulbar conjunctiva at the upper limbus in superior limbic keratoconjunctivitis.*

tion, pain, photophobia, and inability to open the eyes (blepharospasm). The symptoms are variable in degree, and there are remissions and exacerbations that coincide with the signs. When filaments are present, the patient is often extremely symptomatic.

Although superior limbic keratoconjunctivitis occurs in all age groups (ages 4–81), the condition occurs most frequently in patients of middle age or older [17]. Women are more frequently affected than men [4], and the symptoms and signs are more marked in women. In most instances, the condition is bilateral, although one eye may be more involved than the other, and exacerbations may affect only one eye. There is frequently an association with past or present thyroid disease.

The major signs of superior limbic keratoconjunctivitis include papillary hypertrophy of the superior tarsal conjunctiva (Fig. 5-52), sharply circumscribed hyperemia and thickening of the upper bulbar conjunctiva together with thickening and lucidity of the thickened superior limbal conjunctiva (Figs. 5-52 through 5-54), and fine superior epithelial keratitis. The papillae on the upper tarsal conjunctiva are small but numerous. This contrasts sharply with the normal-appearing inferior tarsal conjunctiva. The superior bulbar conjunctiva is hyperemic and thickened and may appear lusterless. The thickening and hyperemia extend from the upper limbus toward the insertion of the superior rectus muscle; the area of involvement is readily delineated with rose bengal stain and less readily shown with fluorescein. The superior limbic conjunctiva adjacent to the involved bulbar conjunctiva is also thickened and often appears lucid because of associated edema. The superior one-third of the corneal epithelium is involved as manifested by a fine or blotchy epithelial

staining of the cornea with fluorescein or rose bengal dye. A superior corneal micropannus is usually associated with the epithelial keratitis.

Multiple corneal and conjunctival filaments may be found on the superior cornea, the limbus, and the palpebral conjunctiva. The filaments are not a constant feature of the disease, but with prolonged observation of the same patient they are usually noted. The filaments are generally stubby. When the filament is removed, corneal staining is noted in the area where the filament was attached.

The natural course of the disease, although usually very prolonged, is gradual, complete clearing. During the course of the disease, short remissions occur, but then gradually the remissions persist for longer periods until the disease spontaneously disappears.

TREATMENT

Topical application of 0.5% or 1.0% silver nitrate to the upper tarsus generally results in relief of symptoms for 4 to 6 weeks. The silver nitrate is generally applied to the anesthetized upper tarsus, and the lid is then allowed to fall over the involved bulbar conjunctiva. Although the silver nitrate is neutralized by the chloride in the tears, the patient frequently notes earlier relief of the symptoms if the conjunctival sac is irrigated with sterile normal saline 1 minute after treatment.

In those instances in which the patient does not note relief of symptoms, silver nitrate can be reapplied after 5 days to 1 week. The silver nitrate can be reapplied to the conjunctiva at 4- to 6-week intervals indefinitely without untoward effects and usually with repeated amelioration of symptoms. Cryotherapy has also been noted to give temporary relief of symptoms, but it offers no advantage over silver nitrate.

Resection or recession of the involved bulbar conjunctiva generally gives immediate and permanent relief of symptoms. The bulbar conjunctiva and underlying Tenon's capsule are either recessed or excised along the limbus from ten to two o'clock extending back towards the superior rectus muscle for 5 to 8 mm. The conjunctiva need not be sutured to the underlying sclera at the point of excision. A dressing is usually applied to the eye for a few hours and the patient asked to return for observation after 1 to 2 days. By that time the patient usually notes marked improvement of symptoms. In rare instances, a recurrence of symptoms and signs occurs; this can again be treated by excision of the involved bulbar conjunctiva or the application of silver nitrate.

SUPERFICIAL PUNCTATE KERATITIS

The term *superficial punctate keratitis* was first coined by Ernst Fuchs [8] to describe the corneal changes that he observed during an epidemic of acute conjunctivitis. In retrospect, the acute keratoconjunctivitis that he observed was probably what we call epidemic keratoconjunctivitis (EKC). After his coining of the name, the term was and still is used to describe many diverse small, discrete lesions of the epithelium, Bowman's membrane, and anterior stroma. Thygeson [19] later used the name for a distinct entity, the morphologic features of which are quite distinctive and quite readily described by

the name superficial punctate keratitis. These features include multiple epithelial lesions limited to the corneal epithelium; a tendency for the lesions to involve the pupillary area preferentially, although they may be scattered throughout the cornea; discrete individual lesions that tend to be grouped into larger lesions; and no associated conjunctivitis.

This section is limited to a discussion of the entity described by Thygeson.

ETIOLOGY

Morphologically, the lesions of superficial punctate keratitis resemble the corneal lesions seen in measles and mumps during the convalescent stage of the infection. The morphologic similarity has led many to speculate that a virus may play a role in the etiology of the disease. In fact, Braley and Alexander [1] recovered a virus from superficial punctate keratitis, and later Lemp and associates [11] reported the isolation of a varicella (herpes zoster) virus from a patient with superficial punctate keratitis. In my studies, however, I have made repeated attempts to isolate a virus and have been unsuccessful. Moreover, serologic studies have not implicated a common virus in patients with superficial punctate keratitis, and epidemiologic studies have not shown a relationship to viral illnesses. The favorable response of the lesions to topical steroids also suggests that if the lesions are caused by a virus, they must at least in part represent an immunologic response to the virus and not just the infectious particle itself.

It appears that the duration of the disease in patients receiving topical steroids has increased, inasmuch as the duration was at first reported to be 2 to 4 years and now with the use of topical steroids for treatment the disease usually persists for much longer periods (10–15 years). This suggests that the topical steroids may have some adverse effect on the natural course of the disease such as one would expect if it were a "slow virus."

This etiology must be considered most likely.

Dyskeratosis has also been suggested as a possible cause of superficial punctate keratitis [25]. The lesions have something of the appearance of a dyskeratotic process. By definition, however, the term *dyskeratosis* means "an abnormal keratinization of epithelial cells," and histologic examination of the cells in superficial punctate keratitis reveals degeneration, not keratinization.

PATHOGENESIS

Since the cause is uncertain, one can only speculate on the pathogenesis of superficial punctate keratitis. Since the lesions have the same clinical picture as the keratitis often seen during the convalescent periods of viral infections such as measles and mumps, the most attractive theory remains that of a slow virus infection. Although we have been unable either by history or serology to determine a common viral denominator, we do know that in many slow virus infections such as verruca and molluscum contagiosum, it is frequently difficult to learn the source of the infection. In addition, in slow virus infections, the time between exposure to the agent and manifest clinical disease is so long that there is little hope of determining the source of the infection. Moreover, serologic studies are often unproductive in infections such as verruca and molluscum contagiosum.

The spontaneous healing of the lesions after 2 to 4 years when steroids have not been used is also compatible with a slow virus infection. In fact, most verruca and molluscum contagiosum nodules heal spontaneously within that time. In addition, the apparent prolongation of the disease by the use of topical steroids is consistent with the fact that immunosuppressive agents tend to prolong infections such as verruca and molluscum contagiosum.

If the disease is caused by a slow virus, the pathogenesis is similar to other diseases caused by slow viruses. The patient is exposed to the virus. In a healthy or, more likely, immunosuppressed host, the virus replicates within the epithelial cells of the cornea, gradually converting the cells' mechanisms to its own use. The viral infection stimulates the cells to divide, and the disease becomes clinically manifest after many months. When the lesions become manifest to the patient, they probably engender a nonspecific inflammatory reaction that causes loss of the grossly infected cells and subsidence of the lesions. Once the lesions subside, the entire process begins anew.

CLINICAL FEATURES
Superficial punctate keratitis has been reported from all parts of the world [13]. It affects the white, black, and Mongoloid races. The sexes are affected with about equal frequency, and all age groups (2½–85 years) may be involved, although patients in the second and third decades of life are most frequently affected.

At the commencement of this disease, patients note the insidious onset of symptoms of foreign-body sensation, photophobia, and tearing. In some instances, they may note a mild redness of the bulbar conjunctiva and blurring of vision. Rarely the symptoms may be so severe as to cause rhinorrhea. The symptoms persist and increase over a 1- to 2-week period and then gradually subside. During periods of remission, the patient is asymptomatic. Remissions tend to last 4 to 6 weeks, and then the symptoms begin anew. Remission and exacerbation occur for 2 to 4 years. The symptoms and signs are generally bilateral but may be more severe in one eye. In some instances, at the end or near the end of the course of the disease, one eye may become entirely asymptomatic while the symptoms persist and recur for a variable period in the other eye.

The disease is manifested by discrete white or gray dots located in the corneal epithelium. The dots tend to be located preferentially within the central epithelium. The dots are microscopic but tend to group into larger oval opacities that are arranged vertically. The larger grouped lesions are readily seen with the slit-lamp or on retroillumination with the retinoscope. The epithelium in areas between the lesions is entirely normal.

During exacerbations, the lesions become slightly elevated, and small punctate foci overlying the lesions stain with fluorescein. The number of lesions varies from one to over 20 at any one time. As the disease subsides and disappears, however, the number of lesions is often markedly reduced during exacerbations. During remissions, one or more or even all of the lesions may disappear completely, or they may merely flatten, becoming even with the surface of the cornea, and fail to stain. During an exacerbation, the lesions may recur in the same area or they may be noted in new areas of the corneal epithelium.

The lesions are entirely epithelial, although during exacerbations some mild edema of the underlying Bowman's membrane may be noted (Fig. 5-55). When IDU or other toxic drugs are used, however, Bowman's membrane underlying the lesions may be damaged, leaving a ghostlike image of the lesion that has been noted to persist for months and even several years after the disease has completely subsided.

The corneal sensation in most instances is normal, but in a few instances I have noted the sensation to be slightly reduced. Vascularization of the cornea is very unusual, but I have noted, in several instances, superficial neovascularization in areas where there have been recurrent lesions located close to the limbus.

Conjunctivitis does not occur at onset or during the course of the disease. In some instances, the patient may note mild circumcorneal hyperemia during exacerbations, however.

In almost all instances of superficial punctate keratitis in which corticosteroids are not used, the unaltered course of the disease has been that of remissions and exacerbations with eventual complete healing within 2 to 4 years [19, 20, 22]. In exacerbations, the symptoms generally begin insidiously, gradually increase in intensity over a 2-week period, and then slowly subside. The remissions generally last 4 to 6 weeks, followed by a new exacerbation. The duration of the exacerbations and remissions varies from patient to patient and also with the duration of the disease. In some instances, the exacerbation may persist for only a few days to be followed by a remission of several months. In other cases, the exacerbation may persist for several months to be followed by only a very short remission. As the disease normally subsides, the exacerbations become milder and shorter, and the remissions last longer and longer.

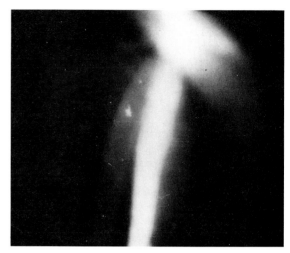

FIGURE 5-55. *Corneal lesions associated with superficial punctate keratitis.*

TREATMENT

Various treatments including removal of corneal epithelium, the use of antivirals such as IDU, soft contact lenses (continuous-wear), and topical steroids have been tried.

In cases in which I have removed the corneal epithelium for cultures, I have found that there appeared to be no effect on the course of the disease. The lesions recurred at approximately the same intervals as previously, often in the same place on the cornea.

IDU appears, if anything, to have a deleterious effect on the lesions. Without the use of IDU, I have seen only several patients who developed ghostlike lesions. Even in those patients who developed ghostlike images without a history of the use of IDU, the history usually indicated that the patient had used drops of an unknown type that may have been IDU.

In almost all cases, I have found that both signs and symptoms respond to topical steroids. I have found that most patients respond to very dilute steroids (e.g. dexamethasone 0.01%) used 1 to 3 times daily for 1 or 2 days. In a few patients, more concentrated steroids may be needed to bring on a remission, and in fact, in 1 patient I found that I had to use full-strength steroids (dexamethasone 0.1%) in a pulsed fashion for several hours to obtain resolution of symptoms. One should be aware, however, that steroids have many potential side effects. Cataracts and ocular hypertension have occurred in patients with superficial punctate keratitis receiving continuous steroid therapy. I have had 1 patient with superficial punctate keratitis develop herpex simplex keratitis resulting in corneal scarring and reduced central vision. In addition, since the introduction of the use of steroids, there seems to have been a change in the total duration of the disease, and even though one cannot state that there is a definite cause-and-effect relationship, one must certainly consider the possibility that the use of topical steroids may well prolong the course of a self-limited disease. Steroids may be used sparingly if at all and in as low a dose and as infrequently as possible to allow the patient to carry on his activities.

Although it is too early to tell what the final outcome will be with the use of soft contact lenses worn on a continuous basis for superficial punctate keratitis, certainly the patient frequently notes relief of symptoms. Therefore this may be a reasonable alternative to the use of topical steroids. The use of continuous-wear soft contact lenses has modified the picture of superficial punctate keratitis. Patients note quite rapid relief of symptoms of the superficial punctate keratitis once the contact lens is applied, but the corneal lesions appear to show little change. (I have had one interesting experience in which a patient was fitted with a continuous-wear contact lens in one eye and noted immediate and continuous relief of symptoms in both eyes. The lesions in the eye without the lens continued to go through the usual pattern of what I felt were exacerbations and remissions without the patient's experiencing symptoms.) What effect the wearing of continuous-wear soft contact lenses will have on the duration of the disease is not known.

NUMMULAR KERATITIS

The word *nummular* is taken from the Latin term *nummulus*, the diminutive of the word *nummus*, meaning "coin." The name distinctly describes the individual lesions characteristically found in nummular keratitis. Nummular keratitis is manifested by the gradual onset of corneal inflammation without associated conjunctivitis. The round, coinlike corneal lesions are quite distinctive and are usually not confused with other forms of keratitis except for the corneal involvement that occurs late in the course of EKC.

ETIOLOGY

The cause of nummular keratitis is unknown. The disease occurs most commonly in agricultural workers or those exposed to irrigation water. Dimmer's original description of the condition [5] and Pillat's more recent observations [12] suggested that initially the condition was limited to a rather narrow agricultural area in the middle of Europe. More recently, however, reports of a similar condition have come from areas such as China, Indochina, the Philippines, South Africa, and the United States [7, 12, 23].

Many authorities suspect that the condition is caused by a virus. In fact, Hofman claimed to have demonstrated inclusion bodies in the epithelial cells of scrapings taken from the cornea of a patient with nummular keratitis (reported in Duke-Elder [7]). He also claimed cultivation of the organism in the chorioallantoic membrane of embryonated hens' eggs and further fulfilled Koch's postulate by the experimental inoculation of the organism into a human, producing similar lesions of nummular keratitis. Unfortunately, no further characterization of the virus was reported.

Other suggested causes include water-borne bacteria such as leptospirae and brucellae and water-borne parasites such as *Hartmannella*; however, serologic studies for virus and water-borne organisms (except for parasites) that might be causal have been negative when performed at the Proctor Foundation. Moreover, cultures, both bacterial and viral, made from the conjunctival sac and the cornea have been unrevealing. It is true, however, that several weeks have usually elapsed between the onset of symptoms and the time that the patient is seen. Valenton's studies have also failed to demonstrate a viral or bacterial agent, although he also speculated that the causal agent is a virus [23].

PATHOGENESIS

Inasmuch as the cause of nummular keratitis is unknown, one can only speculate about the pathogenic mechanisms for the development of the signs and symptoms. The mechanism is probably similar to that postulated for the formation of disciform keratitis in herpes simplex infections of the corneal epithelium [10].

The causal agent (viral, bacterial, or parasitic) infects the corneal epithelium, probably after minor

trauma. The organism may be introduced into the eye at the time of the injury. The organism then replicates within the epithelial cells. During the replication phase and at the time of death of the infected epithelial cells and their loss from the cornea, the toxins or antigens produced by the agent, or the agent itself, are absorbed into the underlying stroma, where they incite a hypersensitivity reaction that results in the production of corneal stromal opacities as well as the symptoms of foreign-body sensation, irritation, and photophobia. The suggestion of a hypersensitivity reaction is substantiated by the favorable effects of topical corticosteroids in about two-thirds of patients with nummular keratitis as reported by Valenton [23]. The corneal opacities appear round and become grossly visible by virtue of the attraction of inflammatory cells to the focal areas where the antigen or organism is located. The resultant hypersensitivity reaction may result in necrosis of the corneal stroma. Neovascularization eventuates in those instances in which necrosis has occurred in lesions located in the peripheral cornea. Corneal facets occur because of contraction of scar tissue and thinning of the cornea, which in turn has resulted from necrosis.

In most cases of nummular keratitis, the clinician is able to obtain a history of exposure to irrigation water within a short period of time before onset of the symptoms and signs. Dimmer, for instance, reported his patients as being farmers working in a rather isolated farming area in Europe [5]. Westoff reported that the keratitis, which he called Sawah keratitis, or keratitis punctata tropica, occurred in epidemics among adult farmers who worked in rice fields (reported in Duke-Elder [7]). Valenton also found his cases occurred in patients who lived in rural areas and primarily in the rice-growing provinces near Manila [23].

In the majority of patients, the lesions are unilateral. The patient often gives a history of mild trauma to the eye or water getting into the eye. The patient frequently dates the onset of the symptoms from the time of trauma, with the time from trauma to onset varying between 1 and 35 days [23].

CLINICAL FEATURES

Patients with nummular keratitis generally complain of symptoms of a foreign-body sensation, photophobia, and blurring of vision. There is typically no history of conjunctivitis. The patient may also complain of white spots in the eye. The symptoms generally persist for 9 to 12 months, and although at onset they are only minimal, they may become more severe as the disease progresses.

The findings are generally limited to the cornea, although the patient may have mild to moderate circumcorneal injection [5]. Depending on the location of the opacities, the visual acuity may be normal or decreased.

Characteristically patients are noted to have multiple, small, round, white, grossly visible lesions within the cornea, which in Dimmer's original cases were located in the anterior stroma, but in later cases were found to be located at any level of the stroma (Fig. 5-56). The lesions are preferentially located centrally but not infrequently are located near the limbus. The number of epithelial opacities is variable but may be as high as 40 or 50 [23]. The nummular lesions measure 0.5 to 1.5 mm in diameter. In some instances, however, they may measure up to 3.0 mm in diameter, and if several lesions become confluent they may be even larger and irregular in shape. When observed with the aid of high magnification, the lesions are noted to be made up of small opacities that are grouped into larger lesions. The lesions are located in one plane of the corneal stroma like a disc. At onset, the epithelium overlying the area where the nummular opacities will appear is elevated and irregular and may take up stain [12]. After a few days, however, the epithelium becomes flattened and appears normal. Epithelial filaments are uncommon but have been reported [23]. The stroma underlying the involved epithelium develops a focal infiltrate surrounded by a halo of inflammatory cells. Eventually the halo disappears, and the nummular lesions are then sharply demarcated from the surrounding clear stroma [5]. As the individual lesions evolve, they may become compressed, giving them a faceted appearance. In rare instances, the central area of opacity may resorb, leaving an anular lesion [12]. In areas where the opacities are located close to the limbus, superficial and deep neovascularization of the cornea often occurs. Epithelial bullae may occur because of endothelial damage [7].

Over the next 1 to 2 years, the infiltrates that make up the disciform nummular lesion are resorbed and replaced by scar tissue, and the facets may become more marked. Over a period of 4 to 6 years, the scars are altered and may be recognized only as faint nebulae, and the facet tends to decrease, perhaps owing to a thickening of the corneal epithelium.

The corneal sensation is generally intact but rarely may be reduced. There is no associated conjunctivitis, and the anterior chamber is optically empty.

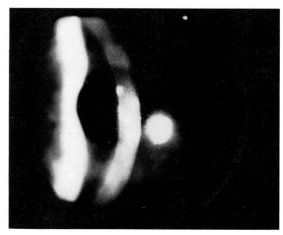

FIGURE 5-56. *Round coinlike lesions seen in nummular keratitis.*

The corneal lesions of nummular keratitis may be confused with those found in the late stages of EKC [12]. Clinicians can usually readily differentiate the two diseases, however, by obtaining a history of conjunctivitis in EKC. Moreover, there is no tendency for faceting or corneal neovascularization in EKC. In addition, the lesions of EKC tend to be more uniform and less dense than those seen in nummular keratitis [12].

Valenton called attention to the frequent association of disciform keratitis with the nummular lesions [23]. The finding of disciform keratitis makes differentiation of the condition from herpes simplex keratitis more difficult. In herpes simplex keratitis, however, the nummular lesions are noted at the time of resolution of the disciform keratitis and usually only when topical corticosteroids have been used. In addition, in herpes keratitis, corneal sensation is absent, and if the lesions are viewed with retroillumination they will be found to be associated with involvement of the intervening stroma.

Nummular lesions of the cornea may be seen in secondary varicella infections. The lesions tend to occur when the crusts overlying the skin lesions begin to disappear. The skin lesions are usually very destructive, however, which helps to differentiate secondary varicella from nummular keratitis.

Both acquired and prenatal syphilis may also cause areas of focal interstitial keratitis. These lesions are generally located in deep stroma, however, and look more like a round ball than a disc. An FTA-ABS test is invariably positive in such cases.

TREATMENT

Nummular keratitis is self-limited, and the symptoms associated with it resolve without treatment within 9 to 12 months. The corneal lesions themselves resolve after 6 to 8 years with a residue of faint nebulae, mild neovascularization, and only minimal decrease in vision.

Topical corticosteroids tend to relieve the symptoms in the majority of patients within 5 to 7 days. Although the topical corticosteroids reduce visual symptoms, they appear to have very little effect on the final visual outcome or the final appearance of the cornea. If topical corticosteroids are to be used, the clinician should attempt to use as low a dosage as possible (e.g., dexamethasone diluted 1 : 2 or 1 : 5) 3 to 4 times daily. If the symptoms are not relieved after 4 to 5 days, one can then increase the dosage. When symptoms are relieved, the clinician should attempt to titrate the level of the corticosteroids to the dosage that gives relief of symptoms, and periodically try to reduce the dosage further until the drug is finally stopped. Generally, treatment must be maintained for a period of 4 to 8 weeks to prevent recurrence of symptoms. The clinician should remember, however, that the final visual outcome is about the same whether topical corticosteroids are used or not.

In cases in which there are severe symptoms and the patient is very photophobic, dilation of the pupil using a mydriatic such as atropine 1% twice daily or cyclopentolate hydrochloride 1% 3 times daily may also be of value.

REFERENCES

1. Braley, A. E., and Alexander, R. C. Superficial punctate keratitis: Isolation of a virus. *A.M.A. Arch. Ophthalmol.* 50:147, 1953.
2. Cher, I. Clinical features of superior limbic keratoconjunctivitis in Australia. *Arch. Ophthalmol.* 82:580, 1969.
3. Collin, B., et al. The fine structure of nuclear changes in superior limbic keratoconjunctivitis. *Invest. Ophthalmol. Vis. Sci.* 17:79, 1978.
4. Corwin, M. E. Superior limbic keratoconjunctivitis. *Am. J. Ophthalmol.* 66:338, 1968.
5. Dimmer, F. A type of cornea inflammation closely related to keratitis nummularis. *Z. Augenheilkunde* 13:621, 1905.
6. Donshik, P. C., et al. Conjunctival resection treatment and ultrastructural histopathology of superior limbic keratoconjunctivitis. *Am. J. Ophthalmol.* 85:101, 1978.
7. Duke-Elder, S., and Leigh, A. G. Diseases of the Outer Eyes. In S. Duke-Elder (Ed.), *System of Ophthalmology.* Vol. 8, Part 2. London: Kimpton, 1965. Pp. 746–751.
8. Fuchs, E. Keratitis punctata superficialis. *Wien. Klin. Wochenschr.* 2:837, 1889.
9. Grayson, M. *Diseases of the Cornea.* St. Louis: Mosby, 1979. Pp. 79–81.
10. Jones, B. R. The clinical features of viral keratitis and a concept of their pathogenesis. *Proc. R. Soc. Med.* 51:13, 1957.
11. Lemp, M. A., Chambers, R. W., Jr., and Lurdy, J. Viral isolation in superficial punctate keratitis. *Arch. Ophthalmol.* 91:8, 1974.
12. Pillat, A. The differential diagnosis of nummular keratitis (Dimmer) and epidemic keratoconjunctivitis. *Am. J. Ophthalmol.* 43:58, 1957.
13. Qusi, M., Diallo, J., and Rogez, J. P. Thygeson's superficial punctate keratitis. *Arch. Ophtalmol. (Paris)* 28:497, 1968.
14. Tenzel, R. R. Comments on superior limbic filamentous keratitis: Part 2 (letter to the editor). *Arch. Ophthalmol.* 79:508, 1968.
15. Theodore, F. H. In discussion of paper by P. Thygeson, and S. J. Kimura, Chronic conjunctivitis. *Trans. Am. Acad. Ophthalmol. Otolaryngol.* 67:514, 1963.
16. Theodore, F. H. Superior limbic keratoconjunctivitis. *Eye Ear Nose Throat Mon.* 42:25, 1963.
17. Theodore, F. H. Superior limbic keratoconjunctivitis: Further studies. Proceedings of the 21st International Congress of Ophthalmology, Mexico, 1970. Pp. 556–669.
18. Theodore, F. H., and Ferry, A. P. Superior limbic keratoconjunctivitis. Clinical and pathological correlation. *Arch. Ophthalmol.* 84:481, 1970.
19. Thygeson, P. Superficial punctate keratitis. *JAMA* 144:1544, 1960.
20. Thygeson, P. Further observations on superficial punctate keratitis. *Arch. Ophthalmol.* 66:158, 1961.
21. Thygeson, P., and Kimura, S. J. Chronic conjunctivitis. *Trans. Am. Acad. Ophthalmol. Otolaryngol.* 67:494, 1963.
22. Thygeson, P. Clinical and laboratory observation on superficial punctate keratitis. *Am. J. Ophthalmol.* 61:1344, 1966.
23. Valenton, M. J. Deep stromal involvement in Dimmer's nummular keratitis. *Am. J. Ophthalmol.* 78:897, 1974.
24. Wander, A. H., and Musukawa, T. Unusual appearance of condensed chromatin in conjunctival cells in superior limbic keratoconjunctivitis. *Lancet* 2:42, 1981.
25. Williams, H. P. Thygeson's Superficial Punctate Keratitis. In F. T. Fraundfelder and F. H. Roy (Eds.), *Current Ocular Therapy.* Philadelphia: Saunders, 1980. Pp. 388–389.
26. Wright, P. Superior limbic keratoconjunctivitis. *Trans. Ophthalmol. Soc. U.K.* 92:555, 1972.

6. IMMUNOLOGIC DISEASES

Ocular Allergies

Mathea R. Allansmith and Mark B. Abelson

DEFINITION OF ATOPY

In 1923, Coca [14] used the word *atopy* (*a* means without, *topos* means place) to indicate a "strange reactivity" in persons with hereditary backgrounds of allergic disease who showed immediate wheal-and-flare skin reactivity to skin-sensitizing antibody (now called IgE) and IgE in their blood that could be transferred to the skin of a normal subject [32]. Unlike other immunoglobulins, which do not attach to skin components, the specific IgE antibodies of atopic patients attach to skin and mast cells or basophils of normal persons. One or two days after the injection of serum IgE into the skin, when the appropriate sensitizing allergen (an antigen causing an IgE response) is injected into the same site, a wheal and flare appear immediately (Prausnitz-Küstner reaction [32]).

The major atopies are seasonal rhinitis (hay fever), perennial rhinitis, bronchial asthma, and atopic dermatitis. The minor atopies include food allergies, urticaria, and nonhereditary angioedema. Atopy can occur in other animal species besides humans [12, 31].

INCIDENCE, HEREDITY, AND ONSET OF ATOPY

Approximately 15 percent of the population show the allergic manifestations described above. Males appear to be more commonly afflicted than females. The disease occurs in families, and histocompatibility (HLA) associations are important in the expression of the disease. Those homozygous for the allergy gene tend to develop allergic disease earlier than do those heterozygous for this gene [35]. Most persons heterozygous for the allergy gene do not develop atopic disease but may transmit the allergy gene to their children [41]. Early onset of disease is associated with severe, long-lasting disease. On the average, three-fourths of asthmatic and hay fever patients have family histories of atopy. Hay fever, asthma, vasomotor rhinitis, and atopic dermatitis are all genetically related.

OCULAR ALLERGIC DISORDERS

HAY FEVER REACTIONS

Hay fever conjunctivitis is a recurrent disease associated with airborne substances such as pollen from grasses and weeds, molds, dust, and danders and characterized by itching, redness, and swelling of the lids and conjunctiva.

SYMPTOMS

The patient complains of mild and occasionally moderate itching. Tearing, burning, and a feeling described as pressure behind or in the eyes may be present. These symptoms wax and wane throughout the year, because in the early spring trees cast their pollen into the winds, in May or June the grasses reach the height of discharge of their pollen, and, after a short respite in the middle of the summer, ragweed (in the eastern portion of the United States) sheds its pollen. At times the symptoms may disappear entirely. If there are corneal dellen, pain, photophobia, and blurred vision may occur.

SIGNS

There may be no clinically observable signs. A patient may complain of itching, hot, tearing eyes and yet the adnexal tissue may appear entirely normal. Research has confirmed that eyes of rats in a model of topical hay fever may appear normal although degranulation of mast cells [8] or microscopic increase in interstitial edema may be present. How to diagnose and differentiate hay fever conjunctivitis from other disease entities (i.e., irritation from air pollutants) in the absence of clinical signs is an unsolved problem.

Most patients have some edema of their conjunctiva, dilation of the ciliary and other conjunctival vessels, or minor swelling of the lids (Fig. 6-1). The edema may occasionally result in pallor of the palpebral conjunctiva. The exudative material is clear or white if the ocular reaction is acute and mucopurulent, thicker, and even stringy if the reaction is chronic. A papillary reaction may occur, but no giant papillae and no opacification of the collagen are apparent. The limbus and cornea are usually normal, but corneal dellen have been seen associated with marked conjunctival chemosis. Corneal edema has been reported as a rare and transient condition accompanying attacks of urticaria or an-

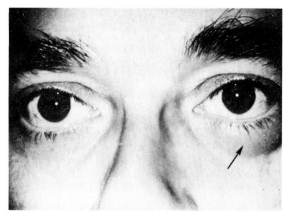

FIGURE 6-1. *Edematous lid* (arrow) *characteristic of hay fever conjunctivitis. (From M. H. Friedlaender and M. R. Allansmith, Ocular allergy.* Ann. Ophthalmol. 7:1171, 1975.)

gioedema but has not been seen in hay fever conjunctivitis per se.

An occasional patient will have an allergen to which they are allergic, such as animal dander, enter directly into the eye. Marked swelling of the lid and conjunctiva will occur. This degree of swelling exceeds that seen in the usual cases of hay fever conjunctivitis.

PATHOGENESIS

There is good evidence that the mechanism by which hay fever conjunctivitis occurs is a type I hypersensitivity response [19]. If serum from an allergic person is transferred to the conjunctiva of a normal person, the normal person responds with an ocular hay-fever-like syndrome on later instillation of the relevant antigen [34]. The immediate swelling, itching, and edema of the conjunctiva in reaction to the instillation of pollen is equivalent to hives of the skin, which are a type I reaction.

The conjunctiva and nasal mucosa are exposed to airborne allergens. These allergens interact with tissue mast cells via the IgE molecules that are tightly bound to the surface of the mast cell.

Mucosal mast cells appear to differ from connective tissue mast cells in that they contain intracytoplasmic IgE as well as the surface IgE that serves as a trigger for mast cell degranulation. It has been assumed that mast cells are armed in situ by IgE from the peripheral blood circulation, and the level of IgE in the blood has been shown to be directly related to the degree of sensitization. Recent work seems to indicate, however, that in the case of allergen challenge at a mucosal surface IgE production appears to occur almost exclusively in the regional lymph nodes [20]. It has been hypothesized that mast cell precursors migrate from the mucosal surface (conjunctiva) to the regional lymph nodes, pick up the IgE as they mature to mast cells, and then home back to the mucosal surface and remain fixed in that site.

The binding of allergen to the IgE–mast cell complex initiates a change in the IgE molecule at its Fc portion, which is the portion of the molecule bound at the mast cell membrane. (See Chapter 3, Immunology, for more details.) This membrane event activates a serine esterase, which in turn causes an intracellular biochemical cascade that results in the release of pharmacologically active mediators. The mediators released include histamine, slow-reacting substance of anaphylaxis (SRS-A or leukotrienes), eosinophil chemotactic factor of anaphylaxis, platelet activating factor, and heparin. These mediators cause vasodilation and an increase in vascular permeability leading to itching, edema, and redness, the hallmarks of hay fever ocular disease.

The mediator released from mast cells and basophils is directly influenced by the levels of adenosine 3',5'-cyclic monophosphate (cAMP) in these cells (elevated levels of cAMP inhibit release) and by the levels of guanosine 3',5'-cyclic monophosphate (cGMP) (elevated levels of cGMP enhance release). Prostaglandins act through membrane-bound adenyl cyclase to increase levels of cAMP. Stimulation of the beta-adrenergic receptor also increases the levels of cAMP. Stimulation of the alpha-adrenergic receptor can reduce the level of cAMP [40]. Phosphodiesterase breaks down cAMP to 5'-adenylic acid. Inhibitors of this action, e.g., aminophylline, theophylline, and caffeine, can elevate the levels of cAMP. The cholinergic receptor, which can be stimulated by acetylcholine or carbachol, leads to elevated levels of cGMP and mediator release. Atropine can block this stimulation. By elevating the level of cAMP or reducing the level of cGMP, the symptoms of allergy caused by the mediators can be alleviated.

Histamine, which stimulates muscle contraction in target tissues through its interaction with specific H-1 receptors, also interacts with H-2 receptors on the surface of reacting target cells. This latter interaction leads to an increase in intracellular cAMP and thus to inhibition of mediator release [27]. This histamine and H-2 receptor interaction is thus the first level of feedback inhibition. H-1 and H-2 receptors are present in the external ocular tissues. Drugs that compete with or block histamine interaction with H-1 or H-2 receptor sites alleviate different symptoms. It would appear from early work [2] that stimulation of the H-1 receptor may be responsible for itching and stimulation of the H-2 receptor the redness.

At the second level of feedback inhibition, eosinophils move into the target area, become immobilized, and accumulate. The eosinophils contain substances that elevate cAMP, inactivate SRS-A and platelet activating factor, and inhibit histamine release [23].

DIAGNOSIS

Seasonal itching, burning, and tearing eyes in a patient with a family or personal history of atopy is helpful in making the diagnosis of hay fever conjunctivitis. Clinical appearance (see above), special tests, and response to the appropriate therapy can help confirm the diagnosis.

These patients have positive reactions to pollens on skin test, but this procedure is generally not performed in the ophthalmologist's office. The skin test is performed as follows: A small amount of the suspected allergen (usually diluted) is applied to a cutaneous scratch or injected intradermally. The rapid appearance, within seconds or minutes, of a wheal and flare indicates a positive reaction. Topical instillation of allergenic substances into the conjunctival sac has also been used diagnostically. A positive response is the nearly immediate onset of swelling and hyperemia of the conjunctiva and itching. These tests may not be innocuous and may indeed be fatal.

Brauninger and Centifanto reported that the tear IgE levels were elevated in 2 of 4 hay fever patients [13]. Tear histamine levels in humans with ocular hay fever were not elevated in the few determinations performed by one of us (M.R.A.). Biopsies have been performed on a few patients with ocular hay fever, and mast cells and eosinophils were not found in the epithelium. A comprehensive study of the light and electron microscopic changes in ocular hay fever conjunctivitis has not been performed.

Since it requires time for eosinophils to enter the tear film and conjunctival epithelium, they may not be present in acute ocular allergic states. When the allergic condition becomes chronic, eosinophils may be noted.

A rapid response to appropriate therapy may be useful in making a correct diagnosis. Epinephrine applied locally or intensive corticosteroid therapy locally often rapidly ameliorates the signs and symptoms of hay fever conjunctivitis. Local and systemic antihistamines require more time to alter the course of the disease.

DIFFERENTIAL DIAGNOSIS

Acute inflammation caused by toxic or irritating substances may result in conjunctival and lid edema and hyperemia, a watery discharge, and a burning sensation. There is no itching, however. The conjunctival response may be follicular, and no eosinophils are found in the conjunctival scraping. Serum and tear IgE and serum eosinophil levels are normal.

A foreign body under the upper lid may cause acute chemosis and hyperemia of the bulbar conjunctiva, lid edema, a watery discharge, and a burning or foreign-body sensation, depending upon the consistency, size, and placement (central placement will more severely involve the cornea) of the foreign body. Linear vertical scratches may be present on the cornea of these patients.

Contact dermatitis of the lids may produce some lid edema, hyperemia, and itching. This process is a cell-mediated reaction, and no alterations of IgE or eosinophil levels are to be expected.

Mild keratitis sicca may result in redness of the bulbar conjunctiva in the palpebral fissure and a burning sensation. Punctate keratopathy in the palpebral fissure area, corneal filaments, and decreased tear flow help differentiate this entity from hay fever conjunctivitis.

TREATMENT
When feasible, an effort should be made to remove the patient from the offending allergen, and if this is logistically impossible, it may be possible to limit exposure to it.

Vasoconstricting agents such as naphazoline hydrochloride 0.05% or 0.10% may be helpful in mild cases. The addition of an antihistamine that competes with histamine for the H-1 receptor site may be helpful. Antazoline phosphate 0.5% is effective topically, and preparations containing this agent and naphazoline are readily available. Disodium cromoglycate has been used in a 2% solution topically. The drops are applied four times a day [35].

The use of systemic or subconjunctival corticosteroids is not warranted in the hay fever type of ocular allergy, but topical corticosteroids may be indicated when the above forms of therapy are ineffective. Low antiinflammatory doses may be very effective. Prednisolone 0.12% bid or tid employed over a short period of time is associated with few complications. High doses of corticosteroids (prednisolone 1% every 2 hours) are immunosuppressive as well as antiinflammatory and are very effective in severe hay fever conjunctivitis.

ATOPIC KERATOCONJUNCTIVITIS
Approximately 3 percent of the population has atopic dermatitis, and some of these persons have ocular manifestations of atopy (atopic keratoconjunctivitis, or AKC). In Hogan's series [22], the patients were men between the ages of 29 and 47. Most had had atopic dermatitis as children. AKC appears in the late teen years and lasts for many years. Most cases improve or "burn out" by the fourth or fifth decade of life.

SYMPTOMS
The symptoms of AKC are usually present all year long, there being minimal association with hot weather. AKC is invariably bilateral. The symptoms include itching, burning, and tearing with a watery to mucopurulent thick, ropy, white discharge. Itching, the most prominent feature, varies from moderate to severe.

SIGNS
The lid margins may be indurated and lichenified (Fig. 6-2). The conjunctiva may be pale and have papillary hypertrophy, most prominently on the inferior palpebral conjunctiva. Conjunctival scarring and shrinkage of the fornix may occur (principally inferiorly). Hyperemia of the palpebral and bulbar conjunctiva may also be present. Limbal abnormalities include gelatinous infiltration, thick opacification (usually superior), Horner's points (Trantas' dots), and true cysts [22]. The corneal changes include pannus, ulceration, scarring, keratoconus, pseudogerontotoxon, and punctate epithelial keratitis. The ulcer tends to be horizontally oval, shallow, and have irregular edges.

In 10 percent of atopic dermatitis cases, cataracts develop [10]. These are usually seen in the most severe forms of the disease. The opacity may be the anterior subcapsular (shieldlike) type or the posterior polar complicated type. Almost 90 percent of the cataracts accompanying AKC are bilateral. They first appear in the teenage years and either progress slowly or mature in a few months. Cataracts developed in atopic dermatitis patients before the introduction of corticosteroids, but there is little doubt that corticosteroids have increased their incidence and severity [35].

PATHOGENESIS
The cause of AKC is not known. Its clinical and histologic appearance (cellular infiltration with mast cells, basophils, eosinophils, and possibly lymphocytes) is quite different from that of ocular hay fever, and thus other forms of hypersensitivity, in addition to the anaphylactic type, are implicated. The cutaneous basophilic hypersensitivity response (nonclassical type of cell-mediated immune response) may play a major role in AKC and vernal keratoconjunctivitis (VKC).

Serum IgE is elevated in atopic conjunctivitis [37];

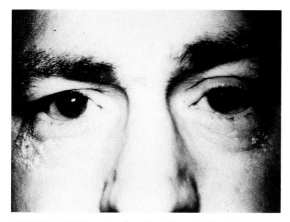

FIGURE 6-2. *Thickened and scaling lids and skin of atopic conjunctivitis. (From M. H. Friedlaender and M. R. Allansmith, The eye in immunologic disease.* Compr. Ther. *2:51, 1976.)*

however, the level may decrease when there is a remission [24]. The numbers of circulating peripheral lymphocytes bearing IgE have been shown to be normal in AKC patients, even though serum IgE is elevated [37]. However, the number of peripheral blood lymphocytes bearing complement has been shown to be increased [30]. In most cases, the serum levels of IgA, IgM, and IgD are normal.

Cellular immune mechanisms are usually deficient in atopic patients. McGeady and Buckley [30] have found that cutaneous type IV delayed hypersensitivity responses to *Candida* and streptokinase-streptodornase antigens may be depressed. Inability to become sensitized to topical dinitrochlorobenzene may also occur [30]. Rachelefsky and colleagues [33] found defective T cell function in patients with atopic dermatitis. These patients' mitogenic T cell response to phytohemagglutinin was found to be significantly depressed. The percentages of peripheral blood T cells were significantly lower in atopic patients than in normal controls. In addition, they found an increase in B cells and eosinophils in the circulating blood. It has been postulated that because of suppressed cell-mediated immune function, these atopic patients are more susceptible to certain fungal and viral diseases [28]. Ocular staphylococcal and herpetic infections are more common than in the nonatopic population.

Important regulators of IgE synthesis have been shown to be T cells. It has been suggested that helper T and suppressor T cells may be responsible for failure to arrest IgE responses. The helper T cell affects the initiation of IgE production, and the suppressor T cell regulates its production. The IgE molecule causes mast cell degranulation and histamine release. Therefore an excess of IgE antibody may cause continual release of histamine and other

mediators, which results in the clinical manifestations of atopic disease.

DIAGNOSIS
The typical clinical picture, a family and personal history of atopy, and the appropriate laboratory test responses help the clinician in diagnosing AKC. Conjunctival scrapings contain eosinophils and some mononuclear cells. Serum and tear IgE levels may be elevated.

DIFFERENTIAL DIAGNOSIS
AKC may be confused with VKC since both entities are probably IgE-mediated, chronic type I and type IV hypersensitivity reactions. Both are associated with itching, local and systemic eosinophilia, possible elevated tear IgE, a personal or family history of atopy, and similar clinical findings. Differentiating points do exist, however. Conjunctival scarring and shrinkage of the fornix occur only in AKC; deep corneal vessels appear more commonly in AKC; AKC affects the lower palpebral conjunctiva principally, whereas VKC mainly affects the upper; AKC is not as seasonal (hot-weather-related) as VKC and may be severe in the winter; AKC lasts longer than VKC and occurs in an older population (teenage years up to fifth decade); AKC patients have fewer eosinophils on their conjunctival scrapings and rarely show free eosinophilic granules; and AKC patients may have atopic dermatitis of their lids.

TREATMENT
Vasoconstrictors and antihistamines applied topically may be beneficial. Systemically administered antihistamines may also ameliorate the symptoms. Disodium cromoglycate 2% applied qid topically may be quite beneficial alone or in combination with other medications (e.g., corticosteroids). Lowering the elevated tear pH with saline irrigation results in some relief of symptoms as does the use of mucolytic agents (e.g. 10% acetylcysteine drops) when a thick, ropy discharge is evident.

The topical use of corticosteroid solutions brings dramatic relief of symptoms. The drops should be used in as low a dose and for as short a time as possible since long-term corticosteroid therapy is fraught with many unacceptable complications such as cataracts, glaucoma, and the enhancement of infections. These patients are more susceptible to infections [9].

Since suppressor T cell deficiency may cause atopic disease, trials with agents that enhance T cell response have been carried out in severe cases of atopy. Transfer factor [16, 38] and levamisole hydrochloride have also been so employed. Results with these latter agents, while still inconclusive, seem to demonstrate a beneficial effect.

VERNAL KERATOCONJUNCTIVITIS

VKC is a seasonally recurrent, bilateral inflammation of the conjunctiva, characterized by giant papillae on the upper tarsal conjunctiva (Fig. 6-3). The distribution of VKC is worldwide although it occurs more frequently in warm climates such as Italy, Greece, Israel, and parts of South America [11]. It is a disease of youth, rarely appearing in patients younger than 3 or older than 25 years of age. Eighty percent of those who develop VKC are less than 14 years of age. In all series, more boys than girls have the disease; the ratio is about 2 : 1. Two-thirds of patients have a family history of atopic allergies. These diseases are present in approximately three-fourths of the patients themselves. VKC lasts an average of 4 to 10 years, the maximum range being 1 to 20 years. The disease is at its worst in the spring and summer in the northern hemisphere; hence the name *vernal* (spring). Many patients have their symptoms year round, with an intensification of the symptoms in the spring.

SYMPTOMS

Itching is the most constant feature. It may be said: no itching, no vernal. The itching can be intense and persistent and precede all tissue changes. It worsens toward evening and may be aggravated by exposure to dust, wind, or bright lights or by physical exertion. Rubbing the involved area can increase the itching.

Tearing may be a problem. Clear tears seep out from the corner of the eye to macerate the skin.

Irritation is a word frequently used by patients to describe the hot, tight, sensitive feeling of the eyes. Photophobia may be marked and indicate that the cornea is involved. The child with VKC may appear in the office with head lowered, sunglasses on, eyes closed, and be almost impossible to examine because of the severe ocular discomfort.

SIGNS

The discharge is characteristic. Several times a day the patient may have to pull a ropy, thick strand of dirty yellow or whitish material from the lids. Accumulation of a similar material at the inner canthus is found in the morning. The lids do not stick together in the morning or become crusted unless a secondary bacterial infection is present.

Two forms of vernal conjunctivitis, palpebral (Fig.

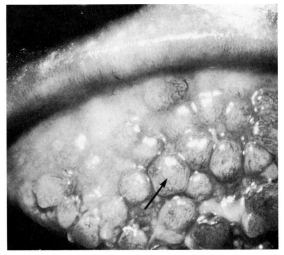

FIGURE 6-3. *Giant papillary excrescenses* (arrow) *resembling cobblestones on the upper palpebral conjunctiva in vernal conjunctivitis. (From M. R. Allansmith, Vernal Conjunctivitis. In T. D. Duane [Ed.], Clinical Ophthalmology. New York: Harper & Row, 1976.)*

6-3) and limbal (Fig. 6-4), usually occur together, although one may predominate. It is not known why the degree to which each area is affected varies. The palpebral form affects the tarsal conjunctiva of the upper lid. In patients with lower lid involvement, the upper lid is also involved and more extensively. The conjunctiva of the upper lid may show only mild papillary hypertrophy. Even in this stage, many eosinophils are present in a conjunctival scraping. Hard, elevated papillae of various sizes develop. They may be discrete or clumped. The most affected area is the superior border of the tarsal plate. Sometimes erythematous, sometimes pale, the papillae crowd together as they develop. They are flat-topped, presumably because of the pressure of the tarsal conjunctiva on the cornea. Eventually they may resemble a mosaic of flat-topped cobblestones (giant papillae). The weight of these may produce a mechanical ptosis of several millimeters.

A milky coating lies over the giant papillae. If a cotton applicator is gently drawn over the surface of the conjunctiva, a stringy material is removed. This fibrin accumulation is enhanced by heat (e.g., examination of the upper tarsal conjunctiva at the biomicroscope may cause formation of this fibrin pseudomembrane [Maxwell-Lyons sign]).

The limbal form of VKC is marked by a thickened, broad, gelatinous opacification of the upper limbus. Occasionally this limbal papilla will extend 360 degrees around the cornea. Its corneal edge is sharp, but the conjunctival edge blends gradually with the

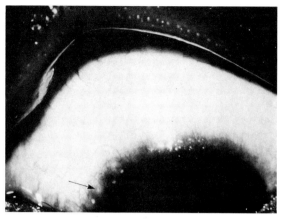

FIGURE 6-4. *Trantas' dots* (arrow) *and papillary hypertrophy of the limbal conjunctiva in vernal conjunctivitis. (From M. R. Allansmith, Vernal Conjunctivitis. In T. D. Duane [Ed.],* Clinical Ophthalmology. *New York: Harper & Row, 1976.)*

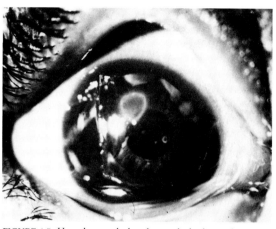

FIGURE 6-5. *Vernal corneal ulcer from palpebral vernal conjunctivitis in a 9-year-old boy. (From M. R. Allansmith, Vernal Conjunctivitis. In T. D. Duane [Ed.],* Clinical Ophthalmology. *New York: Harper & Row, 1976.)*

normal tissue. The color of this opacification may vary from grayish white to pink depending upon the degree of vascularization. Within the raised masses at the limbus, whitish chalklike excrescences may be seen (Horner's points or Trantas' dots) (Fig. 6-4). Composed of concretions of eosinophils, these excrescences may be evanescent, may appear at any stage of the disease, and may be present on the bulbar or palpebral conjunctiva as well. Cysts and minute marginal pits occur. The cysts are ovoid, closely packed in some areas, contain clear, colorless fluid, and appear elevated. They are true cysts. The marginal pits appear as transparent, round to oval glassy spots 1 to 5 mm in diameter on the opaque limbus. They are confined to the superior limbus. They represent areas in which the limbal infiltrate has almost returned to normal. They are not to be confused with the Herbert's peripheral pits of trachoma, which are larger and permanent.

Corneal findings are common and are the cause of the most distressing symptoms in this disease. There may be epithelial keratitis with punctate stippling [17]. The corneal epithelium may contain minute, dull, grayish points that look like flour dusting. The upper part of the cornea is mainly affected, and there is a relative sparing of the periphery. This syncytial pattern has been adequately described [25, 39]. These gray points remain discrete and stain irregularly with fluorescein. Small intraepithelial cysts may be seen.

The vernal ulcer (Fig. 6-5) is, fortunately, a rarer manifestation than the epithelial lesions. The ulcer characteristically is transversely oval and centrally placed in the superior part of the cornea. It is shallow and smooth and usually does not become vas-

cularized. Shaggy grayish white dead epithelium is seen at the edges of the ulcer. The underlying Bowman's layer is slightly grayish, and the superficial stroma shows varying degrees of cellular infiltration. The ulcer is indolent, does not tend to spread, and may persist for weeks. Occasionally, vernal ulcers lead to corneal scarring, plaque formation, or both. The gray-white plaque heals slowly, leaving an oval gray zone in Bowman's layer. The corneal ulcer and plaque seem to occur mainly in the very young.

The most common degenerative change in the cornea is the pseudogerontotoxon. It is an arclike or anular opacity, separated from the limbus by a narrow lucid zone, thereby resembling an arcus senilis. The opacity is yellowish gray. A change in corneal curvature also occurs. There is a steepening of the cornea, resulting in myopic astigmatism and, late in the disease, possibly keratoconus.

PATHOGENESIS
Because of the highly seasonal incidence, the allergens responsible for this disease are most probably the airborne pollens of grass and weeds. Type I hypersensitivity probably plays a role in VKC, but other mechanisms must be implicated in this disease because of the accumulation of certain cells in the upper tarsal conjunctival tissue. Histopathologic study of VKC [7] shows tremendous proliferation of collagen, mast cells in the epithelium, eosinophils and basophils in the epithelium and substantia propria, and lymphocytes in the substantia propria (Fig. 6-6). In addition, by electron microscopy it can

be seen that most of the mast cells are "phantom" mast cells in that they are so depleted of their granules that they would not be recognized as mast cells by light microscopy. Therefore, although the light microscopy counts of mast cells per cubic millimeter can be only slightly above the counts in normals, if one takes into account the enormous number of phantom mast cells, it can be seen that the number of mast cells in VKC is greatly increased over normal counts. The presence of basophils suggest that cutaneous basophil hypersensitivity may, along with type I hypersensitivity, play a role in VKC.

DIAGNOSIS

The typical clinical picture, a family and personal history of atopy, and the appropriate laboratory test results help the physician in diagnosing VKC.

A scraping of the upper tarsal conjunctiva easily reveals eosinophils. More than two eosinophils per high-power field is pathognomonic of vernal conjunctivitis, and this finding reflects the high tissue eosinophilia.

Tear histamine is 4 times normal in VKC [1], whereas it is not elevated in hay fever conjunctivitis (only a few samples were tested) or in contact lens–associated giant papillary conjunctivitis (see below). This again indicates that VKC has mechanisms that sustain the recruitment of eosinophils and the recruitment or cloning of mast cells at a much higher rate than that seen in hay fever conjunctivitis.

DIFFERENTIAL DIAGNOSIS

The differential diagnosis of VKC and AKC was discussed in the previous section.

TREATMENT

The best form of therapy is the elimination of the allergen or a means of decreasing its effect. Moving from a warm climate to a cooler one often is accompanied by a relief from symptoms and a diminution of the signs. In hay fever conjunctivitis, hyposensitization relieves approximately 80 percent of the symptoms 80 percent of the time. Patients with multiple major atopic disease plus VKC seem to receive more benefit from general allergy care and hyposensitization injections of allergens than do those in whom VKC is the only major problem.

Helpful topical therapy may include cold compresses for 10 minutes several times a day. Topical astringents with or without antihistamine provide considerable relief, and several types should be tried. For the mild case not helped by astringents or

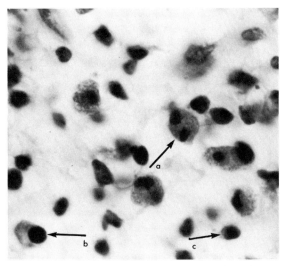

FIGURE 6-6. *Eosinophils* (a), *plasma cells* (b), *and lymphocytes* (c) *found in an 8-year-old boy with vernal conjunctivitis. (From M. R. Allansmith, Vernal Conjunctivitis. In T. D. Duane [Ed.],* Clinical Ophthalmology. *New York: Harper & Row, 1976.)*

antihistamines, a mild antiinflammatory agent (e.g., medrysone) may be tried. These medications may be all that a patient with mild VKC needs. For patients with severer disease, these topical medications are helpful between doses of steroids. Oral antihistamines may be given at bedtime as an adjunct to these therapies.

Disodium cromoglycate has been evaluated in the treatment of VKC in a placebo-controlled clinical trial at Moorfield's Eye Hospital [18]. Applied as a 2% topical solution 4 times a day, it was an effective adjunct to local steroid therapy. Frequently, the corticosteroid therapy could be diminished or even halted. Disodium cromoglycate prevents mast cell degranulation induced by antigen-antibody reactions [15] and thus requires several weeks to produce beneficial clinical results. This drug seems to be effective in assisting in the healing of a corneal ulcer or plaque. In view of the great number of mast cells in the epithelium in VKC, the use of disodium cromoglycate seems theoretically indicated.

Unquestionably, corticosteroids give the sufferer more relief from symptoms than does any other form of therapy, but their complications (glaucoma, cataract formation, infection, and the aggravation of corneal ulcers) are more likely to occur in VKC than in other diseases because of the months or years that treatment may be needed. Once patients have experienced the relief that steroids provide, they wish to continue them; therefore, control must be exercised by the ophthalmologist. Diminution of symptoms, not complete relief, should be sought;

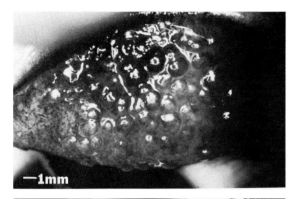

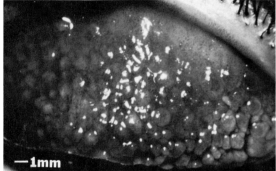

FIGURE 6-7. *Giant papillae in a 23-year-old hard lens wearer (top) and in a 10-year-old boy with vernal conjunctivitis (bottom). (From M. R. Allansmith et al. [3].)*

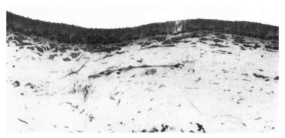

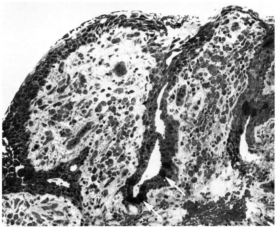

FIGURE 6-8. *Normal conjunctiva (top) (×780) compared with giant papillae from a soft lens wearer (bottom) (×640). Goblet cells are visible (arrows) at the base of papillae. (From M. R. Allansmith et al. [3].)*

patients should be encouraged to tolerate mild discomfort or to depend on less dangerous forms of topical therapy. The use of systemic steroids for 1 or 2 weeks several times a year may provide satisfactory relief in severe cases. At no time should a patient be assigned to long-term use of steroids on a maintenance basis.

For severely affected patients, we have found a pulse of corticosteroid therapy to be successful. This is given as 1 drop of topical prednisolone 1% or dexamethasone 0.1% every 2 hours during the day for 4 days. The symptoms are usually sufficiently suppressed to allow for their control by other forms of therapy for many weeks. When the symptoms again become intolerable, another pulse of steroid may be given. Thus, only one to three courses of steroids may have to be given yearly.

GIANT PAPILLARY CONJUNCTIVITIS IN CONTACT LENS WEARERS

Giant papillary conjunctivitis (GPC) was initially defined as a papillary reaction of the tarsal conjunctiva of the upper lid (Fig. 6-7) in which the papillae reach a diameter of 1 mm or more, are elevated (Fig. 6-8), and are associated with symptoms of mucus or itching or both. But further work showed that papillae over ⅓ mm are abnormal [26].

Although recent work has been concerned with contact lens–associated GPC [3], other agents besides contact lenses have been reported to cause GPC-type reactions. Srinivasan and associates [36] have reported 7 cases of GPC associated with polymethylmethacrylate keratoprostheses and artificial eyes. The rubbing of a lid against a protruding suture end also has been implicated in creating GPC [29].

SYMPTOMS

Four stages of symptoms occur in contact lens–associated GPC [3]. In stage 1 (preclinical), mucus or discharge in the morning is minimal although increased over normal. The eyes itch mildly upon removal of the contact lenses, but lens wear during the remainder of the day is uneventful and vision is good. Symptoms increase through stages 2 and 3 until stage 4, the severe stage, in which mucus is abundant in the morning and the eyelids stick together. There is pain on insertion of the lens in some persons. There is itching while the lens is worn, and upon removal of the lens the itching is mild to severe. The patient has some distress or pain while wearing the lens. The vision with the lens depends on the amount of mucus secretion and deposits on the lens but may be quite blurred. Lens movement is so great that the lens may be pulled off the cornea by a blink.

SIGNS

There are four stages of signs of contact lens–associated GPC [3]; in general, these parallel the four stages of symptoms. In the preclinical stage there are no abnormal signs, and the patient has only symptoms. This is an important stage as it is a particularly difficult one for the physician faced with a complaining contact lens wearer in the absence of signs. Conjunctival biopsies of persons in the preclinical stage show histologic changes. However, this procedure is not recommended for diagnosing the disease.

In stages 1 and 2, the lens is lightly coated with an amorphous, whitish material. The normal papillae are elevated, and there is an initial formation of some giant papillae. Fluorescein stains the top of the giant papillae occurs occasionally; this is an important sign of activity. The procedure used to test for this sign employs ultraviolet light from the biomicroscope, 2% fluorescein added to the tear film, and observation of the conjunctiva with the high power on the slit lamp. There is minimal or no conjunctival hyperemia or edema. Mucus formation is usually minimal on the conjunctiva and more abundant over the papillae. At this stage, the cornea is rarely involved but will on occasion show punctate staining superiorly.

The signs in stage 3 are severer. In stage 4, the severest stage, heavy coating of the contact lens occurs. The papillae show flattening of their apices and increased elevation. The giant papillae can be seen with the naked eye. A greater number of apices of the giant papillae stain with 2% fluorescein. Erythema and edema of the upper tarsal conjunctiva is commonplace. The mucus on the conjunctiva surface appears in heavy sheets, strands, or globs. The superior portion of the cornea occasionally has a white syncytial infiltrate. In advanced forms of the disease, limbal involvement (e.g., gelatinous masses) may occur.

Soft lenses generally result in a greater number of papillae in the conjunctiva of a responder than do hard contact lenses. Hard contact lens papillae are more likely to be in the midtarsal or inferior tarsal area near the lashes, in contrast to the superior tar-

sal involvement seen with soft contact lenses. In GPC associated with hard contact lenses, the papillae are more widely separated and more likely to be flat on top rather than rounded as in soft lens GPC. In soft lens–associated GPC, symptoms generally occur within months of beginning to wear lenses. Most of the patients with difficulties have onset between 3 months and 1 year, with an average of 8 months of lens wear. However, late cases of GPC (i.e., GPC that develops after years of contact lens wear) have been seen (especially in hard lens wearers).

PATHOGENESIS

Two factors seem to work together to produce contact lens–associated GPC: the trauma of the upper lid conjunctiva by the foreign substance and the exposure of the upper lid to allergens on the lens (Fig. 6-9). Both of these factors must be present to produce the disease. The trauma is thought to predispose the conjunctiva to greater absorption of antigens presented by the lens. The deposits on the lens are a complex accumulation of tear proteins, bacteria, and environmental particles. These allergens are rubbed against the upper tarsal conjunctiva approximately ten thousand times a day.

Certain types of inflammatory cells are present in the normal conjunctiva: neutrophils, lymphocytes, mast cells, and plasma cells. Neutrophils and lymphocytes are routinely found in both the epithelium and substantia propria of normal tissues. Mast cells and plasma cells are normally present in the substantia propria but not in the epithelium. Basophils and eosinophils are not normally found in either epithelium or substantia propria; their presence would be considered abnormal [4]. Quantitative histologic studies of the upper tarsal conjunctiva of asymptomatic lens wearers, those with GPC, and clinically normal tissue have been performed. The findings in the normal group and asymptomatic contact lens wearers were the same, with no abnormal infiltration of cells [6]. Thus, in the asymptomatic lens wearer, the trauma to the lid does not result in abnormal cell infiltrate although it does change the surface of the conjunctiva [21]. The distribution of inflammatory cells in GPC associated with contact lens wear differs from the norm and is characterized by mast cells in the epithelium and eosinophils and basophils in the epithelium and substantia propria [5] (Fig. 6-10). About one-third of the total number of mast cells seen by electron microscopy could be classified as phantom, having too few granules to be counted by light microscopy. This is in contrast to VKC, in which 80 to 90 percent of the mast cells were phantom. The number of lymphocytes and plasma cells per cubic millimeter of

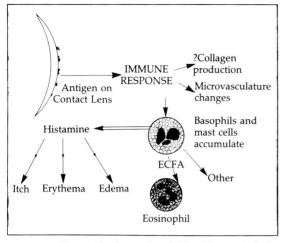

FIGURE 6-9. *Hypothesis of an antigen-initiated immunologically mediated mechanism for giant papillary conjunctivitis.*

tissue from subjects with GPC was not increased. However, the total mass of conjunctiva on the upper tarsal plate in GPC is at least double the norm; the total number of lymphocytes and plasma cells in the total lid conjunctiva is therefore markedly increased. The conjunctiva is so populated with inflammatory cells in the normal state that it is probable that when additional chemotactic cells arrive in GPC there is no place for them, and thus the conjunctiva expands its volume. This expansion is seen clinically as thickening of the conjunctiva and then as giant papillae.

DIFFERENTIAL DIAGNOSIS

VKC must be ruled out. It occurs in a much younger age group, is a far more serious disease, and is not related to contact lens wear. The appearance of the

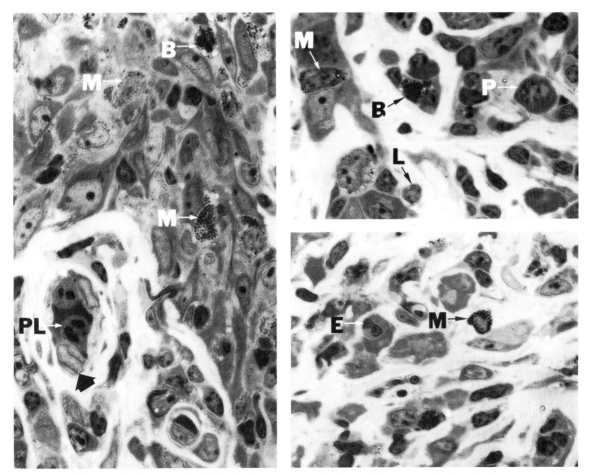

FIGURE 6-10. *Left, Basophils (B), mast cells (M), and polymorphonuclear leukocytes (PL) are present in the epithelium in contact lens-associated giant papillary conjunctivitis. (×1680.) Right, Basophils (B), plasma cells (P), lymphocytes (L), mast cells (M), and eosinophils (E) are present in the substantia propria. (×1520.) (From M. R. Allansmith et al. [3].)*

conjunctiva in the two diseases may be indistinguishable morphologically. GPC has not been associated with corneal ulceration, corneal plaque formation, pseudogerontotoxon, myopic astigmatism, and keratoconus.

Eosinophils are present in scrapings in only about 25 percent of patients with GPC, whereas they are routinely present in VKC. Eosinophilic granules, common to VKC, are not seen in GPC. Tear histamine is not elevated in GPC, whereas it is markedly elevated in VKC.

TREATMENT

The two necessary factors in GPC, trauma of the tarsal conjunctiva and presentation of allergen on the contact lens surface to the upper tarsal conjunctiva, are important to consider in evaluating treatment. The lid trauma may be decreased by reshaping the edge of the contact lens. A lid that is traumatized extensively by one edge type may be able to tolerate another edge type, so that switching to lenses from different manufacturers may be helpful. Changing the soft contact lens to a hard one ameliorates the disease and may be necessary in severer cases. The lens deposits can be decreased by meticulous cleaning with much surface rubbing of the contact lens with cleaners. Papain is very useful to help break up the protein (antigenic) deposits. The use of papain should be approached in a dose-response fashion. In general, once a week is a reasonable preventive use of papain lens cleaner but more frequent use is indicated when symptoms develop. After a lens has been worn a certain period, generally about 1 year, the deposits may not be removed sufficiently by any cleaning treatment and a new lens must be prescribed. The time at which the old lens is no longer usable because of unremovable deposits varies from patient to patient but once a patient is in difficulty the lens lifetime becomes shorter.

Topical steroids have been tried in GPC. The relief afforded by even high levels of strong steroids is not remarkable. In addition, since the wearing of lenses is elective and the lens problem is chronic, the use of steroids is not reasonable. Disodium cromoglycate in a 2% solution used 4 times a day is helpful but not as helpful as it is in VKC. Astringents and astringents with antihistamines have minor usefulness in contact lens–associated GPC. The real resolution of the disease depends on minimizing the lid trauma and reducing the amount of deposits being presented to the upper tarsal conjunctiva. With maximum cooperation by the pa-

tient, approximately 85 percent of contact lens–associated GPC can be satisfactorily handled. Although it is true that removal of the lenses results in almost immediate disappearance of symptoms (and disappearance of papillae after several months or years), patients need not discontinue lenses since the problem will only again arise on reinstituting lens wear.

Contact lens–associated GPC can result in scarring of the palpebral conjunctiva, but no permanent visual loss has been reported to date.

REFERENCES

1. Abelson, M. B., et al. Histamine in human tears. *Am. J. Ophthalmol.* 83:416, 1977.
2. Abelson, M. B., Allansmith, M. R., and Friedlaender, M. H. Effects of topically applied ocular decongestant and antihistamine. *Am. J. Ophthalmol.* 90:254, 1980.
3. Allansmith, M. R., et al. Giant papillary conjunctivitis in contact lens wearers. *Am. J. Ophthalmol.* 83:697, 1977.
4. Allansmith, M. R., Greiner, J. V., and Baird, R. S. Number of inflammatory cells in the normal conjunctiva. *Am. J. Ophthalmol.* 86:250, 1978.
5. Allansmith, M. R., Korb, D. R., and Greiner, J. V. Giant papillary conjunctivitis induced by hard or soft contact lens wear: Quantitative histology. *Trans. Am. Acad. Ophthalmol. Otolaryngol.* 85:766, 1978.
6. Allansmith, M. R., Baird, R. S., and Greiner, J. V. Number and type of inflammatory cells in conjunctiva of asymptomatic contact lens wearers. *Am. J. Ophthalmol.* 87:171, 1979.
7. Allansmith, M. R., Baird, R. S., and Greiner, J. V. Vernal conjunctivitis and contact lens–associated giant papillary conjunctivitis compared and contrasted. *Am. J. Ophthalmol.* 87:544, 1979.
8. Allansmith, M. R., Baird, R. S., and Bloch, K. J. Topical model of ocular anaphylaxis. In preparation.
9. Aly, R., Maibach, H. L., and Shinefield, H. R. Microbial flora of atopic dermatitis. *Arch. Dermatol.* 113:780, 1977.
10. Beethan, W. P. Atopic cataract. *Arch. Ophthalmol.* 24:21, 1940.
11. Beigelman, M. N. *Vernal Conjunctivitis.* Los Angeles: University of Southern California Press, 1950.
12. Bloch, K. J. Immunoglobulin Heterogeneity and Anaphylactic Sensitization. In K. F. Austen and E. L. Becker (Eds.), *Biochemistry of the Acute Allergic Reactions.* Oxford: Blackwell, 1968.
13. Brauninger, C. E., and Centifanto, Y. M. Immunoglobulin E in human tears. *Am. J. Ophthalmol.* 72:558, 1971.
14. Coca, A. F., and Cook, R. A. On the clas-

sification of the phenomenon of hypersensitiveness. *J. Immunol.* 8:163, 1923.

15. Cox, J. Disodium cromoglycate (FPL670) (Intal): A specific inhibitor of reaginic antigen-antibody mechanisms. *Nature* 216:1329, 1967.

16. Dahl, B., et al. Lymphocyte transformation: IgE and T cells in eczema vaccinatum treated with transfer factor. *Acta Derm. Venereol.* (Stockh.) 55:187, 1975.

17. Duke-Elder, S., and Leigh, A. G. Diseases of the Outer Eye. In S. Duke-Elder (Ed.), *System of Ophthalmology,* Vol. 18. St. Louis: Mosby, 1965.

18. Easty, D. L., Rice, N. S. C., and Jones, B. R. Disodium cromoglycate in the treatment of vernal conjunctivitis. *Trans. Ophthalmol. Soc. U.K.* 91:491, 1971.

19. Gell, P. G. H., and Coombs, R. R. A. (Eds.). *Clinical Aspects of Immunology.* Oxford: Blackwell, 1968.

20. Gillon, J. Where do mucosal mast cells acquire IgE? *Immunol. Today* 2:80, 1981.

21. Greiner, J. V., et al. Conjunctiva in asymptomatic contact lens wearers. *Am. J. Ophthalmol.* 86:403, 1978.

22. Hogan, M. J. Atopic keratoconjunctivitis. *Am. J. Ophthalmol.* 36:937, 1953.

23. Hubscher, T. Role of the eosinophil in the allergic reactions. *J. Immunol.* 114:1379, 1975.

24. Johansson, S. G. O., and Juhlin, L. Immunoglobulin E in healed atopic dermatitis and after treatment with corticosteroids and azathioprine. *Br. J. Dermatol.* 82:10, 1970.

25. Jones, B. R. Vernal keratitis. *Trans. Ophthalmol. Soc. U.K.* 81:215, 1961.

26. Korb, D. R., et al. Prevalence of conjunctival changes in wearers of hard contact lenses. *Am. J. Ophthalmol.* 90:336, 1980.

27. Lichtenstein, L. M. Sequential analysis of the allergic response. *Int. Arch. Allergy Appl. Immunol.* 49:143, 1975.

28. Lobitz, W. C., Honeyman, J. F., and Winkler, N. W. Suppressed cell-mediated immunity in two adults with atopic dermatitis. *Br. J. Dermatol.* 86:317, 1972.

29. Mackie, I. A., and Wright, P. Giant papillary conjunctivitis (secondary vernal) in association with contact lens wear. *Trans. Ophthalmol. Soc. U.K.* 98:3, 1978.

30. McGeady, S. J., and Buckley, R. H. Depression of cell-mediated immunity in atopic eczema. *J. Allergy Clin. Immunol.* 56:393, 1975.

31. Patterson, R. Investigation of spontaneous hypersensitivity of the dog. *J. Allergy Clin. Immunol.* 31:351, 1960.

32. Prausnitz, C., and Küstner, H. Studien uber die Ueberemfindlichkeit. *Centralbl. Bakteriol.* 86:160, 1921.

33. Rachelefsky, G. S., et al. Defective T cell function in atopic dermatitis. *J. Allergy Clin. Immunol.* 57:569, 1976.

34. Sherman, H., Feldman, L., and Walzer, M. Studies in atopic hypersensitivity of the ophthalmic mucous membranes. *J. Allergy* 4:437, 1933.

35. Smolin, G., and O'Connor, G. R. *Ocular Immunology.* Philadelphia: Lea & Febiger, 1981.

36. Srinivasan, B. D., et al. Giant papillary conjunctivitis with ocular prostheses. *Arch. Ophthalmol.* 97:892, 1979.

37. Stone, S. P., Muller, S. A., and Gleich, G. J. IgE levels in atopic dermatitis. *Arch. Dermatol.* 108:806, 1973.

38. Strannegard, K., et al. Transfer factor in severe atopic disease. *Lancet* 2, 1975.

39. Tobgy, A. F. Keratitis epithelialis vernalis. *Bull. Ophthalmol. Soc. Egypt* 28:104, 1935.

40. Verulet, D., Vellieux, P., and Charpin, J. Potentiation of cutaneous reactivity and blood leukocyte histamine release by deuterium oxide in human beings. *Acta Allergol.* 31:367, 1976.

41. Wiener, A. S., Zieve, J., and Fries, J. H. The inheritance of allergic disease. *Ann. Eugenics* 7:141, 1936.

Mooren's Ulceration

David J. Schanzlin

Chronic serpiginous ulcer of the cornea, or ulcus rodens, was first described by Bowman in 1849 [cited in 28]. MacKenzie made note of this clinical entity in his book published in 1854 [cited in 28], but the true credit for describing this insidious corneal problem and defining it as a clinical entity goes to Mooren, who published cases in 1863 and 1867 [cited in 28].

In 1902, Nettleship [28] summarized the accumulated reported experience with the disorder in a classic article, in which he reviewed the 67 previously published cases and added 11 new cases from his experience. Although well over 165 cases of Mooren's or Mooren's-like ulcer have been described in the literature since Nettleship's classic review, our understanding of this devastating condition is still vague.

Mooren's ulceration appears to affect both sexes equally and is rare in patients under the age of 20. Although primarily a disease of adults, one case has been reported in a 3-year-old infant [34]. Nettleship [28] found that 75 percent of the cases that he reviewed were in patients over the age of 40 when the first attack occurred. The African cases described below are in a younger population (third decade).

ETIOLOGY

Wood and Kaufman [39] described the two clinical types of Mooren's ulcer (Table 6-1). The first, or limited, type of Mooren's ulcer, responds to relatively conservative medical or surgical therapy. This type is typically unilateral and occurs in older patients. The second type of Mooren's ulcer is relentlessly progressive and unresponsive to any form of therapy. The patients in this group are usually younger, as noted above, and scleral involvement is more frequent. These ulcers are similar to those described by Kietzman [23], who reported 37 progressive Mooren's ulcers in Nigeria. In his series, the disease affected primarily healthy men between the ages of 20 and 30 years, and the clinical course was very rapid with total involvement and destruction of the cornea within 6 weeks. Perforations were frequent, occurring in 36 percent of the patients.

The causes of these two clinical variations may be different. For example, since the description of Kietzman [23] demonstrated a relatively high incidence of Mooren's ulcer in Nigeria, there has been conjecture that this condition may be triggered by exposure to parasitic infections. Reports have suggested that Mooren's ulcer is associated with infections by parasitic worms. Recent reports from Nigeria have demonstrated Mooren's ulcer in young men. In one series [25], helminthiasis was found in 4 of the 5 patients with Mooren's ulcer. In another study [36], 34 cases of Mooren's ulcer were treated over a 5-year period. The cases were divided into groups according to development of the disease. In 14 cases, the progress of the ulceration was arrested by local treatment and simultaneous treatment of systemic helminthiasis (caused by *Ascaris lumbricoides* and *Ancylostoma duodenale*) from which the patients were also suffering. The high incidence of recurrent infection with helminths suggests that these organisms are causally related to Mooren's ulcer. The ulcer may be caused by an antigen-antibody reaction to helminth toxins that may be deposited in the peripheral cornea during the blood-borne phase of the infection.

Mooren's ulcer after ocular surgery (such as cataract extraction) has also been described [2, 22].

TABLE 6-1. *Clinical Features of Two Types of Mooren's Ulcer*

Feature	Mooren's Ulcer	Atypical Mooren's
Age	Old	Young
Sex	M > F (3:2)	M > F (3:1)
Race predilection	None	Black
Laterality	25% bilateral	75% bilateral
Pain	Moderate to severe	Variable
Course	Slow and relentless	Rapid progression
Prognosis	Fair	Poor
Perforation	Rare	One-third
Predisposing factors	Unknown	Injury; other

SOURCE: Modified from K. F. Tabbara, The Role of the Conjunctiva in Peripheral Corneal Disease: Mooren's Ulcer. In G. R. O'Connor (Ed.), *Immunologic Diseases of the Mucous Membrane.* New York: Masson, 1980.

In these cases, it was assumed that the surgical trauma was the exciting factor in the development of these peripheral corneal ulcers.

PATHOGENESIS

It is unlikely that Mooren's ulceration represents a primary immunologic disturbance with the production of autoantibodies against normal conjunctival and corneal tissue. It is possible, however, that the inflammation associated with the antecedent injury or infection mentioned above alters the antigens of the epithelium of the cornea and conjunctiva (the disease remains limited to the anterior portion of these tissues) or releases otherwise sequestered antigens. This may initiate the development of autoantibodies in a person prone to their formation.

Evidence that an autoimmune process plays a major role in the pathogenesis of this disease includes the findings of histologic examinations: a predominance of plasma cells actively producing RNA, polymorphonuclear leukocytes, immunoglobulin, and complement [6, 13]. In 1976, Brown and colleagues [9] reported the presence of many plasma cells in the conjunctiva adjacent to the ulcerated area in cases of Mooren's ulcer, as well as tissue-fixed immunoglobulins and complement (C3) present in the conjunctival epithelium. In 1977, Eiferman and Hyndiuk [12] reported a band of tissue-fixed IgE along the epithelial basement membrane in a patient with Mooren's ulcer.

In 1969, Schaap and associates [31] demonstrated circulating antibodies to corneal tissue in patients suffering from Mooren's ulcer. Circulating antibodies to corneal tissue, however, have been found in many patients who have chronic keratitis [32].

Mondino and coworkers [27] described a series of patients with a clinical diagnosis of Mooren's ulcer who demonstrated positive macrophage migration inhibition (MIF) to corneal tissue. Six of the seven patients diagnosed demonstrated a positive MIF in response to corneal antigens. This suggests that cell-mediated immunity as well as humoral immunity plays a major role in the cause and perpetuation of Mooren's ulceration. In one of the seven patients, MIF was negative when the disease was in an inactive state, but became positive in association with the recurrence of the disease.

In 1972, Brown [5] showed that the conjunctiva adjacent to the area of ulceration exhibited collagenolytic activity. The source of this activity may be the conjunctival epithelium, the abundant polymorphonuclear leukocytes, or both.

CLINICAL FEATURES

Mooren's ulcer is a chronic painful ulceration of the cornea that starts in the periphery and may progress

centrally or circumferentially to involve the entire cornea. The disease is a bilateral process in at least 25 percent of the cases in older people, although the involvement of both eyes may not be simultaneous [28]. In the young black patients in Africa, the disease may occur bilaterally in 75 percent of the cases and run a more acute course as noted above. Clinical experience has shown that cases with bilateral involvement are usually relentless in progression and resistant to treatment [39].

The ulceration always begins in the periphery of the cornea. In most cases, this process begins within the interpalpebral fissure. The ulcerative process begins as a narrow gray infiltration near the limbus that breaks down to form the marginal ulceration within a few weeks (Fig. 6-11). This gray infiltrate may begin in multiple areas that then extend circumferentially and coalesce.

The corneal melting spreads slowly, involving the anterior one-third to one-half of the corneal stroma. The advancing margin of the ulcer undermines the anterior corneal stroma, producing a gray, infiltrated overhanging edge of diseased corneal tissue with an overlying intact epithelium (Fig. 6-12). The ulcerative process only rarely involves the entire crescent of diseased tissue at any one time, and the areas of active ulceration can be easily followed with fluorescein stain. Because of tissue swelling, the exact depth of the undermining is difficult to appreciate unless the overhanging edge is removed. Blood vessels from the conjunctiva eventually cover the remaining deep stroma and Descemet's membrane after the ulcerative process has destroyed the anterior corneal lamella.

Progression of the ulcerative process is usually slow, with the uninvolved area of the cornea remaining clear. The limbus is involved, and there is a contiguous inflammation of the conjunctival, episcleral, or scleral tissue. The ulcerative process may continue for 3 to 12 months if the entire cornea is involved. Perforation may occur, especially if there is trauma.

One of the most debilitating features of Mooren's ulcer is severe pain associated with photophobia and excessive lacrimation. The bulbar conjunctiva is injected adjacent to the area of active ulceration. A mild to moderate anterior uveitis is common in patients with this disease, and secondary glaucoma and cataract may further complicate the course. The resulting visual loss, however, generally corresponds with the involvement of the corneal visual axis. Hypopyon does not usually occur without secondary infection. In severe cases, the ulceration may extend posteriorly to involve the scleral tissue.

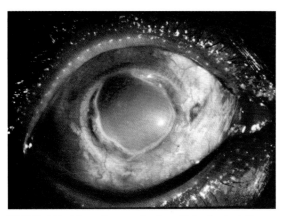

FIGURE 6-11. *Mooren's corneal ulcer. Note the typical gray infiltrate along the active edge of the ulcer. This ulcer has spread circumferentially and involves the peripheral cornea from the 12 to the 10 o'clock position. (Courtesy Stuart I. Brown, M.D.)*

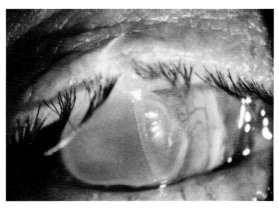

FIGURE 6-12. *Mooren's ulcer at a later stage in the ulcerative process. The entire peripheral cornea is involved, and the superior and inferior undermined edges hamper proper lid movement. (Courtesy Stuart I. Brown, M.D.)*

DIFFERENTIAL DIAGNOSIS

Although the clinical picture in Mooren's corneal ulceration is fairly typical, care should be taken to exclude other diseases that may present similarly (Tables 6-2 and 6-3). These include the collagen disorders rheumatoid arthritis, Wegener's granulomatosis, systemic lupus erythematosus, and polyarteritis nodosa. Terrien's marginal degeneration, pellucid degeneration, and senile marginal degeneration are corneal degenerations that, in some clinical presentations, may be confused with the active melting process of Mooren's ulcer. Less common systemic disorders with corneal changes that may mimic Mooren's ulcer include leukemia, gonorrhea,

syphilis, bacillary dysentery, staphylococcal ring abscess, and food allergy. These disorders usually present with a ring abscess or ulceration of the cornea, but the differentiation from Mooren's ulcer may be subtle in some cases.

LABORATORY STUDIES

The study of any case of Mooren's ulcer should begin with both complete and differential blood cell counts, sedimentation rate, latex fixation, antinuclear antibodies, chest x-ray, liver enzyme, VDRL, FTA-ABS, BUN, and creatinine tests. These blood studies are performed to rule out collagen vascular disease (especially Wegener's granulomatosis), malignancy, or diseases of an ischemic or occlusive etiology. In cases of suspected collagen vascular disease, a thorough medical examination should be performed.

TREATMENT

Numerous medical therapies have been suggested for the management of Mooren's ulcer. Early therapies included carbolic acid, formalin, tincture of iodine, nitric acid [33], curettage, trichloroacetic acid [29], and galvanocautery [10]. Other medical means advocated for the treatment of this condition include chemotherapeutic and antibiotic agents such as cyanide of mercury [21] and subconjunctival injection of bichloride of mercury [1]. Irradiation [38], vitamin B_1 injections, and tuberculin injections

TABLE 6-2. *Autoimmune Diseases* That May Cause Marginal Corneal Infiltration, Ulceration, or Thinning*

Organ-specific
  Ulcerative colitis (colon)
  Mooren's ulcer (cornea)
  Psoriasis (skin)
  Thyroiditis (thyroglobulin)
Generalized or non-organ-specific
  Systemic lupus erythematosus (nuclear antigens)
  Rheumatoid arthritis (IgG)
  Progressive systemic sclerosis (nucleolar, nuclear antigens)
  Wegener's granulomatosis (?)
Organ-specific and generalized
  Sjögren's syndrome (salivary and lacrimal glands, nuclear antigens)
Tissue-specific
  Polyarteritis nodosa (arteries)
  Cogan's syndrome (arteries)
  Myasthenia gravis (acetylcholine receptors)

*Autoantigen in each disease is shown in parentheses.
SOURCE: Modified from K. F. Tabbara, The Role of the Conjunctiva in Peripheral Corneal Disease: Mooren's Ulcer. In G. R. O'Connor (Ed.), *Immunologic Diseases of the Mucous Membrane.* New York: Masson, 1980.

have also been attempted. All of the above therapies today are considered to be ineffective. Paracentesis [17, 26] and delimiting keratotomy [14, 18, 35] have also been tried with limited success.

In recent years, the use of collagenase inhibitors and subconjunctival injections of heparin have been recommended to arrest the progression of this condition [3]; however, the value of these therapies is controversial [19]. It is difficult to assess the effect of any treatment on Mooren's ulcer because the cases are few and varied, and there is occasionally spontaneous healing.

The initial therapy of Mooren's ulcer should consist of topical cycloplegics and a therapeutic soft contact lens. This will often help relieve pain but rarely leads to quiescence of the ulcer. The therapeutic soft contact lens vaults the ridge of diseased corneal tissue, preventing trauma caused by the blinking lid. A vigorous course of topical corticosteroids should be implemented to suppress the iritis, and occasionally, especially in the unilateral form of Mooren's ulcer, this will quiet the ulcerative process. In the bilateral form of the disease, topical corticosteroids are usually ineffective.

The use of systemic corticosteroids, theoretically, should be effective, in view of the evidence for autoimmune mechanism in Mooren's ulcer. However, the efficacy of various dose levels of systemic corticosteroids has not yet been fully established [27]. Similarly, immunosuppressive therapy for Mooren's ulcer has not yet been shown to be efficacious, although the initial experience with cyclophosphamide (Cytoxan) and methotrexate has been favorable [15, 16, 24].

The patient should be carefully monitored after beginning medical therapy. If progression occurs with vigorous medical therapy, surgical excision of 4 mm of perilimbal conjunctiva adjacent to the ulcer has been effective in quieting the ulcerative process. Application of cryotherapy to the perilimbal con-

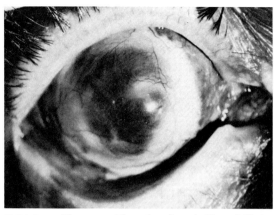

FIGURE 6-13. *The cornea of the patient shown in Figure 6-12 after lamellar keratectomy of the central island of stromal tissue. A therapeutic soft contact lens covers the fibrovascular scar over the posterior corneal lamellae. (Courtesy Stuart I. Brown, M.D.)*

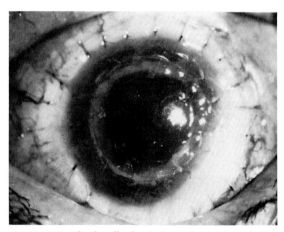

FIGURE 6-14. *After lamellar keratectomy, the eye shown in Figures 6-12 and 6-13 quieted, and a penetrating keratoplasty was performed. Note the 13-mm tectonic graft and the 7.5-mm therapeutic graft. (Courtesy Stuart I. Brown, M.D.)*

junctiva [4] in the area adjacent to the ulceration has similarly been effective. Brown reports that excision of the conjunctiva is successful 50 percent of the time [7]; however, it may be necessary to repeat this procedure three times before a beneficial effect is seen. Most often the disease's progression is only transiently affected by this procedure.

It is speculated that removing conjunctival tissue adjacent to the ulcer removes the source of plasma cells, tissue-fixed immunoglobulin, complement, and collagenase, thus interrupting the ulcerative process long enough for the epithelium to heal over

TABLE 6-3. *Nonautoimmune Diseases That May Cause Marginal Corneal Infiltration, Ulceration, or Thinning*

Systemic disorders
  Syphilis
  Gonorrhea
  Bacillary dysentery
  Leukemia
  Food allergy
Ocular disorders
  Dystrophies and degenerations
    Terrien's marginal degeneration
    Pellucid degeneration
  Staphylococcal corneal infiltrate or ring ulcer

the bed of the ulcer. After conjunctival excision, the patient's eye is patched to encourage epithelial healing. A therapeutic soft contact lens may be used for this purpose as well. The healing of the conjunctiva and the ulcer may take weeks following this procedure.

Other surgical procedures, including lamellar corneal transplants [20, 30, 40] and conjunctival flaps [11, 37], have also been attempted to quiet Mooren's ulcer. In general, when conjunctival excision fails, conjunctival flaps or lamellar transplants also fail [7]. Lamellar keratectomy of the remaining central island of corneal stromal tissue often arrests the ulcerative process, facilitates healing, and speeds up the rehabilitation of the patient [8]. After removal of the central island of the cornea, the conjunctival epithelium and fibrovascular scar cover the posterior corneal lamellae (Fig. 6-13). Many times, visual acuity of 20/200 can be achieved.

Once the active ulceration has ceased and the remaining cornea has been completely opacified and vascularized, it is possible to perform penetrating keratoplasty on these patients [8]. Because of the extreme peripheral corneal thinning, a 13-mm tectonic corneal graft is first sutured in place, and then a 7.5- or 8.0-mm therapeutic graft is performed (Fig. 6-14). Glaucoma and cystoid macular edema have been a problem in these cases, and although the grafts remain clear, the visual result is only rarely better than 20/200.

REFERENCES

1. Andrade, E. Ulcus rodens corneae. Ann. d'Ottal. 29:654, 1900. (Abstract in Ophthamol. Rev. 20:167, 1901.)
2. Arentsen, J. J., Christiansen, J. M., and Maumenee, A. E. Marginal ulceration after intracapsular cataract extraction. Am. J. Ophthalmol. 81:194, 1976.
3. Aronson, S. B., et al. Pathogenetic approach to therapy of peripheral corneal inflammatory disease. Am. J. Ophthalmol. 70:65, 1970.
4. Aviel, E. Combined cryoapplications and peritomy in Mooren's ulcer. Br. J. Ophthalmol. 56:48, 1972.
5. Brown, S. I. Collagenolytic enzymes in corneal pathology. Isr. J. Med. Sci. 8:1537, 1972.
6. Brown, S. I. Mooren's ulcer: Histopathology and proteolytic enzymes of adjacent conjunctiva. Br. J. Ophthalmol. 59:670, 1975.
7. Brown, S. I. Mooren's ulcer. Treatment by conjunctival excision. Br. J. Ophthalmol. 59:675, 1975.
8. Brown, S. I., and Mondino, B. J. Penetrating keratoplasty in Mooren's ulcer. Am. J. Ophthalmol. 89:255, 1980.
9. Brown, S. I., Mondino, B. J., and Rabin, B. S. Autoimmune phenomenon in Mooren's ulcer. Am. J. Ophthalmol. 82:835, 1976.
10. Cronquist, S. Ulcus rodens corneae. Nord. Med. 34:1449, 1947. (Abstract in Ophth. Lit., 1: No. 1279, March 1948, p. 1458.)
11. Dean, A. C. Ulcus rodens of right eye treated by a conjunctival flap operation. Minn. Med. 13:44, 1930.
12. Eiferman, R., and Hyndiuk, R. IgE in limbal conjunctiva in Mooren's ulcer. Can. J. Ophthalmol. 12:234, 1977.
13. Feingold, M. Mooren's ulcer of the cornea. Am. J. Ophthalmol. 4:161, 1921.
14. Ferguson, E., III, and Carreno, O. Mooren's ulcer and delimiting keratotomy. South. Med. J. 62:1170, 1969.
15. Foster, C. S. Immunosuppressive therapy for external ocular inflammatory disease. Ophthalmology (Rochester) 87:140, 1980.
16. Foster, C. S., et al. The immunopathology of Mooren's ulcer. Am. J. Ophthalmol. 88:149, 1979.
17. Fuchs, A. Concerning unusual ulcers of the cornea and their treatment. Br. J. Ophthalmol. 17:193, 1933.
18. Gifford, S. R. Rodent or Mooren's ulcer of the cornea. Arch. Ophthalmol. 10:800, 1933.
19. Goldberg, D., Schanzlin, D. J., and Brown, S. I. Mooren's Ulcer. In F. Fraunfelder and F. H. Roy (Eds.), Current Ocular Therapy. Philadelphia: Saunders, 1980. Pp. 360–361.
20. Grana, P. Therapeutic keratoplasty in Mooren's ulcer. Arch. Ophthalmol. 62:414, 1959.
21. Jones, E. L. Simultaneous bilateral rodent ulcer of the cornea cured by combined curetting, thermocautery, and massive cyanide subconjunctival injection. Br. J. Ophthalmol. 18:579, 1934.
22. Joondeph, H., et al. Mooren's ulcer: Two cases occurring after cataract extraction and treated with hydrophilic lens. Ann. Ophthalmol. 8:187, 1976.
23. Kietzman, B. Mooren's ulcer in Nigeria. Am. J. Ophthalmol. 65:679, 1968.
24. Linn, J., Jr. Chronic serpiginous ulcer of the cornea (Mooren's ulcer)—Etiologic and therapeutic considerations. Am. J. Ophthalmol. 32:691, 1949.
25. Majekodunmi, A. A. Ecology of Mooren's ulcer in Nigeria. Doc. Ophthalmol. 49:211, 1980.
26. Mayou, S. Chronic serpiginous ulceration of the cornea (Mooren's ulcer). Ophthalmoscope 13:438, 1915.
27. Mondino, B. J., Brown, S. I., and Rabin, B. S. Cellular immunity in Mooren's ulcer. Am. J. Ophthalmol. 85:788, 1978.
28. Nettleship, E. Chronic serpiginous ulcer of

the cornea (Mooren's ulcer). *Trans. Ophthalmol. Soc. U.K.* 22:103, 1902.

29. Risley, S. D.   Discussion of DeSchweinitz's paper. *Ann. Ophthalmol.* 20:436, 1911.

30. Rycroft, B. W., and Romanes, G. J.   Lamellar corneal grafts—Clinical report on 62 cases. *Br. J. Ophthalmol.* 36:337, 1952.

31. Schaap, O. L., Feltkamp, T. E., and Breebaart, A. C.   Circulating antibodies to corneal tissue in a patient suffering from Mooren's ulcer (ulcus rodens corneae). *Clin. Exp. Immunol.* 5:365, 1969.

32. Shore, B., Leopold, I. H., and Henley, W.   Cellular immunity in chronic ophthalmic disorders (leukocyte migration inhibition in diseases of the cornea). *Am. J. Ophthalmol.* 73:62, 1972.

33. Stevens, E. W.   Mooren's ulcer of the cornea. *Ophthalmol. Rec.* 17:198, 1908.

34. Taylor, S. J.   Notes of a case of rodent ulcer of the cornea in a child. *Trans. Ophthalmol. Soc. U.K.* 22:98, 1902.

35. Thygeson, P.   Marginal corneal infiltrates and ulcers. *Trans. Am. Acad. Ophthalmol. Otolaryngol.* 121:198, 1946-47.

36. Trojan, H. J.   Aetiology and therapy of Mooren's ulcer (author's translation). *Klin. Monatsbl. Augenheilkd.* 174:166, 1979.

37. Tyrrell, F.   Case of Mooren's ulcer treated with a conjunctival flap. *Trans. Ophthalmol. Soc. U.K.* 37:205, 1917.

38. Ward, R.   Radium in ophthalmology with illustrative cases. *Proc. R. Soc. Med.* 26:1515, 1933.

39. Wood, T., and Kaufman, H.   Mooren's ulcer. *Am. J. Ophthalmol.* 71:417, 1971.

40. Zu, D., et al.   Mooren's ulcer treated by lamellar keratoplasty. *Jpn. J. Ophthalmol.* 23:257, 1979.

Rheumatoid Diseases

Ronald E. Smith and David J. Schanzlin

Many systemic disorders are associated with inflammatory arthritis. Adult rheumatoid arthritis (RA) may be considered the classic example of such diseases, and study of this entity provides the basis for discussing variants of RA.

RA and its variants are part of a larger group of connective tissue disorders that also includes ankylosing spondylitis, psoriatic arthritis, systemic lupus erythematosus (SLE), polyarteritis nodosa, systemic vasculitis, Wegener's granulomatosis, relapsing polychondritis, juvenile rheumatoid arthritis (JRA), scleroderma, polymyositis and dermatomyositis, Reiter's syndrome, and Sjögren's syndrome. Many of these syndromes are discussed in other sections of this text. The purpose of this section is to discuss the systemic and ocular complications (specifically corneal) of RA and its variants, JRA, and relapsing polychondritis. The corneal findings in most of the other listed disorders are discussed elsewhere in this book.

RHEUMATOID ARTHRITIS

For many years, there has been a debate as to whether RA has an immunologic or infectious etiology. Since extensive bacteriologic and virologic studies have failed to detect an organism from synovial fluid, it is generally agreed that an immunologic mechanism plays a vital role in the pathogenesis of RA [34, 52, 57, 80, 81]. It is possible, however, that atypical microbial agents, which are at present not culturable, are important in the etiology of these disorders. There is also the strong possibility that there is a genetic predisposition to the development of RA and other related inflammatory conditions. A combined microbiologic, immunologic, and genetic etiology for RA is probably quite likely [79].

Figure 6-15 outlines a general scheme for the pathogenesis of RA. Rheumatoid factor has been characterized as an antibody to human gamma globulin. Production of this aberrant antibody may occur in the joint with subsequent formation of antigen-antibody complexes (immune complexes), which activates complement and results in a cascade of inflammatory events. Release of destructive enzymes and other factors results in arthritis (or scleritis), tissue destruction, and scarring [26, 34, 36, 57, 79–81].

Even if this proposed pathogenesis is correct, the nature of the exciting antigen that results in production of this atypical antibody to human gamma globulin is still not known. The possibility remains that this antigen is a virus. The possibility of a genetic predisposition to the development of such conditions also remains.

SYSTEMIC MANIFESTATIONS

CLINICAL FEATURES

Adult RA is a generalized, chronic, inflammatory polyarthritis involving almost any peripheral joint, usually in a symmetrical fashion [79]. Women are affected three times more frequently than men. The average age of onset is between 30 and 40 years, and the disease has been known to occur in families. A prodrome of fatigue, malaise, loss of appetite, and weight loss may be noticeable in some patients. This is followed by the gradual onset of morning stiffness, pain, and swelling involving the inter-phalangeal and metacarpophalangeal joints in the fingers and wrists. Larger joints such as knees, ankles, shoulders, and elbows can become inflamed. Almost any joint may be affected. The chronic progressive nature of the arthritis leads to the well-known characteristic joint deformities of this disease (Fig. 6-16).

The course of the disease varies from a short, mild episode of arthritis to a progressive severe process. The longer the activity, the less the likelihood of a remission.

Numerous extra-articular problems are part of the RA syndrome [29]. Cardiac, respiratory, central nervous system, cutaneous, and reticuloendothelial system changes occur (Table 6-4). Pulmonary complications seem to be more frequent in men. These include pleurisy with or without effusion, rheumatoid pneumoconiosis (Caplan's syndrome), non-pneumoconiotic intrapulmonary rheumatoid nodules, and diffuse interstitial pulmonary fibrosis [72]. Peripheral neuropathy with a mixed sensorimotor component occurs in less than 5 percent of the advanced cases. It is probably caused by vasculitis of the vasa vasorum of the peripheral nerves

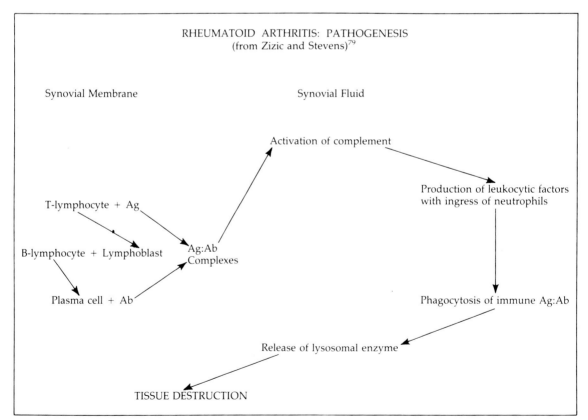

FIGURE 6-15. *Proposed pathogenesis of rheumatoid arthritis. (Ag = antigen; Ab = antibody.) (After T. M. Zizic and M. B. Stevens [79].)*

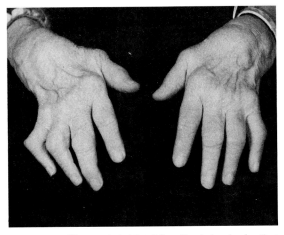

FIGURE 6-16. *Characteristic joint deformities in hands of patient with rheumatoid arthritis.*

TABLE 6-4. *Extra-articular Manifestations of Rheumatoid Arthritis*

Systemic Changes	Frequency
Rheumatoid nodules	Common
Systemic vasculitis	Uncommon
Ocular manifestations	
Keratoconjunctivitis	
sicca	Very common
Keratitis	
Marginal ulceration	Common
Marginal thinning	Common
Sclerosing keratitis	Rare
Keratolysis	Rare
Scleritis	
Diffuse anterior	Common
Nodular anterior	Uncommon
Necrotising anterior	In severe systemic disease
Scleromalacia perforans	In long-standing disease
Posterior	Uncommon
Diffuse nodular	
episcleritis	Uncommon
Uveitis	Rare
Respiratory changes	Uncommon
Cardiac disease	Uncommon
Disease of lymph nodes and	
spleen	Uncommon
Amyloidosis	Common

SOURCE: Modified from Zizic and Stevens [79].

[29, 79]. Cutaneous manifestations include the characteristic subcutaneous nodules that occur in about 25 percent of the patients [79]. Raynaud's phenomenon, erythema nodosum, or ischemic necrosis secondary to vasculitis have also been reported. Generalized lymphadenopathy occurs with splenomegaly in some patients with RA. (Felty's syndrome includes rheumatoid arthritis, splenomegaly, and neutropenia.)

The pathologic features of RA occur primarily in the involved joints and surrounding tissue [24, 29, 34, 52, 53, 79]. These lesions probably begin in the synovial membrane with a proliferation of cells lining the synovium. Giant multinucleated cells can occur in many instances. Inflammatory cells, including plasma cells and mononuclear infiltration, are also characteristic. The lymphocytic infiltrates include mononuclear cells, macrophages, lymphocytes, and plasma cells, and may be extremely dense, forming nodules. An exudative fluid into the synovial space occurs as a result of the inflammatory reaction. The marked inflammatory reaction of the synovial membrane may cause cartilage and periosteal involvement within the joint capsule, resulting in erosion of bone, formation of granulation tissue, and ultimately destruction of the joint itself and replacement by fibrous tissue. Loss of structure and function of the joint results in the characteristic deformities of RA (Fig. 6-16). A rheumatoid nodule contains a central area of devitalized tissue and necrosis surrounded by pallisades of cells including lymphocytes, plasma cells, and some giant cells. These nodules have a characteristic histopathologic appearance whether they are found in the joint, the eye [24, 76], or other extra-articular areas.

LABORATORY FINDINGS

The most characteristic laboratory feature of RA is the presence of rheumatoid factor [66, 79]. There are many such factors, which are actually antibodies to IgG in the patient's serum. They are present in almost 90 percent of patients with RA. Numerous rheumatoid factor tests have been developed. The most commonly used tests include the Waaler-Rose test and the latex test. The first employs sheep red blood cells sensitized with rabbit antibodies to sheep cells. Rheumatoid factor combines with the rabbit IgG, causing agglutination of the sheep red blood cells. Test results are positive in 60 to 70 percent of cases of RA [79]. The latex test involves adsorbing aggregated human 7S IgG on latex particles; rheumatoid factor reacting with IgG causes flocculation of the latex particles. Results are positive in 80 to 90 percent of the cases. An increased frequency of positive test results and higher titers occurs with subcutaneous nodules, RA variants (Felty's, Sjögren's), and systemic disease.

Rheumatoid factor is found in connective tissue diseases other than RA [79]. It is present in up to 20 percent of patients with scleroderma, polyarteritis nodosa, and SLE. However, in ankylosing spondylitis, colitic arthropathy, Reiter's syndrome, and JRA, it is usually not present. It is, therefore, a helpful test in differentiating variants of rheumatoid disorders.

In addition to rheumatoid factor, low-grade anemia and slight elevation of the white cell count may be present. If neutropenia is present, Felty's syndrome may be suspected. An increased sedimentation rate is the rule in patients with active disease. A positive antinuclear antibody response can be seen in about 25 percent of patients with classic RA.

TREATMENT
Treatment of RA and its variants is very difficult and time-consuming and requires a dedicated internist or specialist in these disorders. These patients have chronic problems that require not only medical treatment, but also rehabilitation services and possibly surgery to relieve deforming and incapacitating deformities in joints. Therefore, an internist or rheumatologist should be involved in management.

Almost 25 percent of RA patients respond initially to aspirin alone [79]. Although there are serious side effects, salicylates remain the first drug of choice, and other agents should be added to them. The salicylates inhibit prostaglandin synthesis. Therapeutic serum levels of salicylates are in the range of 20 to 25 mg/100 ml. Enteric-coated aspirin may be required in patients who have gastric intolerance to the 2 to 4 gm of aspirin generally required per day to achieve this serum level. If there is no clinical response to adequate serum levels within several weeks, other agents can be used instead of salicylate. Naproxen (Naprosyn), tolmetin sodium (Tolectin), ibuprofen (Motrin), indomethacin (Indocin), and phenylbutazone, although less effective for RA than for other rheumatoid variants, may also be used. Gold salts [7, 14, 22, 23, 30] and antimalarials are also employed. Antimalarials that are quinoline derivatives have a number of side effects, including some related to the eye. It is important for the ophthalmologist to be aware of the corneal deposits and retinal toxic changes that may occur in the pigment epithelium of patients taking certain quinoline derivatives. Currently, however, the positive effects of these drugs are achieved at a lower dosage than that which usually results in ocular toxicity.

Systemic corticosteroids also have a very potent antiinflammatory effect, relieve pain, and maintain some functional activity of joints in RA patients. However, they do not seem to delay progression of joint destruction, and the conservative therapies outlined above are to be recommended before use of systemic corticosteroids [79]. However, these drugs work rapidly in many patients and can be used initially to allow the slower-acting remittive agents to take effect. Immunosuppressives that may have a similar favorable effect on the inflammation can be considered if all drugs fail to induce a remission. The risk of delayed neoplastic processes after the use of cytotoxic agents such as chlorambucil is real and must be considered in the management of RA, which in itself is a nonfatal disease.

OCULAR MANIFESTATIONS
The ocular manifestations in adult RA patients include keratoconjunctivitis sicca (Sjögren's syndrome), scleritis, episcleritis, peripheral corneal melting (furrows), keratitis, sclerosing keratitis, and keratolysis [26, 49, 67]. Ocular complications may occur in patients with limited systemic disease but are more common in those with marked systemic complications including vasculitis, pericarditis, and rheumatoid nodules.

KERATOCONJUNCTIVITIS SICCA
The most common eye finding in RA is keratoconjunctivitis sicca (KCS) [49, 69]. The complete Sjögren's syndrome is present in some cases. This syndrome is discussed in more detail in Chapter 7. The dry eye associated with RA is indistinguishable from dry eye in the nonrheumatoid patient. However, unexplained xerostomia and RA (or other collagen vascular disease), with or without swelling of the salivary glands, complete the syndrome described by Sjögren. The presence of HLA-DW3 [27], HLA-BW44, and HLA-DRw4 [51], hypergammaglobulinemia, and reduced T-lymphocytes are frequent findings in RA and Sjögren's syndrome [26] and serve to distinguish patients with these ailments from those without RA. Tear lysozyme is deficient or absent in Sjögren's [26].

Clinical manifestations of KCS associated with RA are those of any dry eye, including foreign-body sensation, crusting on the lid margins, mucous threads, and the feeling of dryness and tightness around the eyes, often worse later in the day as tears evaporate [49]. Examination reveals a very thin marginal tear strip, rose bengal staining of the conjunctiva in the interpalpebral area, corneal complications related to dry eye (punctate erosive keratopathy, filaments, loss of luster), and shortened breakup time of the tear film.

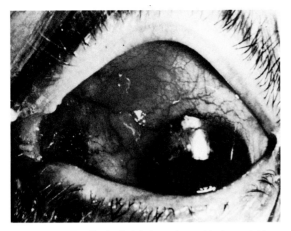

FIGURE 6-17. *Localized scleritis in patient with rheumatoid ar-thritis.*

SCLERITIS AND EPISCLERITIS

Inflammation of the collagenous coats of the eye (sclera and cornea) is a serious complication of RA [40, 43, 44, 46, 76]. Scleritis (Fig. 6-17) is the most common, although episcleritis and corneal changes are features in many patients. Scleral diseases can be classified as nodular or diffuse episcleritis, nodular or diffuse scleritis, scleromalacia perforans, and necrotizing scleritis with inflammation [39, 74, 76].

Patients with scleritis and episcleritis characteristically have severe pain. In scleritis, a deep, boring orbital pain occurs. This type of pain is not present in episcleritis. Episcleral involvement, whether nodular or diffuse, is generally localized to a more superficial location and characterized by a fiery, bright red appearance. If a nodule is present, it may be slightly movable over the underlying sclera. There may be associated conjunctival vascular injection that can be blanched by the use of topical phenylephrine hydrochloride (Neo-Synephrine) or epinephrine. After the overlying vessels are blanched, dilatation of the vessels in the episclera can be observed. As emphasized by Watson [74, 76], the pattern of vessel dilatation (episcleral versus scleral) may be helpful in differentiating episcleritis from scleritis.

In scleritis, there is a violet hue to the inflamed areas owing to the location of the inflammation and the associated vascular dilatation of the deeper layers of sclera. In both episcleritis and scleritis, the involved area is tender; this serves to differentiate these from severe conjunctivitis, which may otherwise mimic episcleritis.

Although the exact pathogenesis of scleral and episcleral inflammation in RA has not been established, it probably has the same cause as the joint inflammation [74, 76]. Immune complexes are prob-

ably deposited in the sclera of patients with rheumatoid scleritis, just as they occur in synovia of joints in RA patients [26, 36]. These antigen-antibody complexes, with complement, trigger the cascade of events leading to scleral (or joint) inflammation (i.e., attraction of polymorphonuclear leukocytes and release of various enzymes and other mediators followed by localized tissue destruction) [76]. In a joint, this sequence leads to arthritis. In the sclera or cornea, scleritis, episcleritis, or sclerokeratitis occurs, depending on the location of the inflammatory event. In addition to the immunologic inflammatory scleral disease involving deposition of antigen-antibody complexes in the sclera, an intrascleral vasculitis may also occur [3, 4]. This may result in deep scleral intravascular coagulation, ischemic necrosis, and scleral melting [4, 76]. Scleral inflammation and vasculitis are probably both present in some cases [76].

The pathologic changes of rheumatoid scleritis include foci of fibrinoid necrosis of the sclera surrounded by palisading fibroblasts and an inflammatory component consisting largely of polymorphonuclear leukocytes, lymphocytes, and plasma cells [24, 62]. The amount of cellular proliferation and necrosis varies, depending on severity and the extent of vascular involvement.

Scleritis and episcleritis occur in approximately 4 to 10 percent of all RA patients [74, 76]. However, when a patient comes to an ophthalmologist with scleritis, RA must be strongly considered, since it is the most common cause of scleritis (and episcleritis). Besides history taking for RA and other collagen disorders that may also be associated with scleritis, certain laboratory tests are recommended. Rheumatoid factors, uric acid, sedimentation rate, FTA-ABS and VDRL, PPD (tuberculosis), and chest x-ray (tuberculosis) are suggested screening tests.

In cases of severe scleritis with a necrotizing and ischemic component, a white-gray area is present in the center of the patch of scleritis. This probably represents ischemic necrosis and is a danger signal, since this area may slough, leaving a scleral defect with bulging uveal tissue. If the intraocular pressure is elevated, as sometimes is the case in active inflammatory disease of the sclera, a pronounced bulge of the uvea may occur (Fig. 6-18). This form of necrotizing scleritis, when associated with severe surrounding scleral inflammation, is quite painful. On the other hand, classic scleromalacia perforans is an equally severe necrotizing and melting process, but it is relatively asymptomatic in an otherwise quiet eye without pain. Slow, progressive

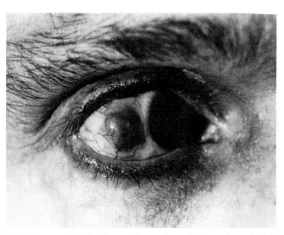

FIGURE 6-18. *Ectatic sclera with uveal staphyloma after scleritis in rheumatoid arthritis.*

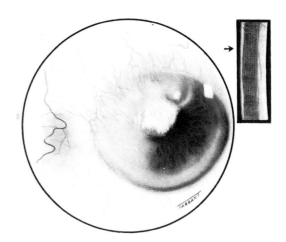

FIGURE 6-19. *Sclerosing keratitis. Diffuse marginal gray thickening is present. Opacity may spread centrally to visual axis, with crystalline changes in corneal stroma behind the advancing edge. Inset shows depth of corneal disease. (From P. G. Watson [74].)*

melting of the sclera with exposure of underlying uveal tract occurs. This form of scleritis has generally been associated with long-standing, severe RA [76]. The inflammatory and painful variety of necrotizing scleritis may be seen in RA as well, but it is also associated with other connective tissue disorders such as Wegener's granulomatosis and periarteritis nodosa [28, 76].

Secondary intraocular inflammation frequently occurs with severe scleritis, including uveitis and serous retinal detachment [76]. Both resolve with improvement of the overlying scleritis.

CORNEAL CHANGES
Corneal changes may be found adjacent to areas of scleral inflammation or as the only ocular complications of RA [74, 76]. Localized infiltration of the cornea followed by development of epithelial defects and frank melting of the cornea may occur. A relatively severe proliferation and infiltration of inflammatory cells with secondary fibrovascular invasion results in peripheral corneal scarring in some cases.

Corneal involvement in rheumatoid arthritis includes keratitis and sclerosing keratitis, peripheral corneal melting (furrows), and keratolysis [74, 76].

When confronted with corneal disease associated with RA, it is most important for the ophthalmologist to be certain that KCS is *not* present, since sterile corneal ulceration and melting may be associated with dry eyes.

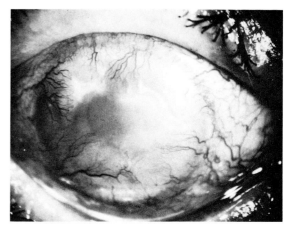

FIGURE 6-20. *Sclerosing keratitis and keratolysis in rheumatoid arthritis patient with scleritis. Note marked vascularization of the cornea with thinning.*

KERATITIS AND SCLEROSING KERATITIS
Sclerosing keratitis is the most common corneal complication of scleritis [74, 76]. By definition, it occurs in association with severe scleral disease and not as an isolated corneal finding [74]. This is in contradistinction to peripheral guttering of the cornea, which may occur without scleral inflammation in patients with long-standing RA.

In sclerosing keratitis, a gradual gray corneal stromal thickening progresses toward the center of the cornea followed by vascularization (Figs. 6-19 and 6-20). The advancing edge may have a striate configuration with crystallinelike changes devel-

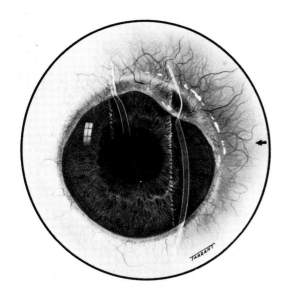

FIGURE 6-21. *Localized thinning in sclerokeratitis. Note thin area in periphery of cornea. (From P. G. Watson [74].)*

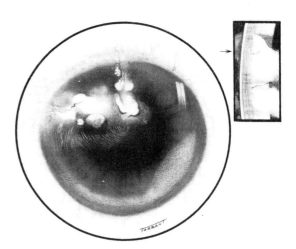

FIGURE 6-22. *Lipid deposition in sclerosing keratitis. Accumulation of lipid occurs in chronic sclerokeratitis. Inset shows level of corneal involvement. (From P. G. Watson [74].)*

oping behind this edge. If this process extends into the visual axis, it causes a marked decrease in vision. If the associated scleritis is nodular, sclerosing keratitis is geneally localized to that quadrant. However, if the scleritis is diffuse, the entire cornea may become white and vascularized. Sclerosing keratitis may lead to perforation as a result of (noninfectious) localized corneal ulceration (Fig. 6-21). Lipid deposition is a late change (Fig. 6-22).

Keratitis alone (sterile corneal inflammation) may also be associated with scleritis and may occur in areas adjacent to the active scleral inflammatory process (Fig. 6-23). Such corneal inflammation has been found in from 30 to 70 percent of patients with scleritis or episcleritis associated with RA [46, 62]. The corneal inflammatory process includes mid-stromal and superficial stromal infiltrates, depending on the nature of the scleritis. The infiltrates may become very diffuse and even result in corneal epithelial breakdown, melting, and frank ulceration. This corneal complication may take a sclerosing configuration, with ingrowth of vessels and connective tissue resulting in peripheral corneal scarring as noted above.

PERIPHERAL CORNEAL MELTING (FURROWS)
Peripheral corneal melting or furrow ulceration occurs with or without associated scleral or episcleral inflammation (Figs. 6-24 and 6-25). Brown and Grayson reported marginal furrows in patients with chronic RA [8]; this is probably a more common

occurrence in RA patients than has been previously reported [38]. The thinned area, usually located inferiorly, may be very superficial at first but progresses rapidly. The peripheral corneal melt or furrow is often associated with a mildly inflamed conjunctiva. This mild contiguous inflammatory process should not be confused with episcleritis. There is usually no vascularization in the bed of the furrow, and the corneal epithelium is intact. Limbal furrowing or guttering [8, 38, 46, 75] may also be seen in association with rheumatoid scleritis, episcleritis, or sclerosing keratitis (Fig. 6-26). Although the majority of these "ulcers" do not progress, others have resulted in marked thinning and descemetocele formation. Perforation is rare but may occur with minor trauma.

The pathogenesis of the corneal lesions is unclear. Collagenase has been found in the conjunctiva and corneal epithelium adjacent to the furrow itself [21]. The pathogenesis of the scleral and corneal disease may be the same as that for joint disease [26]. As indicated earlier, it is postulated that cells associated with synovial tissue (and by analogy, with scleral or corneal collagen) produce an IgG antibody in response to an unknown antigenic stimulus, possibly an atypical virus. The IgG antibody may be altered and no longer recognized as "self." Other immunoglobulins are formed to this "nonself" IgG antibody. Thus, immune complexes are formed with the abnormal IgG, which are then deposited locally

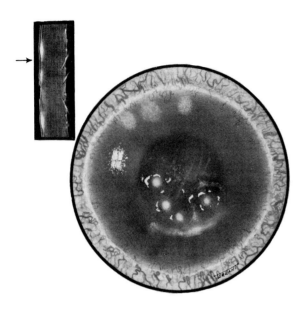

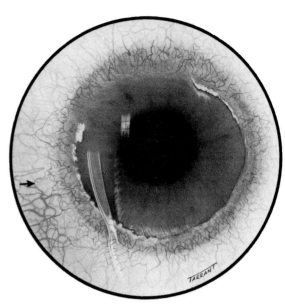

FIGURE 6-24. *Marginal furrow in rheumatoid arthritis. Associated scleritis may also be present. (From P. G. Watson [74].)*

FIGURE 6-23. *Keratitis and scleritis. Cornea is edematous and infiltrated. Inset shows level of corneal disease. (From P. G. Watson [74].)*

in the synovium [8, 26]. These complexes activate the complement cascade, which triggers release of mediators of inflammation, attracts polymorphonuclear leukocytes, and causes tissue destruction and tissue melting. This sequence probably occurs in the sclera and the limbus as well. Destruction of collagen and occlusion of associated vessels results in the scleritis, ischemic necrosis, and melting associated with rheumatoid syndromes.

KERATOLYSIS
Frank melting of clear cornea (Fig. 6-27) may occasionally occur in cases of necrotizing scleritis [74–76]. Although uncommon, it occurs particularly in cases associated with scleromalacia perforans in long-standing RA. The superficial layers of the cornea begin to melt, and a descemetocele may occur in the severest cases. Minor trauma may result in rupture. Keratolysis is almost always associated with severe scleral disease and is not to be confused with limbal guttering, which may be present in the absence of major scleritis.

TREATMENT
The management of KCS includes replacement tear therapy, occlusion of the lacrimal drainage puncta in advanced cases, removal of filaments (if present),

and therapy for associated lid margin infection. (See Chapter 7 for details.)

The treatment of episcleritis and scleritis is directed toward the underlying inflammatory reaction. Initial therapy is frequent topical corticosteroids (every hour to the afflicted eye). Nonsteroid antiinflammatory topical preparations (e.g., topical oxyphenbutazone) are said to be effective but are not available in this country [74, 76]. Unfortunately, topical therapy frequently fails, especially in scleritis; in these cases, Watson and Hazelman suggest oxyphenbutazone as the oral drug of choice in a dosage of 600 mg per day [76]. Early response to therapy includes a dramatic decrease in the deep pain of scleritis, even though the redness remains. Gradual resolution of scleritis occurs over a period of several weeks. Tapering of topical and oral medication is recommended over this period. Prostaglandin inhibitors such as indomethacin can also be used orally as an adjunct. In cases resistant to these drugs, high-dose systemic corticosteroids should be tried (e.g., 100–120 mg prednisone each day). Immunosuppressives (e.g., chlorambucil) have been used in cases resistant to all other forms of therapy and are recommended if all else fails [37]. Active involvement of an experienced internist or rheumatologist is mandatory in the management of such cases, especially when systemic corticosteroids or immunosuppressives are employed. Clues to improvement include rapid relief of pain, decrease in redness, and improvement of vision.

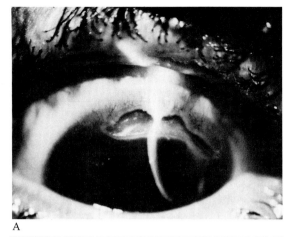

A

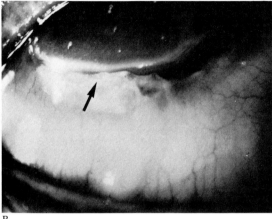

B

FIGURE 6-25. *A. Limbal furrow in rheumatoid arthritis. No associated scleritis. B. Same patient as in A. Note infiltrate* (arrow) *at advancing edge of furrow.*

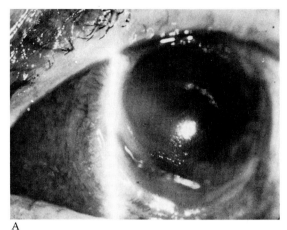

A

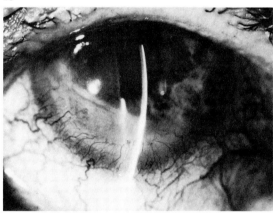

B

FIGURE 6-26. *A. Marginal furrow with scleritis in rheumatoid arthritis. B. Same patient as in A, after local corticosteroid therapy. Note decreased corneal edema and infiltrate and increased neovascularization.*

Therapy for keratitis and sclerosing keratitis includes the use of high-dose topical corticosteroids to prevent progression of the corneal disease and relieve the associated scleritis [4, 74]. Systemic therapy (prostaglandin inhibitors, corticosteroids) as outlined earlier for scleritis is important to treat both the associated scleritis and the corneal disease.

Therapy for marginal furrows associated with RA is controversial. It is important to rule out microbial infection in suspicious cases. If there is no infiltration in the furrow, and a clear zone is present between the limbus and the ulcer, corticosteroids should not be used since there is a danger of perforation [8, 74, 76]. However, if the ulcer resembles a Mooren's ulcer by beginning at the limbus, extending centrally and circumferentially, and having a major infiltrative component, topical steroids may rarely be helpful (Bartley Mondino, M.D., personal communication, 1981). Frequent monitoring is essential since perforation is a definite hazard. Im-

provement and resolution of marginal ulcers with high-dose topical therapy may occur when low-dose and low-frequency therapy have failed.

Topical collagenase inhibitors such as acetylcysteine (Mucomyst 20%) have been used in the treatment of such corneal melting syndromes (five or six times per day) [21]. Hydrophilic bandage lenses may also be effective in creating a structurally intact superficial corneal surface to promote healing. Tissue adhesive (glue) applied in small amounts to the base of the ulcer furrow may be helpful in very thin corneas. In the event that corticosteroid and anticollagenase therapy has no effect, resection of the conjunctiva may be employed [77]. Under local anesthesia, a 3- to 5-mm resection of the conjunctiva is performed to remove inflamed (or uninflamed) conjunctiva adjacent to the furrow itself [77].

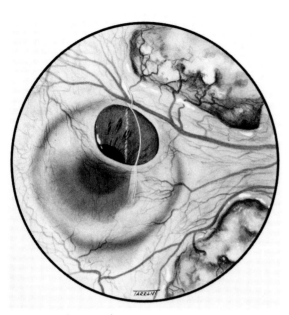

FIGURE 6-27. *Keratolysis in patient with scleritis and keratitis. Superficial layers of cornea have melted away. (From P. G. Watson [74].)*

Aronson, Elliott, and colleagues have recommended heparin to reduce ischemic necrosis secondary to thrombus formation and vascular clotting resulting from severe intrascleral inflammation [3, 4]. Others have not found this to be a successful mode of therapy.

Immunosuppressive therapy has been employed in unusually severe cases in which topical medication did not suffice [37, 74, 76]. Azathioprine, cyclophosphamide, and chlorambucil have been used to treat not only severe rheumatoid systemic disease and severe scleritis, but also the associated corneal melting.

Perforation occurs in the corneal ring ulcer or furrow. If imminent, perforation can be prevented with a ring, patch, or lamellar corneal graft or fascia lata graft [70, 76]. The melting process may involve this graft later [8].

The treatment of keratolysis is directed toward the underlying scleritis and includes frequent administration of topical corticosteroids and systemic prostaglandin inhibitors as outlined in the discussion of scleritis. If a descemetocele has formed, a layover lamellar corneal transplant is indicated [74]. Suturing is difficult because of the thinness of the cornea and sclera. Continued systemic therapy for the underlying scleritis is important in such in-

stances. After therapy for keratolysis, the corneal defects may fill in, but residual irregular thinning of the cornea with permanent scarring is the rule. Penetrating keratoplasty may be necessary for visual purposes at a later date [74, 76].

JUVENILE RHEUMATOID ARTHRITIS

There are several hundred thousand cases of JRA in the United States. It is an important cause of chronic and progressive crippling in childhood in this country. The age of onset is generally between 2 and 4 years, with some cases occurring in preteen years. JRA rarely occurs before the age of 6 months. It occurs a little more frequently in girls than in boys. The iridocyclitis and associated complications are major causes of blindness in children in this country; therefore recognition of this syndrome and accurate classification are important. Band keratopathy is the principal corneal feature of JRA [20, 49, 50].

Classification of the forms of JRA has been clarified over the past several years [9, 10, 12]. There are three relatively distinct forms, and classification is important since ocular inflammation is rare in the more severe systemic form of JRA (Still's). The three types are acute toxic Still's disease, polyarticular JRA, and monarticular (oligoarticular) JRA [9, 10, 12, 60].

CLINICAL FEATURES

Still's disease is the classic febrile, severe illness with large joint involvement, splenomegaly, and lymphadenopathy—a systemic illness [65]. Iridocyclitis (or any other ocular finding) is rare in the Still's category. The polyarticular variety accounts for about 50 percent of patients with JRA and is usually seen in younger children. Fever and lymphadenopathy may occur. The most severely involved group from the ocular standpoint are JRA patients with monarticular onset (one joint involvement) [12, 60]. Although the systemic illness may be very mild in such patients, the ocular complications are very severe and occur in up to 25 percent of patients [12, 60]. Chronic iridocyclitis is the most predominant finding [11, 33, 59, 63, 68]. These patients generally have no systemic illness and may have only vague complaints of arthralgia by history. The presenting symptom may be decreased vision on a routine school examination or the onset of cataract with a white pupil observed by a parent or teacher. Most of these patients do not have acute symptomatic iridocyclitis. By the time they are examined, they may have early band keratopathy, cells and flare in the anterior chamber, dense synechiae with a bound down pupil, secondary cataract, and secondary glaucoma. The disease is usually present bilaterally. Because of the insidious onset and chronic nature of the ocular disease, all patients with known JRA should be examined by an ophthalmologist routinely.

The iridocyclitis is frequently relentlessly progressive, despite corticosteroid therapy, with eventual blindness caused by cataract and glaucoma [42, 64]. Posterior inflammation is uncommon, although lesions of the choroid have been reported. Pathologic findings are nonspecific, with infiltrates (mononuclear cells and lymphocytes) in the ciliary body and iris structures [33]. Synechiae and other secondary complications also occur quite commonly.

A clinical suspicion of JRA is most important in all children with iridocyclitis. Referral to a pediatrician or rheumatologist is mandatory.

Although the most important ocular complication of JRA is chronic iridocyclitis, corneal complications (band keratopathy) also produce visual morbidity. Band keratopathy frequently occurs in young patients with any form of chronic inflammation but is especially prominent in patients with JRA [20]. The keratopathy begins in Bowman's layer, usually at 9 and 3 o'clock, with deposition of calcium crystals. Involvement of the deep layers of the corneal epithelium progresses in a band-shaped fashion across the entire cornea. "Holes" in the calcium deposition give it the characteristic Swiss-cheese appearance in the full-blown clinical pattern. These holes may represent areas where nerves penetrate Bowman's membrane, ending in corneal epithelium.

A number of entities are associated with band keratopathy (Table 6-5). Although it occurs as a secondary change in patients with chronic intraocular inflammation, it also occurs without other major eye problems [13, 19, 25, 31, 49, 54]. In some cases, serum calcium may be elevated [73].

The pathophysiology of the deposition of calcium crystal in Bowman's membrane is unclear. O'Connor has reviewed this problem and proposes the following mechanism [50]: 99 percent of the body's calcium is in the form of bone or hydroxyapatite, a complex crystalline structure with calcium and phosphate ions. Excess calcium favors precipitation as a calcium phosphate under certain local conditions. Doughman and associates felt that evaporation in the interpalpebral area resulted in deposition of calcium salts in a band configuration [18]. In addition to the evaporation, which would favor the precipitation of calcium phosphate, O'Connor also implicated the diffusion of gases with a subsequent increase in local pH [50]. Loss of CO_2, which affects the ionization of carbonic acid, may result in a decrease in the availability of free hydrogen ions and therefore increase the pH specifically in the exposed

TABLE 6-5. *Conditions Associated with Band Keratopathy*

Local degenerative diseases
  Chronic uveitis
  Phthisis bulbi
  Absolute glaucoma
  Juvenile rheumatoid arthritis
  Interstitial keratitis
Trauma
  Chronic exposure to irritants such as mercury fumes, calomel, calcium bichromate vapor
Hypercalcemia
  Hyperparathyroidism
  Excessive vitamin D, as with oral intake, sarcoidosis with liver involvement, osteoporosis
  Renal failure, as with Fanconi's syndrome (cystinosis)
  Hypophosphatasia
  Milk-alkali syndrome
  Paget's disease
  Idiopathic
Discoid lupus erythematosus
Gout (urate crystals)
Tuberous sclerosis
Anterior mosaic dystrophy, primary type
  Labrador keratopathy
Ichthyosis
Rothmund-Thomson syndrome: bilateral cataracts, skin pigmentation, telangiectasis
Idiopathic
Progressive facial hemiatrophy (Parry-Romberg syndrome)

SOURCE: Modified from Roy [54].

area of the cornea (interpalpebral area). Increased gaseous exchange at the surface of the exposed cornea in the interpalpebral area with loss of CO_2 and increase in pH thus would result in deposition of the calcium phosphate crystalline material comprising the band.

O'Connor also performed extensive histopathologic examinations of eyes with band keratopathy, including those from patients with JRA and uveitis [50]. Calcific deposits were found in Bowman's layer, in the basement membrane of the epithelium, and in the superficial stromal lamellae. These were common changes regardless of the cause.

Serum levels of calcium are not elevated in JRA patients; however, it is postulated that in the development of bone in children, there is more circulating calcium ion available for deposition in the form of band keratopathy.

LABORATORY STUDIES

Antinuclear antibody is present in 80 percent of patients with JRA who develop iridocyclitis. It is absent in JRA patients who do *not* develop iridocyclitis [58]. Sedimentation rate is elevated and rheumatoid factor is absent [49, 60]. The knee is the most common joint involved, and a routine knee examination and x-ray is recommended in cases in which JRA is suspected, even in the absence of clinically active arthritis [79].

DIFFERENTIAL DIAGNOSIS

Uveitis in childhood results from a group of diseases that it is important to differentiate. Toxocariasis, pars planitis, and toxoplasmosis are common posterior or diffuse forms of ocular inflammation in children, and it is important to differentiate these entities since therapy and prognosis vary. Sarcoidosis uncommonly occurs in childhood and may mimic JRA. We have seen patients who have been followed for JRA when, in fact, they had sarcoid iridocyclitis. Chest x-ray, skin testing for anergy, and other tests for sarcoidosis are important in the differential diagnosis of suspicious cases of iridocyclitis in children. The presence of joint changes and the typical history help make the diagnosis of JRA. Antinuclear antibody is present in the serum of JRA patients who have iridocyclitis.

TREATMENT

Therapy for the chronic form of iridocyclitis in JRA is often ineffectual [42, 59, 63–65]. Very early cases may present with just a few cells in the anterior chamber and no synechiae. Dilating agents alone are recommended in early cases since such patients are often subject to a long-term chronic course of corticosteroids with little hope for resolution of the process. Corticosteroids are recommended in cases in which the anterior chamber cellular reaction increases and synechiae begin to form. At this stage, topical steroids should be titrated and every attempt made to avoid overuse of this drug. These patients often have a tremendous amount of flare in the anterior chamber at all times, even in the absence of cellular reaction. Flare will be present indefinitely because of the breakdown of the blood-aqueous barrier. Flare alone is *not* an indication for corticosteroid therapy. The presence of numerous cells in the anterior chamber, on the other hand, is an indication for treatment. If topical corticosteroids are not effective and there is marked progression of the disease, then sub-Tenon injections may be necessary. Although topical corticosteroids may be sufficient to suppress the inflammation in the more acute forms, in the chronic form there may be exacerbations requiring systemic corticosteroids. However, the intraocular inflammation tends to be chronic and recurrent, and topical corticosteroids are preferred if the intraocular inflammation can be suppressed. In severe, intractable cases with progressive disease leading to bilateral blindness, immunosuppressives such as chlorambucil may be used [48].

Glaucoma is initially managed as are all forms of secondary glaucoma: medically. Miotics, however, should be avoided. The management of cataract in JRA is a serious problem. Results of standard surgery have been poor [42, 64], and combined lensectomy and vitrectomy may be appropriate in some cases [15, 16]. In cases in which only one eye is involved and the other eye is normal, it is probably best to avoid surgery in the involved eye as long as no retinal complications are present.

It is important to monitor JRA patients closely since they frequently do not complain of photophobia and redness but rather present with far advanced intraocular inflammation, cataract, band keratopathy, and glaucoma. In general, the acute varieties of iridocyclitis associated with JRA do much better with better resolution and fewer recurrences than does the chronic variety, which has a poor prognosis [20, 50].

Therapy for band keratopathy includes the use of chelating agents [20, 50]. A variety of techniques may be employed. In general, a topical anesthetic is applied, the epithelium is removed with an applicator or blade, and dilute (1:50) disodium EDTA (0.37M) is applied with a cotton-tip applicator with vigorous massage of the underlying Bowman's membrane to remove the calcium deposits. After allowing the EDTA to soak into Bowman's layer for several minutes, a knife may be used to scrape the remaining calcium deposits. A cycloplegic agent and antibiotic are instilled and a semipressure patch applied until the epithelium heals. (See Chapter 9 for more details.)

RELAPSING POLYCHONDRITIS

Relapsing polychondritis, an uncommon connective tissue disease, is also known as chronic atrophic polychondritis [1, 32, 41, 71]. Systemically, there is recurrent inflammation of the cartilaginous tissues throughout the body, particularly in the ears and nose. The disease occurs equally in men and women, with onset between the ages of 30 and 50 years.

The pinnae of the ears are the most commonly involved area [17]. The ears become red, swollen, and painful. This gradually subsides over a period of weeks. Resorption of ear cartilage may result in flaccid, drooping ears. Arthritis may also be seen but should not be confused with the disabling and destructive joint disease associated with RA. When nasal cartilage is involved, there is pain on movement of the nose, destruction of cartilage, and deformity of the nose. Aortic, laryngotracheal, and costal cartilages may also be involved. The course of the systemic disease is variable but may be fatal in a low percentage of patients if vital structures, such as the aortic ring or trachea, are seriously involved. Cardiovascular and respiratory complications are the cause of death in such cases [17, 28].

The pathogenesis of relapsing polychondritis is unknown [17]. Antibodies to cartilage have been found in these patients [28]. There are no specific laboratory tests to assist in the diagnosis of relapsing polychondritis. The sedimentation rate is usually elevated. Serum protein abnormalities and leukocytosis occur. Most patients have no rheumatoid factor, no LE cells, and negative results on serum tests for syphilis. However, there may be other associated systemic collagen disorders including vasculitis or SLE. Pathologic examination reveals acute inflammatory changes in the cartilage (early) or atrophy and fibrous replacement of cartilage (late) [28, 41, 71].

Therapy for the systemic disorder includes antiinflammatory agents in high doses to decrease the severe inflammatory involvement of cartilage. Occasionally, immunosuppressive agents such as azathioprine may be necessary.

A variety of ocular findings have been associated with relapsing polychondritis, including episcleritis (40 percent of cases), conjunctivitis (25 percent of cases), iridocyclitis, and keratitis [2, 5, 6, 35, 45, 47, 55, 56]. In fact, episcleritis or conjunctivitis may be the presenting features of relapsing polychondritis in some cases. KCS, abducens nerve palsies, and exophthalmos have also been reported [56].

Localized peripheral corneal infiltrates with moderate progressive thinning have been reported [28]. This may be associated with thinning of the sclera and early staphyloma formation. Normal anterior segment angiograms have been reported with these findings, which suggests that scleral and corneal melting is not caused by underlying vasculitis or an ischemic process [78]. The cause of the corneal complications is not known. The serious ocular complications of relapsing polychondritis are related to peripheral corneal ulcerations (melting), which may, in rare cases, result in corneal perforation and its complications [28, 75].

Therapy for corneal complications of relapsing polychondritis includes high-dose topical corticosteroids and management of the associated systemic

process [28, 74]. Treatment of associated KCS is tear replacement.

ACKNOWLEDGMENT
We thank William Chin, M.D., Assistant Clinical Professor of Medicine, University of Southern California, for critically reviewing this manuscript.

REFERENCES

1. Anderson, B. Ocular lesions in relapsing polychondritis and other rheumatoid syndromes: The Edward Jackson Memorial Lecture. *Am. J. Ophthalmol.* 64:35, 1967.
2. Anderson, B. Ocular lesions in relapsing polychondritis and other rheumatoid syndromes. *Trans. Am. Acad. Ophthalmol. Otolaryngol.* 71:227, 1967.
3. Aronson, S. B., et al. Pathogenetic approach to therapy of peripheral corneal inflammatory disease. *Am. J. Ophthalmol.* 70:65, 1970.
4. Aronson, S. B., and Elliott, J. H. Scleritis. In B. Golden (Ed.), *Ocular Inflammatory Disease.* Springfield, Ill.: Thomas, 1974. Pp. 43–49.
5. Barth, W. F., and Berson, E. L. Relapsing polychondritis, rheumatoid arthritis and blindness. *Am. J. Ophthalmol.* 66:890, 1968.
6. Bergaust, B., and Abrahamsen, A. M. Relapsing polychondritis: Report of a case presenting multiple ocular complications. *Acta Ophthalmol.* 47:174, 1969.
7. Brown, A. J., McLendon, B. F., and Camp, A. V. Epithelial deposition of gold in the cornea of patients receiving systemic therapy. *Am. J. Ophthalmol.* 88:354, 1979.
8. Brown, S. I., and Grayson, M. Marginal furrows: A characteristic corneal lesion of rheumatoid arthritis. *Arch. Ophthalmol.* 79:563, 1968.
9. Bywaters, E. G. L., and Ansell, B. M. Monoarticular arthritis in children. *Ann. Rheum. Dis.* 24:116, 1965.
10. Calabro, J. J., and Marchesano, J. M. Juvenile rheumatoid arthritis. *N. Engl. J. Med.* 277:696, 746, 1967.
11. Calabro, J. J., et al. Chronic iridocyclitis in juvenile rheumatoid arthritis. *Arthritis Rheum.* 13:406, 1970.
12. Calabro, J. J., Parrino, G. R., and Marchesano, J. M. Monarticular-onset juvenile rheumatoid arthritis. *Bull. Rheum. Dis.* 21:613, 1970.
13. Cogan, D. G., Albright, F., and Bartler, F. C. Hypercalcemia and band keratopathy. *Arch. Ophthalmol.* 40:624, 1948.
14. The Cooperating Clinics Committee of the American Rheumatism Association. A con-

trolled trial of gold salt therapy in rheumatoid arthritis. *Arthritis Rheum.* 16:353, 1973.

15. Diamond, J. G., and Kaplan, H. J. Lensectomy and vitrectomy for complicated cataract secondary to uveitis. *Arch. Ophthalmol.* 96:1798, 1978.

16. Diamond, J. G., and Kaplan, H. J. Uveitis: Effect of vitrectomy combined with lensectomy. *Ophthalmology* (Rochester) 86:1320, 1979.

17. Dolan, D. L., Lemmon, G. B., and Teitelbaum, S. L. Relapsing polychondritis: Analytical literature review and studies on pathogenesis. *Am. J. Med.* 41:285, 1966.

18. Doughman, D. J., Olson, G. A., and Nolan, S. Experimental band keratopathy. *Arch. Ophthalmol.* 81:264, 1969.

19. Duke-Elder, S., and Leigh, A. G. Diseases of the Outer Eye. In S. Duke-Elder (Ed.), *System of Ophthalmology.* St. Louis: Mosby, 1965. Vol. 8, Pt. 2, p. 898.

20. Edstrom, G. Band-shaped keratitis in juvenile rheumatoid arthritis. *Acta Rheum. Scand.* 7:169, 1961.

21. Eiferman, R. A., Carothers, D. J., and Yankeelov, J. A., Jr. Peripheral rheumatoid ulceration and evidence for conjunctival collagenase production. *Am. J. Ophthalmol.* 87:703, 979.

22. Empire Rheumatism Council. Gold therapy in rheumatoid arthritis: Final report of a multiclinic controlled trial. *Ann. Rheum. Dis.* 20:315, 1961.

23. Ennis, R. S., Granada, J. L., and Posner, A. S. Effect of gold salts and other drugs on the release and activity of lysosomal hydrolases. *Arthritis Rheum.* 11:756, 1968.

24. Ferry, A. P. The histopathology of rheumatoid episcleral nodules. *Arch. Ophthalmol.* 82:77, 1969.

25. Fishman, R. S., and Sunderman, F. W. Band keratopathy in gout. *Arch. Ophthalmol.* 75:367, 1966.

26. Friedlaender, M. H. Ocular allergy and immunology. *J. Allergy Clin. Immunol.* 63:51, 1979.

27. Fye, K. H., Terasaki, P. I., and Michalski, J. B. Relationship of HLA-DW3 and HLA-B8 to Sjögren's syndrome. *Arthritis Rheum.* 21:377, 1978.

28. Gold, D. H. Ocular Manifestations of Connective Tissue (Collagen) Disease. In T. Duane (Ed.), *Clinical Ophthalmology.* Hagerstown, Md.: Harper & Row, 1980. Vol. 5, Chap. 26, pp. 1–30.

29. Gordon, D. A., Stein, J. L., and Border, I. The extra-articular features of rheumatoid arthritis: A systematic analysis of 127 cases. *Am. J. Med.* 54:445, 1973.

30. Gottlieb, N. L., Smith, P. M., and Smith, E. M. Tissue gold concentration in a rheumatoid arthritic receiving chrysotherapy. *Arthritis Rheum.* 15:16, 1972.

31. Grayson, M., and Keates, R. H. *Manual of Diseases of the Cornea.* Boston: Little, Brown, 1969. P. 293.

32. Hilding, A. C. Syndrome of joint and cartilaginous pathologic changes with destructive iridocyclitis: Comparison with described concurrent eye and joint diseases. *Arch. Intern. Med.* 89:445, 1952.

33. Hinzpeter, E. N., Naumann, G., and Bartelheimer, H. K. Ocular histopathology in Still's disease. *Ophthalmol. Res.* 2:16, 1971.

34. Hollander, J. L., et al. Studies on the pathogenesis of rheumatoid joint inflammation: I. The "R.A. cell" and a working hypothesis. *Ann. Intern. Med.* 62:271, 1965.

35. Hughes, R. A. C., et al. Relapsing polychondritis: Three cases with a clinico-pathological study and literature review. *Q. J. Med.* 163:363, 1972.

36. Immune complexes in rheumatic disease (editorial). *Lancet* 2:79, 1976.

37. Jampol, L. M., West, C., and Goldberg, M. F. Therapy of scleritis with cytotoxic agents. *Am. J. Ophthalmol.* 86:266, 1978.

38. Jayson, M. I. V., and Easty, D. L. Ulceration of the cornea in rheumatoid arthritis. *Ann. Rheum. Dis.* 36:428, 1977.

39. Jayson, M. I. V., and Jones, D. E. P. Rheumatoid arthritis and scleritis. *Trans. Ophthalmol. Soc. U.K.* 91:189, 1971.

40. Jayson, M. I. V., and Jones, D. E. P. Scleritis and rheumatoid arthritis. *Ann. Rheum. Dis.* 30:343, 1971.

41. Kaye, R. L., and Sones, D. A. Relapsing polychondritis: Clinical and pathologic features in fourteen cases. *Ann. Intern. Med.* 60:653, 1964.

42. Key, S. N., III, and Kimura, S. J. Iridocyclitis associated with juvenile rheumatoid arthritis. *Am. J. Ophthalmol.* 80:425, 1975.

43. Lachman, S. M., Hazelman, B. L., and Watson, P. G. Scleritis and associated disease. *Br. Med. J.* 1:88, 1978.

44. Lyne, A. J., and Pitkeathley, D. A. Episcleritis and scleritis: Association with connective tissue disease. *Arch. Ophthalmol.* 80:171, 1968.

45. Matas, B. R. Iridocyclitis associated with relapsing polychondritis. *Arch. Ophthalmol.* 84:474, 1970.

46. McGavin, D. D. M., et al. Episcleritis and scleritis: A study of their clinical manifestations and associations with rheumatoid arthritis. *Br. J. Ophthalmol.* 60:192, 1976.

47. McKay, D. A. R., Watson, P. G., and Lyne, A. J. Relapsing polychondritis and eye disease. *Br. J. Ophthalmol.* 58:600, 1974.

48. Mehra, R., et al. Chlorambucil in the treat-

ment of iridocyclitis in juvenile rheumatoid arthritis. *J. Rheumatol.* 8:141, 1981.

49. Michels, R. G. Ocular Manifestations in Arthritis. In S. J. Ryan and R. E. Smith (Eds.), *The Eye in Systemic Disease.* New York: Grune & Stratton, 1974. Pp. 363–379.

50. O'Connor, G. R. Calcific band keratopathy. *Trans. Am. Ophthalmol. Soc.* 70:58, 1972.

51. Powell, T. R., et al. HLA-Bw44 and HLA-DRw4 in male Sjögren's syndrome patients with associated rheumatoid arthritis. *Clin. Immunol. Immunopathol.* 17:463, 1980.

52. Rawson, A. J., Abelson, N. M., and Hollander, J. L. Studies on the pathogenesis of rheumatoid joint inflammation: II. Intracytoplasmic particulate complexes in rheumatoid synovial fluids. *Ann. Intern. Med.* 62:281, 1965.

53. Restifo, R. A., et al. Studies on the pathogenesis of rheumatoid joint inflammation: III. *Ann. Intern. Med.* 62:185, 1965.

54. Roy, F. H. *Ocular Differential Diagnosis* (2nd ed.). Philadelphia: Lea & Febiger, 1975. Pp. 191–192.

55. Rucker, C. W., and Ferguson, R. H. Ocular manifestations of relapsing polychondritis. *Trans. Am. Ophthalmol. Soc.* 62:167, 1964.

56. Rucker, C. W., and Ferguson, R. H. Ocular manifestations of relapsing polychondritis. *Arch. Ophthalmol.* 73:46, 1965.

57. Ruddy, S., and Austen, K. F. The complement system in rheumatoid synovitis: I. An analysis of complement component activities in rheumatoid synovial fluids. *Arthritis Rheum.* 13:713, 1970.

58. Schaller, J., et al. Antinuclear antibodies (ANA) in patients with iridocyclitis and juvenile rheumatoid arthritis (JRA, Still's disease). *Arthritis Rheum.* 16:130, 1973.

59. Schaller, J., Kupfer, C., and Wedgwood, R. J. Iridocyclitis in juvenile rheumatoid arthritis. *Pediatrics* 44:92, 1969.

60. Schaller, J., Smiley, W. K., and Ansell, B. M. Iridocyclitis of juvenile rheumatoid arthritis (JRA, Still's disease): A follow-up study of 76 patients. *Arthritis Rheum.* 16:130, 1973.

61. Schmid, F. R., et al. Arteritis in rheumatoid arthritis. *Am. J. Med.* 30:56, 1961.

62. Sevel, D. Rheumatoid nodule of the sclera. *Trans. Ophthalmol. Soc. U.K.* 85:357, 1965.

63. Smiley, W. K. Iridocyclitis in Still's disease. *Trans. Ophthalmol. Soc. U.K.* 85:351, 1965.

64. Smiley, W. K. The eye in juvenile rheumatoid arthritis. *Trans. Ophthalmol. Soc. U.K.* 94:817, 1974.

65. Smiley, W. K., May, E., and Bywaters, E. G. L. Ocular presentations of Still's disease and their treatment. Iridocyclitis in Still's disease: Its complications and treatment. *Ann. Rheum. Dis.* 16:371, 1957.

66. Stage, D. E., and Mannik, M. Rheumatoid factors in rheumatoid arthritis. *Bull. Rheum. Dis.* 23:720, 1972–1973.

67. Stanworth, A. The association of ocular and articular disease. *Trans. Ophthalmol. Soc. U.K.* 71:189, 1951.

68. Stewart, A. J., and Hill, R. H. Ocular manifestations in juvenile rheumatoid arthritis. *Can. J. Ophthalmol.* 2:58, 1967.

69. Thompson, M., and Eadie, S. Keratoconjunctivitis sicca and rheumatoid arthritis. *Ann. Rheum. Dis.* 15:21, 1956.

70. Torchia, R. T., Dunn, R. E., and Pease, P. J. Fascia lata grafting in scleromalacia perforans with lamellar corneal-scleral dissection. *Am. J. Ophthalmol.* 66:705, 1968.

71. Verity, M. A., Larson, W. M., and Madden, S. C. Relapsing polychondritis: Report of two necropsied cases with histochemical investigation of the cartilage lesion. *Am. J. Pathol.* 42:251, 1963.

72. Walker, W. C., and Wright, V. Pulmonary lesions and rheumatoid arthritis. *Medicine* 47:501, 1968.

73. Walsh, F. B., and Howard, J. E. Conjunctival and corneal lesions in hypercalcemia. *J. Clin. Endocrinol.* 7:644, 1947.

74. Watson, P. G. Diseases of the Sclera and Episclera. In T. Duane (Ed.), *Clinical Ophthalmology.* Hagerstown, Md.: Harper & Row, 1980. Vol. 4, Chap. 23, pp. 1–39.

75. Watson, P. G., and Hayreh, S. S. Scleritis and episcleritis. *Br. J. Ophthalmol.* 60:163, 1976.

76. Watson, P. G., and Hazelman, B. L. *The Sclera and Systemic Disorders.* London: Saunders, 1976.

77. Wilson, F. M., Grayson, M., and Ellis, F. D. Treatment of peripheral corneal ulcers by limbal conjunctivectomy. *Br. J. Ophthalmol.* 59:675, 1975.

78. Zion, V. M., Brackup, A. H., and Weingeist, S. Relapsing polychondritis, erythema nodosum and sclerouveitis: A case report with anterior segment angiography. *Surv. Ophthalmol.* 19:107, 1974.

79. Zizic, T. M., and Stevens, M. B. Rheumatoid Arthritis and Varients. In S. J. Ryan and R. E. Smith (Eds.), *The Eye in Systemic Disease.* New York: Grune & Stratton, 1974. Pp. 315–339.

80. Zvaifler, N. J. A speculation on the pathogenesis of joint inflammation in rheumatoid arthritis. *Arthritis Rheum.* 8:289, 1965.

81. Zvaifler, N. J. Further speculation on the pathogenesis of joint inflammation in rheumatoid arthritis. *Arthritis Rheum.* 13:895, 1970.

Ocular Manifestations of the Nonrheumatic Acquired Collagen Vascular Diseases

C. Stephen Foster

SYSTEMIC LUPUS ERYTHEMATOSUS

The modern history of systemic lupus erythematosus (SLE) began with the 1939 descriptions by Rose and Pillsbury [83] of disseminated multiorgan involvement in this chronic, progressive disease of unknown etiology. With the publication, in 1941, of the now classic paper, "Pathology of Disseminated Lupus Erythematosus," by Klemperer, Pollack, and Baehr [59], in which the importance of vasculitis was emphasized, research interest in this disease with protean manifestations expanded greatly. SLE is a clinical syndrome of unknown etiology characterized by multisystem involvement and subject to multiple remissions and exacerbations in one or more systems. It is a chronic, often progressive pleomorphic disease. The clinical course of SLE may be mild or severe and continuous or recurrent, with destructive inflammatory processes affecting any organ. The eight organ systems most notably involved in SLE are

System	Involvement
Articular	Arthralgias, arthritis, aseptic bone necrosis
Cutaneous	Rash, alopecia, photosensitivity
Renal	Glomerulonephritis
Hematologic	Anemia, leukopenia, autoantibodies
Pulmonary	Pleurisy, pleural effusion, pneumonitis
Neurologic	Behavioral disturbance, seizures, mononeuritis
Cardiovascular	Raynaud's phenomenon, vasculitis, pericarditis
Ocular	Corneal epitheliopathy, scleritis, retinopathy

INCIDENCE AND PREVALENCE

The estimated incidence (new cases per unit population per unit time) of SLE has increased over the past 30 years from 0.5 in 100,000 in 1950 to between 2.7 and 7.6 in 100,000 in 1974 and 1973 (data from New York and San Francisco, respectively) [29, 87]. How much of this increase is a true increase in disease frequency and how much is the result of improved diagnostic capabilities is unclear, but certainly improved techniques for diagnosing SLE and increased awareness of the disease by physicians have contributed to the increase. The prevalence of SLE (the total number of cases existing in a given period) has similarly increased to between 15.5 and 50.0 cases in 100,000. This increase has resulted from the increased incidence and improved survival of patients with SLE.

Although SLE occurs in both males and females and has been reported to have its onset as early as 1 year of age or as late as age 90, it is found primarily in women of childbearing age. Approximately 90 percent of patients with SLE are women, and most of them experience onset of symptoms between ages 15 and 45. Most studies show no racial predilection for this disease.

PATHOGENESIS

Although the fundamental cause of SLE is unknown, the best available body of scientific evidence today strongly points to a dysfunction in immunoregulation. The most reasonable hypothesis for the pathogenesis of this disease includes a genetic predisposition to the development of defective suppressor T-lymphocyte function, possibly after the perturbation of the immune system by some environmental factor. Defective T cell function then results in inadequately controlled helper T-lymphocyte and B-lymphocyte function, with resultant production of autoantibodies. Autoantigen-autoantibody immune complexes are formed, predominantly in the circulation, and then deposited in certain organs and tissue locations, primarily because of physical factors and molecular sieving restrictions. Activation of the complement pathway, through both classic and alternate routes, then causes, at the site of the immune-complex deposition, chemotaxis of neutrophils and macrophages, release of proteolytic enzymes, and activation of the clotting cascade sequence, as well as the activation of various kinins. It appears that the bulk of the tissue damage occurring in SLE results from these latter reactions and tissue digestion by the proteolytic enzymes, particularly from neutrophils.

Patients with SLE have been shown to have decreased numbers of suppressor T-lymphocytes and those present have been shown to be functionally defective, particularly during periods of major disease activity [1, 3, 26, 67]. There is a pronounced impairment in the ability of suppressor T-lymphocytes from SLE patients to control B-lymphocyte antibody synthesis. Once defective suppressor T-lymphocyte function is triggered, probably by some environmental factor in the genetically predisposed person, antilymphocyte antibodies are manufactured, along with many other autoantibodies. One of the more prominent antilymphocyte antibodies manufactured in these patients is one that is specifically reactive with suppressor T-lymphocytes. The activity of this autoantibody probably further compromises suppressor T-lymphocyte function, with a resultant increase in disease activity.

PREDISPOSING FACTORS
Family studies have provided evidence for both genetic and environmental factors in the development of SLE. Both related and unrelated household contacts of SLE patients have a higher incidence of circulating autoantibodies than the population at large [18], and approximately 5 percent of patients with SLE are found to have family members with the disease as well. The available evidence suggests that both genetic predisposition and environmental stimuli are important in the development of serologic abnormalities and clinically apparent SLE.

GENETIC FACTORS
Strong evidence for a major role of genetic susceptibility in the development of SLE has emerged from family studies, studies of monozygotic and dizygotic twins [8], genetic studies of the composition of the region on chromosome 6 where the putative immune response gene is located, and studies of the New Zealand (NZ) mouse model of SLE.

Genetic studies, primarily those involving HLA typing, have failed to show any relationship between HLA-A/B/C phenotype and SLE susceptibility. But recent evidence suggests that HLA-DW2 or HLA-DW3 may predispose to SLE [38, 80]. There is also an increased incidence of Ia-715 phenotypes in SLE patients compared to those without SLE [80]. Schur [85] has reported a higher incidence of SLE in patients with inherited deficiencies of complement. This is of interest since the gene coding for synthesis of the second component of complement is believed to lie in close juxtaposition to a putative immune response gene on chromosome 6 of humans.

ENVIRONMENTAL FACTORS
A great deal of evidence suggests that, in the genetically susceptible person, certain environmental stimuli, such as viral infection, ultraviolet irradiation, or contact with certain drugs, induce alterations in DNA, immunoregulatory networks, or both, with resultant formation of autoantibodies, including antinuclear antibody. DeHoratius and co-workers [18] showed that unrelated persons in the same household as patients with SLE had an increased frequency of antilymphocyte antibodies, compared with the normal population. In the Nevada study of Chantler and colleagues [11], the impressive prevalence of eight cases of SLE in six different families in a community of less than 3000 over a 15-year period was suggestive of an environmental influence on the development of SLE.

A number of investigators have hypothesized that SLE can be caused by inappropriate immune responses to viral infection. Type C virus (oncornavirus C within the RNA reovirus family) endogenous xenotropic infection is commonly present in NZ mice and is transmitted vertically, during cell division, from parent to offspring. This virus has a particular tropism for thymus cells, and most investigators believe this is at least partially responsible for the thymic dysfunction and disturbed immunoregulation seen in these mice [74]. Viral glycoprotein–antiviral glycoprotein immune-complex deposits are found in the nephritic kidneys of NZB/NZW mice [100]. Conflicting data have been obtained in studies for type C viral antigens in humans [46, 66, 73, 75].

Ultraviolet irradiation is another environmental factor that may trigger the development of, or aggravate, SLE in the genetically susceptible person. Twenty-five to 35 percent of SLE patients are photosensitive (compared with 1 percent of normal persons and 1 percent of patients with rheumatoid arthritis). Tan and Rodnan [93] believe that DNA damage from ultraviolet irradiation may trigger the development of SLE. About one-third of patients with SLE have antibodies against ultraviolet-damaged DNA [94].

A number of drugs are capable of altering DNA and stimulating the production of antinuclear antibodies. Fifteen to 70 percent of those receiving these drugs (hydralazine, procainamide, methyldopa, isoniazid, chlorpromazine, hydantoins, ethosuximide, trimethadione) over a prolonged period will develop antinuclear antibodies. Some people may be more genetically susceptible to development of pathologic changes from the immune complexes that result from antinuclear antibody–DNA reactions or from inappropriate immunoregulatory responses to the development of DNA alterations and the formation of antinuclear antibodies. These may be the patients who develop clinically obvious SLE after ingestion of these drugs.

Hormonal factors may influence the development or clinical expression of SLE. As has been pointed out above, for example, the disease occurs much more commonly in females than in males. And approximately 30 percent of female patients with SLE have a major increase in disease activity during pregnancy [102]. Studies from the NZB/NZW F1 mouse model of SLE also lend support to the notion that hormonal factors may play an important role in the clinical expression of SLE [89]. The evidence suggests that female sex hormones are important in triggering or permitting the immune responses that result in the development of clinically apparent SLE; it may also be that male sex hormones offer some protection against the disease.

CLINICAL FEATURES

OCULAR INVOLVEMENT

Although the ophthalmologist may be the first physician to see the patient with SLE, more commonly the patient is referred to the ophthalmologist for evaluation of ocular symptoms. The most conspicuous findings are those related to the cornea and sclera, but the retinal and choroidal findings frequently serve as a better barometer of the severity and prognosis of the disease.

CORNEAL

The corneal manifestations of SLE are, by and large, confined to the epithelium. Although peripheral ulcerative keratitis has been reported in patients with SLE and keratitis and neovascularization have been described in patients with discoid lupus [44, 48, 51, 79], these lesions rarely occur in SLE. Sicca syndrome is quite common, however, in SLE patients with inadequately controlled systemic disease.

Pillat [77] reported superficial keratitis in 1 of his 16 patients with SLE, and Gold and associates [43] found a 6.5 percent incidence of keratitis in an outpatient population of SLE patients. Spaeth [88] found, in a study of SLE patients hospitalized at the National Institutes of Health, that 88 percent had superficial punctate keratitis with fluorescein corneal staining. He reported that Schirmer test results were normal in these patients, and therefore the issue of whether the superficial punctate keratitis seen in patients with SLE is always truly the result of sicca syndrome or in fact is secondary to corneal epithelial damage associated with lupus disease activity is unclear (Fig. 6-28). Reeves [79] described bilateral deep segmental interstitial keratitis and subsequent recurrent iritis in a patient who 1 year later developed cutaneous, articular, and hematologic manifestations of SLE. Halmay and Ludwig [48] had described similar cases previously, and Grayson [44] mentioned deep stromal keratitis as a rare finding in patients with SLE.

Superficial punctate keratitis can also occur in patients with discoid lupus erythematosus (DLE). Doesschat [20] reported persistent superficial punc-

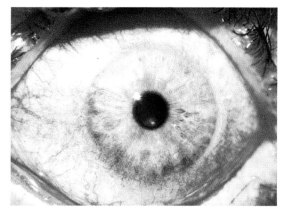

FIGURE 6-28. *Rose bengal staining of conjunctival and corneal epithelium in a patient with systemic lupus erythematosus. The Schirmer values are 12 mm of wetting, OU, after topical anesthesia.*

tate keratitis and recurrent corneal epithelial erosion in a patient with DLE. The corneal lesions were minimal in the superior cornea, where the ocular surface was protected from the environment by the upper lid. Doesschat reported marked improvement in the keratopathy in association with systemic quinacrine hydrochloride therapy. I [31] reported similar findings in a patient with chronic blepharoconjunctivitis and keratitis of 4 years' duration, in whom the diagnosis of DLE was made on the basis of histopathologic study of lid skin; systemic quinacrine hydrochloride therapy resulted in prompt resolution of the ocular lesions. Lid abrasions from SLE may lead to secondary changes such as trichiasis and exposure.

SCLERAL

Episcleritis or scleritis may occur in patients with SLE and may be the initial presenting manifestation of the disease [32]. Scleritis is a reasonably accurate guide to the presence of major systemic activity in the SLE patient. As in the case of retinopathy, it is suggested that any patient who develops scleritis be examined for SLE. Scleritis will resolve with adequate control of systemic disease; it will not respond to topical therapy (Fig. 6-29). Uveitis is an unusual isolated finding in SLE. It may rarely occur in the absence of other ocular lesions but usually is seen in association with severe lupus scleritis.

Finally, iatrogenic ocular lesions occur in SLE patients treated with corticosteroids or antimalarial drugs. Cataract and (rarely) glaucoma may occur with long-term systemic corticosteroid therapy, and the retinopathy secondary to high-dose or prolonged antimalarial drug therapy is well known.

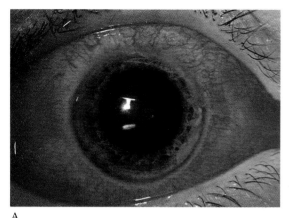

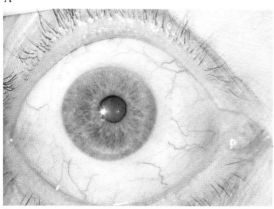

A

B

FIGURE 6-29. A. Diffuse scleritis as the presenting manifestation of systemic lupus erythematosus. Therapy with systemic oxyphenbutazone and topical 1% prednisolone acetate failed to affect the scleral and episcleral inflammation. After confirmation of diagnosis, systemic prednisone therapy was begun. The intense scleritis resolved within 72 hours. B. Same eye, after resolution of the scleritis by treatment with systemic prednisone.

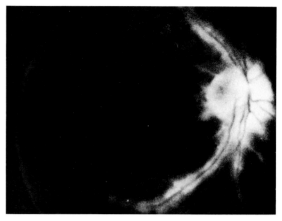

FIGURE 6-30. Fluorescein angiogram of a patient with systemic lupus erythematosus. Note the leakage of fluorescein dye from the retinal vessels, indicating retinal vasculitis.

RETINAL AND CHOROIDAL

A major event early in the development of lupus retinopathy is the appearance of retinal vasculitis, which is evident on fluorescein angiography (Fig. 6-30). Similar findings may occur in iris vessels as well (Fig. 6-31). Subtle macular or disc edema may appear next, followed by intraretinal hemorrhages and cotton-wool spots (Fig. 6-32). These latter changes may be indistinguishable from hypertensive retinopathy; in the SLE patient with idiopathic, renal, or iatrogenic hypertension, it may be impossible for the clinician to decide whether the retinal lesions are secondary to hypertension or to SLE immune-complex vasculitis. A combined posterior segment and anterior segment fluorescein angiographic search for vasculitis may be helpful in this regard.

Gold and coworkers [43] have emphasized that the appearance and disappearance of retinal lesions in SLE patients parallel the systemic clinical course and that effective therapeutic control of the systemic disease is associated with a dramatic decrease in retinal lesions. Although absolute direct proof that the lesions of lupus retinopathy are caused by immune-complex vasculitis is lacking, clinical and experimental evidence to support this assumption does exist. Aronson and associates [5] found immunoglobulin and complement components in the ciliary processes and choroidal vasculature of the eyes of a patient who died of SLE, and immunoglobulins and complement have been demonstrated in the ciliary body and choroidal vasculature of eyes from rabbits in an animal model of serum sickness. This suggests that whenever a patient with SLE develops retinopathy (or whenever existing retinopathy worsens), a thorough study of renal and pulmonary status should be done and the appropriate serologic studies be performed in search of systemic evidence for disease activity, with prompt, aggressive therapy and longitudinal monitoring of the ocular and systemic abnormalities. The therapeutic goal should be to suppress active disease, minimize the amount of tissue damage, and reduce the incidence of clinically important exacerbations over the lifetime of the patient.

SYSTEMIC INVOLVEMENT

The presenting and eventual organ systems involved in SLE are shown in Tables 6-6 and 6-7. In its earliest phases, SLE may be relatively subtle and difficult to diagnose. Any patient exhibiting constitutional symptoms (malaise, anorexia, easy fatigability, and fever) who is found to have antinu-

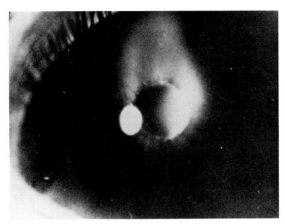

FIGURE 6-31. *Fluorescein angiogram, anterior segment, of the eye shown in Figure 6-30. Note the leak of fluorescein dye from the iris vasculature superiorly, which suggests iris vasculitis.*

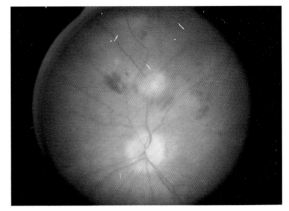

FIGURE 6-32. *Funduscopic photograph of a patient with systemic lupus erythematosus. Note the extensive lupus retinopathy, with blood-dot hemorrhages and cotton-wool spots being the most notable findings. The blood pressure in this patient was normal.*

clear antibodies in the serum should be carefully investigated for multiorgan disease typical of SLE. The benefits of making the diagnosis early stem from adequate therapy, which will decrease tissue damage over the rest of the patient's life.

ARTICULAR

Ninety-five percent of patients with SLE develop arthralgia, articular findings, or both during the course of their disease, and 55 percent of patients experience arthralgia as the initial manifestation of their disease. Some SLE patients (about 10 percent) develop deforming arthritis changes similar to those seen in rheumatoid arthritis; the most commonly affected site is the hands.

CUTANEOUS

Seventy to 80 percent of SLE patients develop skin lesions at some point during their lives [21], and approximately 20 percent have skin lesions as the initial symptom of the disease. The "butterfly rash" across the nose and cheek, occurring in about 30 percent of SLE patients, is one of the more notable rashes occurring in these patients. This rash is edematous and is exacerbated by ultraviolet exposure. It also commonly involves the skin of the chin and ears.

Alopecia occurs in 25 to 40 percent of patients with SLE; it has been emphasized that this finding commonly is associated with clinically active disease in some other organ system. The development of mucous membrane ulcers (nasal septum, larynx, pharynx, palate, vagina), petechiae or purpura, ulcerative lesions of the skin (commonly on the

TABLE 6-6. *Presenting Clinical Manifestations in Systemic Lupus Erythematosus*

Manifestation	Patients with Manifestation (%)
Arthralgia	55
Rash	20
Fever	10
Nephritis	10
Serositis	10
Neurologic changes	5
Anemia	5
Thrombocytopenia	2
Leukopenia	2

fingertips, around the nail folds, and on the ankles and arms), and periungual erythema and telangiectasis signify the development of frank vasculitis.

The skin manifestations seen in DLE, the cutaneous disease that probably represents the benign end of the spectrum of lupus erythematosus, unlike the skin lesions of SLE, are destructive. Hypopigmented scars result from the cutaneous inflammation in DLE, and the alopecia that occurs is permanent.

RENAL

Immune complex deposition in the kidney occurs in virtually all patients with SLE. It has been shown that, even if there is no clinical evidence of renal disease in an SLE patient, kidney biopsy specimens are routinely abnormal when studied by immunofluorescence and electron microscopy. The

American Rheumatism Association criteria
  Four or more of the following:
    Facial rash
    Discoid lupus
    Raynaud's phenomenon
    Alopecia
    Photosensitivity
    Oral or nasopharyngeal ulcer
    Nondeforming arthritis
    ANA or LE cells
    False-positive STS results
    Proteinuria (3.5 gm/day)
    Urinary sediment cellular casts
    Pleuritis and/or pericarditis
    Psychosis and/or convulsion
    Anemia, leukopenia, and/or thrombocytopenia
Hahn's criteria
  ANA (1:5) + score of 7 points

	Points
Butterfly rash	2
Rash biopsy findings compatible with SLE	2
Polyarthritis	2
Serositis	2
Glomerulonephritis biopsy findings compatible with SLE	2
LE cells	2
Rash compatible with SLE, not biopsy-proven	1
Clinical nephritis, no biopsy	1
Organic brain syndrome	1
Localizing neurologic signs	1
Alopecia	1
Raynaud's phenomenon	1
Nail-bed capillary abnormality	1
Arthralgia	1
Fever	1
Retinal cytoid bodies	1
Polymyositis	1
Myocarditis	1
Hemolytic anemia	1
Leukopenia	1
Thrombocytopenia	1
Lymphadenopathy	1
Positive results on direct Coombs' test	1
False-positive STS results	1
Antibodies to DNA	1
Hypergammaglobulinemia	1
Hypocomplementuria	1
Circulating anticoagulant	1

ANA = antinuclear antibody; LE = lupus erythematosus; STS = serologic test for syphilis; SLE = systemic lupus erythematosus. SOURCE. A. S. Cohen et al. [15] for American Rheumatism Association criteria; B. H. Hahn [47].

mesangium is apparently the site of earliest involvement with immune complex deposition.

End-stage renal disease is probably the most common SLE-related cause of death in patients with SLE. Approximately 50 percent of SLE patients develop clinically apparent renal disease, and 10 to 20 percent develop renal failure. It should be emphasized, therefore, that SLE patients should be carefully examined, repeatedly, for evidence of renal disease.

NEUROLOGIC
SLE-related central nervous system (CNS) changes may be the second most common SLE-related cause of death in patients with SLE. The most common neurologic manifestation is behavioral disturbance ranging from anxiety to psychosis; the second most common is grand mal seizures. Recurrent headache and organic brain syndrome can also occur. But in approximately 15 percent of patients with SLE, severe CNS changes occur. Multifocal disease mimicking multiple sclerosis, cranial nerve palsies, transverse myelitis, hemiparesis, and frank cardiovascular accident with paralysis may occur. Hypothalamic, extrapyramidal, and cerebellar dysfunction may occur when the tracts or centers controlling these functions are affected.

CARDIOVASCULAR
Just as there is a high incidence of subclinical renal disease in SLE, 50 percent of patients with SLE have pathologically demonstrable endocarditis, myocarditis, and/or pericarditis. The inflamed endocardium (Libman-Sacks endocarditis) can be secondarily infected.

PULMONARY
Although pulmonary disease is common in patients with SLE (occurring in 50–75 percent of SLE patients), it is usually not fatal. The most common form of pulmonary involvement is pleurisy. Sixty to 70 percent of patients with lupus have abnormal results on pulmonary function tests even if they are asymptomatic from a respiratory standpoint [21]. The most frequent abnormality is an impairment in the diffusion capacity. It is probably reasonable to carefully evaluate the pulmonary status of any patient with SLE periodically.

HEMATOLOGIC
Nearly all patients with SLE develop normochromic anemia. This usually occurs because of impaired utilization of iron by the bone marrow, and it im-

proves in association with improvement in the other systemic manifestations.

DIAGNOSIS AND DIFFERENTIAL DIAGNOSIS

The diagnosis of SLE is based on a combination of clinical and laboratory criteria, which have varied over the past decade. Two of the most useful systems are those proposed by Cohen and associates [15] (and accepted by the American Rheumatism Association) and by Hahn [47] (Table 6-7).

It should be emphasized that any patient exhibiting constitutional symptoms who is found to have antinuclear antibodies in the serum should be carefully investigated for multiorgan disease typical of SLE. We have found that, in addition to using both the Hahn and the American Rheumatism Association diagnostic criteria as guides, the immunofluorescent lupus band test on biopsy specimens of clinically normal skin, circulating antibodies to autologous erythrocytes, and ribonuclease-insensitive acid nuclear protein (anti-Sm) are very helpful in establishing the diagnosis of SLE. Moses and Barland [69] have emphasized the usefulness of these three diagnostic laboratory tests in patients with SLE.

The other collagen vascular diseases may, in their early stages, be difficult to differentiate from SLE. Thus, the patient with rheumatoid arthritis, antinuclear antibodies, Raynaud's phenomenon, and photosensitivity may be believed to have SLE if seen before the typical radiographic joint changes appear. Patients with progressive systemic sclerosis, dermatomyositis, and polymyositis may be similarly misclassified initially. A patient with prominent arthralgia, photosensitivity, antinuclear antibodies, proteinuria, Raynaud's phenomenon, digital pad infarcts, scleritis, and nasal mucosal ulceration (and possibly perforation) may be initially diagnosed as having polyarteritis nodosa. Yet all of these findings can and have occurred in patients with SLE, and it is only with careful longitudinal follow-up and repeated investigations that the correct diagnosis can be made. Chronic active hepatitis and mixed connective tissue disease may also mimic SLE in the early stages.

TREATMENT

OCULAR

Therapy for the ocular surface manifestations of SLE is based on successful control of the underlying disease, as well as local therapy for the keratitis and tear deficiency. The usual therapy for sicca syndrome (tear replacement, soft contact lenses, punctal occlusion) may produce both symptomatic and objective improvement. Topical steroid therapy may be a useful adjunct to systemic steroid therapy in the treatment of the scleritis. The retinopathy resolves only with successful control of the underlying systemic disease.

SYSTEMIC

Many patients with SLE have relatively mild disease, and they will lead relatively normal lives with conservative therapy in the form of adequate rest and nutrition, use of a skin-protective sunscreen when avoidance of sun exposure is impossible, and use of salicylates and other nonsteroidal antiinflammatory agents for control of arthralgia, myalgia, low-grade serositis, and mild constitutional symptoms. Antimalarial therapy (e.g., hydroxychloroquine sulfate) may be the next step employed in arthralgia and arthritis control or in therapy for cutaneous lesions if nonsteroidal antiinflammatory agents have not been effective.

Severe manifestations of SLE require therapy with systemic corticosteroids. Disabling constitutional symptoms and articular, cutaneous, and other systemic manifestations of the disease unresponsive to the aforementioned conservative therapy should be treated with the minimum daily dose of corticosteroid required for adequate control of disease activity. Alternate-day steroid therapy is ineffective in the treatment of SLE, and most patients respond considerably better to divided daily doses (e.g., bid or tid) than to single morning doses of corticosteroid. Severe disease affecting the central nervous, cardiovascular, pulmonary, or renal systems may require initial high-dose (60–300 mg of prednisone per day) steroid therapy, tapered as soon as clinical improvement warrants it. In tapering daily prednisone dosage from the 60 mg per day level, a useful rule of thumb is to decrease the dosage by 10 percent every 3 days until 40 mg per day is reached; then the taper should be slower.

SLE renal or CNS crisis is usually treated with high-dose intravenous steroid therapy (1–2 gm of methylprednisolone per day for 3–6 days) in conjunction with high-dose oral steroid (100–300 mg of prednisone per day). Combination corticosteroid-cytoxic therapy may be helpful in cases of severe lupus and in cases in which the systemic corticosteroids cannot be tapered below toxic levels without exacerbations of clinical disease. Cyclophosphamide may be the most effective cytotoxic agent studied for this purpose. Plasmapheresis for lupus crisis is also under investigation.

POLYARTERITIS NODOSA

Kussmaul and Maier [61] described the clinical characteristics and histopathologic findings in a patient dying of multisystem involvement with the disease they called periarteritis nodosa. The name of this multisystem disease has been changed to polyarteritis nodosa because histopathologic study of the lesions shows that all layers of the involved vessels, rather than just the adventitial layer are involved with inflammatory changes. Over the century since Kussmaul and Maier's description of polyarteritis nodosa, a great many case reports, reviews, and histopathologic studies of patients with systemic vasculitis have been published. Many of the reported cases exhibited features quite different from those in the original description of Kussmaul and Maier, and it has become clear that there is a spectrum of systemic vasculitis. Zeek [101] has proposed a classification of vasculitis that has been found to be quite useful in establishing the diagnosis and formulating a plan of therapy for individual patients (Table 6-8).

Classic polyarteritis nodosa is a systemic necrotizing vasculitis involving small and medium-sized muscular arteries with segmental acute and chronic inflammatory cell infiltration of all layers of the vessel wall and infiltration of the perivascular areas. Granuloma formation with multinucleated giant cells is a histopathologic feature of classic polyarteritis nodosa. The disease is of unknown etiology, has protean manifestations, and can be rapidly fatal.

There are no accurate figures on the true incidence of classic polyarteritis nodosa, but it appears to be fairly rare. It may occur in patients of any age, though is seen most usually in 20- to 40-year-olds. There is a 3:1 male-to-female predilection. There seems to be no racial or geographic association.

TABLE 6-8. *Classification of Systemic Vasculitis*

I. Polyarteritis nodosa group
  A. Classic polyarteritis nodosa of Kussmaul and Maier
  B. Allergic granulomatosis and angiitis of Churg and Strauss
  C. Overlap syndrome of systemic necrotizing vasculitis
II. Hypersensitivity vasculitis
  A. Serum sickness
  B. Schönlein-Henoch purpura
  C. Vasculitis associated with connective tissue disorders
    1. Rheumatoid arthritis
    2. Systemic lupus erythematosus
    3. Polymyositis, dermatomyositis
    4. Progressive systemic sclerosis
    5. Rheumatic fever
  D. Vasculitis associated with malignancy
  E. Vasculitis associated with mixed cryoglobulinemia
  F. Vasculitis associated with gastrointestinal disease (ulcerative colitis, Crohn's disease)
  G. Vasculitis associated with pulmonary disease (Goodpasture's syndrome)
  H. Vasculitis associated with drug or chemical hypersensitivity reactions
III. Wegener's granulomatosis
IV. Lymphomatoid granulomatosis
V. Giant cell arteritis
  A. Temporal arteritis
  B. Takayasu's arteritis
VI. Mucocutaneous lymph node syndrome
VII. Erythema nodosum
VIII. Thromboangiitis obliterans (Buerger's disease)
IX. Miscellaneous
  A. Behçet's syndrome
  B. Cogan's syndrome
  C. Stevens-Johnson syndrome
  D. Eale's disease
  E. Hypocomplementemic vasculitis
  F. Erythema elevatum diutinum
  G. Hypereosinophilic syndromes

PATHOGENESIS

The cause of polyarteritis nodosa is unknown. It has been reported to occur in association with upper respiratory tract infections [84], drug use (particularly methamphetamine) [12], and hepatitis B antigenemia [40]. Sergent and colleagues [86] reported hepatitis B antigenemia in approximately 30 percent of their study population with polyarteritis nodosa. Fye and associates [37] reported circulating immune complexes containing hepatitis B antigen and IgG antihepatitis B antigen in patients with polyarteritis nodosa, and Gocke and coworkers [41] demonstrated hepatitis B antigen, IgM, and complement in the vascular walls of patients with polyarteritis nodosa. These findings, coupled with the observation of decreased serum complement levels in the acute phases of the disease, plus the characteristic histopathologic findings provide strong circumstantial evidence that the disease is caused by an immune complex–mediated vasculitis. The antigen in some cases is probably microbial [95].

Polyarteritis nodosa appears to occur as a complication in hepatitis B virus infection in approximately 1 in 500 cases [78]. The finding that 30 to 50 percent of patients with polyarteritis nodosa are chronically infected with hepatitis B virus is especially intriguing with respect to microbe-induced immune-complex vasculitis as a possible, even probable, mechanism in polyarteritis nodosa. The size and composition of the immune complexes are no doubt critical in determining clinical disease production.

Dixon and colleagues [19] provided a great deal of insight into the pathogenic mechanism of serum sickness vasculitis, a vasculitic syndrome sharing many features with polyarteritis nodosa. They demonstrated that the vasculitic lesions were in fact induced by immune-complex deposition at vascular basement membranes, with activation of complement pathways, chemotaxis of neutrophils and other inflammatory cells, and resultant tissue damage. To be pathogenic, the immune complexes had to be of a certain size, approximately 10^6 daltons. Complexes formed in antibody excess were rapidly cleared by the phagocytic system, and complexes in great antigen excess were typically too small to be sieved and lodged at the basement membrane zone and the internal elastic lamina of arteries. The most toxic complexes were formed in slight antigen excess and were of IgG1 and IgG3 complement-fixing subtypes. These investigations also showed that increased permeability, through IgE-histamine pathways, can enhance immune-complex deposition in arteriolar walls. In patients with the serum-sickness-like prodrome of hepatitis B virus infection, the hepatitis B antigen–antihepatitis B antibody complexes contain the complement-fixing IgG1 and IgG3 subtypes [56]. In contrast, circulating immune complexes in patients with hepatitis B virus infection without the prodromal vasculitic syndrome do not contain these complement-fixing antibodies. A polyarteritislike syndrome occurs in blue foxes (*Alopex lagopus*). It has been shown that this disease is induced by a protozoon, *Encephalitozoon* (*Nosema*) *cuniculi*, and that an immune-complex arteritis accounts for the pathologic lesions [72].

HISTOPATHOLOGIC FINDINGS

In contradistinction to SLE, histopathologic study of ocular tissues of patients with polyarteritis nodosa has been performed by a number of investigators. As early as 1889, Müller [70] described classic histopathologic evidence of choroidal vasculitis in a patient with polyarteritis nodosa. At least nine excellent, well-documented histopathologic reports on choroidal, retinal, and ciliary arteritis have appeared since then. There is a scattered pattern of vasculitic lesions with all stages—acute, chronic, and healing lesions—seen in the involved tissues. Acute lesions show infiltration of the vessel walls and surrounding tissues with neutrophils and eosinophils; monocytes, lymphocytes, and plasma cells surround the vessel. Endothelial swelling and proliferation, with fibrinoid necrosis of the involved vessels, occur, and this process affects all the layers of small to medium-sized arteriole walls. Fibrosis and scarring mark the healed lesions.

The histopathologic features of the scleral, conjunctival, and corneal lesions of polyarteritis nodosa are strikingly nonspecific. Specimens of cornea from areas of active corneal ulceration show almost exclusively a neutrophil infiltrate; this is not surprising, since the major effector cell for collagen degradation in most forms of corneal ulceration appears to be the neutrophil [33, 34]. Specimens of conjunctiva that appears infiltrated adjacent to peripheral ulcerative keratitis lesions show numerous eosinophils, plasma cells, and lymphocytes in the substantia propria. Specimens of sclera from involved areas show neutrophils in areas of frank scleral destruction and necrosis, with surrounding zones of lymphocytes and plasma cells.

The exact mechanism involved, then, in production of the scleral and corneal lesions in polyarteritis nodosa is unclear. A reasonable hypothesis would be the deposition of immune complexes in sclera or corneoscleral limbus, with subsequent activation of complement pathways resulting in chemotaxis and inflammatory cell recruitment to the area of immune-complex deposition.

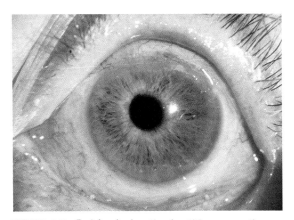

FIGURE 6-33. *Peripheral ulcerative keratitis seen as the presenting manifestation of polyarteritis nodosa. Low-grade anterior scleritis is present in the superior aspect of the globe. Note the deep gutter ulcer superiorly, which extends approximately from 11:00 o'clock clockwise to 2:30 o'clock. This ulcer has progressed circumferentially and centrally in spite of a wide variety of topical therapies, including ulcer debridement and surgical adhesive applications. The ulcer has an undermined area centrally with an overhanging lip of ulcerating cornea. Note also, however, that the sclera at the limbal region has also been involved with the ulcerative process.*

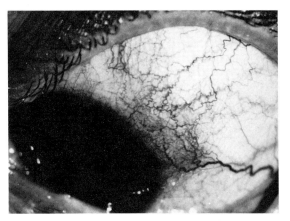

FIGURE 6-34. *Nodular scleritis in a patient with polyarteritis nodosa. Note the very small patch, near the 3 o'clock position of the limbus, of nodular scleritis with scleral edema and injection of the episcleral and conjunctival vessels.*

CLINICAL FEATURES

OCULAR INVOLVEMENT

CORNEAL

Peripheral ulcerative keratitis, morphologically similar to Mooren's ulcer, may occur in polyarteritis nodosa and may be the presenting manifestation of this lethal disease [32, 49, 68, 99]. A clinical characteristic of the keratitis in these cases is corneal ulceration at the limbus that is progressive, both centrally and circumferentially, associated with ocular pain and inflammation and with undermining of the central edge of the ulcer, resulting in an overhanging lip of cornea. Involvement of adjacent sclera has commonly been reported; this may be a distinguishing characteristic from classic Mooren's ulcer (Fig. 6-33). All forms of local therapy for these ulcers have ultimately failed. The importance of diagnosis of the underlying systemic condition and adequate systemic therapy to control it, which affords concomitant control of the destructive ocular lesions, has been emphasized [9, 32, 55].

SCLERAL

The scleral lesions of polyarteritis nodosa are highly destructive and are invariably progressive unless correct diagnosis and control of the underlying systemic disease is achieved. The scleritis is always painful and may be diffuse or nodular (Fig. 6-34). It may eventually progress to a necrotizing scleritis and may be associated with perforation and loss of all visual function.

RETINAL AND CHOROIDAL

Choroidal vasculitis is the most common ophthalmic manifestation in polyarteritis nodosa, and it may be considerably more common than is currently recognized. Repeated longitudinal funduscopic examinations and retinal fluorescein angiograms may be especially helpful in the diagnosis of polyarteritis nodosa. Clinically, symptomatic ocular involvement occurs relatively infrequently (approximately 20 percent of patients). Choroiditis, retinal vasculitis, optic atrophy (possibly secondary to ciliary vasculitis), papilledema, exudative retinal detachment, and central retinal artery occlusion are the most frequent abnormalities found. In addition, one may see Elschnig spots scattered throughout the posterior pole (Fig. 6-35). These are isolated, round, light yellow spots, 1/6 to 1/3 disc diameter in size, with a pigmented center. Such spots are not specific for polyarteritis nodosa, but in fact occur in a variety of systemic vasculitis syndromes. Their appearance is said to be a grave prognostic sign [58]. Hypertensive retinopathy may also obviously occur with the development of renal vascular hypertension secondary to renal involvement in polyarteritis nodosa. The report by Newman and coworkers [71] of repeated episodic monocular constriction of the visual field with sparing of central vision in a patient who was ultimately shown to have polyarteritis nodosa is of particular interest. These episodes of "peephole" vision occurring 3 to 12 times per day in either eye and lasting 4 to 5 minutes were shown by fluorescein angiography to be associated with incomplete choroidal filling until late in the venous phase. Autopsy findings showed impressive vasculitis of the short posterior ciliary arteries, as well as other small and medium-sized orbital arteries.

SYSTEMIC INVOLVEMENT

The clinical manifestations of polyarteritis nodosa are so protean and varied that a classic characteristic description is impossible. The clinical manifestations include fever, malaise, easy fatigability, weight loss, anorexia, myalgia, muscle wasting, and arthralgia. The disease may have an abrupt or gradual onset. The initial clinical manifestations are usually related predominantly to one organ system, frequently the articular or muscular system. The clinical manifestations are usually progressive, without notable remission and exacerbation. The disease may be rapidly or slowly progressive, and as it evolves, multisystem manifestations appear. It may be rapidly fatal; renal involvement is the major cause of death.

RENAL

Polyarteritis with glomerulonephritis, glomerulitis, or both may occur in patients with polyarteritis nodosa. Proteinuria, urinary sediment casts, microscopic hematuria, and progressive renal failure with renal hypertension are the usual sequences. These changes may be rapidly progressive and may be fatal, if untreated, within less than 6 months after the onset of the illness.

CUTANEOUS

Cutaneous lesions in polyarteritis nodosa are relatively uncommon, but the appearance of livedo reticularis, tender subcutaneous nodules, or both is an extremely helpful diagnostic sign when present.

HEMATOLOGIC

Leukocytosis with neutrophilia and sometimes eosinophilia is common in polyarteritis nodosa. Since they are quite uncommon in the other connective tissue diseases with which polyarteritis nodosa may sometimes be confused, these hematologic findings may be diagnostically helpful. Results of rheumatoid factor and antinuclear antibody tests are routinely negative, and immunoglobulin levels are usually normal. Complement levels may be depressed during acute phases of the disease, and circulating immune complexes or cryoglobulins may be present in the serum.

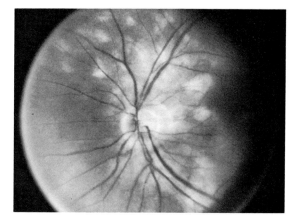

FIGURE 6-35. *Elschnig spots in a patient with polyarteritis nodosa. Note the scattered, light foci of various sizes, some of which have a slightly pigmented center (note in particular the small lesions at 12 o'clock and approximately 11 o'clock just distal to the venule branch). These are areas of ischemic infarct of the choriocapillaris.*

NEUROLOGIC

Peripheral neuropathy commonly occurs in patients with polyarteritis nodosa, and the disease should always be considered in the differential diagnosis of any patient with peripheral neuritis and constitutional symptoms.

PULMONARY

Pulmonary involvement in classic polyarteritis nodosa is quite uncommon. When obvious pulmonary involvement occurs in a systemic syndrome identical to classic polyarteritis nodosa, the more likely diagnosis is either Wegener's granulomatosis or allergic granulomatosis of Churg and Strauss: Granulomatous reactions are typically present in these diseases; granulomatous reactions are not found in histopathologic specimens from patients with classic polyarteritis nodosa.

CARDIOVASCULAR

Cardiovascular disease—myocardial infarction, hypertensive cardiomyopathy, and congestive heart failure—is a major cause of death in patients with polyarteritis nodosa. Segmental coronary arteritis is a very frequent finding at autopsy.

GASTROINTESTINAL

Gastrointestinal manifestations frequently occur in patients with polyarteritis nodosa, and the patient may present with severe abdominal pain mimicking appendicitis or cholecystitis. Superior mesenteric arteritis may produce bowel infarction with subsequent necrosis and perforation. More commonly, however, the gastrointestinal symptoms are less pronounced and usually consist of anorexia, nausea, vomiting, and diarrhea.

Hepatic infarction from vasculitis may occur in up to 50 percent of patients with polyarteritis nodosa. When cases of massive hepatic infarction secondary to surgery are excluded, nearly half of all cases of massive hepatic infarction and necrosis are found to be caused by polyarteritis nodosa.

GENITAL

Testicular or epididymal pain is a frequent finding in male patients with polyarteritis nodosa, and testicular biopsy is likely to reveal the characteristic histopathologic features of polyarteritis nodosa in patients with this symptom.

DIAGNOSIS AND DIFFERENTIAL DIAGNOSIS

The diagnosis of polyarteritis nodosa rests on histopathologic evidence of nongranulomatous vasculitis of small and medium-sized arteries in a patient with multisystem clinical disease compatible with polyarteritis nodosa. There are no laboratory tests or other diagnostic data that can confirm the diagnosis.

Nodular skin lesions, symptomatic muscle, and the testes in men are the appropriate biopsy sites likely to reveal the characteristic histopathologic findings. Electromyography may be helpful in selecting a suitable muscle biopsy site in the absence of muscle symptoms. Blind muscle biopsy is almost never positive. Clinically involved tissue should be biopsied as quickly after the clinically apparent lesion appears as possible. Immunoglobulin and complement components may be degraded rapidly after deposition at tissue sites. Cochrane and Koffler [13] have shown that these components are undetectable 24 to 48 hours after injection into animals. This underscores the crucial importance of obtaining biopsy specimens from clinical lesions as quickly as possible after their appearance in an effort to enhance the likelihood of diagnosis.

TREATMENT

OCULAR

Although none of the ocular lesions can be satisfactorily treated by local means, it is possible to retard progressive corneal destruction in cases of peripheral ulcerative keratitis associated with polyarteritis nodosa through local means while control of the underlying systemic disease is being achieved through systemic therapy. Conjunctival resection, ulcer debridement, application of cyanoacrylate tissue adhesive to the ulcer bed and to a small rim of surrounding normal cornea and sclera, and application of a continuous-wear bandage soft contact lens

may be useful while the patient is being adequately immunosuppressed (Fig. 6-36). The use of topical corticosteroids to inhibit inflammatory cell activity does not seem to be particularly effective and may in fact be harmful because of its inhibitory effect on new collagen formation. Inhibitors of collagenase synthesis, such as 1% medroxyprogesterone acetate drops, and competitive inhibitors of collagenase activity, such as acetylcysteine (20% drops), are other adjunctive forms of topical therapy that may help retard ulcer progression while the disease is being brought under control.

SYSTEMIC

The prognosis of untreated polyarteritis nodosa is extremely grim. The disease is almost invariably relentlessly progressive, with death usually resulting from renal failure, myocardial infarction, congestive heart failure, hepatic failure, bowel perforation, cerebral infarction, or subarachnoid hemorrhage. The five-year survival in untreated cases is approximately 13 percent [36]. High-dose systemic corticosteroid therapy improves the five-year survival rate to approximately 48 percent [36, 76]. A striking increase in five-year survival in patients with polyarteritis nodosa is achieved with a combination of corticosteroid and cytotoxic immunosuppressive therapy. Fauci and associates [24] documented striking complete remissions in patients with advanced polyarteritis nodosa treated with prednisone and cyclophosphamide. Lieb and colleagues [62], in a retrospective longitudinal cohort study of outcome with respect to therapy in patients with polyarteritis nodosa, found a 12 percent five-year survival in untreated patients, a 53 percent five-year survival in patients treated with systemic corticosteroids, and an 80 percent five-year survival in patients treated with both corticosteroid and cytotoxic agent immunosuppression.

WEGENER'S GRANULOMATOSIS

Wegener's granulomatosis is a multisystem disease of unknown etiology, first described by Klinger [60] in 1931 and later characterized as a distinctive syndrome by Wegener [96, 97]. The disease is characterized by glomerulonephritis; necrotizing granulomatous vasculitis of small and medium-sized pulmonary arteries and veins; necrotizing granulomatous lesions of the mucosa of sinuses, nose, and nasopharynx; and generalized necrotizing granulomatous vasculitis of other organs, including the eyes. Although not rare, Wegener's granulomatosis is uncommon. It affects males more commonly than females (3:2) and has been reported in patients of all ages from infancy to the ninth decade but has its peak incidence in the fourth and fifth decades [27]. There are no obvious racial, geographic, or occupational predispositions.

PATHOGENESIS

Although definitive proof is lacking, one of the more popular current hypotheses about the pathogenesis of the tissue destruction that occurs in Wegener's granulomatosis is that it represents immune complex–mediated vasculitis. IgG, complement component C3, and fibrin have been demonstrated in glomerular vessel walls [27, 81], and immunoglobulin and complement have been found in the vascular lesions of skin [54]. Circulating immune complexes have been demonstrated in the sera of patients with Wegener's granulomatosis [25, 53].

HISTOPATHOLOGIC FINDINGS

Lesions from the upper respiratory tract typically show extensive granulomatous inflammation with tissue necrosis and a prominent giant cell reaction. Pulmonary arteries and veins and arteries, arterioles, veins, and venules from other clinically involved organs show a necrotizing vasculitis with acute, chronic, and healing lesions all typically represented in the same organ. Neutrophils predominate in the vascular walls in the acute lesions; mononuclear cells predominate in the more chronic lesions. Fibrinoid necrosis of vascular walls is prominent, and granulomas with multinucleated giant cells may be found in and around involved vessels and scattered in isolated foci within the involved tissue. Focal and segmental necrotizing glomerulonephritis is seen in the kidney; as the disease progresses, proliferative glomerulonephritis is the predominant histopathologic feature in the kidneys. IgG and complement have been demonstrated by immunofluorescence technique in the glomeruli of renal biopsy specimens from some patients with Wegener's granulomatosis [27].

The histopathologic features of conjunctival biopsy specimens from areas adjacent to necrotizing scleritis or peripheral ulcerative keratitis are almost never diagnostic of the underlying disorder. Lymphocytes and plasma cells predominate in the substantia propria, and variable numbers of neutrophils and eosinophils may be seen. The deeper tissues, however (episcleral and superficial sclera), may show a typical granulomatous reaction with

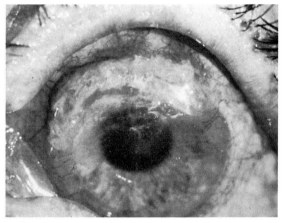

FIGURE 6-36. *Anterior necrotizing scleritis and peripheral ulcerative keratitis in a patient with polyarteritis nodosa. The area of ulcerating cornea has been debrided; the necrotic, overhanging lip of cornea and the conjunctiva adjacent to the area of ulceration have been resected; and a layer of cyanoacrylate surgical adhesive has been applied in a wide area encompassing not only the area of active corneal and scleral degradation but also extending to clinically normal tissue in an effort to effect a tight bond. A soft contact lens has been applied to protect the glue from the trauma of the lid with each blink and to protect the patient against irritation of the tarsal conjunctiva by the glue.*

epithelioid cells and giant cells present. Specimens of ulcerating sclera commonly show neutrophils in the area of active scleral degradation, fibrinoid necrosis, and surrounding granulomatous inflammation, including, in some cases, extensive arrays of multinucleated giant cells. If intrascleral vessels have been obtained in the biopsy specimen, true necrotizing vasculitis with inflammatory cell infiltration into the vascular wall and fibrinoid necrosis of the vessel may be seen. Granulomas of the ciliary body and of the iris have been found, and necrotizing vasculitis of the anterior ciliary arteries as they lie in the rectus muscles has been demonstrated [7, 28, 35].

Biopsy specimens of the overhanging lip of undermined cornea at the edge of a peripheral ulcerative keratitis lesion in these patients commonly show predominantly neutrophil infiltration in the area of active collagen degradation, with variable numbers of lymphocytes. The histopathologic findings abruptly change immediately adjacent to the area of active collagen degradation to granulomatous reaction with vast numbers of plasma cells, lymphocytes, and multinucleated giant cells. It should be emphasized that simply obtaining biopsy specimens of conjunctiva and of ulcer margin is unlikely to yield important clues to the diagnosis.

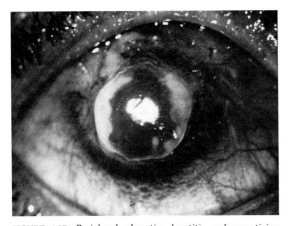

FIGURE 6-37. *Peripheral ulcerative keratitis and necrotizing scleritis in a patient with undiagnosed Wegener's granulomatosis. Note the characteristic intrastromal infiltrates of inflammatory cells in advance of the underlying ulcer with overhanging lip of ulcerating cornea. Note also the extensive involvement of the anterior sclera.*

CLINICAL FEATURES

OCULAR INVOLVEMENT

A review of the reported cases of Wegener's granulomatosis in the world literature reveals that the eye may be involved in 50 to 60 percent of cases. The ocular lesion may be the first major clinical expression of the disease that stimulates the patient to seek medical attention, and hence patients with this potentially lethal disease may have their first contact with the health care system through the ophthalmologist. Table 6-9 lists the approximate frequency of ocular and orbital lesions occurring in the reported cases of Wegener's granulomatosis. External ocular complaints ranging from conjunctivitis and nasolacrimal duct obstruction to proptosis, necrotizing scleritis, and peripheral ulcerative keratitis predominate [14, 50, 90, 98].

TABLE 6-9. *Frequency of Ocular Lesions in Wegener's Granulomatosis*

Lesion	Frequency (%)
Scleritis and/or peripheral ulcerative keratitis	18
Proptosis or pseudotumor	18
Conjunctivitis	15
Retinal vasculitis	8
Uveitis	6
Dacryocystitis	3

CORNEAL

Peripheral ulcerative keratitis, necrotizing scleritis, or both are reported with increasing frequency as the first major clinical manifestation of Wegener's granulomatosis. The peripheral ulcerative keratitis is frequently preceded by localized conjunctivitis or episcleritis, followed by the onset of true scleritis and the development of intrastromal peripheral corneal inflammatory infiltrates. Pain may be mild or severe. Corneal ulceration develops with breakdown of the peripheral corneal epithelium, and the crescentic peripheral corneal ulcer progresses centrally and circumferentially, producing a biomicroscopic appearance quite similar to that of Mooren's corneal ulcer, except that sclera is never involved in the latter (Fig. 6-37).

SCLERAL

Scleral involvement is invariably present in peripheral ulcerative keratitis associated with Wegener's granulomatosis, and this may be helpful in differentiating it from Mooren's ulcer. The corneal and scleral destruction progresses, often slowly but always relentlessly, in spite of all medical and surgical ocular therapy. Topical and systemic corticosteroid therapy is notably ineffective. Before the institution of immunosuppressive therapy for Wegener's granulomatosis, eyes with necrotizing scleritis, peripheral ulcerative keratitis, or both were commonly lost because of perforation and relentless tissue destruction.

SYSTEMIC INVOLVEMENT

PULMONARY

Although patients with Wegener's granulomatosis may have clinical manifestations in any organ system, the most common presentation is with upper respiratory tract symptoms: recurrent epistasis; chronic rhinorrhea; painful, purulent sinusitis; chronic otitis media; hoarseness; dysphagia; cough; or pleurisy. These symptoms may have been present for weeks, months, or even years, with gradual or sudden worsening, or with the sudden onset of fever, malaise, anorexia, weight loss, and weakness.

Physical examination very frequently reveals nasal, nasopharyngeal, or pharyngeal ulcerative lesions. X-rays of the ethmoidal, frontal, or sphenoidal sinus are frequently abnormal, and the chest x-ray may show multiple nodular or cavitary pulmonary lesions.

RENAL
Overt clinical renal symptoms are usually absent in the early phases of the disease, though microscopic hematuria and proteinuria may be found on urinalysis.

HEMATOLOGIC
The erythrocyte sedimentation rate is always elevated, and the patient usually has mild leukocytosis and mild anemia. Mild hypergammaglobulinemia may be present, circulating autoantibodies to smooth muscle may be found, and circulating immune complexes may be detected in the serum. The test for rheumatoid factor frequently has a positive result. Screening for hepatitis B antigen and for antinuclear antibodies typically have negative results. Delayed hypersensitivity skin test reactions may be impaired in patients with Wegener's granulomatosis.

CUTANEOUS
Skin lesions occur in approximately 50 percent of the patients; rash, petechiae, ischemic ulcers, and subcutaneous nodules may all occur.

DIAGNOSIS
The diagnosis of Wegener's granulomatosis rests on demonstration of necrotizing granulomatous vasculitis in biopsy specimens from clinically involved upper or lower respiratory tract lesions in a patient with glomerulonephritis and a clinical history compatible with Wegener's granulomatosis.

There are few consistently abnormal immunologic laboratory test findings in study populations of patients with Wegener's granulomatosis. Most do have a moderate hypergammaglobulinemia, notably IgA hypergammaglobulinemia. Mild anemia, mild leukocytosis, elevated erythrocyte sedimentation rate, and a weakly positive rheumatoid factor (in approximately 60 percent of patients) may be found. Urinalysis generally reveals proteinuria, microscopic hematuria, or granular, hyalin, or red cell casts. Chest x-ray frequently reveals hilar enlargement and multiple nodular or cavitary pulmonary infiltrates. These infiltrates may be extremely evanescent, with changing radiographic patterns occurring rapidly. X-rays of the paranasal sinuses are frequently abnormal. One of the earliest radiologic abnormalities is mucosal thickening of the maxillary antrum. The ethmoidal, frontal, or sphenoidal sinuses are involved in decreasing order of frequency. As sinus involvement progresses, radiographic evidence of sinus clouding, complete opacification, development of air-fluid levels, or bony destruction may appear [23].

Lethal midline granuloma has sometimes been confused with Wegener's granulomatosis. The former, however, lacks pulmonary and renal involvement and commonly has necrotizing lesions of the face as part of its features. The sinus and nasal lesions of Wegener's granulomatosis never erode the skin and face, and therefore it should not be difficult to differentiate these two diseases.

Liebow [63] has described three forms of pulmonary granulomatosis that might be confused with Wegener's granulomatosis. Lymphogranulomatosis may clinically resemble Wegener's granulomatosis, but histopathologic study of clinical lesions in lymphogranulomatosis shows an active atypical lymphoreticular proliferation that is quite distinct from the necrotizing granulomatous vasculitis typical of Wegener's. Necrotizing sarcoid granulomatosis resembles Boeck's sarcoidosis histopathologically by the presence of noncaseating granulomas, but differs from sarcoidosis in that diffuse necrotizing angiitis may also be seen. Bronchocentric granulomatosis may clinically resemble Wegener's granulomatosis of the lung, but histopathologic study in the former reveals the lesions to be centered around the bronchi rather than around the vessels. Extrapulmonary lesions have not been described in this disorder. Goodpasture's syndrome, the other classic pulmonary-renal syndrome, lacks the upper respiratory manifestations of Wegener's granulomatosis and is distinguished by the presence of antiglomerular basement membrane antibody and by the positive linear immunoglobulin staining patterns of glomeruli on fluorescent antibody study of biopsy specimens.

TREATMENT

OCULAR
Local ocular therapy will never cure the ocular lesion without successful treatment of the underlying systemic disease. However, as in the case of polyarteritis nodosa, some measures may be quite helpful in saving the eye from perforation and destruction while systemic immunosuppression is being achieved. The use of topical antibiotics, conjunctival resection, ulcer debridement, cyanoacrylate tissue adhesive, and soft contact lenses, along with anticollagenolytic agents, may be beneficial in this regard. Definitive therapy is systemic immunosuppression [32, 50] (Fig. 6-38).

SYSTEMIC
Wegener's granulomatosis is a fatal disease, and the mean survival time is approximately 5 months after

the onset of renal disease. Corticosteroids alone are ineffective in influencing the long-term prognosis [23]. Systemic immunosuppression with cyclophosphamide, however, is extremely effective in the treatment of this disease, and long-lasting complete remissions of many years' duration have been achieved in patients with far advanced disease in this once universally fatal illness [23, 27].

PROGRESSIVE SYSTEMIC SCLEROSIS (SCLERODERMA)

Progressive systemic sclerosis (PSS) is a multisystem disease characterized by inflammation, fibrosis, and degenerative changes of skin, vessels, synovium, and visceral organs such as the gut, kidney, heart, and lungs. The disease is of unknown etiology, and there is no known cure. The clinical course and prognosis depend on the extent of visceral involvement.

Curzio [16] may have been the first to describe the syndrome that we call scleroderma today. Gintrac [39] was the first to use the term *scleroderma* to describe the syndrome. Visceral involvement in patients with the disease was not emphasized in the medical literature until Matsui [65] did so, and in 1945 Goetz [42] proposed the name *progressive systemic sclerosis* for this multisystem disorder.

The disease appears to affect women 4 times more frequently than men, with an especially high degree of disparity between the two sexes during the third and fourth decades. There is no racial or geographic predilection. There is an unusually high incidence of PSS in miners (both coal and gold miners) and in other workers with major exposure to silica dust [82].

HISTOPATHOLOGIC FINDINGS

Histopathologic study of skin biopsy specimens during the active (as opposed to the fibrotic) phase of sclerodermatous involvement in PSS shows almost an exclusive T-lymphocyte infiltrate [30], vascular endothelial cell proliferation with hyalinization, myxomatous degeneration of arterioles [10], perivascular mononuclear cell infiltration, and greatly increased amounts of immature collagen fibers with resultant thickening of the dermis. Increased melanin is also seen in the basal layers of the epidermis.

PATHOGENESIS

Patients with PSS commonly exhibit hypergammaglobulinemia, and approximately 50 percent will have either circulating immune complexes detectable as cryoglobulins or circulating rheumatoid factor and antinuclear antibody. A speckled pattern on the immunofluorescent test for antinuclear antibody

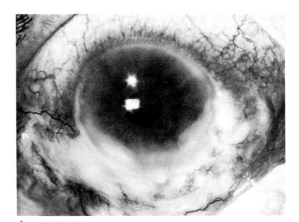

A

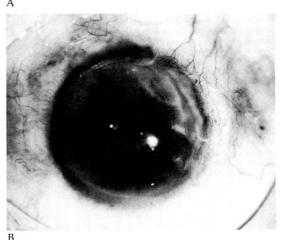

B

FIGURE 6-38. *A. Peripheral ulcerative keratitis and necrotizing scleritis in a patient with Wegener's granulomatosis. The ulcerative process has extended from 8:30 o'clock counterclockwise to 3:00 o'clock. Note the intrastromal inflammatory cell infiltrates as well as the intrascleral nodules of inflammatory cells. B. Same eye, after conjunctival resection, ulcer debridement, cyanoacrylate tissue adhesive application, soft lens application, and systemic immunosuppression with prednisone and cyclophosphamide. Ocular inflammation and progressive corneal and scleral destruction ceased within 4 weeks of institution of systemic immunosuppression. Soft lens and surgical adhesive were removed, the patient was treated with cytotoxic therapy for 18 months, and therapy was then discontinued. He has remained disease-free during a 5-year follow-up period and maintains a visual acuity of 20/20.*

is particularly common in patients with PSS, and an antinuclear antibody that appears to be unique to patients with PSS has recently been described [92]. Approximately half the patients with PSS also have circulating antibodies to nuclear RNA. The relative numbers of circulating T-lymphocytes in the peripheral blood may be modestly reduced, and some patients with PSS have been shown to have circulating lymphocytes that can be stimulated by skin extracts. Biopsy specimens of pathologic tissue from patients with PSS are typically negative for immunoglobulin and complement deposition, with the exception of renal vessels.

These data suggest that a reasonable working hypothesis for pathogenesis of PSS may involve abnormalities in both the immune and the connective tissue systems, with lymphocyte sensitization to skin antigens, migration of lymphocytes into tissues, and liberation of chemotactic factors attractive to dermal fibroblasts, with resultant proliferation of the fibroblasts and overproduction of immature collagen. The vascular changes seen may conceivably be secondary to these phenomena; an alternative hypothesis involves a more active role for the vascular events. It is clear that the vascular system is involved very early in the course of PSS.

CLINICAL FEATURES

OCULAR INVOLVEMENT

CORNEAL
The association of tear insufficiency with PSS has been well established [2, 57]. A high percentage (probably at least 70 percent) of patients with PSS have tear insufficiency, and many become symptomatic with clinical sicca syndrome (Table 6-10). Most patients with PSS also have progressive conjunctival fornix foreshortening. This should not be surprising in a disease characterized by mucosal subepithelial fibrosis. Stucchi and Geiser [91] and Horan [52] have documented and emphasized the frequency of shallow fornices in patients with PSS. Very rare ocular manifestations of PSS include extraocular muscle myositis [4] and keratitis unrelated to keratoconjunctivitis sicca [64].

RETINAL
As in other collagen vascular diseases, retinopathy has, in general, been underemphasized in PSS. The

TABLE 6-10. *Ocular Manifestations in Progressive Systemic Sclerosis*

Manifestation	Frequency (%)
Sicca syndrome	70
Conjunctival shrinkage	70
Choroidal nonperfusion	50
Episcleritis	5

incidence of choroidal vascular abnormalities in patients with PSS is probably considerably higher than that in patients with SLE. Grennan and Forrester [45] found that 50 percent of their study patients with PSS had patchy areas of nonperfusion of the choroidal vasculature; one patient showed abnormalities of the retinal vasculature (microaneurysmal dilatation of the terminal venules in one quadrant). The abnormalities of the choroidal vasculature were extensive and were found in patients without history of hypertension. Findings of routine ophthalmoscopy had appeared normal in all the patients. The choroidal choriocapillaris and arteriolar abnormalities probably relate to the vascular endothelial basement membrane thickening, with deposition of mucopolysaccharide material in the precapillary arteriolar walls; patchy choroidal nonperfusion occurs then on the basis of vascular obliteration [6, 22].

SYSTEMIC
The most common initial clinical manifestation of PSS is the appearance of Raynaud's phenomenon. Well over 95 percent of patients with PSS develop paroxysmal vasospasm of the fingers, earlobes, tongue, or toes. Episodes are characterized by sudden pallor or cyanosis of the involved areas, with concomitant pain and sensations of cold and numbness. Within 10 to 15 minutes the symptoms and signs begin to resolve. Patients with these signs and symptoms have been shown to have up to a 90 percent decrease in nail-bed capillaries, with abnormal, dilated capillary loops.

CUTANEOUS
Symmetrical painless finger edema generally develops at the same time as or shortly after the onset of Raynaud's phenomenon; alternatively, approximately 30 percent of patients may develop arthralgia along with the sausage-shaped digital edematous changes. Skin involvement of the face, forearms, and trunk may then develop, first as edematous, indurated areas of skin, followed by contraction and hardening of tissue and the development of tight, atrophic skin.

GASTROINTESTINAL
Esophageal dysfunction is the most common visceral abnormality in patients with PSS, and it probably develops in well over 90 percent of patients. The obvious clinical symptom is dysphagia, but even in those patients who do not have overt clinical symptoms of esophageal motility dysfunction, fluorometric radiographic studies have shown that nearly all have abnormal esophageal peristaltic activity, particularly in the lower third of the esophagus [17].

ARTICULAR

Articular changes are common in patients with PSS, with joint stiffness and polyarthralgia being the most frequent complaints. Fibrous deposits on tendon sheaths may produce rubs in association with movement of the affected joint, and many patients with PSS develop such creaking rubs in association with knee movement. Calcinosis—the development of subcutaneous and intracutaneous calcium deposits, particularly in the fingertips—may occur in patients with PSS; this is a prominent feature in patients with the so-called CRST (calcinosis, Raynaud's, sclerodactyly, telangiectasia) or CREST (CRST plus esophageal dysfunction) forms of the disease. Such depositions produce quite characteristic radiographic changes. The explanation for the development of these depositions is unclear.

PULMONARY

Pulmonary involvement is nearly a universal finding in patients with PSS, though many are totally asymptomatic. The most common clinical sign of pulmonary involvement is the development of exertional dyspnea. Pulmonary fibrosis has been found in up to 90 percent of PSS patients at autopsy [17].

CARDIAC

The heart may be involved in PSS as well, with autopsy studies disclosing myocardial fibrosis. Cardiac catheterization studies have shown a high frequency of pulmonary hypertension in patients with PSS, but it is the unusual case that progresses to frank cor pulmonale.

RENAL

Renal disease is the single most common cause of death in patients with PSS, and death is usually the result of severe hypertension in the patients who have had severe and rapidly progressive PSS for less than 3 years. Histopathologic study reveals extensive renal arterial and arteriolar pathologic changes as described above, with fibrinoid necrosis and deposition of immunoglobulin and complement in vessel walls.

REFERENCES

1. Abdou, N. I., et al. Suppressor T cell abnormality in idiopathic systemic lupus erythematosus. *Clin. Immunol. Immunopathol.* 6:192, 1976.
2. Alarcon-Segovia, D., et al. Sjögren's syndrome and progressive systemic sclerosis (scleroderma). *Am. J. Med.* 57:78, 1974.
3. Alarcon-Segovia, D., and Ruiz-Arguelles, A. Decreased circulating thymus-derived cells with receptors for the Fc portion of immunoglobulin G in systemic lupus erythematosus. *J. Clin. Invest.* 62:1390, 1978.
4. Arnett, F. C., and Michels, R. G. Inflammatory ocular myopathy in systemic sclerosis (scleroderma). *Arch. Intern. Med.* 132:740, 1973.
5. Aronson, A. J., et al. Immune complex deposition in the eye in systemic lupus erythematosus. *Arch. Intern. Med.* 139:1312, 1979.
6. Ashton, N., et al. Retinopathy due to progressive systemic sclerosis. *J. Pathol. Bacteriol.* 96:259, 1968.
7. Austin, P., et al. Peripheral corneal degeneration and occlusive vasculitis in Wegener's granulomatosis. *Am. J. Ophthalmol.* 85:311, 1978.
8. Block, S. R., et al. Studies of twins with systemic lupus erythematosus: A review of the literature and presentation of twelve additional sets. *Am. J. Med.* 59:533, 1975.
9. Brubaker, R., Font, R. L., and Shepherd, E. M. Granulomatous scleral uveitis: Regression of ocular lesions with cyclophosphamide and prednisone. *Arch. Ophthalmol.* 86:517, 1971.
10. Campbell, P. M., and LeRoy, E. C. Pathogenesis of systemic sclerosis: A vascular hypothesis. *Semin. Arthritis Rheum.* 4:351, 1975.
11. Chantler, S., Hanson, J., and Jacobson, J. Incidence of nuclear antibodies in patients and in related and in unrelated groups from a community with "microepidemic" of systemic lupus erythematosus. *Clin. Immunol. Immunopathol.* 2:9, 1973.
12. Citron, B. P., et al. Necrotizing angiitis associated with drug abuse. *N. Engl. J. Med.* 283:1003, 1970.
13. Cochrane, C. G., and Koffler, D. Immune complex disease in experimental animals and man. *Adv. Immunol.* 16:186, 1973.
14. Cogan, D. G. Corneoscleral lesions in periarteritis nodosa and Wegener's granulomatosis. *Trans. Am. Ophthalmol. Soc.* 53:321, 1955.
15. Cohen, A. S., et al. Preliminary criteria for the classification of systemic lupus erythematosus. *Bull. Rheum. Dis.* 21:643, 1971.
16. Curzio, C. *Discussioni Anatomio-Pratiche di un Raro e Stravagante Morbo Cutaneo in Questo Grande Ospedale Detel Indurabili.* Naples: G. DiSiome, 1753.
17. D'Angelo, W. A., et al. Pathologic observations in systemic sclerosis (scleroderma): A study of 58 autopsy cases and 58 matched controls. *Am. J. Med.* 46:428, 1969.
18. DeHoratius, R. J., Pillarsetty, R., and Messner, R. P. Antinucleic acid antibodies in systemic lupus erythematosus patients and their fam-

ilies: Incidence and correlation with lymphocyte antibodies. *J. Clin. Invest.* 56:1149, 1975.

19. Dixon, F. J., et al. Pathogenesis of serum sickness. *Arch. Pathol.* 65:18, 1958.

20. Doesschat, J. T. Corneal complications in lupus erythematosus discoidus. *Ophthalmologica* 132:153, 1956.

21. Dubois, E. L. *Lupus erythematosus* (2nd ed.). Los Angeles: *University of Southern California Press,* 1974.

22. Farkas, T. G., Sylvester, V., and Archer, D. The choroidopathy of progressive systemic sclerosis (scleroderma). *Am. J. Ophthalmol.* 74:875, 1972.

23. Fauci, A. S. Vasculitis. In C. W. Parker (Ed.), *Clinical Immunology.* Philadelphia: Saunders, 1980. Pp. 473–519.

24. Fauci, A. S., Doppman, J. L., and Wolff, S. M. Cyclophosphamide-induced remissions in advanced polyarteritis nodosa. *Am. J. Med.* 64:890, 1978.

25. Fauci, A. S., Lawley, T., and Frank, M. M. Unpublished observations, 1978.

26. Fauci, A. S., et al. Immunoregulatory aberrations in systemic lupus erythematosus. *J. Immunol.* 121:1473, 1978.

27. Fauci, A. S., and Wolff, S. M. Wegener's granulomatosis: Studies in 18 patients and a review of the literature. *Medicine* (Baltimore) 52:535, 1973.

28. Ferry, A. P., and Leopold, I. H. Marginal (ring) corneal ulcer as presenting manifestation of Wegener's granuloma. *Trans. Am. Acad. Ophthalmol. Otolaryngol.* 74:1276, 1970.

29. Fessel, W. J. SLE in the community: Incidence, prevalence, outcome and first symptoms; The high prevalence in black women. *Arch. Intern. Med.* 134:1027, 1974.

30. Fleischmajer, R., Perlish, J. S., and Reeves, J. R. T. Cellular infiltrates in scleroderma skin. *Arthritis Rheum.* 20:975, 1977.

31. Foster, C. S. Ocular surface manifestations of neurological and systemic diseases. *Int. Ophthalmol. Clin.* 19(2):207, 1979.

32. Foster, C. S. Immunosuppressive therapy in external ocular inflammatory disease. *Ophthalmology* (Rochester) 87:140, 1980.

33. Foster, C. S. Immunosuppressive Therapy for Experimental Corneal Ulceration. In *Immunology of the Eye. Workshop II: Autoimmune Phenomena and Ocular Disorders.* Arlington, Va.: Information Retrieval, 1981. Pp. 91–102.

34. Foster, C. S., et al. Immunosuppression and selective inflammatory cell depletion in a guinea pig model of corneal ulceration after alkali burning. *Arch. Ophthalmol.* 100:1820, 1982.

35. Frayer, W. C. The histopathology of perilim-

bal ulceration in Wegener's granulomatosis. *Arch. Ophthalmol.* 64:58, 1960.

36. Fronert, P. P., and Scheps, F. G. Long-term follow-up study of periarteritis nodosa. *Am. J. Med.* 43:8, 1967.

37. Fye, K. H., et al. Immune complexes in hepatitis B antigen–associated periarteritis nodosa: Detection by antibody-dependent cell-mediated cytotoxicity and the Raji cell assay. *Am. J. Med.* 62:783, 1977.

38. Gibosky, A., et al. Disease associations of the Ia-like human alloantigens: Contrasting patterns in rheumatoid arthritis and systemic lupus erythematosus. *J. Exp. Med.* 148:1728, 1978.

39. Gintrac, E. Note sur la sclerodermie. *Rev. Med. Chir.* (Paris) 2:263, 1847.

40. Gocke, D. J., et al. Association between polyarteritis and Australian antigen. *Lancet* 2:1149, 1970.

41. Gocke, D. J., et al. Vasculitis in association with Australian antigen. *J. Exp. Med.* 134:330, 1971.

42. Goetz, R. H. The pathology of progressive systemic sclerosis (generalized scleroderma) with special reference to changes in viscera. *Clin. Proc.* (Cape Town) 4:337, 1945.

43. Gold, D. H., Morris, D. A., and Henkind, P. Ocular findings in SLE. *Br. J. Ophthalmol.* 56:800, 1972.

44. Grayson, M. *Diseases of the Cornea.* Mosby, St. Louis: 1979. Pp. 314–333.

45. Grennan, D. M., and Forrester, J. Involvement of the eye in SLE and scleroderma. *Ann. Rheum. Dis.* 36:152, 1977.

46. Haase, A. T., et al. Role of DNA Intermediates in Persistent Infections Caused by RNA Viruses. In D. Schlessinger (Ed.), *Microbiology.* Washington, D.C.: American Society of Microbiology, 1977. Pp. 478–483.

47. Hahn, B. H. *Systemic Lupus Erythematosus.* In C. W. Parker (Ed.), *Clinical Immunology.* Philadelphia: Saunders, 1980. Pp. 583–631.

48. Halmay, O., and Ludwig, K. Bilateral band-shaped deep keratitis and iridocyclitis in systemic lupus erythematosus. *Br. J. Ophthalmol.* 48:558, 1964.

49. Harbart, F., and McPherson, S. D. Scleral necrosis in periarteritis nodosa. *Am. J. Ophthalmol.* 30:727, 1947.

50. Haynes, B. F., et al. Ocular manifestations of Wegener's granulomatosis. *Am. J. Med.* 63:131, 1977.

51. Henkind, P., and Gold, D. H. Ocular manifestations of rheumatic disorders: Natural and iatrogenic. *Rheumatology* 4:13, 1973.

52. Horan, E. C. Ophthalmic manifestations of progressive systemic sclerosis. *Br. J. Ophthalmol.* 53:388, 1969.

53. Howle, S. B., and Epstein, W. V. Circulating

immunoglobulin complexes in Wegener's granulomatosis. *Am. J. Med.* 60:259, 1976.

54. Hu, C. H., O'Laughlin, S., and Winkleman, R. K. Cutaneous manifestations of Wegener's granulomatosis. *Arch. Dermatol.* 113:175, 1977.

55. Jampol, L. M., West, C., and Goldberg, M. F. Therapy of scleritis with cytotoxic agents. *Am. J. Ophthalmol.* 86:266, 1978.

56. Juan, J. R., et al. The pathogenesis of arthritis associated with acute hepatitis B surface antigen–positive hepatitis B. *J. Clin. Invest.* 55:930, 1975.

57. Kirkham, T. H. Scleroderma and Sjögren's syndrome. *Br. J. Ophthalmol.* 53:131, 1969.

58. Klein, B. A. Ischemic infarcts of the choroid (Elschnig spots). *Am. J. Ophthalmol.* 66:1069, 1968.

59. Klemperer, P., Pollack, A. D., and Baehr, G. Pathology of disseminated lupus erythematosus. *Arch. Pathol.* 32:569, 1941.

60. Klinger, H. Grenzformen der Periarteritis Nodosa Frankfurt. *Z. Pathol.* 42:455, 1931.

61. Kussmaul, A., and Maier, R. Huber eine bissher nicht beschriebene eigenthümiliche Artereinerkrankung (Periarteritis nodosa die mit Morbus Brightii und rapid fortschreitender allgeiner Muskellähung einhergeht). *Dtsch. Arch. Klin. Med.* 1:484, 1866.

62. Lieb, E. S., Restivo, C., and Paulus, H. E. Immunosuppressive and corticosteroid therapy for polyarteritis nodosa. *Am. J. Med.* 67:941, 1979.

63. Liebow, A. A. Pulmonary angiitis and granulomatosis. *Am. Rev. Resp. Dis.* 108:1, 1973.

64. Manschot, W. A. Generalized scleroderma with ocular symptoms. *Ophthalmologica* 149:131, 1965.

65. Matsui, S. Über die Pathologie und Pathogenese Von Sclerodermia Universalis. *Mitt. Med. Fakult. Kaiserl. Univ. Tokyo.* 31:55, 1924.

66. Mellors, R. C., and Mellors, J. W. Type C RNA virus expression in systemic lupus erythematosus: New Zealand mouse model and human disease. *Arthritis Rheum.* 21:S68, 1968.

67. Messner, R. P., Lundstrom, F. D., and Williams, R. C., Jr. Peripheral blood lymphocyte cell surface markers during the course of SLE. *J. Clin. Invest.* 52:3046, 1973.

68. Moore, J. G., and Sevel, D. Corneoscleral ulceration in periarteritis nodosa. *Br. J. Ophthalmol.* 50:651, 1966.

69. Moses, S., and Barland, P. Laboratory criteria for a diagnosis of systemic lupus erythematosus. *JAMA* 242:1039, 1979.

70. Müller, P. *Festschrift Surz Feier des fünfzigjährigen Besthenes des Stadtkrankenhauses zu Dresden-Friedrichstadt.* Dresden: W. Baensch, 1889. P. 458.

71. Newman, N. M., Hoyt, W. F., and Spencer, W. H. Macular sparing monocular blackouts: Clinical and pathologic investigations of intermittent choroidal vascular insufficiency in a case of periarteritis nodosa. *Arch. Ophthalmol.* 91:367, 1974.

72. Nordstoga, K., and Westbye, K. Polyarteritis nodosa associated with the nosematosis in blue foxes. *Acta Pathol. Microbiol. Scand.* [A]. 84:291, 1976.

73. Panem, S., et al. C-type virus expression in systemic lupus erythematosus. *N. Engl. J. Med.* 295:470, 1976.

74. Phillips, P. E. The role of viruses in SLE. *Clin. Rheum. Dis.* 1:505, 1975.

75. Phillips, P. E. Type-C oncornavirus studies in systemic lupus erythematosus. *Arthritis Rheum.* 21:S76, 1978.

76. Pickering, G., et al. Treatment of polyarteritis nodosa with cortisone: Results after three years. Report to the Medical Research Counsel by the Collagen Diseases and Hypersensitivity Panel. *Br. Med. J.* 1:1399, 1960.

77. Pillat, A. Über das Vorkommen von Choroiditis bei Lupus erythematodes. *Albrecht von Graefes Arch. Klin. Ophthalmol.* 133:566, 1934.

78. Redeker, A. G. Viral hepatitis: Clinical aspects. *Am. J. Med. Sci.* 270:9, 1975.

79. Reeves, J. A. Keratopathy associated with systemic lupus erythematosus. *Arch. Ophthalmol.* 74:159, 1965.

80. Reinertsen, J. L., et al. B-lymphocyte alloantigens associated with systemic lupus erythematosus. *N. Engl. J. Med.* 299:515, 1978.

81. Roback, S. A., et al. Wegener's granulomatosis in a child: Observations on pathogenesis and treatment. *Am. J. Dis. Child.* 112:587, 1966.

82. Rodnan, G. P., et al. The association of progressive systemic sclerosis (scleroderma) with coal miners' pneumoconiosis and other forms of silicosis. *Ann. Intern. Med.* 66:332, 1967.

83. Rose, E., and Pillsbury, D. M. Acute disseminated lupus erythematosus—a systemic disease. *Ann. Intern. Med.* 12:951, 1939.

84. Rose, G. A., and Spencer, H. Polyarteritis nodosa. *Q. J. Med.* 26:43, 1957.

85. Schur, P. H. Complement in lupus. *Clin. Rheum. Dis.* 1:519, 1975.

86. Sergent, J. S., et al. Vasculitis with hepatitis B antigenemia: Long-term observations in 9 patients. *Medicine* (Baltimore) 55:1, 1976.

87. Siegel, M., and Lee, S. L. The epidemiology of systemic lupus erythematosus. *Semin. Arthritis Rheum.* 3:1, 1973.

88. Spaeth, G. L. Corneal staining in systemic

lupus erythematosus. *N. Engl. J. Med.* 276: 1168, 1967.

89. Steinberg, A. D., and Reinertsen, J. L. Lupus in New Zealand mice and in dogs. *Bull. Rheum. Dis.* 28:940, 1978.

90. Straatsma, B. R. Ocular manifestations of Wegener's granulomatosis. *Am. J. Ophthalmol.* 44:789, 1957.

91. Stucchi, C. A., and Geiser, J. D. Manifestations oculares de la sclérodermie généralisée (points communs avec le syndrome de Sjögren). *Doc. Ophthalmol.* 22:72, 1967.

92. Tan, E. M. Sunlight as a Potential Aetiological Factor in Systemic Lupus Erythematosus. In G. R. Hughes (Ed.), *Modern Topics in Rheumatology.* Chicago: Year Book, 1976. Pp. 99–106.

93. Tan, E. M., and Rodnan, G. P. Profile of antinuclear antibodies in progressive systemic sclerosis (PSS) (abstract). *Arthritis Rheum.* 18:430, 1975.

94. Tan, E. M., et al. Deoxyribonucleic acid (DNA) and antibodies to DNA in the serum of patients with systemic lupus erythematosus. *J. Clin. Invest.* 45:1732, 1976.

95. Trepo, C. G., et al. The role of circulating hepatitis B antigen/antibody immune complexes in the pathogenesis of vascular and hepatic manifestations in polyarteritis nodosa. *J. Clin. Pathol.* 27:863, 1964.

96. Wegener, F. Über generalisierte, septische Gefässerkrankungen. *Verh. Dtsch. Pathol. Ges.* 29:202, 1936.

97. Wegener, F. Über eine eigenartige rhinogene Granulomatose mit besonderer Beteiligung des Arteriensystems und der Nieren. *Beitr. Pathol. Anat.* 102:36, 1939.

98. Weiter, J., and Farcas, C. G. Situ tumor of the orbit as a presenting sign in Wegener's granulomatosis. *Surv. Ophthalmol.* 17:106, 1972.

99. Wise, G. N. Ocular periarteritis nodosa. *Arch. Ophthalmol.* 48:1, 1952.

100. Yoshiki, T., et al. The viral envelope glycoprotein of murine leukemia viruses and the pathogenesis of immune complex nephritis in New Zealand mice. *J. Exp. Med.* 140:1011, 1974.

101. Zeek, P. M. Periarteritis nodosa and other forms of necrotizing angiitis. *N. Engl. J. Med.* 18:1764, 1963.

102. Zurier, R. B. SLE in pregnancy. *Clin. Rheum. Dis.* 1:613, 1975.

Corneal Manifestations of Dermatologic Disorders: PEMPHIGUS, PEMPHIGOID, AND ERYTHEMA MULTIFORME

G. Richard O'Connor

Certain disorders of the skin that are presumably autoimmune in origin have their counterparts in diseases of the cornea. The cornea itself is a primary target in some of these. In others, the cornea is affected secondarily because of pathologic changes that have taken place in adjacent structures such as the conjunctiva or lid margin. It is tempting to think that the skin, mucous membranes, and superficial cornea are attacked in common by certain pathologic processes because of their mutual origin from surface ectoderm. This does not seem farfetched when one realizes that identical immunopathologic changes may occur in the basement membrane of the epithelium in cicatricial pemphigoid of the conjunctiva and in bullous pemphigoid affecting the skin. However, the logic of this scheme does not hold up in diseases such as cicatricial pemphigoid of the esophagus or of the rectum that clearly involve structures of endodermal origin.

Because of limitations of space, this section will be limited to three subjects: pemphigus, cicatricial pemphigoid, and erythema multiforme. These may be considered under the broad category of bullous diseases that cause various degrees of ocular morbidity or blindness depending on the amount of scarring that results. Certain of these disorders are also known by multiple names. In each case, the preferred name will be used in the body of the text, and the older synonyms will be indicated in parentheses.

PEMPHIGUS

Pemphigus is a painful disease of the skin and mucous membranes characterized by the formation of intraepithelial bullae. The two principal forms that affect the eye are pemphigus vulgaris and pemphigus foliaceus. Pemphigus vegetans (Neumann type) is a highly reactive vegetating variant of pemphigus vulgaris that produces fungating, discharging granulations from the base of the lesions. Pemphigus erythematosus (Seanear-Usher syndrome) is a localized form of pemphigus foliaceus characterized by a prolonged erythematous stage. The lesions, which primarily affect the skin of the lids, may resemble those of seborrhea.

This work was supported in part by Grant EY-01597 from the National Institutes of Health and by an unrestricted grant from Research to Prevent Blindness, Inc., New York, N.Y.

PEMPHIGUS VULGARIS

This disease affects Jewish people more frequently than any other ethnic group, but it has been documented in all races and ethnic groups. It is primarily a disease of middle age, although all age groups, with the possible exception of young infants, have been affected.

Pemphigus vulgaris occasionally appears to be associated with other autoimmune diseases such as myasthenia gravis, thymoma, and lupus erythematosus. A viral etiology has been postulated for pemphigus vulgaris [11], and some support for this theoretical concept was provided by the fact that the disease seems more common among people who work in the meat or leather industries. However, the viral origin of this disease has not been confirmed.

PATHOGENESIS

Pemphigus vulgaris appears to be a disease of immunoregulation. Polyclonal B cell activation may occur, as indicated by the presence of multiple types of autoantibodies [9]. There is some indication of a defective suppressor T cell mechanism [12]. Regardless of the triggers of this disease, it seems likely that immunogenetic factors may be of great importance; Park and Terasaki [19] were able to show that more than 95 percent of Jewish patients with pemphigus vulgaris have the HLA-DRw4 antigen. It is likely that this antigen, being in close proximity to an immune response gene, may influence the type of autoimmune inflammatory disease expressed by patients with this disorder.

Beutner and Jordan [5] first described autoantibodies to an intercellular substance located in the prickle-cell layer of the epithelium in 1964. These antibodies could be demonstrated in frozen sections of normal mucosal tissues from both humans and other species by an indirect fluorescent antibody technique. When serum from pemphigus patients was incubated with such frozen tissue sections, fixation of immunoglobulins and complement to an intercellular substance believed to be associated with the glycocalyx of the cell membrane could be demonstrated (Fig. 6-39). A disease closely resembling pemphigus vulgaris could be produced in the mucosal tissues of normal animals by passive transfer of serum antibodies from pemphigus patients [27]. In some cases, the severity of the mucosal disease in a given patient could be directly related to the titer of his serum antibodies [6]; in others, no such correlation could be made [26].

The fixation of IgG and C3 to an intercellular substance in the suprabasal layers of the epithelium appears to be followed by acantholysis. The cells in the affected areas become rounded up (Fig. 6-40),

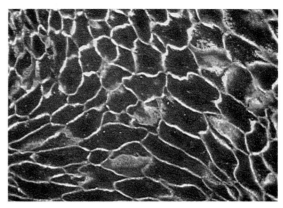

FIGURE 6-39. *Binding of IgG to an intercellular antigen in the buccal mucosa of a patient with pemphigus vulgaris. (UV microscopy, ×1000.)*

and a fluid-filled space entirely within the epithelium produces the bulla so characteristic of the disease (Fig. 6-41). Although the rupture of such bullae is common, an intact layer of basal epithelium attached to a normal basement membrane remains at the base of the bulla. Since the conjunctival stroma is not actually bared of its epithelial covering at any time, there is virtually no tendency to scar formation or symblepharon. In the early phases of the lesion, polymorphonuclear leukocytes, including a substantial number of eosinophils, may be attracted to the lesion site. Later, lymphocytes and macrophages may invade the epithelial lesion and infiltration of the underlying stroma by lymphocytes may be observed. In pemphigus erythematosus, the stromal base of the lesion may remain infiltrated and hyperemic for weeks or months.

The oral mucosa is often the first site of attack. The lesions are painful and generally produce ulcerations that may become secondarily infected. After a certain number of weeks or months, flaccid bullae, usually appearing on an erythematous base, appear on the skin. These rupture easily (Nikolsky's sign), leaving weeping lesions that may cause considerable fluid loss. Healing generally occurs within a few days or a week, leaving some areas of hyperpigmentation but little or no scarring.

CLINICAL FEATURES

The ocular lesions are relatively rare. They affect the palpebral conjunctiva principally (Fig. 6-42) and favor the area near the inner canthus. The lesions consist of intraepithelial bullae of the conjunctiva.

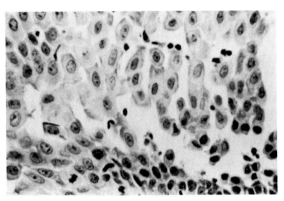

FIGURE 6-40. *Acantholysis and rounding up of suprabasal epithelium in a case of pemphigus vulgaris. (H&E, ×1000.)*

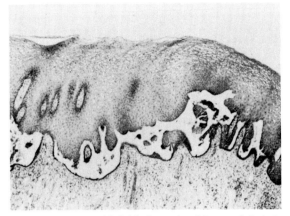

FIGURE 6-41. *Intraepithelial bulla produced by acantholysis in pemphigus vulgaris. (H&E, ×40.)*

Following the rupture of these bullae, scarring is extremely rare except in eyes that have become secondarily infected. The cornea itself is almost never affected except for films of mucopurulent discharge that may briefly obscure vision. Except in rare circumstances, therefore, pemphigus vulgaris is not a very important cause of permanent ocular disability.

TREATMENT
Until recent years, pemphigus vulgaris was almost uniformly fatal. With the advent of corticosteroids, effective control of the bullous lesions was obtained in many patients formerly considered hopeless. Depending on the severity of the case, the initial dose of prednisone was between 180 and 360 mg. The drug was continued until all lesions were fully healed. Many patients took these doses of systemic corticosteroids that produced serious side effects such as demineralization of the bone, hypertension, and cushingoid features. The combined use of cytotoxic immunosuppressive agents, i.e., methotrexate, and corticosteroids has subsequently appeared to be very useful in inducing remissions of the disease or in lowering the maintenance levels of required corticosteroid [20]. Because the effects of circulating autoantibody can be directly correlated with the severity of the lesions in some cases, plasmapheresis has been used in some cases to lower the titer of circulating antibodies in times of pemphigus crisis [2]. This procedure is usually followed by the administration of immunosuppressive agents that inhibit the proliferative responses of B cells in subsequent months.

PEMPHIGUS FOLIACEUS
Pemphigus foliaceus (Cazenave's disease) is a rare member of the pemphigus group that begins in bullous form. Because of the extensive cutaneous involvement, systemic signs and symptoms occur early in the course.

PATHOGENESIS
The immunopathologic changes occurring in pemphigus foliaceus appear to be similar to those of pemphigus vulgaris, but they are different in location, and they appear to be mediated by different antibodies. Fixation of immunoglobulins and complement appears to occur in the intercellular spaces of the more superficial portion of the affected epithelium. Thus, bulla formation takes place in cells that are anterior to the suprabasal epithelium. This being the case, it seems strange that elements of the cornea beneath the epithelial layers should be more profoundly affected in pemphigus foliaceus than in pemphigus vulgaris. In this connection, it is only fair to say that immunopathology of the pemphigus foliaceus has not been adequately studied in the eye.

As is the case with pemphigus vulgaris, in pemphigus foliaceus circulating autoantibodies can be passively transferred. However, when blocking immunofluorescence techniques are used, antibodies from pemphigus vulgaris patients are found to have different specificities from antibodies from pemphigus foliaceus patients, and antisera from the two diseases do not block each other [29]. Bystryn and Rodriguez [8] showed that pemphigus vulgaris antibodies did not bind to intercellular antigens in the lower epidermis from patients with pemphigus foliaceus, but did bind to intercellular antigens in

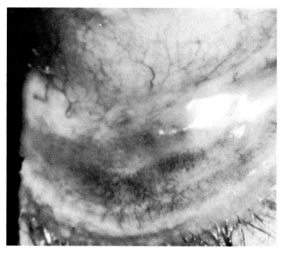

FIGURE 6-42. *Bullous lesion of pemphigus vulgaris affecting the nasal portion of the inferior palpebral conjunctiva. (Courtesy Robert Jordan, M.D.)*

normal skin and in skin from patients with pemphigus vulgaris. Therefore, it seems that the two diseases are different with regard to the site of action of the autoantibody and the ocular manifestations; in addition, there is no cross-reactivity between the antibodies produced by patients suffering from the two maladies.

CLINICAL FEATURES
The ocular manifestations of pemphigus foliaceus have only rarely been encountered in the Northern Hemisphere, and most descriptions of the corneal involvement antedate the development of modern immunofluorescent techniques. This disease is characterized by erythematous, bullous lesions of the skin producing generalized exfoliation, often in a leaflike pattern. The ocular lesions appear to be somewhat different from those of pemphigus vulgaris. In pemphigus foliaceus, the palpebral conjunctiva is usually affected by bulla formation, whereas the bulbar conjunctiva is left intact. This disease may affect the cornea itself, giving rise to cellular infiltration of the superficial stroma, epithelial vesicle formation, pannus, and ultimately facet formation. Thus it may have more direct consequences on vision than does pemphigus vulgaris. Although Rogers and Bourne [22] have indicated that ocular involvement may be limited to lesions of the eyelid and conjunctiva, infiltrative lesions not only of the cornea but also of deeper intraocular structures such as the iris and ciliary body have been described in some cases reported from Brazil, along with cataract [1].

TREATMENT
As in pemphigus vulgaris, corticosteroids administered by mouth seem to be the mainstay of treatment of pemphigus foliaceus. Locally applied steroid drops may modify the extent and severity of the corneal opacities, but the disease is basically a systemic disorder representing an imbalance between helper T and suppressor T elements. It may be that combined corticosteroid and immunosuppressive therapy will offer the best treatment for this disease, as is the case with pemphigus vulgaris.

PEMPHIGOID
Cicatricial pemphigoid has been referred to under various names, including ocular pemphigus, benign mucous membrane pemphigoid, and essential shrinkage of the conjunctiva. All of the above names have now given way to the currently accepted term, *cicatricial pemphigoid,* which seems to express the outstanding feature of the disease, namely, scar formation. This disease produces subepithelial bullae of the conjunctiva, the buccal mucosa, and occasionally the esophagus, vagina, and rectum.

The relationship of cicatricial pemphigoid to bullous pemphigoid of the skin is uncertain. Cicatricial pemphigoid and bullous pemphigoid may be part of a large spectrum of disease.

BULLOUS PEMPHIGOID
Bullous pemphigoid is a chronic disease of gradual onset in the older population characterized by large, tense bullae over wide areas. Usually the abdomen, groin, and flexor surfaces of the forearms have the largest number of lesions. When the bullae break, they have a tendency to heal. Areas of erythema are frequently present too. The involvement of the oral mucosa is mild and may not be present. The eye is only infrequently involved.

CICATRICIAL PEMPHIGOID
Cicatricial pemphigoid affects women much more often than men (2 : 1) and rarely appears before the age of 30. Lesions of the conjunctiva may be the first and only manifestations of the disease, although lesions of the mouth are very common indeed. Twenty to 25 percent of the cases may not show any ocular involvement.

In many patients, the disease seems to take an inexorable course despite all attempts at treatment. The course is generally more severe in women than men, but the reason for this is not understood. Although this disease is usually not associated with the loss of life, it is anything but "benign." Therefore, the older name *benign mucous membrane pemphigoid*, originally used to contrast this disease with pemphigus vulgaris, now seems totally inappropriate.

PATHOGENESIS

It appears that in cicatricial pemphigoid, as well as in bullous pemphigoid of the skin, the basement membrane of the epithelium is under attack by autoimmune processes (Fig. 6-43). By the use of immunofluorescent techniques, C3, IgG, IgM, and IgA have all been found to be localized in the basement membrane zone. This zone consists of four areas: (1) the basal epithelial cell membrane with hemidesmosomes, (2) a lamina lucida with anchoring filaments, (3) an electron-dense basal lamina containing type IV collagen; and (4) a subbasal lamina with anchoring filaments. The deposition of immunoglobulins and complement in cicatricial pemphigoid appears to be located rather specifically in the lamina lucida. As early as 1967, a circulating anti–basement membrane antibody was identified by means of indirect immunofluorescence in the sera of patients with bullous pemphigoid [15]. Although this autoantibody is consistently found in such patients, the titer of the antibody does not seem to correlate with the clinical activity of the lesions, as has been observed in pemphigus vulgaris [10]. The antibody also has rather limited species cross-reactivity; in general, monkey esophageal epithelium is the most reliable substrate for indirect immunofluorescent measurements. Passive transfer of these serum antibodies produces in vivo binding of the antibody in monkeys but no lesions [24]. For reasons that are not well understood, the circulating antibody that is so characteristic of bullous pemphigoid occurs very infrequently among patients with cicatricial pemphigoid. Rogers and colleagues [21] found such antibodies in only 2 of 21 patients.

Although the localization of immunoglobulins and complement in the area of the basement membrane of the epithelium is almost universal in patients with bullous pemphigoid, biopsy specimens from the conjunctiva often fail to show this localization [4]. Thus, although cicatricial pemphigoid may be part of the general spectrum that includes bullous pemphigoid, the two entities seem to differ with regard to sex distribution, the presence of circulating antibodies directed against basement membrane, and preferred sites for attack by a presumably autoimmune process.

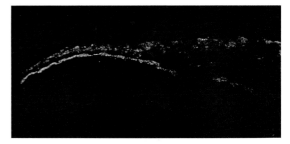

FIGURE 6-43. *Fluorescent antibody detection of C3 in the basement membrane of the epithelium in cicatricial pemphigoid. (UV microscopy, ×1000.)*

As with many other presumably autoimmune diseases, there is some indication of an immunogenetic basis for cicatricial pemphigoid. Mondino and associates [17] found that HLA-B12 was present in 45.0 percent of patients with cicatricial pemphigoid, as opposed to 19.6 percent of the general population ($p < 0.02$). It may be that HLA-B12, and possibly HLA-A3, are genetic markers for the disease, but the figures presented by Mondino and associates, are not nearly as impressive as those that, for example, correlate iritis with HLA-B27–positive ankylosing spondylitis.

CLINICAL FEATURES

In the earliest manifestations, cicatricial pemphigoid may appear to be nothing more than a persistent low-grade papillary conjunctivitis (Fig. 6-44). In the early stages, the disease may affect one eye alone, but eventual bilateral involvement is almost universal. Later in the disease, fine, whitish gray linear opacities appear in the deep conjunctiva (Fig. 6-45). This may be rarely followed, in turn, by bulla formation. In cicatricial pemphigoid, if an ocular bulla forms it is subepithelial; when a bulla ruptures, the raw surface of the underlying tissue is exposed. Because of lack of epithelial continuity over this raw surface, adjacent areas of exposed stroma may fuse, giving rise to a symblepharon (Fig. 6-46). Ultimately, there is loss of the normal fornical spaces. With progressive conjunctival scarring, the epithelium loses its normal goblet cell population and becomes thicker and keratinized. Because of the loss of goblet cells, the tears become deficient in mucus. Eventually, the ductules leading into the superior fornices from the lacrimal glands also become obstructed because of scar formation. When this happens, the tears become deficient not only in mucus but in their aqueous components as well.

With progressive scarring, entropion and trichiasis occur, causing multiple abrasions of the cornea. This, in turn, is a stimulus for neovascularization of the cornea, which ultimately loses its lus-

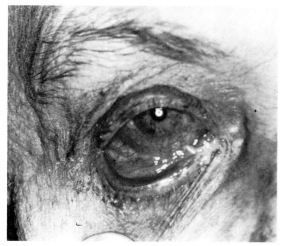

FIGURE 6-44. *Initial stage of cicatricial pemphigoid of the conjunctiva. Changes resemble other forms of papillary conjunctivitis at this stage.*

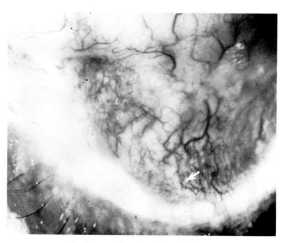

FIGURE 6-45. *Early scarring in cicatricial pemphigoid. Note whitish gray linear streak* (arrow).

ter and transparency because of a combination of dryness and inflammatory infiltrations (Fig. 6-47).

TREATMENT

The treatment of cicatricial pemphigoid has been manifestly unsuccessful in the hands of most practitioners. One study from the Mayo Clinic [14] suggested that the use of subconjunctivally administered depot steroids might halt the course of the disease. This form of therapy has not been universally successful by any means. Locally applied corticosteroid drops may decrease the papillary inflammation that accompanies the early stages of the disease but is of little avail in the later stages. Cicatricial pemphigoid of the conjunctiva is not nearly as responsive to systemic corticosteroids as is pemphigus vulgaris. Recently, however, Foster [13] has shown that cyclophosphamide and prednisone, used in combination, can bring improvement to patients with cicatricial pemphigoid, reversing an otherwise inexorable disease. Rogers and associates [23] recently found that more than 80 percent of patients with cicatricial pemphigoid showed a beneficial response to the oral administration of dapsone. This compound and the closely related sulfone, sulfapyridine, have been found to be effective in the treatment of certain subsets of patients with bullous pemphigoid. The mechanism of action of dapsone remains unclear, but Steñdahl and coworkers [24] have demonstrated that dapsone interferes with the myeloperoxidase-hydrogen peroxide-halide–mediated cytotoxin system of the polymorphonuclear leukocytes. The work of Barranco [3] also indicates that dapsone inhibits the release of lysosomal enzymes. The major complica-

tions of dapsone therapy include hemolytic anemia, skin rashes, and arthralgia. Most patients tolerate 100 mg of dapsone per day without untoward hemolytic effects unless they are deficient in glucose-6-phosphate dehydrogenase or glutathione reductase. Only certain subsets of patients with cicatricial pemphigoid appear to be sensitive to the effects of dapsone; however, one is usually able to detect within 4 weeks whether a patient will or will not respond to this form of therapy. It may also be used as adjunctive therapy with small doses of systemically administered corticosteroids or other antiinflammatory agents.

ERYTHEMA MULTIFORME

Erythema multiforme is a disease characterized by multiple polymorphous skin eruptions with associated lesions of the nails and mucous membranes. The condition is characterized by fever and malaise followed by the development of a papular skin rash and bullae affecting the limbs and face, and by ulcerative lesions of the mucosae, particularly those of the mouth, genitalia, and conjunctivae. The skin lesions may have the appearance of "iris" or "bull's eye" with a deep red center surrounded by a zone of lighter pigmentation.

The disease has traditionally been associated with hypersensitivity to ingested drugs such as sulfonamides or barbiturates. It has been assumed that the offending medication may act as a hapten, combining with autologous tissue protein in such a way as to form an autoantigen. Although drugs have generally been blamed for the development of this dis-

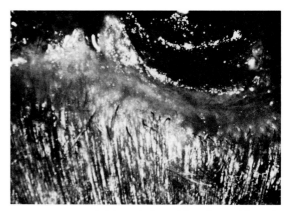

FIGURE 6-47. *Epithelial irregularity and loss of corneal luster in the late stage of cicatricial pemphigoid.*

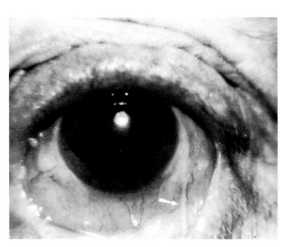

FIGURE 6-46. *Symblepharon formation* (arrow) *in cicatricial pemphigoid.*

ease, it is known to have occurred in the absence of drug therapy. For example, it has developed in the wake of herpes simplex infection [7] and has been observed in association with measles infection, smallpox vaccination, and malignancy [18]. Recurrent cycles of lesions characterize the disease. These generally occur at intervals of about 2 weeks, but most of the lesions will generally have disappeared by the end of 6 weeks.

PATHOGENESIS
It appears likely that erythema multiforme is an immune complex–mediated disease. Recently, Kasmierowski and Wuepper [16] have demonstrated immune complexes in the superficial blood vessels of the skin in patients suffering from erythema multiforme. It appears that this is the stimulus for microthrombus formation, which, in turn, produces necrosis of both the blood vessel wall and the surrounding tissue. Complement is bound to the immune complexes in the blood vessel wall, and this is a powerful attractant to polymorphonuclear leukocytes, which release a number of lytic enzymes.

As in the case of cicatricial pemphigoid, there is localization of immune complexes and complement in the basement membrane of the conjunctival epithelium. Acute inflammatory cells are attracted to the area, and subepithelial bullae may form with frightening rapidity.

The recurrence of symptoms at approximately 2-week intervals is reminiscent of other established immune-complex diseases such as serum sickness. Thus, the iritis discussed by Theodore and Lewson

[26] as a complication of serum sickness recurred almost exactly 2 weeks after the initial attack of the disease. The same periodicity has also been seen in the renal and arthritic complications of the disease.

The ocular lesions of erythema multiforme have not been nearly so well studied from the immunopathologic point of view as have those of pemphigus and pemphigoid. It is tempting to speculate that the lesions of the conjunctiva in erythema multiforme have the same cause as the skin lesions described by Kasmierowski and Wuepper [16]; however, these suggestions await confirmation in ocular tissue biopsy studies.

CLINICAL FEATURES
The ocular signs of erythema multiforme include the formation of conjunctival bullae, which are similar in their appearance to those of pemphigus vulgaris. Ulcerating lesions (Fig. 6-48), often appearing early in the course of the disease, are not infrequently accompanied by secondary infections. The course and histopathologic changes of the disease, however, are much more like those of cicatricial pemphigoid. The bulla is actually subepithelial, and symblepharon formation is frequent. Cicatricial reactions are common, producing extensive scarring of the conjunctiva, dryness of the eyes, and eventual deformities of the lid margins, giving rise to entropion and trichiasis. When these changes occur, ulcerations of the cornea are common. These may become secondarily infected, and the cornea may perforate alarmingly quickly. It is also possible that the peripheral corneal infiltrations occur by mechanisms different from those related to dryness of the eyes and trichiasis. There is a strong indication of immune-complex formation in erythema multiforme; as in other diseases associated with immune-complex formation, the peripheral cornea may be a site of deposit for these substances.

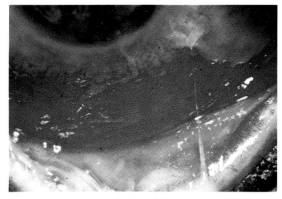

FIGURE 6-48. *Ulcerative lesions of the conjunctiva in Stevens-Johnson syndrome.*

TREATMENT

The early conjunctival lesions of erythema multiforme may be substantially modified by the early use of both systemic and local corticosteroids. Stevens-Johnson syndrome represents a severe, potentially fatal form of erythema multiforme. Because of the serious and potentially fatal nature of this latter disease, corticosteroids are generally administered by systemic routes in any case and have occasionally proven to be lifesaving.

In either erythema multiforme or Stevens-Johnson syndrome irrigation of the conjunctival fornices with balanced salt solutions followed by lysis of any symblephara that have formed (with a sterile glass rod) is generally recommended. The use of local antibiotic preparations to prevent secondary infection is also indicated, provided that the patient has no history of hypersensitivity to the antibiotic. Cultures should be taken of any ulcerating wound before the use of antibiotic solution to establish the species and the antibiotic sensitivities of the pathogen.

The treatment of the disease is difficult and often unrewarding after symblepharon formation has taken place and dryness of the eyes has supervened. Corticosteroids appear to be of no benefit at this stage. Tear substitutes must be used liberally to maintain adequate lubrication of the cornea and remaining conjunctiva. In the late stages of the disease, when shrinkage of the fornices and further damage to the cornea from entropion and trichiasis are feared, limited help may be provided by the wearing of a scleral contact lens.

REFERENCES

1. Amendola, F. Ocular manifestations of pemphigus foliaceus. *Am. J. Ophthalmol.* 32:35, 1949.
2. Auerbach, R., and Bystryn, J. C. Plasma-pheresis and immunosuppressive therapy: Effect on levels of intercellular antibody in pemphigus vulgaris. *Arch. Dermatol.* 115:728, 1979.
3. Barranco, V. P. Inhibition of lysosomal enzymes by dapsone. *Arch. Dermatol.* 110:563, 1974.
4. Bean, S. F., et al. Cicatricial pemphigoid: Immunofluorescent studies. *Arch. Dermatol.* 106:195, 1972.
5. Beutner, E. H., and Jordan, R. E. Demonstration of skin antibodies in sera of pemphigus vulgaris patients by indirect immunofluorescent staining. *Proc. Soc. Exp. Biol. Med.* 117:505, 1964.
6. Beutner, E. H., Jordan, R., and Chorzelski, T. The immunopathology of pemphigus and bullous pemphigoid. *J. Invest. Dermatol.* 51:63, 1968.
7. Britz, M., and Sibulkin, D. Recurrent erythema multiforme and herpes genitalis (type 2). *JAMA* 233:812, 1975.
8. Bystryn, J. C., and Rodriguez, J. Absence of intercellular antigens in the deep layers of the epidermis in pemphigus foliaceus. *J. Clin. Invest.* 61:339, 1978.
9. Chorzelski, T. P., Beutner, E. H., and Jablonska, S. The Role and Nature of Autoimmunity in Pemphigus. In E. H. Beutner, T. P. Chorzelski, and S. F. Bean (Eds.), *Immunopathology of the Skin* (2nd ed.). New York: Wiley, 1979. P. 183.
10. Chorzelski, T. P., Jablonska, S., and Beutner, E. H. Pemphigoid. In E. H. Beutner, T. P. Chorzelski, and S. F. Bean (Eds.), *Immunopathology of the Skin* (2nd ed.). New York: Wiley, 1979. P. 243.
11. Dahl, M. V., et al. Viral studies in pemphigus. *J. Invest. Dermatol.* 62:96, 1974.
12. Diaz, L. A., Glamb, R. W., and Silva, J. A syndrome of multiple immune reactivity: A breakdown in immune regulation. *Arch. Dermatol.* 116:77, 1980.
13. Foster, C. S. Immunosuppressive therapy for external ocular inflammatory disease. *Ophthalmology* (Rochester) 87:140, 1980.
14. Hardy, K., et al. Benign mucous membrane pemphigoid. *Arch. Dermatol.* 104:467, 1971.
15. Jordan, R. E., et al. Basement zone antibodies in bullous pemphigoid. *JAMA* 200:751, 1967.
16. Kasmierowski, J. A., and Wuepper, K. D. Erythema multiforme: Immune complex vasculitis of the superficial cutaneous microvasculature. *J. Invest. Dermatol.* 71:366, 1978.
17. Mondino, B. F., Brown, S. I., and Rabin, B. S. HLA antigens in ocular cicatricial pemphigoid. *Br. J. Ophthalmol.* 62:265, 1978.
18. Ostler, H. B., Conant, M. A., and Groundwater, J. Lyell's disease, the Stevens-Johnson

syndrome, and exfoliative dermatitis. *Trans. Am. Acad. Ophthalmol. Otolaryngol.* 74:1254, 1970.

19. Park, M. S., and Terasaki, P. I. HLA-DRw4 in 91% of Jewish pemphigus vulgaris patients. *Lancet* 2:441, 1979.

20. Roenigk, H. R., and Deodhar, S. Pemphigus treatment with azathioprine. *Arch. Dermatol.* 107:353, 1973.

21. Rogers, R. S., et al. Immunopathology of cicatricial pemphigoid: Studies of complement deposition. *J. Invest. Dermatol.* 68:39, 1977.

22. Rogers, R. S., and Bourne, W. M. Bullous skin diseases with ophthalmic manifestations. *Perspect. Ophthalmol.* 3:195, 1979.

23. Rogers, R. S., Seehafer, J. R., and Perry, H. O. Treatment of cicatricial (benign mucous membrane) pemphigoid with dapsone. *J. Am. Acad. Dermatol.* 6:215, 1982.

24. Sams, W. M., and Gleich, G. J. Failure to transfer bullous pemphigoid with serum from patients. *Proc. Soc. Exp. Biol. Med.* 136:1027, 1971.

25. Stendahl, O., Molin, L., and Dahlgren, C. The inhibition of polymorphonuclear leukocyte cytotoxicity by dapsone: A possible mechanism in the treatment of dermatitis herpetiformis. *J. Clin. Invest.* 62:214, 1978.

26. Theodore, F. H., and Lewson, A. C. Bilateral iritis complicating serum sickness. *Arch. Ophthalmol.* 21:828, 1939.

27. Weissman, V., et al. The correlation between the antibody titers in sera and patients with pemphigus vulgaris and their clinical state. *J. Invest. Dermatol.* 71:107, 1978.

28. Wood, G. W., Beutner, E. H., and Chorzelski, T. P. Studies in immunodermatology: II. Production of pemphigus-like lesions by intradermal injection of monkeys with Brazilian pemphigus foliaceus sera. *Int. Arch. Allergy Appl. Immunol.* 42:556, 1972.

29. Wood, G. W., and Beutner, E. H. Blocking immunofluorescence studies on the specificity of pemphigus autoantibodies. *Clin. Immunol. Immunopathol.* 7:168, 1977.

7. DRY EYES

Keratoconjunctivitis Sicca

David W. Lamberts

This section considers four topics. The first is a rational method for dividing the dry eye syndromes into five categories. The second is the techniques available for diagnosing the dry eye, or sicca syndromes. The third is the currently or potentially available methods useful in treating these diseases. The complications of the dry eye syndromes will be discussed last. A dry eye or keratoconjunctivitis sicca syndrome is said to exist when the quantity or quality of the precorneal tear film is insufficient to ensure the well-being of the ocular epithelial surface.

CATEGORIES OF DRY EYE SYNDROMES

Dividing the dry eye syndromes into five varieties was originally suggested by Holly and Lemp [14]. These divisions are based on specific deficiencies that may have been chosen somewhat arbitrarily; nevertheless, they have excellent clinical applicability. The divisions are as follows: aqueous tear deficiency, mucin deficiency, lipid abnormalities, lid surfacing abnormalities, and epitheliopathies.

AQUEOUS TEAR DEFICIENCY

The aqueous layer forms the greatest bulk of the precorneal tear film. Aqueous tears are produced in the main lacrimal glands, with a lesser contribution from the accessory glands of Wolfring and Krause. Aqueous deficiency is by far the most common of the dry eye syndromes. Various causes share responsibility for the aqueous deficiency syndromes (Table 7-1). In spite of their rather diverse origins, the clinical presentation of these diseases is similar. One entity, Sjögren's syndrome, is such an important disease it is discussed separately in the second section of this chapter.

MUCIN DEFICIENCY

The mucin deficiency diseases are a more compact group of abnormalities than are the aqueous deficiencies (Table 7-2). Mucin is produced primarily by the goblet cells of the conjunctiva. There is some evidence that at least a small amount of mucin is also produced by the main lacrimal gland [16]. With this in mind, it can be said that those illnesses that damage the conjunctiva will result in mucin deficiency. Whether or not the abnormalities seen in these conditions are due to, or only associated with, the mucin deficiency is not yet clear, however.

LIPID ABNORMALITIES

Only in severe anhidrotic ectodermal dysplasia is there a true lipid deficiency. This is extremely rare and occurs when the meibomian glands are congenitally absent. A much more important aspect of lipid abnormality involves the changes found in the meibomian secretion composition in various types of blepharitis. The bacteria that invade the meibomian glands secrete lipases that hydrolyze the normal lipids to produce various types of free fatty acids. These fatty acids are extremely surface active and are capable of rupturing, upon contact, an otherwise stable tear film. Whether these free fatty acids are directly toxic to the corneal epithelium or whether they only damage the epithelium via formation of dry spots is not known. Both mechanisms may play a role in the formation of the superficial punctate staining commonly seen in blepharitis.

LID SURFACING ABNORMALITIES

One of the most important functions of the lid is to resurface the eye with tears constantly through blinking. In a blink, the eyelids sweep the eye's surface, brushing away exogenous contaminates as well as lipid-contaminated mucin strands. Fresh mucin is thereby distributed over the corneal and conjunctival surface. Any break in the integrity of the lid or its close apposition to the ocular surface can produce areas of dryness. Entities in this category are listed in Table 7-3. One of these items, dellen formation (from the German *Delle*, meaning dent or depression), is unique and deserves separate comment. A dellen is an area of locally thinned cornea adjacent to a limbal or conjunctival elevation. Dellen have been associated with muscle surgery, filtering blebs, and limbal and conjunctival tumors. The pathophysiology of dellen formation is shown in Figure 7-1. As the upper lid slides down over the limbal mass, it is unable to touch the adja-

cent "corneal valley." There is a small area that is not resurfaced by the lid and does not receive a rejuvenated layer of mucin with each blink. This area is not able to support a continuous tear film without the benefit of an adequate hydrophilic mucous layer. If allowed to persist, this area of dry cornea will dehydrate to the extent that a shallow crater will appear. This is a dellen (Fig. 7-2). Fluorescein dye will pool in dellen, but the epithelium usually remains intact and will not stain. Most dellen will disappear if the eye is taped shut for 24 to 48 hours. A similar pathophysiology explains the 3-9 o'clock staining syndrome commonly seen in hard contact lens wearers. In this case, the contact lens is the mass that interferes with the lid-globe integrity and thus prevents adequate wetting of the adjacent epithelium. This entity does not progress to the point of stromal thinning, probably because of con-

TABLE 7-1. *Causes of Aqueous Tear Deficiency*

Congenital
  Riley-Day syndrome (familial dysautonomia) [35]
  Anhidrotic ectodermal dysplasia [37]
  Alacrima secondary to congenital absence of the lacrimal gland [5]
  Cri du chat syndrome [15]
  Absence of lacrimal nucleus [46]
  Congenital familial sensory neuropathy with anhidrosis [31]
  Adie's syndrome [7]
  Multiple endocrine neoplasia [2]
Acquired
  Trauma to lacrimal gland
    Surgical removal [39]
    Injury
    Radiation damage
  Inflammation of lacrimal gland
    Sjögren's syndrome (see following section)
    Primary amyloidosis [42]
    Mumps
    Trachoma
  Infiltrations
    Sarcoidosis [41]
    Lymphoma, leukemia [25]
    Amyloidosis
  Drugs
    Antihistamines [17]
    Thiabendazole [8]
    Antimuscarinics
    General anesthetics
  Neuroparalytic hyposecretion
    Brain stem lesions [4]
    Cerebellopontile angle and petrous bone lesions [32]
    Middle fossa floor lesions [46]
    Lesions of the sphenopalatine ganglion [46]

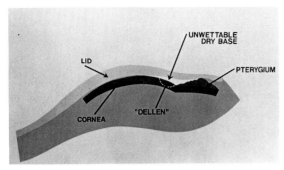

FIGURE 7-1. *In the valley between any limbal mass and the angle of contact of the tear film with the cornea is a zone where the lid cannot wet the epithelium. It is here that a delle forms. (Courtesy F. J. Holly, M.D., M. A. Lemp, M.D., and C. H. Dohlman, M.D.)*

TABLE 7-2. *Mucin Deficiency Diseases*

Goblet cell dysfunction: vitamin A deficiency
Goblet cell destruction
   Alkali burns
   Cicatricial pemphigoid
   Stevens-Johnson syndrome
   Trachoma
Drug-induced
   Practolol [48]
   Echothiophate iodide [28]

TABLE 7-3. *Lid Surfacing Abnormalities*

Lid problems
   Exposure keratitis
   Entropion
   Ectropion
   Symblepharon
   Large lid notches
   Lagophthalmos
   Keratinized lid margin
Surface irregularities
   Dellen formation with limbal lesions
   Three-nine o'clock stain in hard lens wearers
   Topical anesthetic epitheliopathy

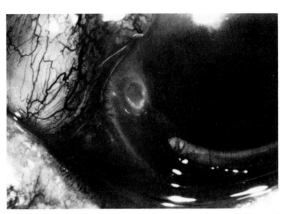

FIGURE 7-2. *A delle inside the limbus, adjacent to a swollen and elevated conjunctival mass. (Courtesy David Donaldson, M.D.)*

sion of dry eye syndromes is the least important. It is included for the sake of completeness and to emphasize the point that the tear film is a fragile structure and subject to variances of the surface on which it rests.

CLINICAL FEATURES

HISTORY

The patient's history is occasionally forgotten in ophthalmology. Nowhere is it more important than in diagnosing dry eye syndromes. Several questions are so basic that they should be part of the routine examination. One such question is, What sorts of things bother your eyes? Dry eye patients are exquisitely sensitive to drafts and winds. Often they will volunteer information regarding their intolerance to air conditioning or driving in the car with the windows rolled down. Reading is often difficult for dry eye sufferers. This probably occurs because the blink frequency decreases during tasks requiring concentration. As the blink frequency goes down, the length of time the eye is left exposed to the atmosphere may become longer than the tear breakup time (discussed below), and so drying may increase. Patients often complain that nighttime or awakening is the worst part of their day. Sleep (like general anesthesia) decreases tear production. If the eye is already compromised with regard to tear flow, further reduction during sleep may be enough to produce nocturnal symptoms. This is especially true if concurrent blepharitis or lagophthalmos is present. Smoke is almost universally intolerable to tear-deficient patients. Since smoke is actually a sus-

tact lens motion, but can be associated with superficial corneal vascularization.

EPITHELIOPATHIES

An intact tear film, because it is very thin, is dependent on a smooth, uninterrupted epithelial surface. Any irregularity in the surface will cause an associated irregularity in the tear film. Such an irregular or elevated area will predispose the tear film to break up instantly at that spot. Since the actual cause of the corneal irregularity (e.g., ulcer, erosion, scar) will usually be of primary concern, clinically this divi-

pension of solid in air, the particulate bombardment of the ocular surface produces discomfort.

Do you have any skin diseases? is a question that should always be asked. Although primary dermatologic illness is rarely the cause of a dry eye problem, looking for such illnesses often provides useful clues. Examples are numerous: scleroderma, scurvy, thrombotic thrombocytopenic purpura, the facial rash in lupus (all these are seen in association with Sjögren's syndrome), skin lesions in pemphigoid, old scars from Stevens-Johnson syndrome, and acne rosacea (associated with lipid abnormalities), to mention a few. An equally important reason for exploring skin problems during history taking is to discover entities that may mimic tear deficiency. A long list of skin disorders is associated with superficial punctate keratopathy and may present a picture that could be confused with sicca. Some of these are seborrheic dermatitis, psoriasis, ichythosis, and keratosis follicularis (Darier's disease).

What medications do you take? should also be asked. Very few adequately contolled double-blind studies have been done to determine the effects of systemic medications on tear flow. Although diuretics and birth control pills have been implicated, neither has been adequately studied. One study of birth control pills produced negative results [9]. At least one drug, chlorpheniramine, was shown by Koffler and Lemp [17] to have a deleterious effect on tear production. Eliciting other types of medication history is of help in learning about the patient's general health.

To ask about the patient's other health problems is perhaps so obvious as not to need mentioning. It should be emphasized, however, that an entity such as Sjögren's syndrome is truly a systemic disease that may involve any organ system, and that ophthalmologists see only a small part of an illness with protean manifestations.

Symptoms described or listed by the patient during the history taking are not particularly helpful in making the diagnosis of sicca. This is obviously due to the fact that there are no "dry receptors" in the cornea. Instead, patients will usually complain of irritation, redness, or a vague discomfort in the eye. Sometimes people will indeed express the specific complaint of dryness, but this is not necessarily indicative of their underlying problem; it is merely another way to describe discomfort. Often a patient with truly dry eyes will complain of tearing or excessive secretion in the eyes. These seemingly paradoxical complaints deserve a word of explanation. First,

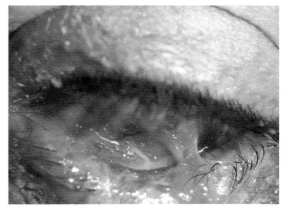

FIGURE 7-3. *In some dry eye patients, as is true with this cicatricial pemphigoid patient, a large amount of lipid-contaminated mucus is one of the major complaints.*

it is possible for the eye to get so dry that it becomes irritated and tears reflexively, much as an eye might do if suffering from a foreign body or abrasion. Secondly, as described in Physiology of the Tear Film in Chapter 1, dry eyes are particularly susceptible to excess mucus precipitation. This can occasionally be such an annoying part of the symptoms that it will be the patient's primary complaint (Fig. 7-3).

PHYSICAL EXAMINATION

The objective physical examination is much more rewarding than the patient's complaints in diagnosing dry eye diseases. The following physical findings will be discussed: filaments, meniscus height, meniscus floaters, mucous strands, and papillary conjunctivitis.

Many factors have been implicated in the formation of filaments (Table 7-4), but by far the most common association is with dryness. Filaments (Fig. 7-4) are short (usually less than 2 mm long) "tails" that hang from the surface of the cornea. Upon sectioning a filament, one finds a PAS-positive central core (mucin) surrounded by epithelium. Although the exact pathogenesis of filament formation is not known, the following represents a reasonable theory (Fig. 7-5): When the cornea dries to a point that is incompatible with a healthy epithelial layer, some surface cells will desiccate and be shed. This creates a small pit on the corneal surface that is hydrophobic compared with the mucus-coated normal surface. Lipid-contaminated mucus will become attached to these pits by hydrophobic bonding. Within a short time, surface epithelium will grow down these mucous cores, and a true filament will thus be born in situ. Because filaments are anchored to epithelial cells, pulling on them is very painful. Unfortunately, this is exactly what happens during blinking, with the resultant symptoms not unlike those produced by a foreign body.

The normal human meniscus height is usually reported to be about 1 mm. In actual fact, normal subjects never have a meniscus height of that magnitude. Rather, a height of 0.2 to 0.3 mm is most common and will be found in about 85 percent of normal subjects [19].

In a large population, no correlation was found between tear meniscus height and subsequent Schirmer test results [19]. In other words, people with a relatively high meniscus (0.4 to 0.6 mm) did not necessarily have higher Schirmer test values. In a smaller study of 9 patients with moderate to severe dry eye (all had keratoconjunctivitis sicca or Sjögren's syndrome confirmed by rose bengal staining and diminished Schirmer test values), 7 had meniscus heights of 0.1 mm and 2 had meniscus heights of 0.2 mm (D. W. Lamberts, unpublished data, 1981). It seems, then, that in normal eyes the tear meniscus height is probably subject to variables other than tear flow. Factors such as the length of the lid, location of the punctum, lid-globe apposition, and the distance of the meibomian glands from the edge of the lid probably play a role in determining meniscus height. If tear flow is reduced beyond a certain level, this apparently is manifested by a reduced meniscus height. In this limited study, a meniscus height of only 0.1 mm was present in 80 percent of the patients tested.

Meniscus floaters are extremely common in dry eye patients. They can be seen as tiny bits of debris being carried along in the upper and lower tear menisci. Floaters probably have two origins. Some are dead epithelial cells that have fallen off the sur-

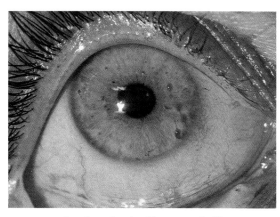

FIGURE 7-4. *Rose bengal stains filaments well. They are sometimes difficult to see without the benefit of the dye. (From D. W. Lamberts, Dry Eye Syndromes. In C. S. Foster (Ed.), Corneal and External Disease. Copyrighted by Year Book Medical Publishers, Inc. In press.)*

face of the cornea, and some are small fibrils of lipid-contaminated mucin. Although almost always present in dry eyes, they are not pathognomonic, because patients with conjunctival infections or blepharitis may also show floaters.

Mucous strands are actually strings of lipid-contaminated mucus that have rolled up and been pushed into the cul-de-sac by the shearing action of the lids. Although common in aqueous-deficient states, they can become rather spectacular in the mucin-deficient diseases (see Fig. 7-3). The proposed dynamics of mucous strand formation are shown in Figure 7-6. If the aqueous layer of tears is thick enough to prevent diffusing lipid from contaminating the mucous layer before a blink, or if mucin is available in excess to absorb the lipid molecules before a blink, then mucous strands will not become a problem. On the other hand, if mucin and excess lipid become intermingled, mucous strands may form.

Papillary conjunctivitis is a rather nonspecific reaction of the conjunctiva to irritation. It is commonly seen in allergic eye disease, infections, and acne rosacea. Its presence in dry eye syndromes is mentioned only to acknowledge its existence; it is of no value in making a diagnosis [23]. Staphylococcal blepharitis, which frequently accompanies a dry eye condition, can also result in punctate keratopathy and papillary hypertrophy of the conjunctiva.

CLINICAL DIAGNOSTIC TESTS

I should openly confess at the start of this discussion that there is no reliable objective test to render

TABLE 7-4. *Causes of Corneal Filaments*

Local
    Keratoconjunctivitis sicca
    Superior limbic keratoconjunctivitis
    Aerosol keratitis
    Beta radiation
    Herpes simplex viral infection
    Recurrent erosions
    Thygeson's superficial punctate keratitis
    Cataract surgery
    Neurotrophic and neuroparalytic keratitis
    Prolonged occlusion of the eyelids
    Retained foreign body beneath the upper lid
Systemic
    Diabetes mellitus
    Psoriasis
    Ectodermal dysplasia
    Atopic dermatitis
    Osler-Weber-Rendu disease

a firm diagnosis of dry eyes. Nevertheless, three tests are in common usage and will be discussed. These are the rose bengal dye test, the measurement of tear breakup time, and the Schirmer test.

ROSE BENGAL STAIN

Rose bengal, a red aniline dye, is a derivative of fluorescein but is different from fluorescein in several important ways. Rose bengal does not stain the precorneal tear film as does fluorescein. Instead, it seems to precipitate at the bottom of the meniscus. Rose bengal does stain devitalized or abraded epithelial cells; this is not true of fluorescein. This is probably due to rose bengal's ability to stain cell nuclei and cell protoplasm. On the other hand, fluorescein is able to permeate through a disrupted epithelial layer and diffuse among the intercellular spaces. Rose bengal also stains mucus and filaments, whereas fluorescein stains only mucus.

Rose bengal application (usually as a 1% solution) is an extremely valuable test in the diagnosis of sicca and deserves to be used more extensively. It has only one disadvantage—irritation upon instillation. The irritation seems to be directly related to the amount of epithelial damage present on the corneal surface and, to some extent, to the size of the drop. It is frequently possible to alleviate some of this pain by dropping the rose bengal onto the wooden end of a cotton-tip applicator and in turn touching the applicator to the inferior cul-de-sac. This decreases the amount of dye instilled in the eye. When using rose bengal in evaluating dry eye patients, it is most helpful to divide each eye into three zones (medial, corneal, lateral) and record the amount of stain in each on a scale of 0 to 3 [44]. In this way, each eye could receive a maximum score of 9 if it stained maximally in all three zones. A score of 3 or more for one eye is considered abnormal. Two false-positives can be seen with rose bengal stain. A small amount of stain over the body of a pterygium or pinguecula is a common and normal finding. Also, if a Schirmer test has been performed before the use of rose bengal stain, the conjunctiva will pick up the dye in the area of contact between the conjunctiva and the paper strip. It is important to remember that

FIGURE 7-5. *A theory of filament formation. As a normal epithelial surface drys (A), some cells die and fall off, leaving a defect (B). Mucin may adhere to this high-energy pit (C), and eventually epithelium may grow down over the mucin to form a filament (D). (From D. W. Lamberts, Dry Eye Syndromes. In C. S. Foster (Ed.), Corneal and External Disease. Copyrighted by Year Book Medical Publishers, Inc. In press.)*

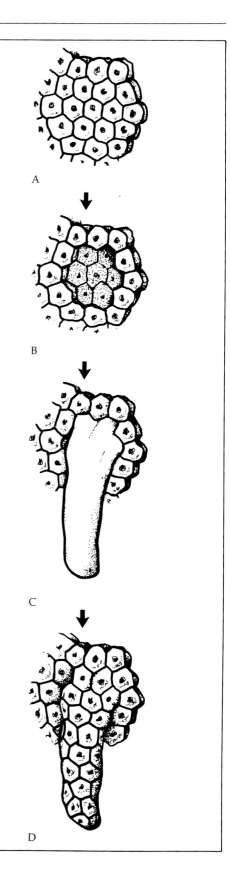

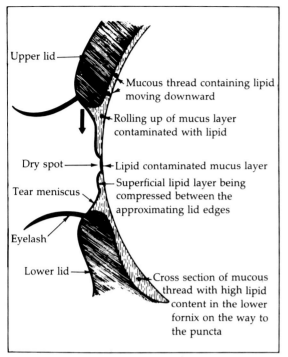

FIGURE 7-6. *Tentative mechanism for the formation of mucus strands. As the tear film thins and breaks, surface lipid may become opposed to the underlying mucin, forming lipid-mucin strands. (From F. J. Holly, and M. A. Lemp [14].)*

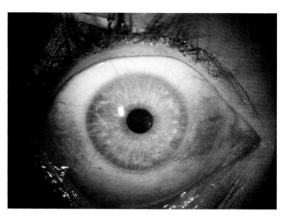

FIGURE 7-7. *The pathognomonic pattern of rose bengal stain in keratoconjunctivitis sicca is two triangles with their bases at the limbus and a band across the central cornea. This left eye has staining with +2 nasally, trace stain on the cornea, and +3 temporally.*

in dry eye syndromes the pattern of the stain, not merely its presence, is important. Anything that can damage the epithelium (infections, trauma, toxic reactions) can cause rose bengal staining, but it is characteristic of sicca to produce the pattern shown in Figure 7-7. This pattern, which is pathognomonic of keratoconjunctivitis sicca, consists of two triangles of stain on the conjunctiva with their bases on the limbus and, in particularly severe cases, a connecting band across the cornea. This area corresponds to the exposed surface of the eye within the palpebral fissure.

TEAR BREAKUP TIME

Tear breakup time (BUT) was originally described in 1969 by Norn [27], who referred to it as corneal wetting time. In this country, the concept of breakup time was popularized by Lemp and Hamill [21] in 1973. Its measurement depends upon the fact that, given enough time, the tear film will thin and eventually rupture. The mechanism of dry spot formation was discussed in Chapter 1. Its clinical measurement is accomplished as follows: A drop of fluorescein is instilled in the eye. The patient is asked to blink 2 or 3 times to distribute the dye. The test is performed at the slit lamp by asking the pa-

tient to stare straight ahead and not blink. Without touching the patient's eyelids, the examiner scans the cornea with the cobalt blue light of the slit lamp, watching for an area of tear film rupture manifested by a black island within the green sea of fluorescein. The breakup time is the time in seconds between the last blink and the appearance of the dry spot. A normal breakup time is considered to be 10 seconds or more. Several points are important when performing the test. First, the examiner must not touch the patient's lids, nor should the patient artificially elevate his lids. These maneuvers tend to expand the interpalpebral fissure and thus artificially shorten the breakup time. Second, the areas of breakup must appear in a random pattern to be counted as tear film breakup. The reason for this is to avoid counting an epithelial irregularity or elevation (which will thin the tear film and cause a rapid breakup) as a representative, random dry spot. Third, the solution in which the fluorescein is dissolved may theoretically play a role in breakup time measurements. Some recent evidence suggests that the preservatives in ophthalmic irrigating solutions and even in the fluorescein paper strip itself may artificially lower the breakup time (F. J. Holly, unpublished data, 1981). Some of these preservatives have detergentlike action and may break up the superficial lipid layer of the tear film, causing it to rupture prematurely. This may help to explain why breakup time has fallen into some disrepute in recent years, since the nature of the fluorescein solution is a variable not usually controlled. It may b better to use a nonpreserved type of fluorescein such as Fluoresoft (Holles Labs, Cohasset, Mass.) or one of the several brands of fluorescein for injection for breakup time measurements. If one uses the latter, caution must be taken to instill a *very* tiny drop (from the tip of a TB syringe, for example), because these solutions are concentrated and burn upon instillation. Because topical anesthetics also contain preservatives that are surface active and capable of rupturing the tear film and adversely affecting the microvilli of the corneal surface [29], they should not be used for the breakup time test.

SCHIRMER TEST

In spite of its notorious variability, the Schirmer test remains the most commonly performed clinical test for sicca. For such a ubiquitous examination, remarkably little basic science has been done to explore the variabilities of the Schirmer test.

It has been demonstrated in vitro that the volume of water in milliliters applied to a paper strip has a linear relation to the length of wetting of the strip in millimeters. In vivo, the relationship is not so clearcut. Figure 7-8A represents a graph of the wetting kinetics of Schirmer strips in normal human volunteers. Figure 7-8B is a companion graph of the rate of tear secretion plotted against time. The striking conclusion obtained from studying these curves is that tear production is extremely high in the first two minutes of the Schirmer test but levels off to a steady state at 4 to 5 minutes. To be more explicit, these flow rates exponentially decrease from a high reflex secretion rate to a lower, final secretion rate. The initial slope of the wetting length-time curve is proportional to the initial secretion rate, and the steady state value is proportional to the final secretion rate. In between these two limiting values, the course of the curve is defined by the magnitude of the secretion rate decay constant, which is in fact characteristic of the subject's response to ocular irritation. The clinical implications of this type of study are interesting grounds for speculation. Perhaps one should ignore the first 5 minutes of the Schirmer strip and measure the advance of wetting during the following 5 minutes, since this is really representative of the patient's "baseline" tear secretion rate. Or perhaps the strip should be made longer and allowed to rest in the patient's eye until the advancing edge stops moving. By knowing how long a column of fluid the patient could "push" out onto the Schirmer strip, the tear secretion rate could be calculated. At present these points are only food for thought, since clinical studies have not been done.

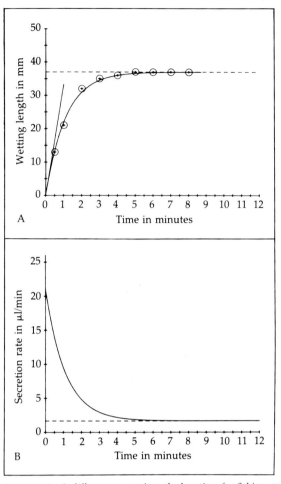

FIGURE 7-8. *A. When one examines the kenetics of a Schirmer test in vivo by plotting the wetting length versus time, one is struck by the rapid outflow of tears in the first 3 or 4 minutes and by the leveling off to a steady state after this time. B. If one plots rate of secretion of tears (in vivo) versus time, one is again impressed by the precipitous fall in secretion after the strip has been in the eye for 4 or more minutes. (Courtesy F. J. Holly, M.D.)*

When conducting the Schirmer test in a general clinical situation, any proposed rose bengal staining should be performed first. Historically, a wide variety of paper types have been used for the Schirmer test (filter paper, litmus paper, cigarette paper, blotting paper). In 1961, Halberg and Berens [12] described their standardized Schirmer paper strip manufactured from No. 589 Black Ribbon filter paper (similar to Whatman No. 41 paper) and prepared in precut strips, 5 mm and 35 mm (SMP Division, Cooper Laboratories, San Germán, Puerto Rico). The strip for the right eye has one corner cut off. A notch is present 5 mm from the other end (actually both strips are notched). The strip is bent at the notch, and the 5 mm end is inserted into the lower fornix. It probably is not important whether the medial or lateral canthal area is used, so long as the strip is not placed in the center of the lid where it might rub against the cornea. It is important to insert the short end of the strip into the fornix all the way to the notch. This assures a constant surface size in the lid available to absorb tears. The 30-mm segment is left to hang over the lower lid. In 5 minutes, the strip is removed, the wetted length measured, and the strip marked and taped in the patient's chart.

Although several normal values have been cited in the literature, most people use van Bijsterveld's value of 5.0 mm wetting in 5 minutes [44]. Some variations in Schirmer testing exist and merit some comment. For years, people have argued over whether the Schirmer test should be done with or without topical anesthesia. Those who do Schirmer tests without anesthesia argue that this is actually more physiologic, that a dry eye is indeed an irritated eye, and that this state of affairs is altered by topical anesthesia. On the other hand, those who use anesthesia argue that without it one is not measuring physiologic tear flow parameters but merely the patient's response to discomfort. Some general facts are known about the mean responses of populations to the Schirmer test done with and without anesthesia. When a large group of normal subjects were tested without anesthesia, the mean wetting value was 20 mm. When the same volunteers were tested with anesthesia, the mean value was 12 mm. Thus it can be concluded that topical anesthesia tends to decrease Schirmer values by about 40 percent when mean values of large populations are compared. Unfortunately, wide individual variation exists, and so this decrease is not realized in every single patient. Another way to look at this statistic is to compare individual wetting of the two groups. In the nonanesthetized patients, about 15 percent had wetting of 5 mm or below (15 percent false-positives). In order to achieve this same level of specificity with anesthesia, a cutoff value of 3 mm wetting (15 percent false-positives) must be used [19].

It is appropriate at this point to clear up an area of confusion in the literature. The terms *Schirmer type I* and *Schirmer type II* are common but are often used incorrectly. What was originally described by Schirmer [40] as his first test was the standard Schirmer test, without anesthesia, as described above. For his second test, he anesthetized the eye with 4% cocaine and then used a camel's hair brush to irritate the nasal mucosa. A Schirmer type II or second test is not generally performed any more in this country. It is more accurate to refer to the Schirmer test as done with or without topical anesthesia.

Should the Schirmer test be done with the eyes open or closed? A study involving a large number of volunteers was recently conducted in an effort to answer this question [20]. Some patients were tested first with closed eyes, and some were tested first with open eyes. In the second half of the test, the order was reversed. When the means were compared, there was no difference in Schirmer test values with eyes open or closed. Interestingly, the order in which the test was conducted turned out to be very important. Whichever test was conducted second was highly likely to show less wetting than the test performed first, regardless of eyelid position. In fact, if a Schirmer test is repeated in the same patient within a few minutes' time, there is only a 10 percent chance that its value will be higher than that of the first Schirmer. Whether this is due to "exhaustion" of the tear flow or merely some type of adaptation on the part of the patient is not known.

LABORATORY TESTS
There are a number of laboratory tests, not readily available in a clinical setting, used for diagnosing sicca patients. Of these, the following will be discussed: fluorescein dilution tests, tear mucin measurement, goblet cell counts, tear osmolality, and tear lysozyme measurements.

FLUORESCEIN DILUTION TESTS
There are many minor variations on the fluorescein dilution test, but all share these basic fundamentals: A small, nonirritating fluorescein drop of known volume is placed in the eye and mixed with tears, and the subsequent levels of fluorescence are used to calculate the tear volume. As the fluorescence diminishes with time because of dilution with new tears, the tear turnover rate can be calculated. The equipment required consists of a slit lamp with a light source passed through an exciting filter and a photometric microscope. Light from the fluorescent solution passes back through a window and a barrier filter to a photomultiplier. The photomultiplier signal is amplified and eventually passed into a microammeter. This is an ingenious method of measurement and, with subtle differences, has been used by numerous investigators. There are, however, some inherent inaccuracies. First, one must assume complete mixing of the dye with the tears, including the tears under the lids and in the fornices. Second, one must assume that no fluorescein is lost through the cornea or conjunctiva. This is not likely to be an important factor if the epithelial barrier remains intact. Third, fluorescein unfortunately does not confine itself to the tear film. It is sequestered in mucous strands, crustations, and the debris around the base of the lashes. This fluorescein is

then available to diffuse back into the tear film, which would result in an underestimation of tear flow.

TEAR MUCIN MEASUREMENT

Dohlman and coworkers [6] described a method of measuring the hexosamine content (one of the principal moieties of mucus) of human tears in normal and presumed mucin-deficient eyes. They collected tear samples from patients with Sjögren's syndrome, cicatricial pemphigoid, and Stevens-Johnson syndrome as well as from normal volunteers. The data showed that patients with cicatricial pemphigoid or Stevens-Johnson syndrome did indeed have a diminished level of hexosamine in their tears, although some hexosamine was present even in eyes in which goblet cells were absent. Thus it seems that there is some source of mucus for the eye other than goblet cells. Perhaps the main lacrimal gland, which does contain some mucus-secreting cells [16], is this additional source. Patients with Sjögren's syndrome had normal tear hexosamine levels.

GOBLET CELL COUNTS

Virchow [45] was the first to describe a technique of measuring goblet cell density in the normal human conjunctiva. He reported 10 goblet cells per square millimeter in specimens from the upper orbital and tarsal areas, and 15 goblet cells per square millimeter from the lower orbital and tarsal regions. In 1975, Ralph [33] reported a study of goblet cell densities (read from biopsy specimens) of the deep tarsal portion of the inferior nasal conjunctival fornix in normal subjects and in patients with keratoconjunctivitis sicca, Stevens-Johnson syndrome, cicatricial pemphigoid, and acute alkali burns. He found the average goblet cell count in normal subjects to be 8.84 (± 4.66) per square millimeter. Interestingly, patients with keratoconjunctivitis sicca (not generally considered a mucus-deficient disease) showed a decreased count of 2.11 (± 0.78) cells per square millimeter. Patients with Stevens-Johnson syndrome and cicatricial pemphigoid had less than 1 cell per square millimeter. As expected, in patients with acute alkali burns no goblet cells could be found (their conjunctiva was destroyed by the alkali).

TEAR OSMOLALITY

Mishima and coworkers [26] were the first actually to demonstrate that sicca patients have a significant increase in the osmolality of their tears. They found an average increase of about 25 mOsm/L in 6 keratoconjunctivitis eyes, compared with normal eyes. More recently, Gilbard and associates [11] studied the osmolality of tear samples obtained from 36 normal eyes, 30 keratoconjunctivitis sicca eyes, and 8 eyes with conjunctivitis. They found that all but 1 of the dry eye patients had tear osmolalities of about 311 mOsm/kg, and all but three of the normals had osmolalities below 311 mOsm/kg (2 of these 3 had particles of eye makeup in their menisci). All of the conjunctivitis patients had osmolalities below 311 mOsm/kg. Whether this phenomenon is a cause of the epithelial pathology observed in sicca patients or merely an incidental finding is not yet known. Some findings have indicated that such small (5–10 percent) increases in tear osmolality has no deleterious effect on the epithelium.

TEAR LYSOZYME MEASUREMENTS

Lysozyme is an easily measurable component of human tears, and tear lysozyme levels may be of diagnostic value in certain diseases. Although decreased lysozyme levels are usually mentioned in reference to dry eye syndromes, the finding is not specific for these disorders. Decreased tear lysozyme levels have been reported in Sjögren's syndrome [1], keratoconjunctivitis sicca [24], smog irritation [38, 46], herpes simplex infection [36], bacterial conjunctivitis [34], and protein-calorie malnutrition [47].

Lysozyme is able to attack the cell walls of certain bacteria and probably functions as one of the eyes' antibacterial defenses. Although a great many ways have been designed to measure tear lysozyme, one of the most popular methods is that of agar diffusion. This method uses an agarose gel slab containing a uniform suspension of *Micrococcus lysodeikticus*, an organism whose cell wall is destroyed by lysozyme. Into the gel is cut a small hole to function as a well to hold the tear sample. The gel with the tear sample is then allowed to incubate, either at room temperature or at 37°C. The enzyme molecules diffuse radially through the agarose gel layer and lyse the bacterial cell walls, thus forming a zone of clearing around the well. The greater the concentration of the enzyme in the solution, the greater the diameter of the cleared zone (after incubation for a given time). Copeland and colleagues [3] have demonstrated that the method of collection of the specimen can lead to errors because of adsorption of the lysozyme on the filter paper or sponge used. Fortunately, techniques of lysozyme testing not employing cellulose sampling methods have still shown that dry eye patients have decreased lysozyme concentration in their tears.

SUPPLEMENTATION OF TEARS

Essentially three types of tear substitutes are currently marketed: drops, ointments, and inserts. Artificial tear drops remain the mainstay of the treatment for sicca (Table 7-5). It has been known for years that the retention time of a low-viscosity (i.e., saline) drop in the eye is very short, with a half-life measured in seconds. In 1945, Swann [43] first described the use of methylcellulose, an inert substance of relatively high viscosity, in an artificial tear. In 1964, Krishna and Brown [18] described polyvinyl alcohol as another drug with good artificial tear potential because of its "film-forming properties." Unfortunately, the picture has since become much more complex. Even on basic premises, such as increasing ocular retention by increasing viscosity, one will find the literature in conflict. Numerous studies have been done comparing the retention properties of the cellulose esters and polyvinyl alcohol. Because the studies are in conflict with one another, the clinician finds no hard evidence to favor one type of drop over another.

In more recent years, two newer drops, Adsorbotear (Burton, Parsons, Washington, D.C.) and Tears Naturale (Alcon, Fort Worth, Tex.) have been marketed. Although these drops contain different polymers, both are reported to be mucomimetic in the sense that they are capable of binding at multiple sites to corneal epithelium, much as does natural mucin, producing a hydrophilic layer. In this

way, these polymers may be able to provide the cornea with an artificial mucous layer that will stabilize the tear film.

Clinically, choosing an artificial tear is a rather arbitrary, nonscientific exercise. In general, there are two schools of thought. One is that since there are no hard data to recommend one drop over another, the patient can be supplied with an assortment of drops to take home and experiment with as he or she chooses. A variation on this "patient selects" technique is to give the patient one drop for the right eye and a different drop for the left eye. Even if both eyes are similarly affected, the patient will often find one drop more comfortable than the other. The second school of thought is that this indiscriminate treatment is a blatant confession of ignorance and that it is better to prescribe one drop for the patient's use and then change it if it is found unsatisfactory. The reader may choose for himself the approach with which he feels comfortable.

Recently, some interest has been generated in the use of eye drops of low osmolality, based upon the observation that dry eye patients tend to have hyperosmotic tears. Hypotears (CooperVision, San Germán, Puerto Rico), a drop with an osmolality of about 220 mOsm/L, was recently marketed as a way to reduce the tonicity of the tear film. There are two problems with this approach. One is that it has never been demonstrated that a moderate increase in tear osmolality is indeed important in the pathophysiology of sicca. It may be a result and not a cause of the changes seen in dry eye patients. Second, the effect on the tonicity of tears from nonisotonic drops is extremely brief. Even drops having extreme nonisotonicity of 0 or 1000 mOsm/L are able to affect tear tonicity for only 60 to 90 seconds [13]. Despite these misgivings, Hypotears has been well received by dry eye patients. It may exert its beneficial action through mechanisms not understood.

In July 1981, a new product, the Lacrisert (Merck Sharp & Dohme, West Point, Pa.), was marketed. Formerly known as the SR-AT (slow-releasing artificial tear), the Lacrisert is a small 5-mg pellet of hydroxypropyl cellulose in cylinder form. When dry, it looks like a grain of rice. The pellet is placed in the inferior cul-de-sac with a plastic inserter (Fig. 7-9A). It is important that the insert be placed below the inferior edge of the tarsal plate, because this location tends to trap the insert and prevent it from popping out. Within a short time, the Lacrisert absorbs tears and becomes a soft, gelatinous blob (Figure 7-9B). During the course of several hours, it

TABLE 7-5. *Polymeric Composition of Tear Substitutes*

Methylcellulose and derivatives
  Bro-Lac (Riker Labs)
  Isopto-Tears (Alcon)
  Lacril (Allergan)
  Methulose (Softcon)
  Murotears (Muro)
  Tearisol (CooperVision)
  Ultratears (Alcon)
Hydroxyethyl cellulose
  Lyteers (Barnes-Hind)
Polyvinyl alcohol
  Pre-Sert (Allergan)
  Liquifilm Tears (Allergan)
  Liquifilm Forte (Allergan)
Polyvinyl alcohol and hydroxycellulose
  Neo-Tears (Barnes-Hind)
  Tears Plus (Allergan)
Polyethylene oxide, polyvinylpyrrolidone, and hydroxyethyl cellulose
  Adsorbotear (Alcon)
Dextran and hydroxypropyl methylcellulose
  Tears Naturale (Alcon)

slowly dissolves and releases its polymer into the tear film. Patients generally use the insert once or twice daily. Sometimes it is helpful to use an artificial tear concurrently to help dissolve the pellet. The Lacrisert has been a valuable addition for the treatment of some dry eye patients. The two most common problems with it has been inadvertent loss of the insert and blurred vision. The latter is quite common and stems from the fact that the insert, as it dissolves, greatly thickens and enlarges the lower tear meniscus. When patients look through this meniscus (particularly upon down gaze) they report blurred vision. Some patients are also annoyed by feeling the presence of the insert.

PRESERVATION OF EXISTING TEARS

Several ingenious methods of tear preservation have been described in the literature. They include swimmers' goggles, clear food wrap shields, silicone rubber shields, moist chamber spectacles, lid taping, bandage contact lenses, and punctal occlusion. The goggle-type treatments all share the common goal of trying to eliminate evaporation by creating moisture traps in front of the eye. One of their drawbacks is lack of social acceptability, although if used at home, especially for reading, they can be helpful. Swimmers' goggles have been invaluable for comatose patients with exposure keratitis. They are tight enough to be truly moisture-proof and protect the eye without the need for tape. Swimmers' goggles have saved me from doing several bedside tarsorraphies.

Bandage contact lenses occupy a unique place in the treatment of sicca. They are most helpful in three situations: filamentary keratitis, mucin-deficient dry eyes with an adequate aqueous phase, and exposure keratitis. In filamentary keratitis, they are the treatment of choice. Relief from pain is almost instantaneous, and the filaments seem to melt away under the bandage lens, not to reappear while the lens is in place. It is important to realize that soft lenses are not completely innocuous in dry eyes (see Chapter 17, Therapeutic Soft Contact Lenses). The risk of infection is increased in dry eyes, and the use of prophylactic antibiotic drops (i.e, chloramphenicol drops twice daily) is recommended. Perhaps more important is that the patient be aware of the possibility of infection and be well educated in what to watch for. Patients must be told that any increase in pain or redness or any decrease in vision may mean that the lens needs to be removed and should prompt them to seek medical attention. Bandage lenses in dry eye patients must be kept moist, and

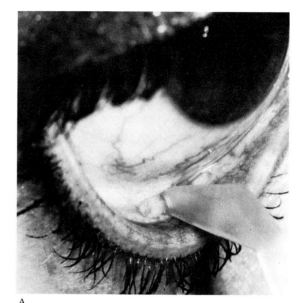

A

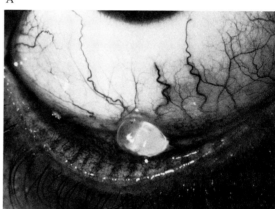

B

FIGURE 7-9. A. A soft plastic insertion aid is used to push the hydroxypropyl cellulose insert (Lacrisert) deep into the lower fornix. B. After a few minutes, the insert forms a soft, gelatinous blob.

the concurrent use of artificial tears is usually recommended. Even with such therapy, more deposits seem to form on lenses in these patients than in normals, and the rate of lens replacement is higher.

Punctal occlusion has been attempted by solid gelatin rods, poly(hydroxyethylmethacrylate) plugs, cyanoacrylate adhesives, silicon plugs, and electrocautery. Electrocautery occlusion is irreversible but is used most commonly. It has generally been taught that punctal occlusion by electrocautery should only be performed on extremely dry eyes with consecutive Schirmer test values below 2 mm in a symptomatic patient. What one often finds in such cases is very little difference in the subjective and objective findings before and after closure. This may be due to the fact that patients with this severity of dryness do not lose tears down their puncta since so little fluid is being formed by the lacrimal glands. Indeed, there is a recent trend to be more aggressive in the use of punctal occlusion, and this philosophy may well be appropriate. A prospective study on punctal occlusion remains to be done.

Temporary punctal occlusion can be attained by placing a heated spatula on the punctum for a second. This procedure will close the punctum for a week or 2 only, but will predict the results to be expected from permanent occlusion. If epiphora results, obviously the eyes are not as dry as had been thought, and permanent occlusion should be avoided.

Permanent occlusion of the puncta is best achieved by electrocautery and is done as follows:

1. Lidocaine hydrochloride 1% (Xylocaine) is used to infiltrate the lid adjacent to the punctum and nasally toward the nasolacrimal sac adjacent to the canaliculus.
2. A topical anesthetic is instilled in the cul-de-sac.
3. The electrocautery (Hyfrecator, Birtcher Corp., Los Angeles, Calif.) is plugged in and the cord inserted into the low-voltage hole.
4. A fine, needle-type epilation tip is placed in the handle.
5. The tip is threaded into the punctum and along the canaliculus for a distance of 10 to 12 mm.
6. With the power setting at 15 to 20, the foot pedal is depressed while the conjunctival side of the canaliculus is observed. A blanching of the conjunctiva signifies cauterization. When this occurs, the tip is pulled 1 to 2 mm out of the canaliculus and the pedal is again depressed.
7. As the tip is withdrawn, the power is continuously decreased. As the tip approaches the punctum, the power should be low (below 5). Caution must be exercised at this end point, because a small amount of power will produce a large amount of burn once the tip is near the lid surface.

It should be noted that the power setting varies depending on the instrument. Only one eye should be done at a time, in the remote event that epiphora should result unexpectedly.

The silicon punctum plug, although not yet on the market, remains an appealing alternative to electrocautery occlusion. Originally described by Freeman [10], these plugs have flanges on the top and bottom (Fig. 7-10A) and are partially hollow. Just before implantation, the punctum is dilated using a special dilator with a maximum diameter of 1.2 mm. This is the minimum opening required for insertion of the plug. A thin metal probe is then placed in the partial hollow in the plug, and the

plug is gently forced into the punctum, leaving the top exposed on the lid surface (Fig. 7-10B). Either one or both puncta may be closed in this manner. The obvious advantage of these ingenious devices is their ease of removal if epiphora ensues or if no improvement is noted. Complications have not been major except in the rare instance in which the plug turns inward and rubs on the nasal conjunctiva. Spontaneous expulsion occurs but is very uncommon. The punctum plug offers exciting possibilities for studying the dynamics of tear flow. Since the plugs are extremely easy to insert (only topical anesthesia is required) and can be switched from punctum to punctum, patients could serve as their own controls and be entered into crossover studies.

STIMULATION OF TEARS
A relatively unexplored area of dry eye therapy is the stimulation of the lacrimal gland to produce more tears. Several medications have been tried in this regard, including bromhexine, eledoisin, and physalaemin. The medications have been rather widely used in Europe but very rarely in this country. They are discussed in Physiology of the Tear Film in Chapter 1.

DISPERSAL OF MUCIN
Occasionally one encounters a patient in whom the production of mucous strands is the most prominent complaint (see Fig. 7-3). In these cases, acetylcysteine at a 20% or 10% level in aqueous solution (Mucomyst) may be used as an eye drop to break up the large mucin molecules into more soluble components. Acetylcysteine is generally administered as fine nebulae for patients with bronchopulmonary disease and inspissated mucus. The medication can be administered as a drop, three or four times daily, directly from the bottle. Disadvantages include its somewhat unpleasant sulfurous odor and burning after administration.

SURGERY
Several surgical procedures have been developed to help with certain aspects of dry eye diseases. Tarsorrhaphy is used basically for only one indication in dry eye patients: after facial nerve paralysis with subsequent exposure keratitis. A temporal tarsorrhaphy, closing 50 percent of the fissure, is usually adequate to protect the cornea and still provide a view of the globe. After trigeminal nerve lesions, neurotrophic keratitis may ensue as a surgical complication. Tarsorrhaphy is frequently performed in

these cases, not because of dryness, but because the protection afforded the eye by the upper lid may be of value in preventing epithelial breakdown (see Chapter 8, Corneal Manifestations of Neurologic Diseases). Other indications for tarsorrhaphy are generally within the realm of the plastic surgeon. Transplantation of the parotid duct was in vogue several years ago but is rarely performed anymore. The parotid gland responds to entirely different stimuli from the lacrimal gland, and the parotid's secretion is rather copious in comparison with the lacrimal gland's. For these reasons, and for the more mundane problem of locating a surgeon willing to undertake the chore, the operation has for the most part been abandoned in this country.

Other procedures such as corneal transplantation, fornix reconstruction, and keratoprosthesis are more heroic measures used to treat the severe complications of sicca syndromes, but they are frequently unsuccessful in preserving vision (see Therapeutic Keratoplasty in Chapter 15 and Chapter 16, Conjunctival Surgery for Corneal Disease).

COMPLICATIONS OF DRY EYE SYNDROMES

Although treating the problems associated directly with decreased tear production is challenging enough, one must also be aware of the complications and sequelae of the sicca syndromes. The following will be discussed: (1) sterile stromal ulcers, (2) blepharitis and conjunctivitis, (3) band keratopathy, (4) keratinization, and (5) psychologic effects.

STERILE STROMAL ULCERS

Pfister and Murphy [30] have recently written an excellent synopsis of the association between keratoconjunctivitis sicca and stromal melting. The cause of stromal melting is not known, but clinically the cases are monotonously similar. Interestingly, men seem to be affected almost as often as women. The patients invariably have rheumatoid arthritis. The melt is typically an oval, noninfiltrated ulcer situated at or just below the visual axis with its longest dimension horizontal (Fig. 7-11). These lesions are sterile but tend to progress quickly and often perforate. The most important facet of treatment appears to be covering up the defect, either with a bandage lens or cyanoacrylate adhesive. In some cases, especially if perforation has occurred, a corneal graft may be necessary. If perforation is prevented, the ulcers eventually heal, either with or without vascularization.

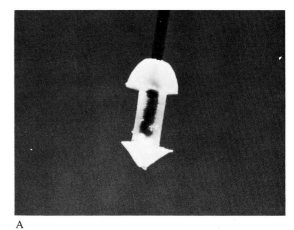

A

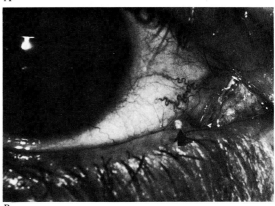

B

FIGURE 7-10. *A silicon punctum plug impaled on its wire inserter, ready to be placed into a punctum. B. With the plug in place, the mushroom-shaped top* (arrow) *is visible above the surface of the skin.*

BLEPHARITIS AND CONJUNCTIVITIS

Infections are more common in dry eye patients than in the normal population. One can speculate that this is true because of the loss of the defense mechanisms provided by the normal flow of tears and their bactericidal components. Not only do the tears stagnate in sicca patients, but the level of lysozyme (and perhaps some of the other bactericidal components of tears) is decreased. The loss of these capabilities puts the eye at increased risk of infection, especially with *Staphylococcus aureus.*

BAND KERATOPATHY

In 1977, Lemp and Ralph [22] described the rapid development of band keratopathy within epithelial defects on dry corneas. The cause of the band keratopathy was not known. The patients had in common the presence of sicca, a precedent epithelial defect, and the frequent use of artificial tears. I

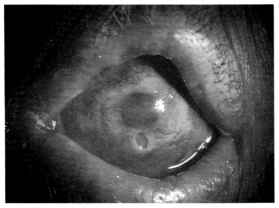

FIGURE 7-11. *A sterile melt in the cornea of a patient with severe dry eye syndrome. The lesion healed after application of a bandage lens.*

had the occasion to see a very similar case of band keratopathy in a 78-year-old woman who had previously received a corneal transplant because of aphakic bullous keratopathy. She suffered from mild keratoconjunctivitis sicca and used artificial tears several times daily. While wearing an aphakic bandage lens, a soft, gelatinous layer of white debris formed on the epithelial surface of the right eye. This was gently scraped off with a blade, and the lens was replaced. Two days later, she returned with a dense, gritty calcium plaque in the area where the epithelium had been scraped. It was subsequently removed with EDTA.

KERATINIZATION
Any of the entities that are capable of harming the conjunctival goblet cells (vitamin A deficiency, cicatricial pemphigoid, alkali burns, Stevens-Johnson syndrome, trachoma) can lead to keratinization of the cornea and conjunctival epithelium. It is as if epithelial keratin formation is a phenomemon associated with abnormal mucous membrane and mucus deficiency. Clinically, keratinization of the epithelium is important for two reasons: it is uncomfortable, and, if severe enough, the cornea may be involved, with subsequent loss of vision. Keratinization of the palpebral conjunctiva is most common and is easily seen on slit lamp examination. Keratinized epithelium has a peculiar pearly white sheen, quite unlike the normal pink, shiny epithelium. Keratinized epithelium also has a rough, slightly elevated surface that fluorescein does not cover because the surface does not wet well with tears. Scrapings from the conjunctiva may reveal these keratinized cells. It is the rough surface that is irritating, and so soft bandage lenses may

sometimes help. Final state cicatricial pemphigoid is notorious for forming dense, keratinized membranes over the corneal surface. These membranes can easily be stripped off, and a remarkably clear cornea may be found underneath the pannus. Unfortunately, the pannus tends to recur eventually. Only in the case of vitamin A deficiency has the keratinization process been demonstrated to be reversible.

PSYCHOLOGIC EFFECTS
With rare exception, the dry eye syndromes are chronic diseases that plague their victims for the duration of their lives. Some of the illnesses, such as cicatricial pemphigoid, are blinding; others, such as Sjögren's syndrome, are not; all are persistent. This puts the physician in a discomfiting position, since we are more or less powerless to cure those who seek our aid. For these reasons, many dry eye patients become extremely dependent upon their physicians and require at least as much compassion as medication. It is important to emphasize that although the disease causing the sicca cannot be eliminated, a great many things can be done to alleviate the symptoms, and essentially all patients can be made more comfortable. Because of the chronic nature of the problem, most patients go through periods of despondency and depression. Unfortunately, this can lead to major changes in lifestyle, including divorce and loss of employment. Ophthalmologists must recognize this part of the illness and actively encourage their patients to continue to pursue their normal activities. A bottle of artificial tears dispensed as a matter of routine may do well in treating the eye, but it is woefully neglectful of the needs of the patient.

REFERENCES
1. Avisar, R., et al. Lysozyme content of tears in patients with Sjögren's syndrome and rheumatoid arthritis. *Am. J. Ophthalmol.* 87:148, 1979.
2. Baum, J. L., and Adler, M. E. A variant of the pheochromocytoma, medullary thyroid carcinoma, multiple mucosal neuroma syndrome. *Arch. Ophthalmol.* 87:574, 1972.
3. Copeland, J. P., Lamberts, D. W., and Holly, F. J. Investigation of the accuracy of tear lysozyme determination by the Quantiplate method. *Invest. Ophthalmol. Vis. Sci.* 10:103, 1982.
4. Crosby, E. C., and DeJonge, B. R. Experimental and clinical studies of central connections

and central relations of the facial nerve. *Ann. Otolaryngol.* 72:735, 1963.

5. Davidoff, E., and Friedman, A. H. Congenital alacrima. *Surv. Ophthalmol.* 22:113, 1977.
6. Dohlman, C. H., et al. The glycoprotein (mucus) content of tears from normals and dry eye patients. *Exp. Eye Res.* 22:359, 1976.
7. Esterly, N. B., et al. Pupillotonia, hyporeflexia, and segmental hypohidrosis: Autonomic dysfunction in a child. *J. Pediatr.* 73:852, 1968.
8. Fink, A. I., and Mackay, S. S. Sicca complex and cholangiostatic jaundice in two members of a family probably caused by thiabendazole. *Ophthalmology* (Rochester) 86:1892, 1979.
9. Frankel, S. H., and Ellis, P. P. Effect of oral contraceptives on tear production. *Ann. Ophthalmol.* 10:1585, 1978.
10. Freeman, J. M. Punctum plug: Evaluation of a new treatment for dry eyes. *Trans. Am. Acad. Ophthalmol. Otolaryngol.* 79:874, 1975.
11. Gilbard, J. P., Farris, R. L., and Santamaria, J., II. Osmolarity of tear microvolumes in keratoconjunctivitis sicca. *Arch. Ophthalmol.* 96:677, 1978.
12. Halberg, G. P., and Berens, C. Standardized Schirmer test kit. *Am. J. Ophthalmol.* 51:840, 1961.
13. Holly, F. J., and Lamberts, D. W. Effect of nonisotonic solutions on tear film osmolality. *Invest. Ophthalmol.* 20:236, 1981.
14. Holly, F. J., and Lemp, M. A. Tear physiology and dry eyes. *Surv. Ophthalmol.* 22:69, 1977.
15. Howard, R. Ocular abnormalities in the cri du chat syndrome. *Am. J. Ophthalmol.* 73:949, 1973.
16. Jensen, O., et al. Mucosubstances of the acini of the human lacrimal gland (orbital part): I. Histochemical identification. *Acta Ophthalmol.* 47:605, 1969.
17. Koffler, B. H., and Lemp, M. A. The effect of an antihistamine (chlorpheniramine maleate) on tear production in humans. *Ann. Ophthalmol.* 12:217, 1980.
18. Krishna, N., and Brown, F. Polyvinyl alcohol as an ophthalmic vehicle. *Am. J. Ophthalmol.* 57:99, 1964.
19. Lamberts, D. W., Foster, C. S., and Perry, H. D. Schirmer test after topical anesthesia and the tear meniscus height in normal eyes. *Arch. Ophthalmol.* 97:1082, 1979.
20. Lamberts, D. W., Perry, H. D., and Holly, F. J. Der Schirmer test bei offenen und geschlossen Augen. *Contactologia* 2D:115, 1980.
21. Lemp, M. A., and Hamill, J. Factors affecting tear film breakup in normals. *Arch. Ophthalmol.* 89:103, 1973.
22. Lemp, M. A., and Ralph, R. A. Rapid development of band keratopathy in dry eyes. *Am. J. Ophthalmol.* 83:657, 1977.
23. Mackie, I. A., and Seal, D. V. The questionably dry eye. *Br. J. Ophthalmol.* 65:2, 1981.
24. McEwen, W., and Kimura, S. Filter-paper electrophoresis of tears: I. Lysozyme and its correlation with keratoconjunctivitis sicca. *Am. J. Ophthalmol.* 39:200, 1955.
25. Meyer, D., Yanoff, M., and Hanno, H. Differential diagnosis in Mikulicz's syndrome, Mikulicz's disease and similar disease entities. *Am. J. Ophthalmol.* 71:516, 1971.
26. Mishima, S., Kubota, Z., and Farris, R. L. The tear flow dynamics in normal and in keratoconjunctivitis sicca cases. In M. P. Solanes (Ed.), Proceedings of the 21st International Congress of Ophthalmology, Mexico, March 8–14, 1970. Amsterdam: Excerpta Medica, 1971. Pt. 2, pp. 1801–1805.
27. Norn, M. S. Desiccation of the precorneal tear film: I. Corneal wetting time. *Acta Ophthalmol.* (Copenh.) 47:865, 1969.
28. Patten, J. T., Cavanagh, H. D., and Allansmith, M. R. Induced ocular pseudopemphigoid. *Am. J. Ophthalmol.* 82:272, 1976.
29. Pfister, R. R., Holly, F. J., and Kuwabara, T. Factors affecting cell wall morphology of corneal epithelium. Read at the meeting of the Association for Research in Vision and Ophthalmology, Sarasota, Fla., 1972.
30. Pfister, R. R., and Murphy, G. E. Corneal ulceration and perforation associated with Sjögren's syndrome. *Arch. Ophthalmol.* 98:89, 1980.
31. Pinsky, L., and DiGeorge, A. M. Congenital familial sensory neuropathy with anhidrosis. *J. Pediatr.* 68:1, 1966.
32. Pulec, J. L., and House, W. F. Facial nerve involvement and testing in acoustic neuromas. *Arch. Otolaryngol.* 80:685, 1964.
33. Ralph, R. A. Conjunctival goblet cell density in normal subjects and in dry eye syndromes. *Invest. Ophthalmol.* 14:299, 1975.
34. Regan, E. The lysozyme content of tears. *Am. J. Ophthalmol.* 33:600, 1950.
35. Riley, C. M., et al. Central autonomic dysfunction with defective lacrimation: Report of five cases. *Pediatrics* 3:468, 1949.
36. Ronen, D., Romano, A., and Smetana, O. Lysozyme tear level in patients with herpes simplex virus eye infections. *Invest. Ophthalmol. Vis. Sci.* 16:850, 1977.
37. Rook, A., Wilkinson, D. S., and Ebling, F. J. G. *Textbook of Dermatology.* Philadelphia: David, 1968. Vol. 1, p. 53.
38. Sapse, A. T., and Bonavida, B. Preliminary study of lysozyme levels in subjects with smog eye irritation. *Am. J. Ophthalmol.* 66:79, 1968.
39. Scherz, W., and Dohlman, C. H. Is the lac-

rimal gland dispensable? *Arch. Ophthalmol.* 93: 281, 1975.

40. Schirmer, O. Studien zur Physiologie und Pathologie der Tranenabsonderung und Tranenabfuhr. *Arch. F. Ophthalmol.* 56:197, 1903.

41. Siltzbach, L. Sarcoidosis: Clinical features and management. *Med. Clin. North Am.* 51:483, 1967.

42. Simon, B. G., and Moutsopoulas, H. M. Primary amyloidosis resembling sicca syndrome. *Arthritis Rheum.* 22:932, 1979.

43. Swann, K. C. Use of methylcellulose in ophthalmology. *Arch. Ophthalmol.* 33:378, 1945.

44. van Bijsterveld, O. P. Diagnostic tests in the sicca syndrome. *Arch. Ophthalmol.* 82:10, 1969.

45. Virchow, H. Conjunctiva. In *Handbuch der Augenheilkunde.* Leipzig: W. Englemann, 1910. 2 Aufl., Band I, Abt. 1, 3 Abschnitt, p. 431.

46. Walsh, F. B., and Hoyt, W. F. *Clinical Neuroophthalmology* (3rd ed.). Baltimore: Williams & Wilkins, 1969. Pp 555–557.

47. Watson, R. R., Reyes, M. A., and McMurray, D. N.: Influence of malnutrition on the concentration of IgA, lysozyme, amylase, and aminopeptidase in children's tears. *Proc. Soc. Exp. Biol. Med.* 157:215, 1978.

48. Wright, P. Untoward effects associated with practolol administration: Oculomucocutaneous syndrome. *Br. Med. J.* 15:595, 1975.

Sjögren's Syndrome

Khalid F. Tabbara

Sjögren's syndrome is a chronic autoimmune disorder with multisystem abnormalities. The disease is characterized by mononuclear infiltration of the lacrimal and salivary glands leading to destruction of the ductal and acinar structures and resulting in deficiency of tears and saliva. The condition leads to keratoconjunctivitis sicca (dry eyes) and xerostomia (dry mouth). Sjögren's syndrome may occur alone but is often accompanied by other autoimmune diseases [3, 19, 21].

HISTORY

The first to describe filamentary keratitis was Leber in 1882 [11]. Hadden in 1888 reported the association of dry eyes and dry mouth with filamentary keratitis and introduced the term *xerostomia* for dryness of the mouth [9]. Hadden's patient was a 63-year-old woman with dryness of the nasal mucosa, and Hadden could not stimulate tear production in her with ammonia. The association of arthritis and filamentary keratitis was noted by Fisher in 1889 [6]. Mikulicz in 1892 reported on a 42-year-old German farmer with bilateral swelling of the lacrimal and parotid glands [14]. The patient died of a ruptured appendix and bacterial peritonitis a few months later; microscopy revealed the extensive lymphocytic infiltration of the lacrimal and salivary glands now recognized as the pathologic hallmark of Sjögren's syndrome. The names *Mikulicz's syndrome* and *Mikulicz's disease* were later used to refer to various clinical conditions causing salivary and lacrimal gland enlargement—irrespective of their cause and with no regard for the histopathologic features of the glands. Since both the pathologic features and the systemic manifestations were the same in the two groups of patients, it became apparent that Mikulicz's disease and Sjögren's syndrome were the same entity [15].

The association of hypofunction of lacrimal gland and filamentary keratitis was noted by Fuchs in 1919 [7]. In 1925, Gougerot, a French ophthalmologist, described three patients with dryness of the eyes and recognized that this was only one manifestation of a more generalized condition in which dryness of the mouth, larynx, nose, and vagina occurred [8]. The disease is sometimes referred to as the Gougerot-Sjögren syndrome. The most comprehensive paper on the subject was presented by the

Swedish ophthalmologist Henrik Sjögren in 1933 [20]. In his classic monograph, Sjögren concluded that keratoconjunctivitis sicca (KCS) was a local phenomenon of a more generalized disorder affecting menopausal women. He also stressed the fact that arthritis was a major feature of the disease.

EPIDEMIOLOGY

Women are more frequently affected by Sjögren's syndrome than men in a ratio of 9:1 [3, 19, 21]. The disease may be encountered in approximately 25 percent of patients with rheumatoid arthritis [19]. The true prevalence of Sjögren's syndrome is unknown. It is considered to be a common autoimmune disorder second only to rheumatoid arthritis in prevalence. The onset of the disease is frequently between the age of 40 and 60. The disease has been reported to occur during childhood and adolescence, but this is rare.

PATHOGENESIS

A genetic, inborn abnormality of the suppressor T-lymphocyte may allow unrestricted proliferation of B cells with the production of non-organ-specific autoantibodies. Exogenous antigenic insult (such as a virus), local tissue factors, or a hormonal imbalance may augment or precipitate the immunologic disorder [18]. The chronically activated lymphocytes, for unknown reasons, home to the exocrine glands such as the lacrimal and salivary glands and participate in destruction and damage of the tissues that lead to hypofunction of the glands.

CLINICAL FEATURES

CLINICAL TYPES OF SJÖGREN'S SYNDROME

KCS and xerostomia in patients with Sjögren's syndrome are the result of chronic mononuclear cell infiltration of the major and accessory lacrimal and salivary glands. The infiltration ultimately damages the glandular structures irreversibly and leads to exocrine gland dysfunction characterized by reduced or absent tears and saliva.

The classic clinical triad of Sjögren's syndrome included KCS, xerostomia (Fig. 7-12), and a connective tissue disease, usually rheumatoid arthritis. There are certain shortcomings in such a restrictive clinical definition. At present, two clinical types of Sjögren's syndrome are recognized [17]: *primary*—sicca syndrome alone or combined with xerostomia—and *secondary*—sicca syndrome (KCS, xerostomia, or both) associated with other connective tissue disorders. Recent clinical studies have demonstrated that there are definite genetic [4], im-

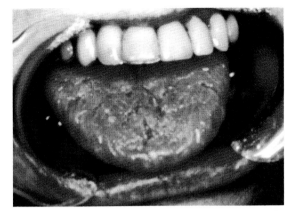

FIGURE 7-12. *Xerostomia. Note the atrophy of the papillae, the fissuring, and the beefy appearance of the tongue.*

munopathologic [10], serologic [2, 12], and clinical [5, 10, 21] differences between the primary and secondary syndromes (Table 7-6).

The autoimmune diseases frequently associated with KCS and xerostomia include rheumatoid arthritis, systemic lupus erythematosus, progressive systemic sclerosis, Hashimoto's thyroiditis, polymyositis, polyarteritis nodosa, and Waldenström's macroglobulinemia. Furthermore, patients with primary or secondary Sjögren's syndrome have a higher risk of developing lymphoma or other lymphoproliferative disorders than does the general population [1, 17].

SIGNS AND SYMPTOMS

The signs and symptoms found in dry eye patients are also found in Sjögren's syndrome patients (Figs. 7-13 through 7-15). In addition, peripheral corneal changes are seen in Sjögren's syndrome.

Peripheral corneal infiltration in Sjögren's syndrome occurs in approximately 10 percent of the patients. Patients complain of acute redness, pain, and photophobia. Biomicroscopy reveals typical single or multiple foci of peripheral corneal whitish gray subepithelial infiltrate with a lucid interval. The foci of infiltration may rarely coalesce, forming a linear or arcuate infiltration in the periphery. The overlying epithelium may remain intact or may break down after a few days, leaving a small ulcer. The corneal sensation remains intact. The peripheral corneal infiltrate in Sjögren's syndrome represents a local deposition of immune complexes in the corneal periphery, in the terminal capillary loops of the limbal vessels, or both; it is similar to the deposition of immune complexes in the glomerular capillaries. Chemotactic factors are released, leading to local infiltration of the cornea with polymorphonuclear cells. Scrapings of these infiltrates show polymorphonuclear cells and no organisms. Peripheral corneal infiltrates in Sjögren's syndrome respond to a short course of topical steroids, which should be discontinued as soon as the lesions improve.

Other peripheral corneal changes may occur in Sjögren's syndrome. Peripheral corneal ulceration, thinning, and perforation similar to changes seen in rheumatoid arthritis may be observed in some patients with primary or secondary Sjögren's syndrome (Fig. 7-16).

DIAGNOSTIC TESTS

Most of the diagnostic tests for the dry eye syndromes are discussed in the foregoing section, Keratoconjunctivitis Sicca. Those described below are more specific for Sjögren's syndrome.

PAROTID FLOW RATE

Determination of the parotid flow rate can be helpful in the diagnosis of xerostomia [5, 13]. Radionuclide scan of the parotid glands and parotid glands sialography [5] are other diagnostic techniques for the assessment of salivary gland function.

BIOPSY OF THE ACCESSORY SALIVARY GLANDS

The histopathologic change in the lacrimal gland of patients with Sjögren's syndrome is mononuclear cell infiltration with lymphocytes and occasionally plasma cells and macrophages (Fig. 7-17). Although a lacrimal gland biopsy may contribute greatly to the diagnosis of Sjögren's syndrome, the possibility of serious complications precludes its use. In contradistinction, a biopsy of accessory salivary glands through a labial incision is a simple surgical technique without serious complications. Like lacrimal gland tissue, the labial accessory salivary glands are affected by a mononuclear cell infiltrate that leads to

atrophy of the glandular tissues. In a clinical study at the University of California in San Francisco, my colleagues and I examined the lymphocytic infiltration of the labial accessory salivary glands and correlated our findings with the degree of ocular pathologic changes observed in patients with Sjögren's syndrome [21]. We assessed the number of lymphocytes per 4 mm^2 of labial salivary gland tissue as follows: grade 0 = absent; grade 1 = slight infiltrate; grade 2 = moderate infiltrate or less than one focus (an aggregate of 50 or more lymphocytes, plasma cells, and macrophages); grade 3 = 1 focus; grade 4 = 2 or more foci. Normal labial salivary gland tissue could be either grade 0 or grade 1. There was a high degree of correlation between the severity of KCS in patients with Sjögren's syndrome and the degree of lymphocytic infiltration of the labial salivary gland tissues. Patients with grade 4 labial biopsy specimens had clinical evidence of severe KCS. Of the patients with grade 4 lymphocytic infiltration of the labial salivary gland tissues, more than 90 percent had reduced or absent tear lysozyme. A labial salivary gland biopsy is, therefore, an important diagnostic procedure for the definitive diagnosis of Sjögren's syndrome and for assessing the severity of the disease.

LABORATORY FINDINGS

HEMATOLOGIC AND SEROLOGIC

Patients with Sjögren's syndrome may show evidence of anemia and leukopenia. Approximately 50 percent of patients with Sjögren's syndrome, primary or secondary, show evidence of elevated sedimentation rate. Hypergammaglobulinemia is

TABLE 7-6. *Differences Between Primary and Secondary Sjögren's Syndrome*

Finding	Primary[a]	Secondary[b]
Severe keratoconjunctivitis sicca[c] [5]	61%	18%
Salivary gland swelling [17]	81%	14%
Mean duration of symptoms [5]	4.5 yr	2.9 yr
Parotid flow rate [5]	1.2 ml/min	3.6 ml/min
Average number of foci/4 mm^2 of labial salivary gland tissue [13]	6	3.5
Salivary beta-2-microglobulin (μg/ml) [13]	4.99 ($\pm$ 1.97)	2.18 ($\pm$ 0.8)
Antisalivary duct antibodies	10%	67%
Serum immune complexes [17]	85%	15%
Antinuclear antibodies [10]	68%	5%
HLA-DW3 [4]	94%	6%

[a]Keratoconjunctivitis sicca and/or xerostomia.
[b]Keratoconjunctivitis sicca and/or xerostomia with associated connective tissue disorder.
[c]Corneal filaments, keratitis > 3 quadrants; Schirmer test value < 5 mm/5 minutes.

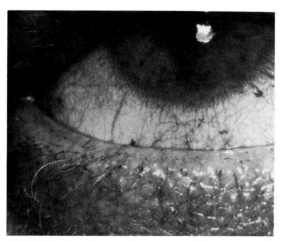

FIGURE 7-13. *Absent tear meniscus on lower lid in a patient with Sjögren's syndrome.*

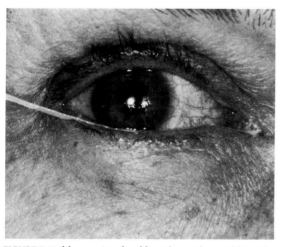

FIGURE 7-14. *Mucous strand and loss of normal corneal luster in a patient with Sjögren's syndrome.*

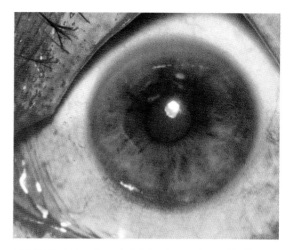

FIGURE 7-15. *Rose bengal staining in a patient with Sjögren's syndrome. Note absence of bulbar conjunctival staining in upper portion, which is normally covered by the upper eyelid.*

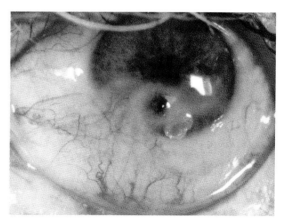

FIGURE 7-16. *Corneal perforation in a patient with Sjögren's syndrome. (Courtesy R. Biswell, M.D.)*

seen in 50 to 90 percent of the patients [11]. Immune complexes may be elevated in patients with Sjögren's as determined by the ^{125}I C1q binding assay or by the RAJI cell radioassay [17]. Serum beta-2-microglobulin is elevated in 30 to 50 percent of patients with Sjögren's syndrome [13].

TISSUE TYPING

Eighty-five percent of patients with rheumatoid arthritis and secondary Sjögren's syndrome have an association with HLA-DW4. It is also interesting that this same group have a decreased frequency of HLA-DW2 when compared with the general population. In contrast, patients with primary Sjögren's syndrome have an increased frequency of HLA-DW2, HLA-DW3, or both [4, 12].

MANAGEMENT OF KERATOCONJUNCTIVITIS SICCA

The management of dry eyes is discussed in the foregoing section. However, because of the lymphocytic infiltration of the major and minor lacrimal glands in patients with Sjögren's syndrome, it has been suggested that the use of antiinflammatory or immunosuppressive agents, or both, may help to inhibit this infiltration and serve to improve the function of the salivary and lacrimal glands. The use of immunosuppressive agents late in the disease, that is, after atrophy and cicatrization of the glandu-

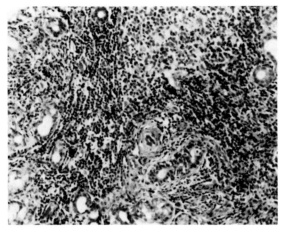

FIGURE 7-17. *H&E-stained section of lacrimal gland from a 38-year-old woman with Sjögren's syndrome. Note the lymphocytic infiltration and destruction of the acinar structures. (× 100.)*

lar structures, would provide no major symptomatic relief, and patients would not be expected to have dramatic improvement in tear production. Furthermore, the hazards and risks of the long-term use of immunosuppressive agents precludes their administration. In the early stages of Sjögren's syndrome, however, and specifically in young patients, systemic steroids may modulate the immunologic reaction before the irreversible destruction of the glandular tissue and before the onset of permanent scarring and fibrosis. Sicca syndrome alone is not a life-threatening disorder, and we must always weigh the potential risk along with the benefits when steroid therapy is contemplated. Michalski and coworkers [13] described two patients with Sjögren's syndrome treated with prednisone in whom clinical improvement was associated with a definite reduction in the salivary beta-2-microglobulin concentration. Moutsopoulos and colleagues [16] reported on three patients with Sjögren's syndrome with immune-complex glomerulonephritis. In all three, moderate daily doses of prednisone (20–30 mg) produced rapid improvement in renal function, and in two of the three the level of the immune complexes was reduced. Systemic steroid therapy may be considered in young patients with early primary Sjögren's syndrome. I have found that a short course of prednisone, 40 mg orally every other day, has minimum side effects and in the early stages of the disease can produce rapid improvement. The consideration of such treatment therefore seems to be justified for patients with early Sjögren's syndrome in whom the diagnosis has been confirmed histologically by labial accessory salivary gland biopsy.

REFERENCES

1. Anderson, L. G., and Talal, N. The spectrum of benign to malignant lymphoproliferation in Sjögren's syndrome. *Clin. Exp. Immunol.* 9:199, 1971.
2. Anderson, L. G., Tarpley, T. M., and Talal, N. Cellular-versus-humoral autoimmune responses to salivary gland in Sjögren's syndrome. *Clin. Exp. Immunol.* 13:335, 1973.
3. Bloch, K. J., et al. Sjögren's syndrome: A clinical, pathological, and serological study of sixty-two cases. *Medicine* 44:187, 1965.
4. Chused, T. M., et al. Sjögren's syndrome association with HLA-DW3. *N. Engl. J. Med.* 296:895, 1977.
5. Daniels, T. E., et al. The oral components of Sjögren's syndrome. *Oral Med.* 39:875, 1975.
6. Fisher, E. Über Fädchenkeratitis. *Graefes Arch. Ophthal.* 35:201, 1889.
7. Fuchs, A. Ein Fall von Fehlen der Tränen und Mundspeichersekretion. *Zschr. Augerh.* 42:253, 1919.
8. Gougerot, H. Insuffisance progressive et atrophie des glandes salivaires et muqueuses de la bouche, des conjonctives (et parfois des muqueuses nasale, laryngee, vulvaire). *Bull. Soc. Fr. Dermatol. Syphiligr.* 32:376, 1925.
9. Hadden, W. B. On "dry mouth" or suppression of the salivary and buccal secretions. *Trans. Clin. Soc. Lond.* 21:176, 1888.
10. Kassan, S. S., and Gardy, M. Sjögren's syndrome: An update and overview. *Am. J. Med.* 64:1037, 1978.
11. Leber, F. Über die Entstehung der Netzhautablösung. *Klin. Mbl. Augenheilk.* 20:165, 1882.
12. Manthorpe, R., et al. Sjögren's syndrome: A review with emphasis on immunological features. *Allergy* 36:139, 1981.
13. Michalski, J. P., et al. Beta-2-microglobulin and lymphocytic infiltration in Sjögren's syndrome. *N. Engl. J. Med.* 293:1228, 1975.
14. Mikulicz, J. Ueber eine eigenartige symmetrische Erkrankung der Thranen und Mundspeicheldruse. *Beitr. Chir. Festchrift Billroth* 2:610, 1892.
15. Morgan, W. S., and Castleman, B. A clinicopathologic study of Mikulicz's disease. *Am. J. Pathol.* 29:471, 1953.
16. Moutsopoulos, H. M., et al. Immune complex glomerulonephritis in sicca syndrome. *Am. J. Med.* 64:955, 1978.
17. Moutsopoulos, H. M., et al. Sjögren's syndrome (sicca syndrome): Current issues. *Ann. Intern. Med.* 92:212, 1980.
18. Roubinian, J. R., Papoian, R., and Talal, N. Androgenic hormones modulate autoantibody

responses and improve survival in murine lupus. *J. Clin. Invest.* 59:1066, 1977.

19. Shearn, M. A.   Sjögren's Syndrome. In L. H. Smith (Ed.), *Major Problems in Internal Medicine,* Vol. 2. Philadelphia: Saunders, 1971.

20. Sjögren, H.   Zur Kenntnis der keratoconjunctivitis sicca (keratitis filiformis bei hypofunktion der Tränendrüsen). *Acta Ophthalmol.* (Copenh.) 11:1–151, 1933.

21. Tabbara, K. F., et al.   Sjögren's syndrome: A correlation between ocular findings and labial salivary gland histology. *Trans. Am. Acad. Ophthalmol. Otolaryngol.* 78:467, 1974.

8. CORNEAL MANIFESTATIONS OF NEUROLOGIC DISEASES

C. Stephen Foster

Abnormalities of the cornea and conjunctiva may occur in association with systemic or localized neurologic disease. The keratopathy seen in association with systemic neurologic diseases, such as Wilson's disease (hepatolenticular degeneration), the Riley-Day syndrome (familial dysautonomia), or Cogan's syndrome (nonluetic interstitial keratitis), is only a part of the abnormalities seen in these conditions. In the case of specific cranial nerve dysfunction, however, the findings are limited to the eye alone. In seventh nerve lesions, the primary abnormality is failure to blink and failure to close the eyes during sleep. Abnormalities of the fifth nerve produce tissue damage by mechanisms less obvious, perhaps related to a lack of trophic substances or a lack of neurotransmitters such as acetylcholine.

The surface of the eye is particularly vulnerable to the effects of fifth and seventh nerve dysfunction. For example, inadequate lid function and constant corneal exposure from seventh nerve palsy lead rapidly to corneal epithelial desiccation and eventually to corneal ulceration. Loss of fifth nerve function with resultant corneal anesthesia also leads primarily to changes in the epithelium, even in the absence of decreased tear production.

The terminology pertaining to corneal pathologic changes secondary to dysfunction of cranial nerves V and VII is inconsistent and often imprecise in the literature. The term *neuroparalytic keratitis* is confusing, since some authors use it to describe fifth nerve dysfunction whereas others employ it for seventh nerve palsy. *Exposure keratitis* is the most appropriate term for keratitis associated with seventh (facial) nerve palsy. The term *neurotrophic keratitis* should be reserved for corneal damage secondary to fifth (trigeminal) nerve damage.

INNERVATION OF THE ORBIT AND GLOBE

SENSORY INNERVATION

The cornea, conjunctiva, and ocular adnexa derive their sensory innervation from the fifth cranial, or trigeminal, nerve (Figs. 8-1, 8-2, 8-4). The trigeminal

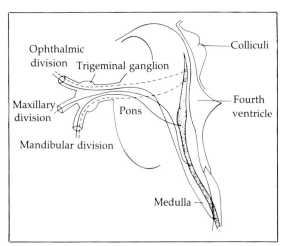

FIGURE 8-1. *Fifth cranial nerve tracts. (From R. Warwick (Ed.), Wolff's Anatomy of the Eye (7th ed.). London: Lewis, 1976.)*

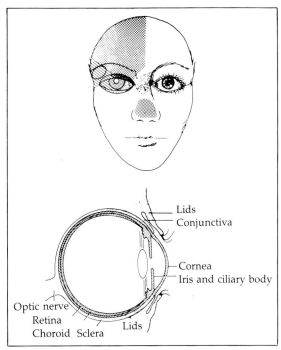

FIGURE 8-2. *Innervation by fifth cranial (trigeminal) nerve. The lacrimal branch (parallel lines) of the ophthalmic division of the fifth cranial nerve innervates the lateral conjunctiva, the skin of the temple, and the lacrimal gland. The frontal branch (cross-hatching) innervates the superior conjunctiva, the upper lid, and the skin of the forehead. The nasociliary branch divides into the long ciliary nerves (dots on cornea and, in transverse section, on ciliary body and iris), which innervate the ciliary body, the iris, and the cornea; the infratrochlear nerve (shading), which supplies the medial conjunctiva, the caruncle, the lacrimal canaliculus and lacrimal sac, and the skin over the bony part of the nose; and the anterior ethmoid nerve (dots on nose), which supplies the skin over the cartilaginous part of the nose.*

nerve arises from the trigeminal nucleus in the pons, pierces the dura under the cerebellum, and joins the trigeminal (gasserian) ganglion, which lies in a small bony fossa in the apex of the temporal bone just above the root of the zygoma. The middle meningeal artery lies lateral to the ganglion, and the cavernous sinus lies medial to it. The first of the three divisions of the fifth nerve emerging from the trigeminal ganglion, the ophthalmic division, splits into three branches: the lacrimal, the frontal, and the nasociliary. This branching occurs just behind the superior orbital fissure, and these three branches enter the orbit through the superior orbital fissure.

The lacrimal branch of the ophthalmic division of the trigeminal nerve runs along the upper border of the lateral rectus muscle before proceeding to the lacrimal gland. The frontal branch travels forward adjacent to the levator palpebrae superioris and divides into supraorbital and supratrochlear branches, which supply sensory innervation to the superior conjunctiva, upper lid, and skin of the forehead.

The nasociliary branch of the ophthalmic division of the trigeminal nerve enters the orbit through the anulus of Zinn and travels forward and medially, giving off five branches: the sensory root of the ciliary ganglion, the long ciliary nerves, the posterior ethmoidal nerve, and the infratrochlear nerve. The sensory root of the ciliary ganglion travels to the ciliary ganglion. The long ciliary nerves pierce the sclera, travel between sclera and choroid, and provide sensory fibers to ciliary body, iris, and cornea; motor fibers to the iris dilator muscles are

also present. The posterior ethmoidal nerve supplies innervation to the posterior ethmoidal and the sphenoidal sinuses. The infratrochlear nerve supplies medial conjunctiva, caruncle, lacrimal canaliculus and lacrimal sac, and skin over the bony part of the nose. The anterior ethmoidal nerve supplies the skin over the cartilaginous part of the nose down to the tip.

MOTOR INNERVATION

The seventh cranial (facial) nerve arises from the facial nucleus, which is anterior and lateral to the sixth or abducens nucleus in the pons. The facial nerve fibers course around the sixth nerve nucleus and emerge from the pons lateral to the corticospinal tract. The fibers enter the internal auditory meatus with the acoustic nerve, bend acutely downward and anteriorly, enter the facial canal, run in this canal through the middle ear, and emerge from the skull through the stylomastoid foramen. The

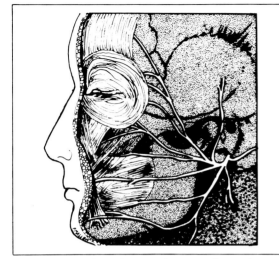

FIGURE 8-3. *Peripheral divisions of the seventh cranial nerve. (From R. Warwick (Ed.), Wolff's Anatomy of the Eye (7th ed.). London: Lewis, 1976.)*

major portion of the nerve then runs forward into the parotid gland, dividing into five or more branches; many of these branches are still clustered rather closely together as they emerge from the parotid gland and as they lie just posterior to the superior posterior ramus of the mandible (Fig. 8-3). The zygomatic branch of the facial nerve supplies the motor fibers that control the frontalis, orbicularis oculi, and corrugator supercilii muscles.

AUTONOMIC INNERVATION
Visceral (parasympathetic) motor fibers supplying the salivary and lacrimal glands leave the facial

nerve in the facial canal, just distal to the geniculate ganglion. These visceral motor fibers travel to the sphenopalatine ganglion and eventually supply the lacrimal gland via the greater superficial petrosal nerve (Fig. 8-4). Parasympathetic innervation to the globe arises in the brainstem, courses along the third nerve, and passes to the ciliary ganglion. After synapsing there, fibers travel with the short ciliary nerves and penetrate into the sclera, supplying vessels and the constrictor muscle fibers in the iris. Although high levels of acetylcholine are found within corneal epithelial cells, there is no direct evidence of parasympathetic innervation to the cornea.

Sympathetic innervation for the globe originates in the superior cervical ganglion and travels along the vessels to the long and short ciliary nerves, and thence to the globe. Adrenergic receptors have been found on corneal epithelial cells, which suggests that sympathetic innervation is present in the cornea.

PRIMARY CRANIAL NERVE ABNORMALITIES
SEVENTH (FACIAL) NERVE PALSY
PATHOGENESIS
Lesions of the facial nerve may occur at any level between the facial nucleus in the pons and the individual branches of the nerve and may be traumatic or nontraumatic. Intrapontine lesions affecting the facial nerve also typically involve the abducens, the corticospinal tract, or both. The usual causes of le-

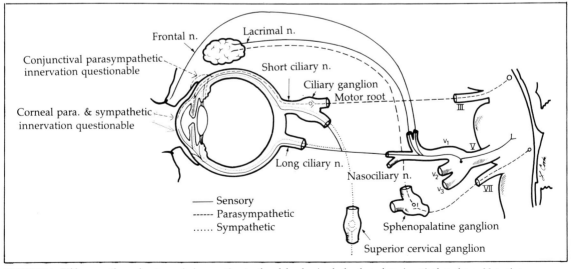

FIGURE 8-4. *Fifth, seventh, and autonomic innervation to the globe, lacrimal gland, and conjunctival surfaces. Note that parasympathetic and sympathetic innervation to the cornea are questionable.*

sions in the pons include cerebrovascular accidents, aneurysms, and tumors. Thus, occlusion of the anterior inferior cerebellar artery produces a lateral inferior pontine syndrome, whereas a tumor in the region of the facial nucleus typically produces facial paralysis, abducens palsy, and contralateral hemiplegia, or the Millard-Gubler syndrome. In the latter condition, facial nerve palsy is only a part of the patient's total neurologic deficit.

Lesions of the facial nerve in the internal auditory meatus also usually affect the eighth nerve, with resultant hyperacusis, deafness, tinnitus, or dizziness. If the geniculate ganglion, which is in close proximity to the facial nerve as it passes through the inner ear, is affected, decreased parasympathetic innervation to the lacrimal gland and hyposecretion of tears will also occur.

Lesions of the facial nerve as it lies in the facial canal will produce on the affected side typical facial paralysis with drooping of the corner of the mouth, lower lid ptosis, and loss of forehead skin furrowing as well as loss of taste in the anterior two-thirds of the tongue. Leprosy, acute polyneuritis, sarcoidosis, tumors, and viral infections (most notably herpes zoster) can produce facial nerve lesions in the facial canal and in the inner ear. The Ramsey Hunt syndrome, for example, probably results from herpes zoster in the geniculate ganglion, with vesicle formation in the external auditory canal, along with seventh and eighth nerve neuritis.

The results of surgical interruption of the facial nerve fibers also depend on the level of interruption, as described above. Thus, the nerve may be damaged during surgery for tic douloureux or for tumor resection. Interruption of the facial nerve fibers at the stylomastoid foramen produces only facial paralysis without loss of taste.

Paralysis of the facial muscles occurs in all of the lesions described above, nuclear or peripheral. However, there is some variation in the degree to which the various facial muscles are paralyzed. For example, in supranuclear lesions, the frontalis and orbicularis muscles are involved considerably less than the muscles of the lower face, since the upper facial muscles receive dual innervation from both sides of the cerebral cortex.

The most common facial nerve palsy is Bell's palsy. Its cause is unknown, although most investigators speculate that it is due to a neuritis of the seventh nerve near the stylomastoid foramen. Bell's palsy typically develops acutely and generally lasts 3 to 20 weeks, with gradual recovery of most or all seventh nerve function in approximately 80 percent

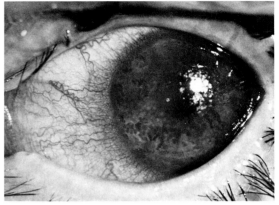

FIGURE 8-5. *Exposure keratitis secondary to seventh nerve palsy. Note the corneal epithelial irregularity caused by drying and the secondary external ocular inflammatory reaction.*

of patients. Varying degrees of more lasting seventh nerve dysfunction are seen in the remaining 20 percent of patients.

One additional, rare cause of facial nerve palsy, which may be of special interest to the ophthalmologist, is Heerfordt's syndrome, or uveoparotid fever. This syndrome, which is caused by sarcoidosis, involves the parotid gland, the uveal tract (with granulomatous uveitis), and the facial nerve, with resultant facial nerve palsy.

CLINICAL FEATURES AND DIAGNOSIS
The corneal damage seen in facial nerve paralysis is an exposure keratitis caused by the desiccation of the corneal epithelium (Fig. 8-5). The exposed epithelium becomes dry from tear evaporation, and the epithelial cell membranes are subsequently damaged, which leads to cell death. Exposure, desiccation, membrane damage, and cell death of the underlying layers of ocular surface epithelium follow. Through this process, multiple small epithelial defects develop on the ocular surface in the exposed area, most noticeably on the cornea itself. Persistence of these epithelial defects eventually results in the development of more extensive areas of defects in the epithelium, and corneal stromal ulceration and neovascularization follow. Secondary infection of the ulcerating cornea is common, and keratinization of the remainder of the ocular surface can occur if exposure persists.

The diagnosis of seventh nerve dysfunction presents no particular problem, since the patient's inability to move the parts of the face supplied by the affected nerve is quite obvious. The diagnosis of exposure keratitis can be made when attempted closure of the eyelids results in little or no movement of the affected lids; the eye on the affected side may rotate upward on attempted closure (Bell's phenom-

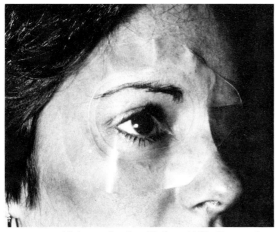

FIGURE 8-6. *Moisture chamber (Guibor shield, Concept Inc., Clearwater, Florida). There is firm adhesion between the adhesive backing of the shield and the skin all around, so that evaporation of moisture from the ocular surface is retarded.*

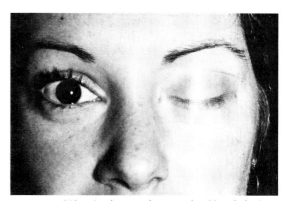

FIGURE 8-7. *Lid taping for seventh nerve palsy. Note the horizontal placement of the tape and the firm attachment to the skin of the upper and lower lids.*

enon). Instillation of 1% rose bengal dye into the inferior cul-de-sac of the affected eye, followed by gentle manual lid closure and examination by slit lamp biomicroscopy (examination with a red-free filter is especially helpful) demonstrates the earliest clinically detectable pathologic changes in exposure keratitis. Epithelial cells with damaged cell membranes will stain with this vital dye, and the examiner will observe a punctate staining pattern of the affected areas. Fluorescein dye (1%) will stain areas of frank epithelial cell loss.

TREATMENT

If the seventh nerve palsy is likely to be temporary (as in Bell's palsy), management may consist of ocular lubrication with appropriate ointments, the use of moisture chambers (Fig. 8-6), and lid taping (Fig. 8-7). Lid taping at bedtime is especially important for prevention of nocturnal lagophthalmos. Daytime taping may be useful as well in patients who do not respond to daytime lubrication. The correct application of tape is essential if one is to avoid not only exposure but possible damage to the ocular surface from tape rubbing on the cornea. The placement of tape shown in Figure 8-7 is particularly useful. The application of ointment should be avoided in the hours close to bedtime, and the skin of the lids should be carefully cleaned of any residual petrolatum or oily products before applying the tape. Transpore tape is particularly effective, since moisture beneath the tape escapes through it without interfering with the adhesion.

If the paralysis of the seventh nerve is expected to be permanent or prolonged, a broad tarsorrhaphy is indicated (Fig. 8-8). The tarsorrhaphy may be cen-

tral, lateral, or lateral and medial. It may be done by simple lid margin shaving (Fig. 8-9), or a tongue-and-groove tarsorrhaphy may be performed (Fig. 8-10).

Ocular lubricants should be used even after tarsorrhaphy, and the ophthalmologist should continue to examine the patient regularly for evidence of pathologic changes of the epithelium, tear insufficiency, or infection.

FIFTH (TRIGEMINAL) NERVE PALSY

CAUSES

In 1892, Rose [33] described five patients on whom he performed trigeminal ganglionectomies for tic douloureux. As a result of the operation, three of

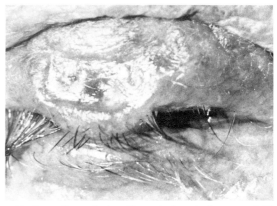

FIGURE 8-8. *Tarsorrhaphy. The protective plastic pegs and lid sutures have just been removed from this eye after a freshly performed tarsorrhaphy. A firm adhesion between the two lids now exists. The eye can still be examined with gentle separation of the lids medially and laterally.*

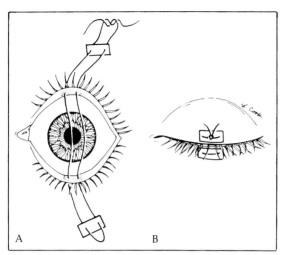

FIGURE 8-9. *Simple marginal shaving tarsorrhaphy. A. Complementary sites on the upper and lower lid margins are prepared by a very superficial shaving of a small area. A double-arm 6-0 black silk suture is placed through a No. 40 silicone band and positioned through the skin of the lid, out the lower lid margin, into the prepared bed in the upper lid margin, and out of the skin of the upper lid. B. Tightening this suture results in firm apposition between the two shaved areas prepared in the margin of each lid.*

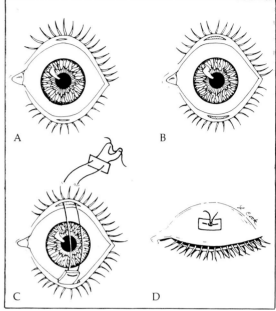

FIGURE 8-10. *Tongue-and-groove tarsorrhaphy. A. An incision is made in complementary sites in the margin of the upper and lower eyelids. B. A dissection pocket is created by blunt dissection with scissors. C. A tongue of tarsus and conjunctiva is then mobilized at the dissection site in the lower lid by making two vertical relaxing incisions in the posterior aspect of the dissected pocket. A double-arm 6-0 black silk suture is placed through the upper third of this tongue of tissue and passed up into the dissection pocket in the upper lid and out of the skin of the upper lid. D. Pulling up this suture results in the drawing of the tongue of tarsus and conjunctiva from the lower lid into the dissection pocket in the upper lid, thereby creating a tongue-and-groove tarsorrhaphy.*

the five developed severe keratitis and disruption of the ocular surface. This clinical observation has been confirmed repeatedly, and today's neurosurgeons recognize corneal anesthesia and keratitis as the most serious complications of trigeminal nerve surgery [37]. The reported incidence of corneal anesthesia after such surgery has been in the range of 15 to 18 percent for the past 30 years [27–29].

Numerous nonsurgical conditions may also cause fifth nerve palsy. These include multiple sclerosis; tumors (e.g., neurofibroma of the nerve or meningioma in the posterior fossa); aneurysms; and cerebrovascular accidents, such as blockage of the short circumferential artery with a resultant lateral midpontine syndrome. Infection, particularly from herpes zoster and herpes simplex virus, may lead to profound damage of various portions of the fifth cranial nerve. Radiation therapy can also produce diffuse or segmental damage to peripheral twigs of the trigeminal nerve with resultant corneal anesthesia.

PATHOGENESIS OF CORNEAL ABNORMALITIES
It is unclear why the corneal epithelium becomes abnormal in the absence of normal innervation. However, once the innervation becomes abnormal, epithelial cell death frequently occurs, and the re-

sultant epithelial defects commonly persist unless the ocular surface is protected against the environment.

The corneal epithelium can become abnormal in the anesthetic eye even in the absence of desiccation, infection, or trauma [3]. Available evidence suggests that maintenance of the normal structure and function of tissues may be regulated by trophic substances transmitted by intact, functioning neurons. These substances move down the nerve axis to the periphery, in the case of motor neurons; in sensory nerves, flow may occur retrograde to the movement of the electrical stimulus, so that sensory nerves may influence the environment from which their sensory impulses originate. Axoplasmic flow can exert dramatic trophic influences on the cells supplied by these nerves [1, 2, 21]. Substances in axoplasm are known, for example, to maintain the form and function of taste buds and other sensory cells [1].

The mediators of the trophic influence, if any, of the trigeminal nerve on corneal epithelium are unknown. Numerous substances have been postulated as playing this secondary, supportive role in epithelial metabolism. For example, Magendie [22], more than 60 years before Rose's report [33], published his observation on corneal degenerative changes after trigeminal nerve interruption in rabbits. He hypothesized that the changes resulted from ablation of specific sympathetic trophic fibers. However, more likely mediators include acetylcholine, proteins, amino acids, cyclic nucleotides, and perhaps substances similar to epidermal growth factor.

Whatever the cause, lack of innervation in many cases leads to epithelial dysfunction. After fifth nerve ablation in animals, respiratory and glycolytic activity are markedly reduced in corneal epithelial cells, which become very permeable [35]. Decreased amounts of acetylcholine [16] and acetylcholine transferase are also found in the corneal epithelial cells of both animals and patients with fifth nerve sensory dysfunction. Patients with familial dysautonomia whose sympathetic innervation is abnormal have similar findings [24].

In addition to these metabolic changes, lack of innervation has also been shown to have an adverse effect on normal epithelial mitosis rates [23, 34].

The net result of the metabolic abnormalities produced by lack of sensation is epithelial cell loss. This leads to the development of epithelial defects, which can in turn lead to stromal ulceration, infection, and perforation. The stromal ulceration results from proteoglycan and collagen degradation from proteolytic and collagenolytic enzymes. These enzymes may be elaborated by damaged corneal epithelial cells, by conjunctival epithelial cells, by corneal fibroblasts, and by inflammatory cells (see Chapter 2, Morphology and Pathologic Response of the Cornea to Disease).

CLINICAL FEATURES AND DIAGNOSIS
The typical clinical picture in patients with neurotrophic keratitis includes initial vasodilation of the vessels of the upper eyelid, subsequent injection of the deeper perilimbal vessels, development of edema of the upper eyelid and conjunctiva, and eventual development of corneal epithelial edema. At this point, the damaged corneal and conjunctival epithelial cells (typically in the interpalpebral fissure zone of exposure) stain with rose bengal dye. Epithelial cell death results in punctate epithelial defects that stain with fluorescein. These punctate defects then coalesce into larger areas of epithelial cell loss (Fig. 8-11). An associated iritis with flare and inflammatory cells in the anterior chamber is usually seen when the persistent epithelial defect or defects have developed. In fifth nerve lesions

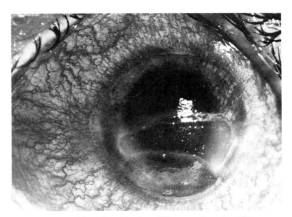

FIGURE 8-11. *Neurotrophic keratitis secondary to fifth nerve palsy. Note the large, horizontally oriented trophic epithelial defect with gray, rolled up edges and extensive ocular inflammation.*

caused by herpes zoster, the associated iritis may be extremely severe. The typical vesicular skin lesions along the ophthalmic division of the trigeminal nerve would, of course, accompany these findings in a patient with acute herpes zoster (Fig. 8-12).

In neurotrophic keratitis secondary to herpes zoster ophthalmicus with trigeminal nerve damage, severe keratitis with corneal ulceration may persist even years after resolution of the acute phases of the disease. In such cases, the patient may have evidence of skin scarring from the previous zoster lesions, but sometimes these findings are minimal or even absent. The corneal sensation is markedly impaired, however, in all cases of neurotrophic keratitis, regardless of the cause. In the most extreme cases, one will find total anesthesia of the ocular surface.

The neurotrophic keratitis seen in patients who have had herpes simplex keratitis is usually more localized than that seen in patients with a history of herpes zoster or with other lesions of the trigeminal nerve. The so-called metaherpetic keratitis lesion is a persistent trophic epithelial defect, in the absence of active viral infection, in a patient who has previously had one or more episodes of infectious herpes keratitis (see Herpetic Diseases in Chapter 5, Infectious Diseases). The trophic defect may be the result of damage to the epithelial basement membrane zone from the previous episodes of infectious keratitis, localized corneal anesthesia from fifth nerve twig damage from previous infectious keratitis, or both these phenomena. In any case, the trophic defect has the typical heaped-up border of gray epithelial cells, and 1% rose bengal dye stains the epithe-

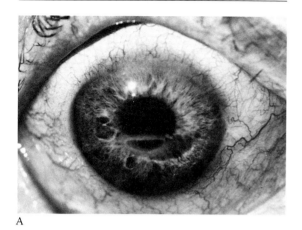

A

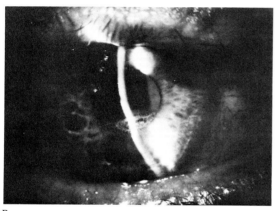

B

FIGURE 8-12. *A. Neurotrophic keratitis secondary to herpes zoster ophthalmicus. Note the horizontally oriented trophic defect with gray, rolled up edges of epithelium. B. Slit lamp photograph of eye shown in A. Note that the trophic defect is accompanied by superficial stromal ulceration.*

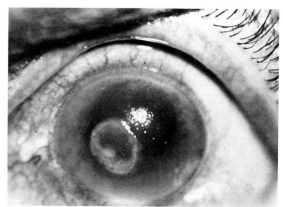

FIGURE 8-13. *Neurotrophic keratitis secondary to herpes simplex, or "metaherpetic keratitis." This nonhealing epithelial defect in a patient with previous episodes of infectious keratitis persists in spite of ocular lubricants and soft lens therapy and in the absence of evidence of active viral infection.*

lial cells at the edges of the defect in a random, nondescript way (Fig. 8-13). This is in sharp distinction to the reasonably regular, punctate arrangement of epithelial cell staining around the edge of the defect in a patient with active, infectious herpetic keratitis.

Regardless of the cause of the fifth nerve damage and neurotrophic keratitis, the longer the epithelial defect persists, the higher the likelihood that corneal stromal ulceration will develop (Fig. 8-12B).

TREATMENT
Since the primary pathologic defects at the level of the neuron and the epithelial cell are untreatable at present, the first goal should be to prevent disruption of the delicate ocular surface. Pathologic changes of the epithelium, as evidenced by ocular surface staining with rose bengal dye, should be treated with ocular lubricants (ointments are particularly useful for this purpose). Nocturnal lagophthalmos, if present, should be treated by lid taping at bedtime, as described above (p. 221).

Development of epithelial defects that stain with fluorescein warrants more aggressive therapy. Although soft lens therapy may sometimes be successful in neurotrophic keratitis, the use of this therapy can be complicated. Not infrequently, the application of a continuous-wear soft lens to an anesthetic eye results in the development, usually very quickly, of a hypopyon. The clinical picture can be alarming (Fig. 8-14) and can suggest infection. In my experience this occurs when the anesthetic eye with the continuous-wear soft lens has not been treated with a cycloplegic. The use of a cycloplegic (1% cyclopentolate hydrochloride 3 times daily) usually prevents this complication.

Anesthetic eyes with epithelial defects are certainly susceptible to infection, particularly when soft lenses are used. If tear insufficiency is present as well, the risk of ocular surface infection is so great that prophylactic topical antibiotics (0.5% chloramphenicol drops twice daily) should be used in conjunction with the lens.

Many practitioners would choose to perform a tarsorrhaphy rather than try a soft lens if epithelial defects develop in a patient with neurotrophic keratitis. In spite of the biochemical and histopathologic abnormalities of the surface epithelium of the anesthetic eye, the surface does not become grossly disrupted if it is protected from the environment by tarsorrhaphy [3, 36]. Over 40 years ago, Jaffee [18] hypothesized a probable explanation for the development of epithelial defects in anesthetic eyes: "In neurotrophic keratitis the abnormal metabolism of the epithelial cells puts them in a posi-

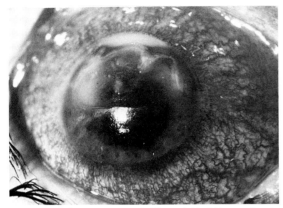

FIGURE 8-14. *Same eye as seen in Figure 8-11, 24 hours after the application of a continuous-wear bandage soft lens. Note that the epithelial defect has enlarged, more ocular inflammation is present, and a hypopyon has developed.*

tion in which they fail to resist the effects of trauma, drying, or infection." The tarsorrhaphy appears to act as a shield for the cornea to prevent trauma and drying. As in the case of seventh nerve lesions, the tarsorrhaphy need not be complete. If a central slit is left open, the patient can still use the eye if the vision is good, and the ophthalmologist can observe the cornea for the development of any complication.

In many cases, the cornea may have deep ulceration before the patient or physician is aware of it. The rapidity with which a corneal ulcer can progress to corneal perforation in an anesthetic eye is astonishing. It is not possible to make specific recommendations for the treatment of this problem. The degree of ulceration, the individual circumstances of the patient, and the past experiences of the ophthalmologist should govern the clinical decision on how to proceed. Such ulcers should routinely be scraped for smears and bacterial and fungal cultures, since secondary bacterial and fungal infection is an ever-present possibility.

Once infection is found (and treated with appropriate antimicróbial agents), or eliminated as a causal agent, the usual measures for treatment of stromal ulceration should be instituted, keeping in mind that protection of the anesthetic cornea by a tarsorrhaphy is ultimately a very worthwhile therapeutic maneuver. Collagenase inhibitors, such as N-acetylcysteine (20% drops given hourly), collagenase synthetase inhibitors, such as medroxyprogesterone (1% drops given four times a day), cyanoacrylate tissue adhesive and soft contact lens application to the ulcer and surrounding cornea, and conjunctival flap are modalities which may be exploited in the management of these challenging cases (see Ocular Manifestations of the Non-

rheumatic Acquired Collagen Vascular Diseases in Chapter 6, Immunologic Diseases).

SYSTEMIC NEUROLOGIC DISEASE

The three most common systemic neurologic diseases that affect the cornea are Wilson's disease, Cogan's syndrome, and the Riley-Day syndrome. Although the corneal abnormalities associated with these diseases may not lead to major visual loss, they may be extremely important in establishing the diagnosis. The ophthalmologist's role may be pivotal in this respect, and hence it is extremely important that every ophthalmologist be aware of these syndromes and of their ocular consequences.

WILSON'S DISEASE (HEPATOLENTICULAR DEGENERATION)

PATHOGENESIS

Wilson's disease [40] is an autosomal recessive inborn error of metabolism. The precise defect responsible for the disease is not known, but most of the abnormalities found can be ascribed to abnormalities in copper metabolism. Many investigators believe that an intrahepatic defect in copper metabolism is responsible for impaired excretion of copper through the bowel, with resultant increased copper storage in the liver. Liver cell poisoning secondary to the elevated copper levels leads to cell necrosis and subsequent cirrhosis. At the same time, there is deposition of copper in other tissues, including kidney, brain, and Descemet's membrane of the cornea [19].

Manifestations of the abnormal metabolism of copper include decreased plasma levels of ceruloplasmin, the protein that carries copper in the blood, as well as elevated levels of copper itself in the blood and urine.

CLINICAL FEATURES

SYSTEMIC FINDINGS

Wilson's disease usually has its onset before age 30. It is progressive and, until relatively recently, was routinely fatal within 5 to 10 years. The condition usually involves the basal ganglia, liver, and kidneys to varying degrees. The initial symptoms usually (approximately 60 percent of cases) are in the form of personality changes or behavioral abnormalities. Patients presenting in this way are commonly misdiagnosed until more obvious pathologic changes in the central nervous system or liver appear.

Some patients with hepatolenticular degeneration

have the signs of lenticular degeneration, with major dysfunction of the basal ganglia. This is an uncommon, severe form of the disease, which has its onset in childhood, as early as the age of 4 years. Spasticity, dysarthria, dysphrasia, tremor, ataxia, and incoordination are the presenting manifestations. Clinical evidence of liver dysfunction is minimal or absent in this form of Wilson's disease, although histopathologic evidence of liver involvement is invariably present.

Some patients with Wilson's disease have cirrhosis. This presentation is very common in patients afflicted with the disease before age 10. Wilson's disease has been found to be such a common cause of hepatic dysfunction in children with cirrhosis that Wilson's disease should be suspected in any child with cirrhosis until proved otherwise.

Many patients with Wilson's disease have kidney dysfunction because of renal tubular damage secondary to copper deposition in the renal tubular epithelium. Urinalysis will reveal glycosuria, aminoaciduria, and a variety of other renal tubular defects.

OCULAR FINDINGS AND DIAGNOSTIC FEATURES
The Kayser-Fleischer ring is said to be the single most important diagnostic sign of Wilson's disease. It is invariably present in patients with overt neurologic disease and is commonly present in patients with other forms of the disease as well. Detection of the Kayser-Fleischer ring is easiest with slit lamp biomicroscopy, although it may sometimes be seen grossly as a golden brown, green, or ruby red band in the peripheral cornea (Fig. 8-15A). The ring typically appears first superiorly between ten and two o'clock, then inferiorly between five and seven o'clock, then medially, and finally laterally. It develops as a pigment deposition band in Descemet's membrane beginning at the limbus and gradually extending centrally and circumferentially [13, 25, 38]. Early in the disease, the Kayser-Fleischer ring may be difficult to detect, even by slit lamp biomicroscopy. Gonioscopy permits visualization of the pigment in the peripheral Descemet's membrane; this diagnostic procedure should be performed in any patient suspected of having Wilson's disease (Fig. 8-15B).

TREATMENT
Without treatment, Wilson's disease is invariably fatal. The cause of death may be from hepatic, renal, or central nervous system lesions. D-Penicillamine therapy, however, is highly effective. D-Penicillamine is a chelating agent that removes cop-

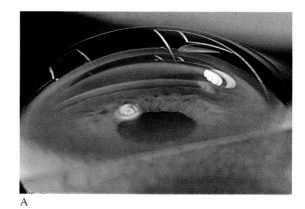

A

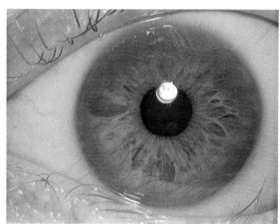

B

FIGURE 8-15. A. Wilson's disease. Note the prominent deposition of copper in the peripheral area of Descemet's membrane, producing the characteristic Kayser-Fleischer ring. B. Goniophotograph. Note the deposition of copper in the most peripheral parts of Descemet's membrane, easily seen by gonioscopy.

per from the patient's tissues. Efficacy of therapy is monitored by the disappearance of the Kayser-Fleischer ring, by a decrease in serum and urine copper levels, by improvement in renal status with disappearance of glycosuria and aminoaciduria, and by improvement in central nervous system and liver function.

COGAN'S SYNDROME
PATHOGENESIS
In 1945 and 1949 Cogan [7, 8] described eight patients who presented with interstitial keratitis and vestibuloauditory symptoms. None of the patients had positive serologic test results for syphilis, and there was no clinical evidence of luetic disease. Since that time, over 50 cases of Cogan's syndrome have been reported. Although the cause of this syndrome, which occurs predominantly in young adults, is unknown, its frequent association with signs and symptoms of systemic vasculitis suggests

a viral or autoimmune pathogenesis. Norton and Cogan [26] reported on the long-term follow-up of 13 patients with Cogan's syndrome in 1959. Two of these 13 developed occlusive vascular disease of the retina, with subsequent optic atrophy and profound visual loss. Eleven developed severe hearing loss and loss of labyrinth function; one, congestive heart failure; three, occlusive vascular disease extraocularly; and three, severe hypertension. Two, though they recovered from the acute phase of Cogan's syndrome, later developed acute fulminating illnesses that were fatal. Norton and Cogan concluded that the oculovestibular portion of Cogan's syndrome was probably only one phase of a systemic disturbance related to the cardiovascular system.

Since Oliner and associates [27] reported Cogan's syndrome in a patient who developed polyarteritis nodosa, many other reports of polyarteritis or other clinical syndromes of vasculitis in association with Cogan's syndrome have been published [5, 6, 9, 10, 12, 14, 15, 17, 30]. In their review of 53 cases of Cogan's syndrome, Chesson and colleagues [6] emphasized the strong association of this syndrome with systemic vasculitis.

CLINICAL FEATURES AND DIAGNOSIS

Cogan's syndrome apparently has no gender, racial, or geographic predilection but is commonly seen in young adults, with the mean age of patients in reported cases being 29 years. The disease typically begins either with the onset of ocular pain and redness and photophobia, or with the abrupt onset of vertigo, tinnitus, and hearing impairment [11]. Regardless of which of these manifestations appears first, the others begin soon after. Corneal findings usually include patchy deep stromal infiltrates, commonly in the midperiphery, but of rapidly changing intensity and distribution. Alternatively, there may be a generalized, fulminating illness, with diffuse infiltration of the corneal stroma with inflammatory cells, producing a diffuse patina (Fig. 8-16). Corneal stromal neovascularization frequently develops, but the vessels typically regress with ultimate resolution of the keratitis, leaving relatively little impairment of visual acuity. The effects on the auditory system are more severe, however, with marked hearing impairment or even rapid progression to complete nerve deafness and nonresponsive labyrinths.

The diagnosis of Cogan's syndrome is based on clinical signs in a patient with negative results of serologic tests (including the fluorescent treponemal antibody absorption test) for syphilis. The differential diagnosis of keratitis, scleritis, or both in a patient with vestibuloauditory symptoms would include syphilis, polyarteritis nodosa, Wegener's

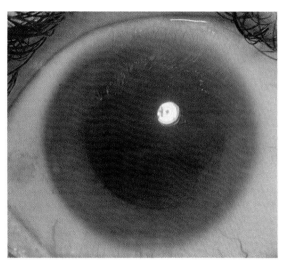

FIGURE 8-16. *Acute Cogan's syndrome. Note the diffuse patina of inflammatory cells in the corneal stroma, as well as the more prominent patches of dense inflammatory cell infiltration.*

granulomatosis, sarcoidosis, and atopic keratoconjunctivitis with eighth nerve disease. Patients with Vogt-Koyanagi-Harada disease or with sympathetic ophthalmia may typically have pain or photophobia, often in association with vestibuloauditory symptoms. However, the ocular findings in these patients are those of severe uveitis and not interstitial keratitis. Although patients with Cogan's syndrome usually have leukocytosis during the acute phase of their illness and sometimes exhibit peripheral eosinophilia, they do not have the other generalized manifestations of polyarteritis nodosa, nor do they typically have the severe constitutional symptoms of that disease. Patients with interstitial keratitis and vestibuloauditory symptoms in association with Wegener's granulomatosis would have clinically detectable lesions in the sinus, respiratory tract, or kidney. Patients with sarcoidosis, interstitial keratitis, and vestibuloauditory symptoms would show other evidence of sarcoidosis, including an elevated serum level of angiotensin-converting enzyme and a positive gallium scan, with enhanced uptake of gallium in the hilar regions of the lungs, lacrimal glands, or parotid glands.

TREATMENT

The keratitis of Cogan's syndrome frequently responds to topical corticosteroid (0.1% dexamethasone phosphate, 1 drop every 2 hours, for 7–14 days). Ocular inflammation subsides, the inflammatory cell patina or stromal infiltrates disappear, and the photophobia vanishes. Systemic steroids are apparently of little benefit for the eighth nerve involvement. If the syndrome occurs in association with polyarteritis nodosa or Wegener's granulomatosis, the treatment of choice is systemic immunosuppression.

FAMILIAL DYSAUTONOMIA (RILEY-DAY SYNDROME)

PATHOGENESIS

Familial dysautonomia, or the Riley-Day syndrome, is an inborn error of metabolism inherited in autosomal recessive fashion found almost exclusively in Ashkenazi Jews. The disease is associated with partial or complete absence of plasma dopamine-beta-hydroxylase activity [39]. This enzyme catalyzes the conversion of dopamine to norepinephrine. A deficiency in this enzyme therefore results in a deficiency of norepinephrine and epinephrine, and at the same time leads to excessive amounts of homovanillic acid in plasma and urine, since the excess dopamine at nerve terminals and the adrenal gland is converted to this substance via alternative metabolic pathways.

CLINICAL FEATURES AND DIAGNOSIS

SYSTEMIC FINDINGS

Familial dysautonomia is characterized by autonomic vasomotor instability; extreme emotional lability; paroxysmal hypertension; excessive sweating and salivation; deficient lacrimation; corneal hypesthesia; deep tendon hyporeflexia; absence of fungiform tongue papillae; episodic bilateral symmetric rash of face, shoulders, and thorax; relative indifference to pain; and motor incoordination. Other manifestations include cyclic vomiting, paroxysmal fever, mental retardation, frequent pulmonary infections, urinary frequency, convulsions, postural hypotension, disturbed speech, failure to develop the usual erythematous flare response around the intradermal wheal induced by intradermal injection of 1:1000 histamine, and abnormal sensitivity to miosis induction by methacholine chloride [31, 32]. Most patients with familial dysautonomia die before the age of 10 years. Aspiration pneumonia and renal failure secondary to hypertension are the leading causes of death.

OCULAR FINDINGS

The corneal manifestations of familial dysautonomia may be severe and may lead to blindness from corneal ulceration, scarring, and vascularization. Pronounced corneal hypesthesia and tear insufficiency are constant features of the disease, and neurotrophic keratitis is very common (Fig. 8-17)

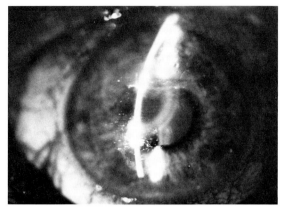

FIGURE 8-17. *Riley-Day syndrome. Note the neurotrophic corneal ulcer and the very dry ocular surface.*

[4]. In some patients the keratopathy is severe, with eventual corneal ulceration and perforation [20].

DIAGNOSIS

If the clinical features are characteristic of familial dysautonomia, the diagnosis can be confirmed by demonstrating decreased levels or absence of dopamine-beta-hydroxylase in the patient's plasma. Other highly suggestive, corroborating findings include increased levels of homovanillic acid in the urine, along with decreased levels of vanillylmandelic acid and 3-methoxy-4-hydroxyphenylethyleneglycol in the urine; failure to develop the typical flare surrounding the wheal produced by intradermal injection of 1:1000 histamine; prompt miosis after installation of 2.5% methacholine chloride (Mecholyl); development of clinically obvious tearing after subcutaneous administration of betamethacholine chloride; and demonstration by fluoroscopy of lower esophageal hypomotility.

The differential diagnosis of familial dysautonomia may vary, depending on the age of the patient. In infancy, frequent pulmonary infection and pulmonary radiographic changes may suggest cystic fibrosis, and peripheral vascular disturbances may suggest acrodynia. In somewhat older children, slow motor development may suggest brain damage or cerebral palsy. The eventual development of episodic hypertension may suggest pheochromocytoma, and behavioral outbursts may suggest childhood schizophrenia. Some patients with familial dysautonomia have had surgery for a nonexistent pheochromocytoma. Patients with the Riley-Day syndrome are at special risk for general anesthesia. They exhibit exquisite intolerance to thiopental sodium (Pentothal), and severe hypotension and cardiac arrest during general anesthesia are common complications. If surgery is necessary in a patient with familial dysautonomia, local anesthesia should probably be employed if at all possible.

TREATMENT

Treatment for familial dysautonomia is predominantly symptomatic. Treatment of the ocular surface should routinely include the use of tear supplements and lubricants, lid taping for nocturnal lagophthalmos, tarsorrhaphy for neurotrophic keratitis, and other therapy for neurotrophic keratitis as discussed earlier in this chapter.

REFERENCES

1. Aguilar, C. E., Bisby, M. A., and Diamond, J. Impulses and the transfer of trophic factors in nerves. *J. Physiol.* (Lond.) 226:60P, 1972.

2. Albuquerque, E. X., et al. Effects of vinblastine and colchicine on neural regulation of the fast and slow skeletal muscles of the rat. *Exp. Neurol.* 37:607, 1972.

3. Alper, M. G. The anesthetic eye: An investigation of changes in the anterior ocular segment of the monkey caused by interrupting the trigeminal nerve at various levels along its course. *Trans. Am. Ophthalmol. Soc.* 72:323, 1976.

4. Boruchoff, S. A., and Dohlman, C. H. The Riley-Day syndrome: Ocular manifestations in a 35-year-old patient. *Am. J. Ophthalmol.* 63:523, 1967.

5. Boyd, G. G. Cogan's syndrome: Report of two cases with signs and symptoms suggesting periarteritis nodosa. *Arch. Otolaryngol.* 65:24, 1957.

6. Chesson, B. D., Blaning, W. Z., and Alroy, J. Cogan's syndrome: A systemic vasculitis. *Am. J. Med.* 60:549, 1976.

7. Cogan, D. G. Syndrome of nonsyphilitic interstitial keratitis and vestibuloauditory symptoms. *Arch. Ophthalmol.* 33:144, 1945.

8. Cogan, D. G. Nonsyphilitic keratitis and vestibuloauditory symptoms: Four additional cases. *Arch. Ophthalmol.* 42:42, 1949.

9. Cogan, D. G., and Dickersin, G. R. Nonsyphilitic interstitial keratitis with postvestibuloauditory symptoms: A case report with fatal aortitis. *Arch. Ophthalmol.* 71:172, 1964.

10. Crawford, W. J. Cogan's syndrome associated with polyarteritis nodosa: A report of 3 cases. *Penn. Med. J.* 60:835, 1957.

11. Donald, R. A., and Gardner, W. J. Keratitis with deafness. *Am. J. Ophthalmol.* 33:889, 1950.

12. Eisenstein, B., and Taubenhause, M. Nonsyphilitic interstitial keratitis with bilateral deafness (Cogan's syndrome) associated with cardiovascular disease. *N. Engl. J. Med.* 258:1074, 1958.

13. Ellis, P. P. Ocular deposition of copper in hypercupremia. *Am. J. Ophthalmol.* 68:423, 1969.

14. Fisher, E. R., and Helstrom, H. R. Cogan's syndrome and systemic vascular disease: Analysis of pathologic features with reference to its relationship to thromboangiitis obliterans (Buerger). *Arch. Pathol.* 72:572, 1961.

15. Gilbert, W. S., and Talbot, F. J. Cogan's syndrome: Signs of periarteritis nodosa and cerebral venous sinus thrombosis. *Arch. Ophthalmol.* 82:633, 1969.

16. Hallermann, W. Zur Lokalbehandlung des Auges mit Acetylcholin. *Klin. Monatsbl. Augenheilkd.* 121:397, 1952.

17. Heinemann, M. H., Soloway, S. M., and Lesser, R. L. Cogan's syndrome. *Ann. Ophthalmol.* 12:667, 1980.

18. Jaffee, M. Neuroparalytic keratitis. *Arch. Ophthalmol.* 20:688, 1938.

19. Kortsak, A., and Bearn, A. G. Hereditary disorders of copper metabolism: Wilson's disease (hepatolenticular degeneration) and Menkes' disease (kinky-hair or steely-hair syndrome). In J. B. Stanbury, J. B. Wyngaarden, and D. S. Fredrickson (Eds.), *The Metabolic Basis of Inherited Disease* (4th ed.). New York: McGraw-Hill, 1978. P. 1098.

20. Liebman, S. D. Ocular manifestations of Riley-Day syndrome: Familial autonomic dysfunction. *Arch. Ophthalmol.* 56:719, 1956.

21. Luco, J. V., and Eyzaguirre, C. Fibrillation and hypersensitivity to acetylcholine in denervated muscle: Effect of length of degenerating nerve fibers. *J. Neurophysiol.* 18:65, 1955.

22. Magendie, J. De l'influence de la cinquieme paire de nurfs sur la nutrition et les fonctions de l'oeil. *J. Physiol.* (Paris) 4:176, 302, 1824.

23. Mishima, S. The effects of the denervation and the stimulation of the sympathetic and the trigeminal nerve on the mitotic rate of the corneal epithelium in the rabbit. *Jpn. J. Ophthalmol.* 1:56, 1957.

24. Mittag, T. W., Mindel, J. S., and Green, J. P. Trophic functions of the neuron. V. Familial dysautonomia. Choline acetyltransferase in familial dysautonomia. *Ann. N.Y. Acad. Sci.* 228:301, 1974.

25. Murphree, A. L., and Maumenee, I. H. *The Eye in Genetic Disease: An Atlas.* St. Louis: Mosby, in press.

26. Norton, E. W. D., and Cogan, D. G. Syndrome of nonsyphilitic interstitial keratitis and vestibuloauditory symptoms: A long-term follow-up. *Arch. Ophthalmol.* 61:695, 1959.

27. Oliner, L., et al. Nonsyphilitic interstitial keratitis and bilateral deafness (Cogan's syndrome) associated with essential polyangiitis (periarteritis nodosa): Review of syndrome with consideration of possible pathologic mechanism. *N. Engl. J. Med.* 248:1001, 1953.

28. Pannabecker, C. L.   Keratitis neuroparalytica: Corneal lesions following operations for trigeminal neuralgia. *Arch. Ophthalmol.* 32:456, 1944.

29. Peet, M. M., and Schneider, R. C.   Trigeminal neuralgia: A review of 689 cases with follow-up study on 65% of group. *J. Neurosurg.* 9:367, 1952.

30. Quinn, F. B., and Falls, H. F.   Cogan's syndrome: Case report and a review of the etiology concepts. *Trans. Am. Acad. Ophthalmol.* 62:716, 1958.

31. Riley, C. M.   Familial autonomic dysfunction. *JAMA* 149:1532, 1952.

32. Riley, C. M., Day, R. L., et al.   Central autonomic dysfunction with defective lacrimation: I. report of 5 cases. *Pediatrics* 3:468, 1949.

33. Rose, W.   Surgical treatment of trigeminal neuralgia. *Lancet* 1:295, 1891.

34. Sigelman, S., and Friedenwald, J. S.   Mitotic and wound-healing activities of the corneal epithelium: Effect of sensory denervation. *Arch. Ophthalmol.* 52:46, 1954.

35. Simone, S. de   Ricerche sul contenuto in acqua totale ed in azoto totale della cornea di coniglio in condizioni di cheratite neuroparalytica sperimentale. *Arch. Ottalmol.* 62:151, 1958.

36. Stookey, B., and Ransohoff, J.   *Trigeminal Neuralgia: Its History and Treatment.* Springfield, Ill.: Thomas, 1959.

37. Sweet, W. H., and Wepsic, J. G.   Controlled thermocoagulation of trigeminal ganglion and routlets for differential destruction of pain fibers: I. Trigeminal neuralgia. *J. Neurosurg.* 40:143, 1974.

38. Walshe, J. M.   The eye in Wilson's disease. *Birth Defects* 12(3):187, 1976.

39. Weinshilboum, R. M., and Axelrod, J.   Reduced plasma dopamine-β-hydroxylase activity in familial dysautonomia. *N. Engl. J. Med.* 285:938, 1971.

40. Wilson, S. A. K.   Progressive lenticular degeneration: A familial nervous disease associated with cirrhosis of the liver. *Brain* 34:295, 1912.

9. DYSTROPHIES AND DEGENERATIONS

Gilbert Smolin

There are many kinds of corneal degenerations and dystrophies that the general ophthalmologist encounters in the course of his practice, and a corresponding number of questions, some of them bothersome, that he should be prepared to answer. Which of the various degenerations or dystrophies is this? What caused it? What is its natural course? And, if the course is unfavorable, can it be altered for the better?

In this chapter, I hope to answer these and related questions with respect to most of the corneal degenerations and dystrophies. I am limited, of course, both by space and by what is currently known. For this reason, the rarest diseases—those least often seen by the practitioner—are not included. Also, as will be seen, not all of the questions pertaining to even the more common degenerations and dystrophies can yet be answered.

It is important to differentiate between degenerations and dystrophies because of differences in their causes, the courses they run, their prognoses, and their treatment. Unfortunately for such differentiation, what appear to be points of difference are sometimes questionable and sometimes more suggestive than definitive. The problem is further complicated by misleading classifications applied in the past to diseases that belong in the other group (e.g., Salzmann's nodular dystrophy is a degenerative process), and by lack of agreement, owing to inadequate knowledge or conflicting ideas about pathogenesis, on how to classify new diseases (e.g., "gelatinous drop–like dystrophy" may be a degenerative process).

Although there are numerous exceptions, as will become apparent, corneal degenerations are usually unilateral, and the lesions are asymmetric, located peripherally or at least eccentrically, and accompanied by vascularization. There is usually no inheritance pattern or genetic (HLA) predisposition, the onset is in middle life or later, and the lesions are progressive. Most important, they are secondary to such compromising processes as aging, inflammation, trauma, or systemic disease. Dystrophies, on the other hand, are usually both bilateral and symmetric, centrally located, avascular, hereditary (usually autosomal dominant), early in onset, only slowly progressive, and unrelated to any systemic or local disease or condition.

DEGENERATIONS

Because there are no natural classifications of corneal degenerations, artificial classifications must be made. For the purposes of this discussion, the degenerations will be grouped according to their location in the cornea (central or peripheral) and whether they are caused primarily by aging or by other processes.

CENTRAL DEGENERATIONS

DEGENERATIONS CAUSED BY AGING

There is often a fine line between normal physiologic senile changes and primary degenerations, especially since the normal changes caused by aging may progress until they cause enough visual impairment to be recognized by the patient.

Advancing age causes a flattening of the vertical meridian (the patient may need plus cylinder at the 180-degree axis), a loss of corneal transparency and luster, a generalized thinning of the cornea (most prominent at the periphery), an increase in the refractive index (oblique light reflects more strongly), and occasionally increased visibility of the corneal nerves. These physiologic senile changes are *not* usually recognized by the patient.

CORNEA FARINATA

Cornea farinata is a speckling of the posterior part of the corneal stroma (usually in the pupillary area) with fine, dustlike, flourlike opacities. Although they are usually bilateral, cases of unilateral cornea farinata have been reported. The deposits may be composed of lipofuscin, a degenerative pigment that accumulates in old cells [35]. (This pigment has been found in pre-Descemet's dystrophy, a condition that resembles cornea farinata clinically.) Conspicuous cornea farinata is sometimes a family trait (dominant inheritance), but the opacities neither reduce vision nor alter corneal sensation.

MOSAIC SHAGREEN OF VOGT

The mosaic (crocodile) shagreen of Vogt consists of grayish white, polygonal opacities separated by relatively clear spaces. It is most often located centrally in the anterior segment of both corneas, less often in the posterior segment. There is no vascularization

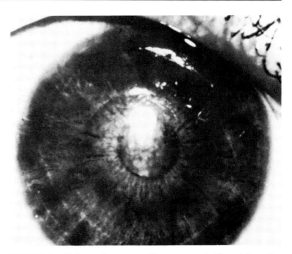

FIGURE 9-1. *Polygonal gray opacities are seen in the axial portion of the corneal stroma in mosaic shagreen of Vogt.*

or diminished sensation; however, the visual acuity may be reduced, necessitating lamellar keratoplasty.

The arrangement of the prominent collagen lamellae of the anterior stroma that enter Bowman's layer obliquely can lead to the mosaic pattern if the normal tension on Bowman's layer is relaxed, and trauma, prolonged hypotension, and aging can relax the normal tension. Ridges form, indenting the epithelium and producing the mosaic pattern (Fig. 9-1). Calcium may be deposited at the apices of these ridges [151], and there may be ruptures in Bowman's layer, with fibrous tissue interposed between the Bowman's layer and the epithelium.

A juvenile form of mosaic shagreen occurs in patients with megalocornea, peripheral calcific band keratopathy, or iris malformations.

DEGENERATIONS NOT CAUSED BY AGING

CALCIFIC BAND KERATOPATHY

In calcific band keratopathy, the calcific band is largely in the palpebral fissure and separated from the limbus by a clear zone. There are numerous holes where corneal nerves penetrate Bowman's layer. The band begins in the corneal periphery and affects the central area last (Fig. 9-2). The calcium, principally hydroxyapatite, is deposited in Bowman's layer, in the basement membrane of the corneal epithelium, and in the most superficial lamellae of the stroma, leaving the remainder of the cornea clear.

Calcific band keratopathy can be distinguished from calcareous degeneration of the cornea since the latter usually affects the deep layers as well as the anterior layers. Furthermore, calcareous degen-

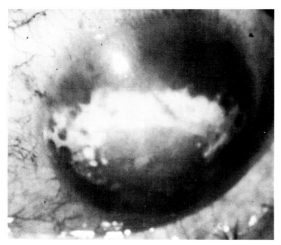

FIGURE 9-2. *Calcific band keratopathy occurs in the interpalpebral fissure area of the cornea. Small holes are present in the band.*

eration of the cornea as seen in seriously injured eyes, phthisis bulbi, and necrotic neoplasms is often accompanied by bone formation elsewhere in the globe [117].

The earliest histologic change in calcific band keratopathy consists of basophilic staining of the basement membrane of the corneal epithelium. This is followed by similar staining in the most anterior part of Bowman's layer. As the lesion develops, Bowman's layer becomes calcified through its entire thickness. Possibly because of its brittleness, Bowman's layer breaks up into many tiny islands or plaques, and the corneal epithelium often becomes detached from the underlying plaque. Concomitantly, masses of eosinophilic amorphous connective tissue insinuate themselves between the fragments of calcified Bowman's layer and the overlying epithelium, and there is patchy calcification of the anterior lamellae of the stroma. Calcium is also deposited in areas where there are signs of fibroblastic proliferation [116].

The pathogenesis of this process of calcium deposition is not clearly understood, but it is known that calcium and phosphate are present in blood and interstitial fluids at levels that nearly exceed the level at which they are soluble. Precipitation can therefore be triggered easily by elevation of the pH, evaporation, or an increase in the concentration of either calcium or phosphate at a given site [6, 24], e.g., in hyperparathyroidism [6], sarcoidosis [155], nephrocalcinosis [154], and vitamin D intoxication [24].

The evaporation of water and subsequent concentration of calcium salts favor precipitation of the cal-

cium in the interpalpebral fissure. The loss of CO_2 at this site increases the pH, and this too favors calcium salt precipitation. The lack of blood vessels in the cornea minimizes the blood's buffering effect on the pH. Initially, the deposition of calcium may be limited to the anterior layers where there is an accumulation of lactic acid; the pH in the deep stroma is lower and calcium precipitation less or absent.

Calcific band keratopathy can be treated successfully with EDTA. An 0.05 M, 1.5% solution of neutral disodium EDTA is effective, and removal of the epithelium facilitates removal of the calcium. A 4% cocaine or lidocaine hydrochloride (Xylocaine) solution may be effective in removing the epithelium and anesthetizing the eye. Since EDTA is quite irritating, I use a water bath over the cornea and put the EDTA into it. This limits ocular exposure to the drug. (Resting a cellulose sponge that has been saturated with EDTA on the cornea is a method that has been used by others [138].) The solution is removed from the water bath with a syringe, the bath is then removed, and the surface of the cornea is gently scraped with a sterile scalpel. Cycloplegics, antibiotics, and patching are used until the cornea has re-epithelialized.

Calciphylaxis [39] is a condition of induced systemic hypersensitivity in which tissues respond to appropriate challenging agents with local calcification. It takes place, for example, in uveitis in children, in calciferol administration, and in induced uveitis in rabbits [68].

CORNEAL AMYLOIDOSIS

Amyloid deposits are amorphous, eosinophilic, glassy, and hyalinlike. They do not provoke an inflammatory response and appear to have little deleterious effect except when they reduce vision or cause recurrent erosions. Amyloid stains metachromatically with crystal violet or methyl violet, produces secondary fluorescence with thioflavine [131], and, when viewed with a polarizing microscope after Congo red staining, shows a unique red-green birefringence.

The amyloid protein, of which there are several types, can be produced by genetically defective cells or by cells under stress. It is possible that one type is of immunoglobulin origin and derived from the polymerized fragments of immunoglobulin light chains [26]. Antisera to amyloid of this type cross-react with Bence Jones protein and have an identical amino acid sequence. Nomenclature remains a problem, but recently it has been suggested that this immunoglobulin type of amyloid protein be called

A$_k$ [28], that tissue-derived, nonimmunoglobulin amyloid protein be called AA, and that serum-derived amyloid protein have an S added as a prefix (i.e., SAA) [27].

Amyloidosis is primary or secondary, systemic or localized. Secondary systemic amyloidosis does not affect the cornea, and primary systemic amyloidosis does so only rarely.

Primary localized corneal amyloidosis is usually the result of direct extension from the conjunctiva. Recently a primary type of the disease has been described in Japan. It is called gelatinous drop–like dystrophy, and in its early stages the patients complain of foreign-body sensation, photophobia, lacrimation, and blurred vision. In its later stages, the corneal lesions are raised, yellowish gray, gelatinous masses with mulberrylike surfaces (Fig. 9-3) [113]; they are bilateral and central, and the peripheral cornea remains clear and free of vascularization. In the very late stages, however, neovascularization does occur. Similar lesions have been reported recently in the United States [125]. Some cases have been sporadic, others have followed an autosomal recessive inheritance pattern, and some patients have had siblings who suffered from various types of dystrophies (e.g., lattice dystrophy, which is discussed later in this chapter).

Histopathologic examination of tissue from this primary localized disease shows a thinned epithelial layer and amyloid deposits. Microscopic studies suggest that the amyloid fibrils are produced by the keratocytes in the stroma.

Total deep lamellar keratoplasty seem to be the preferred treatment of the primary disease because the affected cornea is quite fragile. After a matter of years, unfortunately, a transplanted cornea often develops the same condition.

Secondary localized amyloidosis of the cornea is not unusual. Indeed, not only corneal trauma but a number of other ocular disorders—trachoma, neoplasms, lipoid proteinosis, leprosy, phlyctenulosis, lipoidal degeneration, and keratoconus [31, 140]—may be accompanied by amyloid deposits. According to one group of observers [107], secondary localized amyloidosis was present in 35 percent of all corneal specimens submitted to their pathology laboratory.

There are three kinds of amyloid deposits: subepithelial masses resembling degenerative pannus, lamellar deposits occurring only in the deep stroma, and perivascular deposits associated with corneal vascularization. The clinical appearance of the lesions is influenced by the primary disease, but a

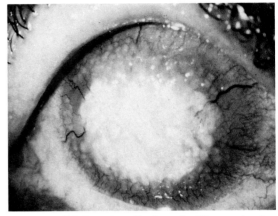

FIGURE 9-3. *Gelatinous drop–like dystrophy. The corneal surface has a mulberry appearance. The opacification is quite dense, and vascularization is present in this severe late stage.*

yellowish gray opacification and vascularization are features common to all of the lesions.

The treatment of secondary localized corneal amyloidosis is also surgical, but surgery should be performed only when vision is impaired. Because of the vascularization of the lesion, there is more than the usual risk of corneal graft rejection. Unfortunately, too, recurrences of the amyloidosis are to be expected.

SALZMANN'S NODULAR DEGENERATION

Salzmann's nodular degeneration has been reported as a late sequela to such corneal disease as phlyctenulosis, trachoma, vernal keratoconjunctivitis, measles, various other viral diseases, and scarlet fever [89, 133]. The antecedent eye disease usually occurs in childhood.

The lesions, which are bluish gray nodules, vary in number from one to nine and are elevated above the surface of the cornea. They occur either in the area scarred by the earlier disease or at the edge of the transparent cornea, and they are either central or peripheral (Fig. 9-4). The degeneration is bilateral in 80 percent of the cases and occurs more often in women than in men.

Histopathologic examination of the lesions shows degenerative changes in the corneal epithelium. The epithelium, whose thickness varies, often consists of only a single layer over the nodular areas. Bowman's layer is missing over the nodules, and in this zone there is excessive secretion of a basement membrane–like material. Hyaline degeneration of collagen, cellular debris, and electron-dense hyaline deposits in the collagen of the nodules are also present [153].

There is usually no need for treatment. Sometimes the associated problems of severe lacrimation,

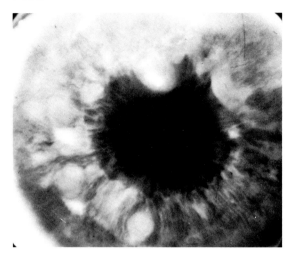

FIGURE 9-4. *Saltzmann's nodular degeneration. Several elevated opacified lesions are present in the midperiphery.*

photophobia, or diminished vision require simple excision of the nodule, but even when the nodules are central, keratoplasty is seldom needed to improve vision.

KELOID FORMATION

Keloids can form in a scarred cornea, but they rarely do [42]. They are a result of exuberant fibrocytic activity that usually originates in the stromal cells. Corneal keloids are white, probably because of the relative paucity of blood vessels. Keratoplasty is indicated in some cases [118].

HYALINE DEGENERATION

Hyaline degeneration of the cornea resembles Saltzmann's nodular degeneration, climatic droplet keratopathy, and granular dystrophy. It has been described as a nodular, yellowish brown, granular opacification that appears in the lower half of the cornea in the shape of a band. There is no vascularization, and the limbal area is clear. Histologically, the opacities have proved to be rounded masses of hyalin beneath the epithelium [15, 41]. Because this type of degeneration occurs in certain geographic areas, it has been assumed that it is related to climatic conditions and may be a form of climatic droplet keratopathy (discussed later in this chapter). Treatment, if necessary, is by lamellar keratoplasty.

LIPID DEGENERATION

Lipid degeneration of the cornea is primary or secondary, the secondary lipid deposits being much more common than the primary ones. Lipid deposits can be laid down after necrosis and vascularization of the cornea, and certain diseases (e.g., herpes zoster) seem especially conducive to their development. In primary lipid degeneration, the deposits can be, and usually are, bilateral, central, and avascular; there may be no history of antecedent corneal disease; and the serum lipid levels may be normal [45]. Occasionally the cholesterol level is elevated [156].

The opacity created by the corneal deposits is dense and yellowish white and has feathery edges; cholesterol crystals can occasionally be seen at its edges (Fig. 9-5). The lesion consists largely of neutral fats [23] but contains phospholipids and cholesterol as well [5].

The pathogenesis of lipid degeneration remains uncertain, but according to some hypotheses, the disease is due to enhanced permeability of the corneoscleral limbal blood vessels, to an excess production of lipids, or to an inability of the corneal cells to metabolize lipids. The opacity can be removed by penetrating keratoplasty, but there are sometimes recurrences in the donor tissue [59].

COAT'S WHITE RING

Coat's white rings, usually related to injuries caused by metallic foreign bodies, are iron deposits and are found at the level of Bowman's layer or in the superficial stroma.

PIGMENTARY DEGENERATIONS

IRON. Iron can be deposited in the cornea as a ring (Coat's white ring), as a line, or diffusely. Iron lines can occur as follows: (1) after an epithelial breakdown (Hudson-Stähli line) [62, 114], (2) around a cone in keratoconus (Fleischer ring) [46, 85], (3) in front of a pterygium (Stocker-Busacca line) [141], (4) near a filtering bleb (Ferry line) [43], or (5) in association with superficial scars. An iron ring can occur in congenital spherocytosis [36] and after an iron foreign body has entered the eye.

The pathogenesis of the iron deposition, except in the case of the iron foreign body, remains obscure. The source of the iron may be the perilimbal blood vessels, and tear transferrin and corneal transferrin may help to carry it to its destination. It has been suggested that enzymes and environmental factors also play a role in causing this degeneration [11].

MELANIN. Melanin can be deposited in the corneas of patients receiving phenothiazides or chloroquine systemically. In patients receiving phenothiazides, the fine stippling of melanin particles begins at the level of Descemet's membrane. The overlying stroma, and even Bowman's layer, can be involved. It has been suggested that ultraviolet light assists the precipitation of the melanin [19]. After the use of chloroquine, there may be a whorllike pattern of melanin near Descemet's membrane [66]. Epinephrine can lead to the deposition of adrenochrome in the region of Bowman's layer and the anterior stroma [44, 126].

METALS. Metallic foreign bodies and heavy metals used therapeutically or industrially (copper, silver, gold, iron) can also be deposited in the cornea.

PERIPHERAL DEGENERATIONS
DEGENERATIONS CAUSED BY AGING

WHITE LIMBAL GIRDLE OF VOGT
The white limbal girdle of Vogt is a narrow, crescentic, chalky white line in the nasal and temporal limbal areas of the cornea in the interpalpebral fissure. It is composed of flecks or short lines lying immediately beneath the epithelium and is probably related to exposure to sunlight. It is present in 55 percent of all patients between the ages of 40 and 60 [147].

Histologically, the limbal girdle of Vogt is an elastotic degeneration of the subepithelial collagen and has no clinical importance. The early literature described it as a type II degeneration and listed another entity, which was probably an early-stage calcific band keratopathy, as type I.

DELLEN
Dellen are depressions in the peripheral cornea caused by desiccation (see Keratoconjunctivitis Sicca in Chapter 7, Dry Eyes). They occur most often at the temporal limbus. Although usually transient (lasting only 24–48 hours), dellen in rare cases may last for weeks and lead to scarring. They are often found where corneal wetting is reduced because of edematous limbal tissue (e.g., after muscle or cataract surgery), lagophthalmos, long-term administration of cocaine eye drops, or the poor wetting ability of tears in the elderly.

Histologically, a dellen is a thinning of the corneal epithelium, Bowman's layer, and the superficial stroma; it can usually be overcome by double patching and the application of a bland ointment.

ARCUS SENILIS
Arcus senilis (corneal arcus) is found in 60 percent of people between the ages of 40 and 60, and in

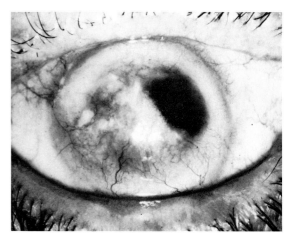

FIGURE 9-5. *In lipid degeneration, dense lipid deposition is present in the peripheral and central portion of the cornea. Vascularization is minimal.*

almost all people over the age of 80. It is more frequent in blacks than in other races.

Corneal arcus is a yellowish white deposit that occurs first in the inferior and then in the superior aspect of the peripheral cornea and eventually encircles the entire cornea. There is a lucid interval (first described by Vogt) between the sharp peripheral border of the arcus and the limbus. The lucid interval is in some way due to the limbal vasculature. The inner border of the arcus has a diffuse edge, and crisscrossing dark lines are sometimes observed within the arcus. The arcus itself consists of cholesterol, cholesterol esters, phospholipids, and triglycerides. The lipids are found extracellularly in the corneal stroma in an hourglass pattern.

The formation of the arcus is related to increasing age, the proximity of blood vessels to the peripheral cornea, the high degree of the vessels' permeability, and hypercholesterolemia. The limbal vessels become increasingly permeable with age, and this allows low-density lipoproteins to pass into the cornea and to carry lipids into the eye [157]. Corneal arcus and atherosclerosis are broadly related to the level of low-density lipoprotein in the plasma.

If a young patient (less than 30 years of age) develops a corneal arcus, his plasma lipid levels should be tested. Juvenile arcus occurs in children with familial lipidemia, megalocornea, or blue sclera. (See Chapter 10.)

HASSALL-HENLE BODIES
Descemet's membrane increases in thickness throughout life. Localized nodular thickenings appear in the peripheral area, disturbing the regular mosaic of the endothelial cells. These thickenings,

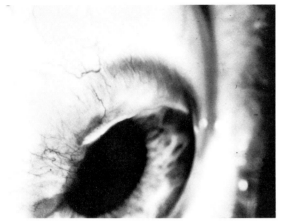

FIGURE 9-6. *Peripheral thinning, vascularization, and lipid deposition at the axial border of the gutter in an eye with Terrien's marginal degeneration.*

known as Hassall-Henle bodies or Descemet's warts, extend toward the endothelium and are microscopically visible in the area of specular reflection where they appear as small, round, dark areas within the normal endothelial mosaic. Occasionally, they become confluent and microscopically visible. The thickenings are due to an overproduction of hyalin by endothelial cells. In appearance these changes are identical to the changes associated with endothelial decompensation and corneal edema that are seen centrally in cornea guttata.

PELLUCID MARGINAL DEGENERATION

Pellucid marginal degeneration begins in the inferior portion of the cornea near the limbus [134]. There is an uninvolved area between the thinned section of the cornea and the limbus, there is no vascularization or lipid deposition, and the corneal sensation remains normal. This rare entity is sometimes associated with keratoconus [49] and may actually be an anomaly of the connective tissue. (It has been seen in patients with skeletal abnormalities.) The pathogenesis is possibly a depolymerization of the mucopolysaccharides in the cornea.

TERRIEN'S MARGINAL DEGENERATION

Terrien's marginal degeneration occurs at any age and most often in men. It is often bilateral, and when unilateral the other cornea eventually becomes thin. The degeneration begins superonasally with the development of fine, white, subepithelial, peripheral opacities that spare the limbus. The opacities may coalesce, and where they are there is progressive thinning of the cornea that also spares the limbus. The epithelium usually remains intact,

but the floor of the gutter becomes increasingly thin. The opacities and the thinning of the gutter floor may progress circumlimbally, and there may be yellowish white (lipid) deposits in the center of the gutter (Fig. 9-6).

Even slight trauma can lead to perforation of the markedly thinned cornea, which is tilted forward, causing astigmatism. In some cases, the eye remains white and quiet, but in the form of the disease that occurs in young people, there is often inflammation, necrosis, and neovascularization of the peripheral cornea.

Histologically, Bowman's layer and the corneal lamellae may be split or fibrillated [148]. Whether or not there is vascularization and inflammation [86] depends on the form of the disease. The cause of Terrien's degeneration remains unknown.

If the thinning becomes extreme and reconstructive surgery is indicated, a full-thickness or lamellar corneoscleral graft, often hand-fashioned to fit the defect, may be necessary. Conjunctival flaps are usually unsuccessful.

Interestingly, atypical pterygium can occur in Terrien's degeneration [65]. (Marginal degenerations associated with systemic diseases are discussed in the section entitled Rheumatoid Diseases in Chapter 6.)

MOOREN'S ULCERATION

Mooren's ulceration is discussed in detail in Chapter 6. The discussion here is limited to those features that serve to differentiate Mooren's ulceration from Terrien's marginal degeneration.

Mooren's ulceration is a chronic, progressive, marginal, nonpurulent ulcer that begins as an infiltrate in the anterior stroma adjacent to the limbus, destroys the epithelium overlying the stroma, and then spreads circumlimbally and axially. In about 30 percent of affected patients, it is bilateral. There is no unaffected area between the corneal lesion and the limbus, differing in this respect from Terrien's degeneration. The conjunctiva adjacent to Mooren's lesion is often hyperemic.

Mooren's ulceration usually starts in the medial and lateral quadrants. Typically, its gross features are a gray, overhanging edge on its axial border, involvement of the anterior one-third to one-half of the anterior cornea, and minimal cicatrization. Some of the ulcerated areas are active and inflamed while others seem to be healing. The ulcer runs a course of from 3 to 12 months and has been known to recur. The course is often severe and may leave the patient with a severely damaged cornea and virtually no vision. Pain starts early, becomes severe as the lesion develops, and is sometimes helped by a therapeutic soft lens. In some cases, the ulceration responds to immunosuppressive agents (e.g., cyclophosphamide [Cytoxan], methotrexate [149]).

There is a type of Mooren's ulceration that is seen in young blacks in Africa [91]. It occurs more often in men than in women, is usually bilateral (75 percent), runs a rapid course with possible perforation of the cornea, and has a very poor prognosis. It also seems less responsive to treatment than are other types of Mooren's ulceration [91].

PERIPHERAL DEGENERATIONS NOT CAUSED BY AGING

CLIMATIC DROPLET KERATOPATHY

Climatic droplet keratopathy has been given a variety of other names, including Labrador keratopathy, spheroidal degeneration, chronic actinic keratopathy, oil droplet degeneration, keratinoid corneal degeneration, elastoid degeneration, hyaline degeneration, degeneratio sphaerularis elaidoes, fisherman's keratopathy, Nama keratopathy, and proteinaceous keratopathy.

The cause of climatic keratopathy is unknown, but certain factors—solar radiation; aging; low humidity; microtrauma from wind, sand, and ice; and possibly extremes of temperature and previous corneal inflammation—seem to be related to its progress. These factors, plus others that are possibly genetic, cause an elastotic degeneration of the collagen in the cornea and conjunctiva [15, 94] and deposits that consist of an exudate of fibroblastic cells of the cornea and conjunctiva.

Fraunfelder and Hanna [55, 56] describe two types of climatic droplet keratopathy. There is, first, a primary corneal type that is bilateral and related to aging—not to corneal disease of any kind. The other type is secondary, bilateral or unilateral, and related to corneal disease or climate or both.

The problem with this classification is that climatic droplet keratopathy is not well defined, and any division into types is likely to be somewhat arbitrary. Climatic factors certainly influence the type occurring in the aged, though they are probably less influential in old than in young patients. Local corneal inflammation may act to enhance the predilection to deposit the material.

Climatic droplet keratopathy most often affects men who work outdoors. The changes begin with subepithelial accumulation of opalescent droplets that coalesce to form a yellowish gray band beneath

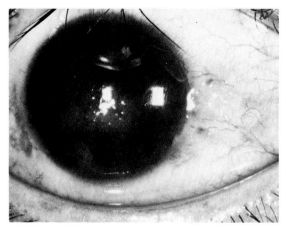

FIGURE 9-7. *Climatic droplet keratopathy. Note the deposits in a band configuration in the interpalpebral portion of the cornea.*

the epithelium. Larger aggregates of droplets accumulate later and elevate the corneal epithelium (Fig. 9-7). Three grades of severity have been described: grade 1, in which only the peripheral, interpalpebral zone of the cornea is affected; grade 2, in which the opacity spreads to the pupillary area, reducing vision to 20/100; and grade 3, in which large, yellowish, opalescent nodules elevate the epithelium and reduce vision to less than 20/200 [58].

Histologically, the deposits are found at the level of Bowman's layer and below. They are extracellular and autofluorescent. The severest cases require surgery.

PIGMENTARY DEGENERATIONS (PERIPHERAL)

STRIATE MELANOKERATOSIS. Subepithelial growth of melanotic cells into the cornea from the limbus is unusual in the white race. In blacks, however, pigment-bearing cells often penetrate far into the cornea in response to a variety of stimuli such as corneal trauma, infection, or epithelial breakdown. The pigmentation, which is permanent, sometimes occurs in a whorl-like pattern [33].

DYSTROPHIES

EPITHELIAL DYSTROPHIES

JUVENILE HEREDITARY EPITHELIAL DYSTROPHY
Juvenile hereditary epithelial dystrophy (Meesmann's epithelial dystrophy) was first described comprehensively by Meesmann [108] and later in the American literature by Stocker and Holt [143]. It has an autosomal dominant inheritance pattern with incomplete penetrance. The penetrance can be as low as 60 percent [80].

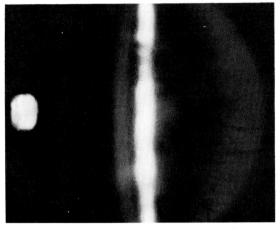

FIGURE 9-8. *Clear cysts are scattered diffusely throughout the corneal epithelium of this eye with juvenile hereditary epithelial dystrophy.*

CLINICAL FEATURES

This bilateral, symmetric disease begins in the first decade of life as tiny, round (or somewhat irregular), clear vesicles in the epithelium. There may be some surface irregularities, but the cornea between the vesicles remains clear. The vesicles are located in the interpalpebral area of the cornea but may appear in a crescentic arrangement near the upper limbus, in a swirl pattern, or in a wedge-shaped pattern [109]. The lesions can be seen by direct illumination or retroillumination. When viewed by retroillumination, they look like cysts (Fig. 9-8). With time, the entire cornea may become involved, and in the later stages of the disease fine, sinuous lines and small gray opacities, subepithelial and amorphous, appear [143].

The patient remains asymptomatic until the fourth or fifth decade when there may be irregular astigmatism and transient blurred vision. The cysts can break through to the surface causing the patient passing discomfort, lacrimation, and photophobia.

PATHOLOGY

An intracytoplasmic "peculiar substance" is the most characteristic ultrastructural finding of juvenile hereditary epithelial dystrophy. This is a focal collection of fibrillogranular material that is either the result of a primary degeneration of cytoplasmic filaments or secondary to a more generalized disturbance of the cytoplasmic ground substance [98]. Although the initial disturbance is probably in the cytoplasmic ground substance in the basal cells, it is followed by homogenization of these basal cells and by the formation of cysts that contain cytoplasmic debris.

The basement membrane is thickened and sometimes pedunculated. The epithelium is thickened and apparently disordered. The transition from basal cells to superficial cells during the maturation process is ill defined. The intraepithelial cysts are most numerous in the anterior epithelial layers.

TREATMENT

Since the symptoms of juvenile hereditary epithelial dystrophy are usually minimal and visual loss is extremely rare, treatment is seldom required. Removal of the epithelium is followed closely by the reappearance of the pathologic changes in the new epithelium [17]. Superficial lamellar keratectomy can be curative but is rarely warranted.

EPITHELIAL BASEMENT MEMBRANE DYSTROPHY

Epithelial basement membrane dystrophy (also called Cogan's microcystic epithelial dystrophy, fingerprint-map-dot dystrophy, dystrophic recurrent erosion) was first described by Cogan and colleagues in 1964 [25] and is probably the most common anterior membrane corneal dystrophy. No definitive hereditary pattern has been recognized, but the disease can be dominantly inherited [96].

CLINICAL FEATURES

This dystrophy seems most often to affect white women over the age of 30, but a few cases have been reported in patients in their first decade of life. The initial symptoms—severe pain on waking in the morning, photophobia, and slightly reduced visual acuity—can be related to recurrent erosions, which often occur in these patients. The lesions are usually concentrated in one area of the cornea, either centrally or eccentrically. There may be dots, maps, and fingerprint opacities, all of which tend to come and go spontaneously. If a recurrent erosion has just occurred, there is loose epithelium and the lesion looks like a "slipped rug." The erosions diminish in frequency with time.

The maps are diffuse, gray lesions that contain clear, oval areas and vary greatly in size; the dots are large gray cysts or fine blebs (Fig. 9-9); the fingerprints are refractile lines that branch or intersect each other and usually appear in groups in the center of the cornea. The maps and dots in combination are seen most often, and the maps alone next most often. Fingerprints in combination with maps or dots are rarely seen, and dots alone are never seen.

PATHOLOGIC CHANGES

Epithelial basement membrane dystrophy is probably a result of the synthesis of abnormal basement membrane. This causes a thickening of the membrane with extensions into the epithelium and with fibrillar material between the membrane and Bowman's layer.

In the map pattern, a thickened epithelial basement membrane with extension into the epithelium is the principle histopathologic change. Collagen may be present in the epithelium. The epithelial cells on top of the abnormal basement membrane do not form hemidesmosomes, which probably accounts for the recurrent erosions. The dots are intraepithelial cysts that contain cytoplasmic debris, nuclear debris, and lipid. They form along with the abnormal tissue that extends into the epithelium. The fingerprint pattern is a result of the deposition of a fine fibrillogranular substance and the reduplication and thickening of the basement membrane [12].

TREATMENT

Although epithelial basement membrane dystrophy rarely causes symptoms or reduces vision, the recurrent erosions require treatment. Hypertonic solutions (e.g., 5% sodium chloride) every 3 or 4 hours during the day, and hypertonic ointment at night, are recommended for mild cases. For other cases, double patching the eye for 48 hours so that the defect will epithelialize, followed by a bland hypertonic ointment at bedtime for weeks to months, can sometimes be effective. In severe recurrent cases, it is usually effective to remove the redundant epithelium mechanically with a cotton-tip applicator after instilling a topical anesthetic, to follow this with a cycloplegic and an antibiotic, and then to patching both eyes for 48 hours. In recalcitrant cases or cases with frequent recurrences, a thin, loosely fitting, high-water-content, soft contact lens can be applied gently and worn continuously for several months. The use of hypertonic eye drops in conjunction with the contact lens may be helpful. Careful observation is indicated in order to minimize the chance of corneal infection.

BLEBLIKE DYSTROPHY

Bleblike dystrophy is probably a variant of epithelial basement membrane dystrophy.

VORTEX DYSTROPHY

Vortex dystrophy is probably a degenerative change caused by toxic keratopathy. It may be that the vor-

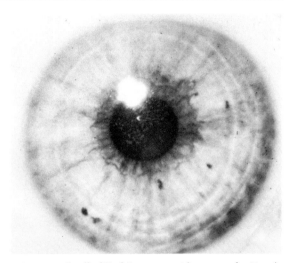

FIGURE 9-9. *Small white dots are present in a grouped pattern in the corneal epithelium in this case of epithelial basement membrane dystrophy.*

tex pattern is formed by the abnormal epithelial cells after they enter the cornea from the limbus. Vortex dystrophy can be caused by chloroquine, indomethacin, quinacrine hydrochloride (Atabrine), chlorpromazine, or amiodarone (Fig. 9-10). A similar cornea verticillata pattern is seen in Fabry's disease (sphingolipidosis).

BOWMAN'S LAYER DYSTROPHY

REIS-BÜCKLERS DYSTROPHY

Reis-Bücklers dystrophy was first described by Reis in 1917 as an anular corneal dystrophy with geographic, chart-shaped opacities [127], and some years later (1949) was described by Bücklers [16] in more detail. It has an autosomal dominant inheritance pattern with strong penetrance [76].

CLINICAL FEATURES

Reis-Bücklers dystrophy is bilateral, symmetric, and axial. It usually appears in the first decade of life as a reticular, superficial corneal opacification associated recurrently with painful epithelial erosions. The erosions usually occur up to three or four times a year and cause severe pain, photophobia, and ocular hyperemia. By the fourth decade, they become less frequent, possibly owing to the replacement of Bowman's layer by scar tissue. Corneal sensation eventually decreases, lessening the pain associated with the attacks of erosion. The corneal surface is rough and irregular. The bluish white opacities, which may be ring- or crescent-shaped, alveolar or polycyclic, or like a geographic chart, frosted glass, a fishnet, or curdled milk [81] (Fig. 9-11), are either isolated or grouped. The densest opacities are in the

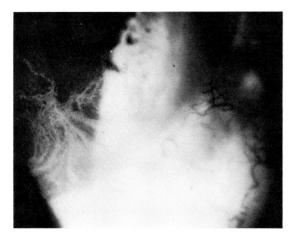

FIGURE 9-10. *Vortex dystrophy in patient taking amiodarone.*

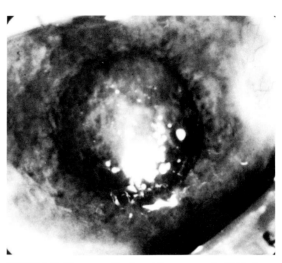

FIGURE 9-11. *Dense opacification of the cornea and a highly irregular surface are present in this eye with Reis-Bücklers dystrophy.*

midperiphery, the extreme periphery almost always remaining clear.

Vision is usually affected by the third or fourth decade of life because of the irregular corneal surface and the opacification. In some of the clinical variants, e.g., Grayson-Wilbrandt dystrophy [70] and honeycomb dystrophy [150], the visual acuity is not severely affected.

PATHOLOGIC CHANGES

There are degenerative changes in the epithelium, especially the basal layers, in Reis-Bücklers dystrophy. Many epithelial cells show cytoplasmic vacuolization, mitochondrial swelling, and clumping of nuclear chromatin. The basement membrane is absent or irregular, and Bowman's layer, also absent, is replaced [72] by masses of disoriented, collagenlike fibrils. This fibrous tissue, which contains cells resembling fibroblasts, interdigitates with the anterior stroma. There are no hemidesmosomes.

The basic disorder is probably in the superficial keratocytes that produce abnormal fibrils. These fibrils replace Bowman's layer. The recurrent erosions may aggravate the scarring.

It has been suggested that Reis-Bücklers dystrophy is a form of lattice dystrophy, but recent evidence to the contrary is convincing [87, 129].

TREATMENT

The recurrent erosions of Reis-Bücklers dystrophy can be treated initially with hypertonic drops during the day and hypertonic ointment at night, double patching of the affected eye and occasionally of the unaffected eye, and debridement or soft contact lenses or both. In severe cases, however, this therapy will not suffice, and the subepithelial fibrous tissue must be peeled off by blunt dissec-

tion. This can improve vision to 20/50 or 20/40 and stop the recurrent erosions [160]. Although both lamellar and penetrating keratoplasties have been performed [69, 105], recurrences in the donor buttons have been reported [18, 119].

STROMAL DYSTROPHIES

GRANULAR DYSTROPHY

Granular dystrophy (bread-crumb dystrophy, Groenouw I dystrophy) was first described by Groenouw in 1898 [73]. Its hereditary pattern is usually autosomal dominant [2, 136].

CLINICAL FEATURES

White opacities appear in the superficial stroma of the central cornea in the first decade of life. Since the stroma between the lesions remains clear and the epithelium regular, most young patients have very few symptoms. As the condition progresses, the opacities enlarge, increase in number, coalesce, and extend into the deep layers of the stroma. The disease is bilateral and symmetric, and the peripheral cornea remains free of lesions. In severe cases, the vision may deteriorate to 20/200 by the fourth decade of life, and there may be recurrent erosions.

There are several variants of the usual course. Sometimes when the lesions have the appearance of bread crumbs (Fig. 9-12), they do not progress in later life. In another variant (progressive dystrophy of Waardenberg and Jonkers), the lesions progress as they do in Reis-Bücklers dystrophy [47].

PATHOLOGIC CHANGES

The substance that accumulates in the stromal lesions in granular dystrophy is hyalin—a noncollagenous protein containing tyrosine, tryptophan, arginine, and sulfur-containing amino acids [61]. There are also phospholipids in the stromal lesions. These hyaline areas stain intensely red with Masson trichrome stain, weakly positive with PAS stain, and not at all with the Verhoeff stains.

Although the epithelium is rarely affected, the basement membrane of the epithelium may be irregular in thickness or absent in some areas [106], and Bowman's layer may be thinner than usual or absent. The hemidesmosomes are rarely affected.

Electron-dense, rodlike deposits of an amorphous substance have been seen with the electron microscope [75, 97]. It has been postulated that these deposits are produced by abnormal keratocytes in the anterior layer of the stroma.

TREATMENT

No treatment is required early in granular dystrophy since the patients are asymptomatic. As the disease progresses, penetrating keratoplasty may be necessary to restore vision. Since affected corneas are avascular and structurally sound aside from the deposits, the prognosis is excellent after keratoplasty. Unfortunately, however, there may be recurrences in the donor graft [146, 152].

If recurrent erosions occur, they should be treated appropriately. (See Treatment under Reis-Bücklers Dystrophy.)

LATTICE DYSTROPHY

Lattice dystrophy (Biber-Haab-Dimmer dystrophy), first described by Biber, Haab, and Dimmer in the 1890s [7], has an autosomal dominant inheritance pattern. The expression of the gene is often so subtle [77] that the disease can be detected in only a few members of an affected family [124]. Some members of the family may show only some dystrophic recurrent erosions with little or no clinically observable opacification. Opacification, when it occurs, is usually symmetric and bilateral, though unilateral cases have been reported [123, 128].

CLINICAL FEATURES

Small refractile lines, white dots, and a faint central haze in the anterior stroma may appear in the first decade of life. The translucent, refractile lines (lattice lines) slowly develop into larger, thicker, more radially oriented lines with a ropy appearance (Fig. 9-13). With time the lines become more opaque,

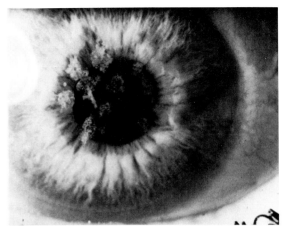

FIGURE 9-12. *Opacities resembling bread crumbs are present in the corneal stroma of an eye with granular dystrophy. Areas between these opacities remain totally clear.*

fewer, and less distinct. The stroma between them is clear early in the course of the disease but becomes progressively hazy.

The discrete white dots between the lattice lines are flakelike and fluffy. The central, grayish white, disc-shaped opacity becomes dense with time and eventually obscures both lattice lines and dots. It is this central or paracentral opacity that eventually causes marked reduction in vision.

Recurrent erosions, accompanied by pain, photophobia, and redness, occur early and often in patients with lattice dystrophy. The erosions remain a serious problem to the patient until the third or fourth decade when their frequency diminishes; at the same time the corneal sensation also diminishes. Vascularization is rare but is sometimes secondary to erosion-induced cellular necrosis of the cornea.

PATHOLOGIC CHANGES

The deposits in lattice dystrophy are amyloid [50, 137, 139], which is an extracellular complex of chondroitin, sulfuric acid, and protein. The staining characteristics and various types of amyloid were described in the section on degeneration. Recent work has shown protein AA and protein AP in the stromal deposits of lattice dystrophy. Fluorescent staining of these deposits does not show any kappa chains, lambda chains, IgG, IgA, or IgM. Thus, the immune type of amyloid may not be present in lattice dystrophy [111].

The origin of the amyloid material is unknown. It may be produced by collagen degeneration (the release by abnormal keratocytes of lysosomal enzymes causing degeneration of stromal collagen or glycosaminoglycans) [49, 52] or by abnormal kerato-

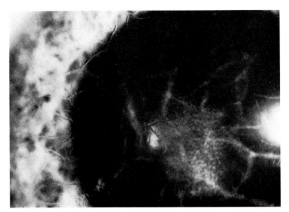

FIGURE 9-13. *Lattice dystrophy. Note lattice pattern of refractile lines and dense diseased central opacification.*

cyte synthesis [93, 121]. The latter theory is the one most favored. It has been assumed that there is no relationship between lattice dystrophy and systemic amyloidosis, but several patients with both systemic amyloidosis and mild lattice dystrophy have been described [110].

The epithelium may vary in thickness; the basement membrane may be fragmented and lack hemidesmosomes [161]; Bowman's layer may be thin, thick, or absent; and the superficial stromal lamellae and Bowman's layer may contain a great many amyloid structures, collagen fibrils, and fibroblasts. Late in the course of the disease, the amyloid deposits extend deeply into the stroma and may be in Descemet's membrane [92].

TREATMENT

The recurrent erosions of lattice dystrophy should be treated by the therapeutic methods listed above in the section on Reis-Bücklers dystrophy. Penetrating keratoplasty has a good prognosis, but recurrences in the graft occur more commonly than in either granular or macular dystrophy [78, 100]. A nonamyloid, pale gray opacification of the donor graft has been described.

MACULAR DYSTROPHY

Macular dystrophy (Groenouw II dystrophy) was first described in 1890 by Groenouw [74]. The hereditary transmission is autosomal recessive. Since asymptomatic carriers are unaware that they carry the gene and may marry each other, the disease can appear in offspring having no family history of it.

CLINICAL FEATURES

Macular dystrophy is a bilateral, symmetric disease that appears in the first decade of life and affects the central portion of the anterior layers of the stroma with diffuse, grayish white spots with indistinct edges. By the third decade, the diffuse stromal opacity with its ground-glass appearance extends posteriorly to the endothelium and laterally to the limbus, and within it are small, irregular, white patches that continue to expand, enlarge, and become more confluent (Fig. 9-14). Late in the course of the disease, Descemet's membrane becomes opacified and there are endothelial guttate changes. The epithelium remains smooth until the late stages of the disease when the subepithelial opacities cause elevations and irregularities of the corneal surface. In the late stages, the vision is also reduced, and there are recurrent erosions and decreased corneal sensation.

PATHOLOGIC CHANGES

Macular dystrophy is a localized form of acid mucopolysaccharide deposition, although a very few cases with an accompanying systemic mucopolysaccharidosis have been reported [112]. Fibrillar material and material resembling basement membrane accumulate beneath the epithelium in Bowman's layer. Both basal cell degeneration and focal areas of epithelial thinning occur over the areas where these materials have accumulated.

The opacities in the stroma correspond to accumulations of glycosaminoglycan (possibly keratan sulfate I) [95] in the keratocytes and among the collagen fibrils. The endothelial cells contain vacuoles and glycosaminoglycan. The deposits stain for acid mucopolysaccharide, i.e., with alcian blue (which stains them blue) or with colloidal iron stain.

This dystrophy appears to be a genetically determined disorder of the corneal keratocytes. It is possible that there are defective catabolic enzymes that affect the metabolism of the glycosaminoglycan, causing it to accumulate excessively in the keratocyte. When the keratocyte eventually dies, the glycosaminoglycan is released into the extracellular spaces of the stroma. The endothelial cells may have the same enzymatic defect.

TREATMENT

Recurrent erosions are infrequent. Visual impairment by the fourth decade of life may necessitate penetrating keratoplasty, but the disease sometimes recurs in the donor graft [102, 130].

CENTRAL CRYSTALLINE DYSTROPHY

Central crystalline dystrophy (Schnyder's crystalline dystrophy) was first described in 1924 and subsequently by Schnyder in 1929 [135]. Although there is an autosomal dominant inheritance pattern [88], a few isolated cases have also been described.

The crystals are not present at birth but appear bilaterally during the first decade of life. The principal feature of this dystrophy is a round, oval, discoid, or anular central opacity composed predominantly of fine, needle-shaped, polychromatic crystals (Fig. 9-15). Five morphologic types of this opacity have been described: (1) a discoid central opacity lacking crystals; (2) a discoid, crystalline lesion with a garlandlike margin; (3) a discoid, central, crystalline opacity with an ill-defined edge; (4) an anular opacity with fine crystals and a clear center; and (5) an anular opacity with crystalline agglomerations and a clear center. There can be any combination of these types in the same family [37], and the clinical appearance of any specific type may vary greatly according to the severity of the opacity. After the second or third decade of life, the disease no longer progresses.

The opacification occurs typically in the anterior portion of the stroma, but deep deposits in pre-Descemet's membrane have also been seen. Aside from the opacity, the stroma is apparently normal except for a dense corneal arcus and limbal girdle. These appear in 80 percent of the cases by the third or fourth decade [13], but the epithelial surface remains smooth, recurrent erosions are rare, and visual impairment is usually minor.

Central crystalline dystrophy is frequently associated with two systemic conditions, hyperlipidemia and genu valgum. Serum cholesterol and triglycerides may be elevated. Members of a single family may have only crystalline dystrophy, only the dystrophy and hyperlipidemia, or only the hyperlipidemia [14, 103]. Genu valgum is also familial [103] but may be an independently inherited trait.

Xanthelasma has been seen in patients with central crystalline dystrophy.

Although the epithelium is usually normal, its basement membrane is sometimes disrupted by focal aggregations of glycogen. In the stroma there are rectangular cholesterol crystals randomly located among the normal collagen fibrils, and there are sometimes small clumps of electron-dense material adjacent to the crystals. There is widespread distribution of neutral fats throughout the stroma and Bowman's layer and noncrystalline cholesterol deposits.

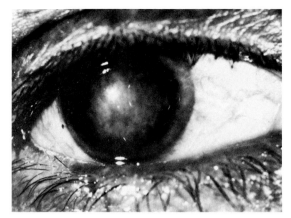

FIGURE 9-14. *Macular dystrophy. The central corneal stroma appears totally opacified. The edges of the opacity are hazy and blend into the unaffected peripheral cornea.*

The blood of one patient with crystalline dystrophy was labeled with ^{14}C-cholesterol 2 weeks before corneal transplantation. When the levels of radioactivity in the blood and in the removed cornea were compared, a higher level of cholesterol was found in the cornea than in the blood. The inference is that the cornea is an active depot for the deposition and turnover of blood cholesterol in patients with central crystalline dystrophy (R. Burns, personal communication, 1979).

Treatment is rarely indicated. Penetrating keratoplasty may occasionally be required, but there may be recurrences in the graft. Hyperlipidemia may be present, and fasting serum cholesterol and triglyceride levels should be determined.

Fleck dystrophy (speckled dystrophy), which was first described by Francois and Neetans [52] in 1956, has an autosomal dominant inheritance pattern [3]. It occurs in the first decade of life and may even be congenital. Although usually bilateral, it may be unilateral, and the lesions may be either symmetric or asymmetric. It is characterized by small, discrete, gray white, dandrufflike specks in the stroma. The opacities can vary in size, shape, and depth, and are often wreathlike with clear centers and distinct margins. All layers of the stroma and the peripheral cornea are affected. This dystrophy is often seen in association with central cloudy corneal dystrophy [53], keratoconus [122], limbal dermoid [122], pseudoxanthoma elasticum [122], lenticular opacities, and reduced corneal sensation [87]. Because of the frequency with which some of these entities oc-

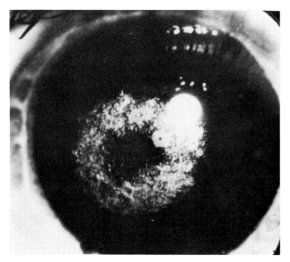

FIGURE 9-15. *A crystalline anular opacity is present in the central corneal stroma of this eye with central crystalline dystrophy.*

cur, one must question whether they are accidental or causally related.

There are no recurrent erosions, vision is not affected, and the dystrophy is not progressive. The stroma and most of the keratocytes in eyes with fleck dystrophy are normal. Isolated keratocytes contain excessive amounts of both glycosaminoglycan and lipids. The pathogenesis of the dystrophy is not known. No treatment is required.

CENTRAL CLOUDY DYSTROPHY
Central cloudy dystrophy was first described by Francois in 1956 [48]. It has an autosomal dominant inheritance pattern [10, 145], but sporadic cases have been reported. The lesions probably occur early in life, but because of the minimal pathologic changes in the cornea, they have been first recognized any time from the first to the ninth decade. The lesions are small, cloudy, gray areas without definite structure or distinct margins. The opacification is located deep in the central third of the corneal stroma. Visual acuity is rarely affected. The histopathology has yet to be defined. No treatment is required.

PRE-DESCEMET'S DYSTROPHY
In 1924, Kraupa first described pre-Descemet's dystrophy as gray flecks in the deep stroma that looked like snowflakes and were associated with ichthyosis. Later, Maeder and Danis [104] described an entity of similar appearance. The inheritance pattern is autosomal dominant.

Pre-Descemet's dystrophy appears between the fourth and seventh decades of life as one or another

of several clinical types [29]. In the usual type, central, anular, or diffuse opacities appear in the pre-Descemet's membrane area. They are usually bilateral and symmetric, and they may vary morphologically in the same cornea, i.e., they may be anular, stellate, comma-shaped, or worm-shaped. Waring and coworkers [158] divides the disease into four clinical types: (1) the pre-Descemet's dystrophy described above; (2) a polymorphic stromal dystrophy that affects the midstroma and deep stroma with punctate and filamentous focal gray opacities; (3) cornea farinata (discussed in the section on degenerations), which is a normal aging change; and (4) the pre-Descemet's dystrophy associated with ichthyosis and occasionally with pseudoxanthoma elasticum.

The opacities may accompany posterior polymorphous dystrophy [71], keratoconus [71], central cloudy corneal dystrophy [30], and epithelial basement membrane dystrophy [71].

Some of the keratocytes anterior to Descemet's membrane contain a PAS-positive material that stains lipids. An accumulation of neutral fats and phospholipids in this area suggest an association with aging [35].

The late onset of pre-Descemet's dystrophy and its infrequent appearance in affected families makes one suspect that, in truth, it is a degenerative change and not a true dystrophy. Treatment is not required.

POLYMORPHIC STROMAL DYSTROPHY
Polymorphic stromal dystrophy is bilateral, symmetric, occurs late in life, and has no definite inheritance pattern. It can be distinguished from pre-Descemet's dystrophy by the midstromal extension of the puncture and filamentous opacities in the polymorphic disorder. There is no visual impairment.

Although there is very little information regarding this disorder, what information there is suggests that it, too, may be a degenerative process associated with aging. The deposits may contain amyloid.

POSTERIOR AMORPHOUS CORNEAL DYSTROPHY
Posterior amorphous corneal dystrophy was originally described in 1977 [20] in several members of three generations of one family. It has an autosomal dominant inheritance pattern and is bilateral and symmetric. It appears in the first decade of life as irregular sheetlike areas of opacification in the deep layers of the corneal stroma. Descemet's membrane is involved, and occasionally there are alterations in

the endothelial mosaic. There is corneal thinning, but the visual acuity remains good, and no treatment is indicated.

CONGENITAL HEREDITARY STROMAL DYSTROPHY
Congenital hereditary stromal dystrophy, an autosomal dominant disease, was described by Witschel and associates [159] in 1978. The dystrophy appears at birth as a bilateral, symmetric, nonprogressive clouding of the central superficial corneal stroma. The epithelium is unaffected, and the stromal opacity is flaky, feathery, and diffuse, fading in intensity as it approaches the periphery. Visual impairment may lead to nystagmus and esotropia.

In congenital hereditary stromal dystrophy, the entire stroma is composed of two types of abnormal collagen lamellae that contain small collagen fibrils and form alternating layers. One type consists of uniformly aligned, compact collagen fibrils that resemble normal corneal fibrils; the other consists of haphazardly arranged, loosely packed collagen fibrils.

The pathogenesis of this disorder is unknown. Theoretically, very early penetrating keratoplasty would offer the infant the possibility of reasonably good vision. (See Chapter 10 for further comments.)

ENDOTHELIAL DYSTROPHIES

POSTERIOR POLYMORPHOUS DYSTROPHY
Posterior polymorphous dystrophy (Schlichting) was first described by Koeppe in 1916 [96] and has an autosomal dominant inheritance pattern with good penetrance. Some reports indicate a recessive inheritance pattern also [22].

CLINICAL FEATURES
The dystrophy can be congenital or develop early in life. The lesions are usually bilateral and can be asymmetric. Clusters of 2 to 20 small, discrete, round lesions that look like vesicles are surrounded by a diffuse gray halo. They can appear anywhere in the posterior cornea and may either remain stationary or progress slowly. There may also be larger geographic lesions in which the vesicles are less obvious and the gray opacification is much denser (Fig. 9-16). Sinuous, broad bands and gray, thickened areas of Descemet's membrane can also be seen. In some cases, when viewed by retroillumination the entire posterior cornea has the *peau d'orange* appearance of beaten metal. In severe cases, there can be stromal and epithelial edema.

The following disorders are found in association

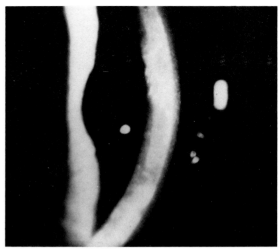

FIGURE 9-16. *Posterior polymorphous dystrophy. Note the nebular, indistinct opacification diffusely present near Descemet's membrane.*

with this dystrophy: broad peripheral iridocorneal adhesions [21], elevated intraocular pressure in 15 percent of the patients [67], anterior chamber cleavage syndrome, calcific band keratopathy, abnormal iris processes, corectopia, deposition of hydroxyapatite in the deep stroma [80], cornea guttata, posterior keratoconus, and epithelialization of the corneal endothelium [9, 80, 132].

PATHOLOGIC CHANGES
The basic characteristic of posterior polymorphous dystrophy is the appearance on the posterior cornea of cells that look like epithelial cells. The association of iris adhesions, anterior cleavage syndrome changes, and glaucoma indicates a mesenchymal dysgenesis. The cause of this dysgenesis remains unknown.

In addition to the multilayered epitheliallike cells on the posterior corneal surface, there can be other corneal changes. Hogan and Bietti [80] examined grossly the corneas of patients with this dystrophy and described four types of lesions: (1) nodules in the deep stroma, (2) ridges that form an anular pattern in the deep stroma, (3) a gray haziness of the deep corneal lamellae, and (4) cornea guttata. Microscopic examination showed multiple guttate changes and calcium in the stromal nodules. Other investigators have failed to find any calcium deposition. In severe cases, stromal and epithelial edema can be seen, and the basement membrane of the epithelium may thicken and fragment.

TREATMENT
The visual acuity remains normal in most cases of posterior polymorphous dystrophy. Mild epithelial

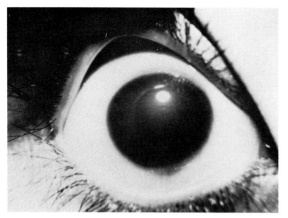

FIGURE 9-17. *A diffusely edematous, normal-sized cornea in a newborn child with congenital hereditary endothelial dystrophy. The stroma has a ground-glass appearance.*

edema may be reduced by the use of hypertonic solutions, hypertonic ointments, and hair dryers. Severe cases may require penetrating keratoplasty; no recurrences have been reported in the donor graft. In cases accompanied by glaucoma, iris adhesions, or both, the prognosis for the maintenance of a clear graft is not as good.

CONGENITAL HEREDITARY ENDOTHELIAL DYSTROPHY

Congenital hereditary endothelial dystrophy was first described by Laurence [101] in 1863. It seems to have an autosomal dominant and recessive inheritance pattern with a variable expressivity ranging from minimal posterior corneal changes to severe corneal edema. The recessive type is present at birth, remains stationary, and is accompanied by nystagmus. The dominant type, which occurs within the first few years of life, is slowly progressive and symptomatic, and is not accompanied by nystagmus.

CLINICAL FEATURES

Epithelial and stromal edema are the hallmark of this dystrophy. The entire cornea is involved, the epithelium shows a diffuse roughness, and the stroma has a ground-glass appearance (Fig. 9-17). Local stromal macular opacities and discrete white dots sometimes appear. Descemet's membrane appears thickened and gray and has a *peau d'orange* texture. The endothelial mosaic may be absent or irregular.

To prevent unnecessary surgery, it is crucial to differentiate this disease from congenital glaucoma without buphthalmos. If inflammation and photo-

phobia are absent bilaterally, and if there is no corneal enlargement or elevated intraocular pressure, a mistaken diagnosis of glaucoma is unlikely.

The differentiation of congenital hereditary endothelial dystrophy from macular dystrophy, congenital hereditary stromal dystrophy, mucopolysaccharidosis, and posterior polymorphous dystrophy is much less crucial since these diseases require the same surgical therapy—keratoplasty (usually within the first 2 months of life). (See Chapter 10 for more details.)

PATHOLOGIC CHANGES

The basic problem in congenital hereditary endothelial dystrophy seems to be degeneration or defective formation of the endothelium in utero [90]. Descemet's membrane is poorly formed, stromal and epithelial edema are widespread, and the structural changes to be expected in the layers with chronic edema are present.

TREATMENT

In mild cases, hypertonic drops and ointments and a hair dryer treatment may be effective. Keratoplasty yields variable results because of the clouding of the grafts and amblyopia present, but it may be the only assistance we can offer.

CORNEA GUTTATA

In cornea guttata, the inheritance pattern is either undeterminable or autosomal dominant. The lesion of this bilaterally symmetric dystrophy makes its first appearance as a golden hue on the posterior surface of the central cornea. Eventually, the entire cornea takes on a bronzed, powdered appearance. Viewed with a slit lamp, the endothelium has a typical beaten-metal appearance with scattered pigment (Fig. 9-18). On specular reflection, the endothelial warts are seen as dark guttate spots, and the endothelium itself is disturbed. The cells are irregular in size and shape.

Secondary cornea guttata may be associated with trauma, inflammation, or degenerative corneal diseases.

The excrescences on Descemet's membrane, which resemble drusen, are both central and peripheral. Some of the endothelial cells are degenerating and are very attenuated over the excrescences; others are as much as 5 times their normal size.

Treatment is usually not required.

FUCHS' DYSTROPHY

When Fuchs first described epithelial-endothelial dystrophy in 1910 he called it an epithelial degeneration [60]. The inheritance pattern has not been clearly defined but is occasionally autosomal dominant [34]. The disease occurs 3 or 4 times more often in women than in men.

CLINICAL FEATURES

Fuchs' dystrophy (or epithelial-endothelial dystrophy) is a bilateral, often asymmetric disease that affects the central corneas of elderly people. There are sometimes several phases [142]. In the first phase, the patient is asymptomatic, but pigment dusting and guttate excrescences appear in the posterior cornea. Descemet's membrane is opaque and thickened. In the second phase, the patients experience glare and hazy vision as the edema worsens. At first, the stromal edema is just anterior to Descemet's membrane and posterior to Bowman's layer, but as it progresses the entire stroma is affected. The epithelial edema appears initially as small, clear cysts in the epithelium, and there is a roughening of its surface (bedewing). Eventually, large epithelial bullae start to appear (Fig. 9-19). These can rupture, causing severe pain. The visual acuity deteriorates during this phase and is at its worst when the patient wakens in the morning. In the third phase, growth of subepithelial connective tissue is accompanied by decreased epithelial edema and less rupturing of the bullae. The patient is therefore more comfortable, but vision may be quite poor in this last phase, and corneal sensation may be reduced or absent. Complications in this phase are elevated intraocular pressure, peripheral neovascularization, and corneal epithelial erosions.

No systemic diseases are associated with this dystrophy.

Essential iris atrophy is a disease of unknown etiology characterized by a slow progressive atrophy of the iris and the development of glaucoma. A concomitant endothelial dystrophy that resembles Fuchs' dystrophy may occur. This entity is significantly more frequent in women, is usually unilateral, and becomes apparent in the third decade of life. The pathogenesis of this entity has not been clearly defined.

PATHOLOGIC CHANGES

In Fuchs' dystrophy, endothelial cells produce new collagenous tissue that has the clinical appearance of a thickened Descemet's membrane. The new collagen tissue may be 4 to 5 μ thick and Descemet's

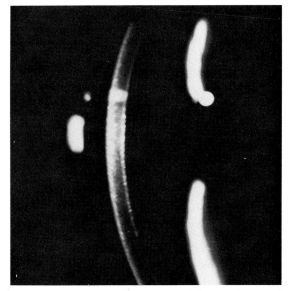

FIGURE 9-18. *Beaten-metal appearance of the posterior corneal surface in cornea guttata.*

membrane 8 to 10 μ thick. The thickening of this new collagen appears as discrete excrescences that correspond to clinically visible cornea guttata in four possible patterns [83]: (1) simple excrescences that protrude into the anterior chamber, (2) multilamellar excrescences, (3) excrescences buried within the multilamellar collagen tissue, or (4) multilamellar collagen tissue without excrescences. The excrescences can push the endothelial nuclei into unusual shapes by thinning the overlying endothelial cells and by producing irregular cell borders. The endothelial cells may increase in size to 1500 μ and lose their characteristic hexagonal shape. Despite the condition of the endothelium, it usually remains intact over the posterior surface of the cornea.

Stromal edema disrupts the normal architecture of the collagen lamellae and widens the interfibrillar spaces.

Bowman's layer usually remains intact except for a few breaks filled with connective tissue [84]. The avascular, subepithelial connective tissue, consisting of active fibroblasts, collagen fibrils, and basement membrane–like material, can reach a thickness of 350 μ; in some areas it extends into the epithelium and forms septae.

The epithelial edema first appears intracellularly in the basal cells. As it increases, the cells may rupture, causing intercellular edema. This edema may eventually form large lakes of fluid that look clinically like bullae. Later, the epithelium may become detached, and subepithelial bullae may appear. The epithelium itself usually remains intact but becomes thickened and irregular as the disease progresses.

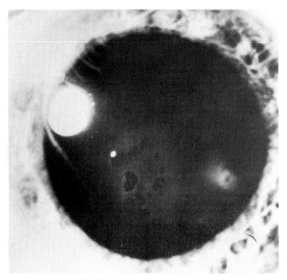

FIGURE 9-19. *Epithelial bullae and diffuse bedewing in an eye with epithelial-endothelial dystrophy.*

TREATMENT

If there is only slight epithelial edema, hypertonic drops during the day and a hypertonic ointment (5% sodium chloride) at night is the usual treatment. Warm, dry air from a hair dryer held at arm's length from the corneal surface may also help. Since the edema is at its worst when the patient wakes in the morning, this is the best time to apply the warm air [38]. This treatment can be repeated two or three times during the day.

The application of a loosely fitted, thin, high-water-content, soft contact lens may be effective in reducing the pain associated with rupturing of the epithelial bullae. If the eye has poor vision from another cause, or if good vision is not a requirement of this patient and keratoplasty is contraindicated, then removal of the epithelium and cauterization of Bowman's layer may be advisable to prevent the formation of epithelial bullae.

Since elevated intraocular pressure (measured by the MacKay-Marg applanometer) may further compromise the poorly functioning endothelial cells, it seems that reducing the pressure with medication might also be advisable. Unfortunately, however, this form of therapy is not usually very helpful.

Penetrating keratoplasty is indicated when the visual acuity is reduced to an unacceptable level. This level will vary with each patient, and such arbitrary criteria as 20/80 vision or worse in both eyes or 20/400 or less in a one-eyed patient, should be applied judiciously. The short-term prognosis is good: In one study, 80 percent of the transplanted corneas remained clear for 2 years [4]. Unfortunately, how-ever, the duration of graft clarity seems to be limited [144], perhaps owing to the poor condition of the remaining endothelial cells. The best results are obtained when the edema is limited to the central cornea.

When keratoplasty is performed on eyes with narrow angles, the lens should be removed to prevent angle closure caused by the formation of peripheral anterior synechiae. Donor grafts can be made slightly larger than their recipient beds.

In patients with epithelial-endothelial dystrophy and advanced lenticular opacities, combined operations can be performed. The visual results are as good as when the keratoplasty is followed later by lens extraction [4], but when the two procedures are combined, there is sometimes cystoid macular edema.

ANTERIOR KERATOCONUS

Anterior keratoconus (conical cornea) was first adequately described in 1854 [115]. It has a dominant or recessive inheritance pattern or no definitive pattern.

CLINICAL FEATURES

Keratoconus may be congenital but usually appears at puberty or shortly thereafter. It is more common in women (2 : 1) and is usually bilateral. Forme fruste can be found in the other eye of a seemingly unilateral case and in family members. The ectasia progresses slowly for 6 or 7 years and then is usually arrested. Sometimes the condition may remain stationary for a time, only to progress again later in life. In the early stages, the cone may be difficult to see, but later it is easily discernible. If the upper lid is raised and the patient looks down so that the free margin of the lower lid bisects the cone horizontally, the lid conforms to the cone, and a distinctive, cone-shaped curve results (Munson's sign). As the condition progresses, the central area develops a slight but progressive translucency. Corneal sensation is sometimes reduced [40].

There may be thinning of the cornea at the apex to one-half its normal thickness. Vertical lines appear in the deeper layers of the stroma, perhaps caused by stretching; the visibility of the corneal nerves, which form a network of gray lines, is increased; and at the base of the cone, there may be an incomplete pigment ring (Fleischer ring), which is an iron deposit [85].

Ruptures occurring in Bowman's layer produce linear scars that may interfere with vision. There may also be ruptures in Descemet's membrane that can lead to acute hydrops or acute ectasia. The rupture may occur suddenly, with an increase in corneal clouding caused by the ensuing edema (Fig. 9-20). Visual acuity becomes markedly decreased and the eye mildly irritable. The condition clears in 8 to 10 weeks, although some scars or chronic edema may remain. Contraction of the scars may lessen some of the optical aberrations by flattening the cone.

In its final state, the cone may be round or oval [120] and is usually confined to the central portion of the cornea, its apex located eccentrically, inferiorly, and nasally. If the ectasia affects the entire cornea, there may be keratoglobus (Fig. 9-21). The height of the cornea is approximately 2.5 mm and the height of the cone up to 2 mm more.

Other ophthalmic disorders such as blue sclera, vernal keratoconjunctivitis, ectopia lentis, congenital cataracts, aniridia, microcornea, and retinitis pigmentosa may be associated with keratoconus [32, 63], as may such systemic diseases as atopy [32], Down's syndrome, Marfan's syndrome, hypothyroidism, osteogenesis imperfecta [64], Apert's syndrome, Ehlers-Danlos syndrome, Noonan's syndrome, Crouzon's disease, Little's disease [64], Laurence-Moon-Biedl syndrome [64], and van der Hoeve's syndrome.

PATHOLOGIC CHANGES
In the area of the cone, there is fragmentation and fibrillation of Bowman's layer and basement membrane. Fibroblastic activity also occurs in the area. Electron microscopic studies suggest that the early changes may be in the basal cells of the epithelium. The basal cells degenerate, releasing proteolytic enzymes that destroy the underlying tissues. Keratocytes near the cone also show degenerative changes, and there is degeneration of endothelium with localized overproduction of Descemet's membrane. The pathogenesis of keratoconus is still unclear.

TREATMENT
Keratoconus patients should wear corrective spectacles as long as they are helpful, but when they no longer correct the vision adequately, hard contact lenses can be tried. (Some ophthalmologists believe that such lenses can aggravate the keratoconus.) Toric lenses are required and must be fitted with great care and great patience [79]. Eventually, however, the lens is likely to touch the center of the cornea and lead to scarring.

Thermokeratoplasty has many drawbacks as a

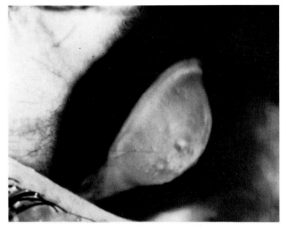

FIGURE 9-20. *Keratoconus. Marked edema is present in the central cone-shaped portion of the cornea.*

treatment of keratoconus. The complications include stromal scarring, recurrence of the steep cone, delayed re-epithelialization, and persistent epithelial defects. The major benefit of this procedure is a possible diminution of corneal sensation, improving the patient's chance of using contact lenses successfully.

Penetrating keratoplasty may be needed if a patient cannot tolerate the contact lens or if the visual correction it provides is inadequate. To ensure success, the graft should be performed before there is too much thinning of the stroma. Although recurrence of keratoconus in the graft has been reported [1], the prognosis of penetrating keratoplasty is extremely good.

If acute hydrops occurs, it should be treated conservatively and the patient assured that it almost always gradually improves. A pressure patch applied during the day to halt the swelling is of limited value. Cycloplegics may be helpful if there is any inflammation.

The edema usually subsides in 8 to 10 weeks, occasionally leaving a residual scar. Topical steroids have been recommended to lessen the scarring, but any agent that might retard healing should be used with extreme caution.

Keratoconus does not cause perforation of the cornea.

POSTERIOR KERATOCONUS
Posterior keratoconus is a nonprogressive entity that seems to have no definitive inheritance pattern but usually occurs in females. There may be a localized, craterlike defect on the posterior corneal surface with the concavity toward the anterior chamber. Descemet's membrane is absent, the stroma is thin, and there is stromal opacification

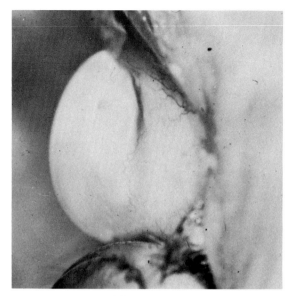

FIGURE 9-21. *Ectasia of the cornea in keratoglobus. The entire cornea is involved.*

over the area. The cause of this dystrophy is obscure but is presumed to be a defect of mesodermal development. (See Chapter 10.)

REFERENCES

1. Abelson, M. B., et al. Recurrent keratoconus after keratoplasty. *Am. J. Ophthalmol.* 90:672, 1980.
2. Akiya, S., and Brown, S. Granular dystrophy of the cornea. *Arch. Ophthalmol.* 84:179, 1970.
3. Aracena, T. Hereditary fleck dystrophy of the cornea. *J. Pediatr. Ophthalmol.* 12:223, 1975.
4. Arentsen, J. J., and Laibson, P. R. Penetrating keratoplasty and cataract extraction. *Arch. Ophthalmol.* 96:75, 1978.
5. Baum, J. L. Cholesterol keratopathy. *Am. J. Ophthalmol.* 67:372, 1969.
6. Berkow, J. W., Fine, B. S., and Zimmerman, L. E. Unusual ocular calcifications in hyperparathyroidism. *Am. J. Ophthalmol.* 66:812, 1969.
7. Biber, M. Über einige seltene Hornhautkränkugen. Thesis, Zurich, 1890.
8. Birndorf, L. A., and Ginsberg, S. P. Hereditary fleck dystrophy associated with decreased corneal sensitivity. *Am. J. Ophthalmol.* 73:670, 1972.
9. Boruchoff, S. A., and Kuwabara, T. Electron microscopy of posterior polymorphous degeneration. *Am. J. Ophthalmol.* 72:879, 1971.
10. Bramsen, T., Ehlers, H., and Baggessen, L. H. Central cloudy corneal dystrophy of Francois. *Acta Ophthalmol.* 54:221, 1976.
11. Broderick, J. D. Pigmentation of the cornea. *Ann. Ophthalmol.* 11:855, 1979.
12. Broderick, J. D., Dark, A. J., and Peace, G. W. Fingerprint dystrophy of the cornea. *Arch. Ophthalmol.* 92:483, 1974.
13. Bron, A. J., and Williams, H. P. Lipaemia of the limbal vessels. *Br. J. Ophthalmol.* 56:343, 1972.
14. Bron, A. J., Williams, H. P., and Carruthers, M. E. Hereditary crystalline stromal dystrophy of Schnyder. *Br. J. Ophthalmol.* 56:383, 1972.
15. Brownstein, S., et al. The elastotic nature of hyaline corneal deposits. *Am. J. Ophthalmol.* 75:799, 1973.
16. Bücklers, M. Über eine weitere familiare Hornhautdystrophie. *Klin. Monatsbl. Augenheilkd.* 114:386, 1949.
17. Burns, R. P. Meesmann's corneal dystrophy. *Trans. Am. Ophthalmol. Soc.* 66:530, 1968.
18. Caldwell, D. R. Postoperative recurrence of Reis-Bücklers' corneal dystrophy. *Am. J. Ophthalmol.* 85:577, 1978.
19. Cameron, M. E. Ocular melanosis with special reference to chlorpromazine. *Br. J. Ophthalmol.* 51:295, 1967.
20. Carpel, E. F., Sigelman, R. J., and Doughman, D. J. Posterior amorphous corneal dystrophy. *Am. J. Ophthalmol.* 83:629, 1977.
21. Cibis, G. W., et al. Iridocorneal adhesions in posterior polymorphous dystrophy. *Trans. Am. Acad. Ophthalmol. Otolaryngol.* 81:770, 1976.
22. Cibis, G. W., et al. The clinical spectrum of posterior polymorphous dystrophy. *Arch. Ophthalmol.* 95:1529, 1977.
23. Ciccarelli, E. C., and Kuwabara, T. Experimental aberrant lipogenesis. *Arch. Ophthalmol.* 62:125, 1959.
24. Cogan, D. G., Albright, F., and Bartter, F. C. Hypercalcemia and band keratoplasty. *Arch. Ophthalmol.* 40:624, 1948.
25. Cogan, D. G., et al. Microcystic dystrophy of the corneal epithelium. *Trans. Am. Ophthalmol. Soc.* 62:213, 1964.
26. Cohen, A. S. Amyloidosis. *N. Engl. J. Med.* 277:522, 1967.
27. Cohen, A. S., et al. Nomenclature, Amyloidosis. In O. Wegelius and A. Pasternack (Eds.), *Amyloidosis.* New York: Academic Press, 1976. P. 9.
28. Cohen, A. S., and Wegelius, O. Classification of amyloid. *Arthritis Rheum.* 23:644, 1980.
29. Collier, M. Les dystrophies prédescemétiques. *Bull. Soc. Ophtalmol. Fr.* 63:53, 1963.
30. Collier, M. Dystrophie nuageuse centrale et

dystrophie pontiforme prédescemétique dans une même famille. *Bull. Soc. Ophtalmol. Fr.* 66:575, 1966.

31. Collyer, R. J. Amyloidosis of the cornea. *Can. J. Ophthalmol.* 3:35, 1968.

32. Copeman, P. W. M. Eczema and keratoconus. *Br. Med. J.* 2:977, 1965.

33. Cowan, T. H. Striate melanokeratosis in negroes. *Am. J. Ophthalmol.* 59:443, 1964.

34. Cross, H. E., Maumenee, A. E., and Cantolino, S. J. Inheritance of Fuchs' endothelial dystrophy. *Arch. Ophthalmol.* 85:268, 1971.

35. Curran, R. E., Kenyon, K. R., and Green, W. R. Pre-Descemet's membrane corneal dystrophy. *Am. J. Ophthalmol.* 77:711, 1974.

36. Dalgleish, R. Ring-like corneal deposits in a case of congenital sperocytosis. *Br. J. Ophthalmol.* 49:40, 1965.

37. Delleman, J. W., and Winkelman, J. E. Degeneratio corneal cristallinea hereditaria. *Ophthalmologica* 155:409, 1968.

38. Devoe, A. G. The management of endothelial dystrophy of the cornea. *Am. J. Ophthalmol.* 61:1084, 1966.

39. Doughman, D. J., et al. Experimental band keratoplasty. *Arch. Ophthalmol.* 81:264, 1969.

40. Duke-Elder, S. S., and Leigh, A. G. Diseases of the Outer Eye. In S. S. Duke-Elder (Ed.), *System of Ophthalmology*, Vol. 8, Pt. 2. St. Louis: Mosby, 1965. Pp. 964–974.

41. Etzine, S., and Kaufman, J. C. E. Band-shaped nodular dystrophy of the cornea. *Am. J. Ophthalmol.* 57:760, 1964.

42. Farkas, T., and Znajda, J. Keloid of the cornea. *Am. J. Ophthalmol.* 66:319, 1968.

43. Ferry, A. P. A new iron line of the superficial cornea. *Arch. Ophthalmol.* 79:142, 1968.

44. Ferry, A. P., and Zimmerman, L. E. Black cornea. *Am. J. Ophthalmol.* 58:205, 1964.

45. Fine, B. S., Townsend, W. M., and Zimmerman, L. E. Primary lipoidal degeneration of the cornea. *Am. J. Ophthalmol.* 78:12, 1974.

46. Fleischer, B. Über Keratoconus und eigenartige figuren Bildung in der Cornea. *Munchen Med. Wochenschr.* 53:625, 1906.

47. Francois, J. Heredo-familial corneal dystrophies. *Trans. Ophthalmol. Soc. U.K.* 86:367, 1966.

48. François, J. Une nouvelle dystrophie hérédofamiliale de la cornée. *J. Genet. Hum.* 5:189, 1956.

49. Francois, J., et al. Dégénérescence marginale pellucide de la cornée. *Ophthalmologica* 155:337, 1968.

50. Francois, J., and Feher, J. Light microscopy and polarization optical study of the lattice dystrophy of the cornea. *Ophthalmologica* 164:1, 1972.

51. Francois, J., Hanssens, M., and Teuchy, H. Ultrastructural changes in lattice dystrophy of the cornea. *Opthalmol. Res.* 7:321, 1975.

52. Francois, J., and Neetans, A. Nouvelle dystrophie hérédofamiliare du parenchyme cornéen. *Bull. Soc. Belg. Optal.* 114:641, 1956.

53. Francois, J., and Neetans, A. L'hérédodystrophie mouchetée du parenchyme cornéen. *Acta Genet. Med. Gemellol.* (Roma) 4:387, 1957.

54. Francois, J., and Victoria-Francoso, V. Histopathogenic study of the lattice dystrophy of the cornea. *Ophthalmol. Res.* 7:420, 1975.

55. Fraunfelder, F. T., and Hanna, C. Speroidal degeneration of the cornea and conjunctiva. *Am. J. Ophthalmol.* 74:821, 1972.

56. Fraunfelder, F. T., and Hanna, C. Speroidal degeneration of the cornea and conjunctiva. *Am. J. Ophthalmol.* 76:41, 1973.

57. Fredrickson, D. S. Hereditary Systemic Diseases of Metabolism That Affect the Eye. In F. A. Mausolf (Ed.), *The Eye and Systemic Disease*. St. Louis: Mosby, 1975.

58. Freedman, A. Climatic droplet keratopathy. *Arch. Ophthalmol.* 89:193, 1973.

59. Friedlaender, M. H., et al. Bilateral central lipid infiltrates of the cornea. *Am. J. Ophthalmol.* 84:781, 1977.

60. Fuchs, E. Dystrophia epithelialis corneal. *Albrecht Von Graefes Arch. Klin. Exp. Ophthalmol.* 76:478, 1910.

61. Garner, A. L. Histochemistry of corneal granular dystrophy. *Br. J. Ophthalmol.* 53:799, 1969.

62. Gass, J. D. The iron lines of the superficial cornea. *Arch. Ophthalmol.* 71:348, 1964.

63. Gasset, A. R. Fixed dilated pupil following penetrating keratoplasty in keratoconus. *Ann. Ophthalmol.* 9:623, 1977.

64. Geeraets, W. *Ocular Syndromes.* Philadelphia: Lea & Febiger, 1976.

65. Goldman, K. N., and Kaufman, H. E. Atypical pterygium. *Arch. Ophthalmol.* 96:1027, 1978.

66. Grant, W. M. *Toxicology of the Eye.* Springfield, Ill.: Thomas, 1962. P. 150.

67. Grayson, M. The nature of hereditary deep polymorphous dystrophy of the cornea. *Trans. Am. Ophthalmol. Soc.* 72:516, 1974.

68. Grayson, M. *Diseases of the Cornea.* St. Louis: Mosby, 1979. P. 187.

69. Grayson, M., and Keates, R. H. *Manual of Diseases of the Cornea.* Boston: Little, Brown, 1969. P. 60.

70. Grayson, M., and Wilbrandt, H. Dystrophy

of the anterior limiting membrane of the cornea. *Am. J. Ophthalmol.* 61:345, 1966.

71. Grayson, M., and Wilbrandt, H. Predescemet's dystrophy. *Am. J. Ophthalmol.* 64:276, 1967.
72. Griffith, D. G., and Fine, B. S. Light and electron microscopic observations in a superficial corneal dystrophy. *Am. J. Ophthalmol.* 63:1659, 1967.
73. Groenouw, A. Knötchenförmige Hornhauttrübungen. *Albrecht Von Graefes Arch. Klin. Exp. Ophthalmol.* 46:85, 1898.
74. Groenouw, A. Knötchenförmige nethauttrübungen. *Arch. Augenheilkd.* 21:281, 1890.
75. Haddad, R., Font, R. L., and Fine, B. S. Unusual superficial variant of granular dystrophy of the cornea. *Am. J. Ophthalmol.* 83:213, 1977.
76. Hall, P. Reis-Bücklers' dystrophy. *Arch. Ophthalmol.* 91:170, 1974.
77. Hammerstein, W. Genetische Beratung, bei hereditaeren Hornhautkrankungen. *Ophthalmologica* 172:90, 1976.
78. Herman, S. F., and Hughes, W. F. Recurrence of hereditary corneal dystrophy following keratoplasty. *Am. J. Ophthalmol.* 75:689, 1973.
79. Hoefle, F. B., Kooerman, J. J., and Buxton, J. The use of contact lenses in patients with keratoconus. *Contact Lens Med. Bull.* Sept. 4, 1972, p. 52.
80. Hogan, M. J., and Bietti, G. Hereditary deep dystrophy of the cornea. *Am. J. Ophthalmol.* 68:777, 1969.
81. Hogan, M. J., and Wood, I. Reis-Bücklers corneal dystrophy. *Trans. Ophthalmol. Soc. U.K.* 91:41, 1971.
82. Hogan, M., and Wood, I. Corneal dystrophies. Pending publication.
83. Hogan, M. J., Wood, I., and Fine, M. Fuchs' endothelial dystrophy of the cornea. *Am. J. Ophthalmol.* 78:363, 1974.
84. Iwamoto, T., and Devoe, A. G. Electron microscopic studies on Fuchs' combined dystrophy. *Invest. Ophthalmol.* 10:9, 1971.
85. Iwamoto, T., and Devoe, A. G. Electron microscopical study of the Fleischer ring. *Arch. Ophthalmol.* 94:1579, 1976.
86. Iwamoto, T., Devoe, A. G., and Farris, R. L. Electron microscopy in cases of marginal degeneration of the cornea. *Invest. Ophthalmol.* 11:241, 1972.
87. Kanai, A., Kaufman, H. E., and Polack, F. M. Electron microscopic study of Reis-Bücklers' dystrophy. *Ann. Ophthalmol.* 5:953, 1973.
88. Karseras, A. G., and Price, D. C. Central crystalline corneal dystrophy. *Br. J. Ophthalmol.* 54:659, 662, 1970.
89. Katz, D. Salzmann's nodular corneal dystrophy. *Acta Ophthalmol.* 31:377, 1953.

90. Kenyon, K. R., and Maumenee, A. E. The histological and ultrastructural pathology of congenital hereditary corneal dystrophy. *Invest. Ophthalmol.* 7:475, 1968.
91. Kietzman, B. Mooren's ulcer in Nigeria. *Am. J. Ophthalmol.* 65:679, 1968.
92. Klintworth, G. K. Lattice corneal dystrophy. *Am. J. Pathol.* 50:371, 1967.
93. Klintworth, G. K. Current concepts on the ultrastructural pathogenesis of macular and lattice corneal dystrophies. *Birth Defects* 7:27, 1971.
94. Klintworth, G. K. Chronic actinic keratopathy. *Am. J. Pathol.* 67:327, 1972.
95. Klintworth, G. K., and Smith, C. F. Macular corneal dystrophy. *Am. J. Pathol.* 89:167, 1977.
96. Koeppe, L. Angeborene Dellenbildung der Hornhauthinterfläche im klin Beobachtungen mit der nerst Spaltlampe in dem Hornhautmikroskop. *Albrecht von Graefes Arch. Klin. Exp. Ophthalmol.* 91:375, 1916.
97. Kuwabara, Y., Akiya, S., and Obazawa, H. Electron microscopic study of granular dystrophy, macular dystrophy, and gelatinous droplike dystrophy of the cornea. *Folia Ophthalmol. Jpn.* 18:463, 1967.
98. Kuwabara, T., and Ciccarelli, E. C. Meesmann's corneal dystrophy. *Arch. Ophthalmol.* 71:676, 1964.
99. Laibson, P. R., and Krachmer, J. H. Familial occurrence of dot, map, fingerprint dystrophy of the cornea. *Invest. Ophthalmol.* 14:397, 1975.
100. Lanier, J. D., Fine, M., and Togni, B. Lattice corneal dystrophy. *Arch. Ophthalmol.* 94:921, 1976.
101. Laurence, G. Z. Corneitis interstitialis in utero. *Klin. Monatsbl. Augenheilkd.* 1:351, 1863.
102. Lorenzetti, D. W. C., and Kaufman, H. E. Macular and lattice dystrophies and their recurrences after keratoplasty. *Trans. Am. Acad. Ophthalmol. Otolaryngol.* 71:112, 1967.
103. Luxenberg, M. Hereditary crystalline dystrophy of the cornea. *Am. J. Ophthalmol.* 63:507, 1967.
104. Maeder, G., and Danis, P. Sur une nouvelle forme dystrophie cornéenne. *Ophthalmologica* 114:246, 1947.
105. Malbran, E. S. Corneal dystrophies: A clinical, pathological, and surgical approach. *Am. J. Ophthalmol.* 74:771, 1972.
106. Matsuo, N., Fujiwara, H., and Ofuchi, Y. Electron and light microscopic observations of a case of Groenouw's granular corneal dystrophy and gelatinous droplike dystrophy of the cornea. *Folia Ophthalmol. Jpn.* 18:436, 1967.
107. McPherson, S., et al. Corneal amyloidosis. *Am. J. Ophthalmol.* 62:1025, 1966.

108. Meesmann, A. Über eine bisher nicht beschriebene, dominant verebte Dystrophia epithelialis corneae. *Ber. Zusammenkunft. Dtsch. Ophthalmol. Ges.* 52:154, 1938.

109. Meesmann, A., and Wilke, F. Klenische und anatomische Untersuchungen uber eine bisher unbekannte, dominant verebte Epitheldystrophie der Hornhaut. *Klin. Monatsbl. Augenheilkd.* 103:361, 1939.

110. Meretojo, J. Familial systemic paramyloidosis with lattice dystrophy of the cornea. *Ann. Clin. Res.* 1:314, 1969.

111. Mondino, B. J., et al. Protein AA and lattice corneal dystrophy. *Am. J. Ophthalmol.* 89:377, 1980.

112. Morgan, G. Macular dystrophy of the cornea. *Br. J. Ophthalmol.* 50:57, 1966.

113. Nagataki, S., Tanishima, T., and Sakimoto, T. A case of primary gelatinous drop–like corneal dystrophy. *Jpn. J. Ophthalmol.* 16:107, 1972.

114. Norn, M. S. Hudson-Stähli line of the cornea. *Acta Ophthalmol.* 46:106, 1968.

115. Nottingham, G. *Practical Observations on Conical Cornea.* London: 1854.

116. Obenberger, J., Ocumpaugh, D. E., and Cubberly, M. G. Experimental corneal calcification in animals treated with dihydrotachysterol. *Invest. Ophthalmol.* 8:467, 1969.

117. O'Connor, G. R. Calcific band keratopathy. *Trans. Am. Ophthalmol. Soc.* 70:58, 1972.

118. O'Grady, R. B., and Kirk, H. Q. Corneal keloids. *Am. J. Ophthalmol.* 73:206, 1972.

119. Olson, R. J., and Kaufman, H. E. Recurrence of Reis-Bücklers' corneal dystrophy in a graft. *Am. J. Ophthalmol.* 85:349, 1978.

120. Perry, H. D., Buxton, J. N., and Fine, B. S. Round and oval cones in keratoconus. *Trans. Am. Acad. Ophthalmol.* 87:905, 1980.

121. Pouliquen, Y., Dhermy, P., and Tallebourg, O. Étude en microscope électronique d'une dystrophie grillagée de Haab-Dimmer. *Arch. Ophtalmol.* (Paris) 33:485, 1973.

122. Purcell, J. J., Krachmer, J. H., and Weingeist, T. A. Fleck corneal dystrophy. *Arch. Ophthalmol.* 95:440, 1977.

123. Raab, M. F., Blodi, F., and Boniuk, M. Unilateral lattice dystrophy of the cornea. *Trans. Am. Acad. Ophthalmol. Otolaryngol.* 78:440, 1974.

124. Ramsey, M. S., and Fine, B. S. Localized corneal amyloidoses. *Am. J. Ophthalmol.* 75:560, 1972.

125. Ramsey, R. M. Familial corneal dystrophy, lattice type. *Trans. Am. Ophthalmol. Soc.* 60:701, 1957.

126. Reinecke, R. D., and Kuwabara, T. Corneal deposits secondary to topical epinephrine. *Arch. Ophthalmol.* 70:170, 1963.

127. Reis, W. Familiare, fleckige Hornhautentartung. *Dtsch. Med. Wochenschr.* 43:575, 1917.

128. Reshmi, C. S., and English, F. P. Unilateral lattice dystrophy of the cornea. *Med. J. Aust.* 1:966, 1971.

129. Rice, N. S. C., et al. Reis-Bücklers' dystrophy. *Am. J. Ophthalmol.* 72:549, 1971.

130. Robin, A. L., et al. Recurrence of macular corneal dystrophy after lamellar keratoplasty. *Am. J. Ophthalmol.* 84:457, 1977.

131. Rodrigues, M. M., et al. Epithelialization of the corneal endothelium in posterior polymorphous dystrophy. *Invest. Ophthalmol. Vis. Sci.* 19:832, 1980.

132. Rogers, P. R. Screening for amyloid with thioflavine T fluorescent material. *Am. J. Clin. Pathol.* 44:59, 1965.

133. Salzmann, M. Über eine abart der knötchenförmigen Hornhautdystrophie. *Z. Augenheilkd.* 57:92, 1925.

134. Schaeppi, V. La dystrophi marginale inférieure pellucide de la cornée. *Probl. Actuels Ophtalmol.* 1:672, 1975.

135. Schnyder, W. F. Scheibenformige Kristalleinlagerungen in der Hornhautmitte als Erbleiden. *Klin. Monatsbl. Augenheilkd.* 103:494, 1939.

136. Schutz, S. Hereditary corneal dystrophy. *Arch. Ophthalmol.* 29:523, 1943.

137. Seitelberger, F., and Nemetz, U. R. Patologia de la amiloidosis. *Arch. Fund Roux Ocefa* 2:135, 1968.

138. Selye, H. *Calciphylaxis.* Chicago: University of Chicago Press, 1962.

139. Smith, M. E., and Zimmerman, L. E. Amyloid in corneal dystrophies. *Arch. Ophthalmol.* 79:407, 1968.

140. Stafford, W., and Fine, B. S. Amyloidosis of the cornea. *Arch. Ophthalmol.* 75:53, 1966.

141. Stocker, F. W. Eine pigmentierte Hornhautline bei Pterygium. *Schweiz. Med. Wochenschr.* 20:19, 1939.

142. Stocker, F. W. *The Endothelium of the Cornea and Its Clinical Implications* (2nd ed.). Springfield, Ill.: Thomas, 1971. Pp. 79–109.

143. Stocker, F. W., and Holt, L. B. Rare form of hereditary epithelial dystrophy. *Arch. Ophthalmol.* 53:536, 1955.

144. Stocker, F. W., and Irish, A. Fate of successful corneal graft in Fuchs' endothelial dystrophy. *Am. J. Ophthalmol.* 68:820, 1969.

145. Strachan, I. M. Cloudy central corneal dystrophy of Francois. *Br. J. Ophthalmol.* 53:192, 1969.

146. Stuart, J. C., et al. Recurrent corneal granular dystrophy. *Am. J. Ophthalmol.* 79:18, 1975.

147. Sugar, H. S., and Kobernick, S. The white limbal girdle of Vogt. *Am. J. Ophthalmol.* 50:101, 1960.

148. Süveges, M. D., Levai, G., and Alberth, B. Pathology of Terrien's disease. *Am. J. Ophthalmol.* 74:1191, 1972.

149. Tabbara, K. F. Mooren's Ulcer. In G. R. O'Connor (Ed.), *Immunologic Diseases of the Mucous Membranes.* New York: Masson, 1980. Pp. 119–126.

150. Thiel, H. J., and Behnke, H. Eine bisher unbekannte subepitheliale hereditäre Hornhautdystrophie. *Klin. Monatsbl. Augenheilkd.* 150: 862, 1967.

151. Tripathi, R. C., and Bron, A. J. Secondary anterior crocodile shagreen of Vogt. *Br. J. Ophthalmol.* 59:59, 1975.

152. Tripathi, R. C., and Garner, A. Corneal granular dystrophy. *Br. J. Ophthalmol.* 54:361, 1970.

153. Vannas, A., Hogan, M. J., and Wood, I. Salzmann's nodular degeneration of the cornea. *Am. J. Ophthalmol.* 79:211, 1975.

154. Wagener, H. P. The ocular manifestations of hypercalcemia. *Am. J. Med. Sci.* 231:218, 1956.

155. Walsh, F. B., and Howard, J. E. Conjunctival and corneal lesions in hypercalcemia. *J. Clin. Endocrinol.* 7:644, 1947.

156. Walton, K. W. Studies on the pathogenesis of corneal arcus formation. *J. Pathol.* 111:263, 1973.

157. Walton, K. W. Studies on the pathogenesis of corneal arcus formation. *J. Pathol.* 114:217, 1974.

158. Waring, G. O., Rodriques, M. M., and Laibson, P. R. Corneal dystrophies: I. Dystrophies of the epithelium, Bowman's layer and stroma. *Surv. Ophthalmol.* 23:71, 1978.

159. Witschel, H., et al. Congenital hereditary stromal dystrophy of the cornea. *Arch. Ophthalmol.* 96:1043, 1978.

160. Wood, T. O., Fleming, J. C., and Dotson, R. S. Treatment of Reis-Bücklers' corneal dystrophy by removal of subepithelial fibrous tissue. *Am. J. Ophthalmol.* 85:360, 1978.

161. Yanoff, M., et al. Lattice corneal dystrophy. *Arch. Ophthalmol.* 95:651, 1977.

10. CONGENITAL ANOMALIES

Fred M. Wilson II

This chapter deals mainly with disorders that are the result of abnormal development of the cornea or associated tissues during embryonic or fetal life. Congenital anomalies of the cornea generally manifest themselves as alterations in the gross morphology of the tissue and are evident at the time of birth. These features are in contradistinction to those of corneal dystrophies, which are more likely to affect the biochemical function of the cornea and which seldom become apparent until several years after birth. Similarly, most systemic diseases that affect the cornea do not do so clinically until sometime after birth and so will be mentioned only briefly here. Corneal degenerations are changes that occur in previously normal tissue, as the result of long-standing disease, and are not discussed in this chapter. Primary congenital glaucoma is a major cause of a cloudy cornea at birth; but it, too, will be given only passing consideration because it involves mainly the anterior chamber angle and affects the cornea only secondarily.

The clinician can usually differentiate these various kinds of corneal problems, but some blurring of distinctions is inevitable. To understand well the causes of the cloudy cornea in infancy, the reader should study also the material in those chapters pertaining to corneal dystrophies and degenerations (Chapter 9) and deposits secondary to systemic disease (Chapter 11).

ABSENCE OF THE CORNEA
Agenesis of the cornea is unknown as an isolated abnormality, but the cornea may fail to develop, or may seem not to have developed, in the disorders discussed below.

AGENESIS OF THE ANTERIOR SEGMENT
In this very rare abnormality, the optic vesicle forms and invaginates to form the optic cup, but the anterior segment fails to differentiate [11]. The result is a scleral shell lined with choroid, retinal pigment epithelium, and retina but lacking cornea, anterior chamber, iris, ciliary body, and lens. This aberration

may be considered to be a form of microphthalmos because it occurs after the formation of the optic vesicle and because the affected eye is usually small.

CRYPTOPHTHALMOS

True cryptophthalmos (ablepharon) is the result of a failure of formation of the eyelid folds (Fig. 10-1) [6, 11, 40]. The cornea undergoes metaplasia to skin and so appears to be absent. Because of the lack of appearance of the lid folds, the brows and lashes are absent. This feature allows for easy differentiation of cryptophthalmos from pseudocryptophthalmos (total ankyloblepharon, discussed below), in which brows and lashes are present. In true cryptophthalmos, the lacrimal gland and puncta are likely to be missing as well, and the anterior segment of the globe is usually disorganized [9].

Cryptophthalmos is usually transmitted as an autosomal recessive trait and may be unilateral or bilateral. When it is unilateral, the other eye may have symblepharons or coloboma of the eyelid. Males and females are affected equally.

Associated systemic abnormalities are common: syndactyly, genitourinary anomalies, and craniofacial anomalies (most common); spina bifida, deformed ears or teeth, cleft palate or lip, laryngeal or anal atresia, ventral hernias, cardiac anomalies, displacement of the nipples or umbilicus, basal encephaloceles, and mental retardation (less common). Cryptophthalmos with extraocular abnormalities is referred to as the *cryptophthalmos syndrome* [6, 9, 20, 30]. Renal agenesis has been reported in siblings of patients with this syndrome [9].

Cryptophthalmos is rare, only about 50 cases having been reported. Affected patients have a layer of skin extending from the forehead to the malar region. An *incomplete form* is recognized, in which only the nasal aspect of the lid fold is involved. Still another presentation is the *abortive form*, in which the upper eyelid is replaced by a fold of skin that is adherent to the upper third of the cornea; the lower eyelid is normal [9]. Even in the complete form, the underlying eye moves and may even show some reaction to bright light in the form of contractions of the periocular skin; but the skin *is* the surface of the eye, so any attempt to incise the overlying integument will only result in entry into a malformed eye. When brows and lashes are absent (indicating the presence of true cryptophthalmos), cutaneous incision will be useless except that it may provide some slight cosmetic benefit.

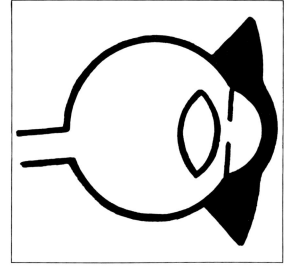

FIGURE 10-1. *True cryptophthalmos. Eyelid folds fail to form, and exposed cornea and conjunctiva undergo metaplasia to skin* (black shaded area). *The skin is continuous above and below with that of the forehead and malar regions, respectively. Note that the cornea is not covered by skin but is actually transformed into skin.*

TOTAL ANKYLOBLEPHARON

In some cases, the eye really is covered by skin (rather than by metaplastic cornea and conjunctiva), and an underlying cornea is present [11, 47*]. If so, the lid folds have formed but have undergone complete fusion. Brows and lashes are present. Incision may be of some value, although the newly formed lids tend to close again.

ABNORMALITIES OF SIZE

MEGALOCORNEA

The term *megalocornea* refers to an enlarged cornea (not secondary to glaucoma) that measures 13 mm or more in horizontal diameter (Fig. 10-2) [6, 11, 40]. The ciliary ring and lens are often enlarged as well (*anterior megalophthalmos*) [59]. The cornea is clear and histologically normal. It should be remembered that the final, adult size of the cornea cannot be determined until about 1 year of age.

Some patients with megalocornea are myopic because of increased corneal curvature, although the curvature may also be normal. With-the-rule astigmatism is often present when the corneal curvature is increased.

The condition is usually harmless except for three

---

*The case reported in reference 47, in which cutaneous incision was apparently of value, was reported as cryptophthalmos but might better be referred to as ankyloblepharon; lashes and brows were present, as were underlying corneas.

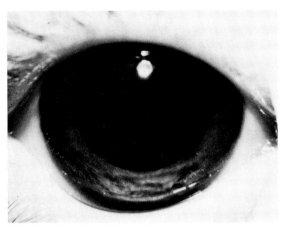

FIGURE 10-2. *Megalocornea. The cornea measures 14 mm in horizontal diameter but is otherwise normal. Glaucoma is not present. The dilated pupil is the result of drops used for examination.*

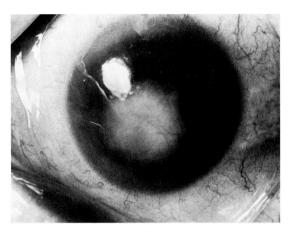

FIGURE 10-3. *Microcornea, in this case associated with the mesodermal form of Peters' anomaly, as evidenced by the corneal leukoma to which strands of iris are attached. The cornea measures 10 mm in horizontal diameter. The clearly defined limbus indicates the presence of true microcornea. The limbus would be indistinct if the cornea were only apparently small from mild sclerocornea.*

TABLE 10-1. *Abnormalities Associated with Megalocornea*

Ocular
  Myopia
  Astigmatism
  Arcus juvenilis
  Krukenberg's spindle
  Mosaic corneal dystrophy
  Hypoplasia of iris stroma
  Miosis (hypoplasia of iris dilator)
  Prominent iris processes
  Pigmentation of trabecular meshwork
  Open-angle glaucoma
  Congenital glaucoma (rare)
  Cataract (usually posterior subcapsular)
  Ectopia lentis
Systemic
  Marfan's syndrome
  Craniosynostosis

complications that may appear later in life: ectopia lentis; glaucoma secondary to associated anomalies of the angle; and cataract, which is usually posterior subcapsular but may be nuclear or peripheral. Other associated abnormalities, most of which are uncommon, are listed in Table 10-1 [6, 11, 40, 51, 70].

Megalocornea is almost always X-linked recessive, and 90 percent of cases are in males. It is occasionally dominant and still less often recessive. Megalocornea is usually bilateral, but it is possible, although rare, for an individual to have megalocornea in one eye and congenital glaucoma in the other [11]. Because congenital glaucoma can also cause enlargement of the cornea, it is always man-

datory to be sure that glaucoma is not present before making a diagnosis of megalocornea. Megalocornea and congenital glaucoma can also occur in different members of the same family [39, 51].

Megalocornea is probably the result of a failure of the anterior tips of the optic cup to grow sufficiently close to one another, the remaining space being taken up by the cornea. Other possible explanations are that it represents an exaggeration of the normal tendency for the cornea to be large, relative to the rest of the eye, from embryonic life to the age of 7 years; an atavistic regression to the tendency for nonhuman mammals to have larger corneas relative to their globes; or spontaneously arrested congenital glaucoma.

MICROCORNEA
A microcornea is one that has a horizontal diameter of less than 11 mm (Fig. 10-3) [11, 40]. It can occur as an isolated anomaly, and it is in this context that it is discussed here. If the whole anterior segment is small, the term *anterior microphthalmos* applies. *Nanophthalmos* indicates an eye that is small but otherwise normal, and *microphthalmos* refers to a small eye that is also malformed in other ways.

Patients with microcornea are likely to be hyperopic because their corneas are relatively flat, but any kind of refractive error is possible owing to variations in length of the globe. Open-angle glaucoma

TABLE 10-2. *Abnormalities Associated with Microcornea*

Ocular
  Hyperopia (other refractive errors possible)
  Cornea plana
  Corneal leukoma
  Mesodermal remnants in angle
  Uveal coloboma
  Corectopia
  Persistent pupillary membrane
  Congenital cataract
  Microphakia
  Open-angle glaucoma
  Angle-closure glaucoma
  Congenital glaucoma
  Microblepharon
  Small orbit
Systemic
  Weill-Marchesani syndrome or similar habitus
  Ehlers-Danlos syndrome
  Meyer-Schwickerath and Weyers syndrome
  Rieger's syndrome
  Partial deletion of long arm of chromosome 18

develops later in life in 20 percent of patients, and some predisposition to narrow-angle glaucoma also exists because of the shallow anterior chamber. Congenital glaucoma coexists occasionally. An eye with microcornea (or microphthalmos) is sometimes misinterpreted as being normal in comparison to its fellow (actually normal) eye, which is thought erroneously to have corneal enlargement from congenital glaucoma. Table 10-2 lists other problems that are sometimes associated with microcornea [11, 18].

Microcornea is thought to be caused by an overgrowth of the anterior tips of the optic cup, leaving less than normal space for the cornea. It may be transmitted as a dominant or recessive trait, the former being more common.

ABNORMALITIES OF SHAPE

HORIZONTALLY OVAL CORNEA

Actually, it is normal for the cornea to have a horizontally oval shape when it is viewed from the front, although it is round when seen from the back. The oval appearance is caused by greater scleral encroachment above and below than in the horizontal meridian. An exaggeration of the normal oval shape usually indicates the presence of some degree of sclerocornea (discussed below) [11, 40].

VERTICALLY OVAL CORNEA

A vertically oval cornea sometimes occurs in association with iris coloboma, Turner's syndrome (ovarian dysgenesis, XO karyotype), or intrauterine keratitis (usually from congenital syphilis) [11, 18, 40, 55, 65]. It is interesting that the luetic interstitial keratitis can appear before or after the observation of the abnormal shape of the cornea.

ABNORMALITIES OF CURVATURE

CORNEA PLANA

Cornea plana (flat cornea) is seldom an isolated entity. It is more often seen in association with microcornea or sclerocornea [11, 14, 40, 60]. The sclerocornea is likely to be more prominent above and below, so that the cornea appears to be horizontally oval as well. The limbus in cornea plana is usually indistinct, whereas it is typically well defined in simple microcornea.

Cornea plana often produces hyperopia, but the refractive error is unpredictable because the length of the globe varies. The cornea itself must have a radius of curvature of less than 43 diopters if it is to be designated as a cornea plana, but measurements of 30 to 35 diopters are more common. A keratometry reading of as low as 23 diopters has been reported [14]. A corneal curvature that is the same as that of the sclera is almost pathognomonic for cornea plana. The cornea is even flatter than the sclera in some cases. The anterior chamber is shallow, and angle-closure glaucoma is not uncommon. The incidence of open-angle glaucoma is also increased. Other possible abnormalities are listed in Table 10-3 [11, 14, 40, 60].

Cornea plana is thought to be the result of a developmental arrest in the fourth month of fetal life, when the corneal curvature normally increases relative to that of the sclera. The heredity may be dominant or recessive. The recessive form is more severe and can be complicated by the presence of central corneal opacities. Cornea plana is especially likely to occur in patients of Finnish extraction [14].

ANTERIOR KERATOCONUS AND KERATOGLOBUS

Anterior keratoconus usually develops during the first two decades of life and is only rarely evident at birth. Keratoglobus (globular cornea) is not infrequently congenital; but it, too, can appear after birth. Both of these corneal ectasias are usually classified as corneal dystrophies (see Chapter 9) and so will not be discussed here, although some of their features are summarized in Table 10-4.

GENERALIZED POSTERIOR KERATOCONUS

In this condition, the entire posterior surface of the cornea has an increased curvature, i.e., it has a shorter radius of curvature and so is more strongly curved, while the contour of the anterior surface remains normal [11, 23, 31, 49]. The differential features of anterior keratoconus, keratoglobus, generalized posterior keratoconus, and circumscribed posterior keratoconus (discussed later) are given in Table 10-4 [23, 31, 40, 49].

Generalized posterior keratoconus is the least common of the four disorders. It probably represents a developmental arrest, as the posterior surface of the cornea is normally more curved during fetal life [49]. Generalized posterior keratoconus is usually unilateral. All examples have been in women, but there is no evidence of hereditary transmission. Central corneal thinning is present, but the condition is nonprogressive, and the vision is normal unless there is associated clouding of the cornea, which seldom occurs.

KERATECTASIA

Keratectasia is characterized by the presence of a bulging, opaque cornea that protrudes through the palpebral aperture [11, 37, 40]. Most cases are unilateral and are probably the result of intrauterine keratitis; corneal perforation in utero causes the cornea to undergo metaplasia to tissue resembling skin (dermoid transformation). The metaplasia involves only the cornea and does not extend over the entire eye to the area of the lids as occurs in cryptophthalmos.

Some examples of keratectasia may be caused by a failure of mesoderm to migrate into the developing cornea, resulting in subsequent corneal thinning, bulging, and metaplasia, with or without preceding perforation.

CONGENITAL ANTERIOR STAPHYLOMA
Congenital anterior staphyloma differs from keratectasia only in that the staphyloma is, by definition, lined by uveal tissue [11, 37, 40].

CORNEAL ASTIGMATISM
Corneal astigmatism is usually just a variation, i.e., a common and minor deviation from normality, although Duke-Elder considered radii of curvature of less than 6.75 mm or greater than 9.25 mm to be deformities [11, 40].

Corneal astigmatism is nearly always dominant. Autosomal or X-linked recessive transmission is rare but may occur, especially with high degrees of astigmatism. The approximate amounts, and even the axes, of astigmatism are often remarkably similar in related individuals [40, 60].

ABNORMALITIES OF STRUCTURE

ANTERIOR SEGMENT MESODERMAL DYSGENESIS
Mesodermal dysgenesis (anterior chamber cleavage syndrome) should be thought of as a spectrum in which any of several abnormalities may exist alone or in various combinations [1, 11, 23, 37, 46, 51, 62]. Some of the more frequently occurring combinations are given eponymic designations such as Rieger's syndrome, Peters' anomaly, and others. All of these problems are the result of abnormal differentiation or persistence of anterior segment mesoderm, sometimes with associated ectodermal abnormalities.

In trying to understand this subject, it is helpful to review briefly some of the embryology of the anterior segment of the eye [12, 23, 40]. After separation of the lens vesicle, the surface ectoderm forms a layer that becomes corneal epithelium. Three waves of mesoderm then move in behind the surface ectoderm: The first wave gives rise to corneal endothelium, the second forms corneal stroma, and the third becomes iris stroma. During early development, there is no anterior chamber, the entire area being filled with mesoderm. This gradually recedes, and its remnant in the form of the pupillary membrane begins to undergo atrophy at about the sev-

TABLE 10-3. *Abnormalities Associated with Cornea Plana*

Ocular
  Hyperopia (other refractive errors possible)
  Blue sclera
  Sclerocornea
  Microcornea
  Arcus juvenilis
  Nonspecific corneal opacities
  Mesodermal dysgenesis
  Absence of normal iris markings and collarette
  Uveal and retinal coloboma
  Aniridia
  Congenital cataract
  Ectopia lentis
  Retinal and macular aplasia
  Angle-closure glaucoma
  Open-angle glaucoma
  Pseudoptosis (Streiff's sign)
Systemic
  Osteogenesis imperfecta
  Hurler's syndrome (mucopolysaccharidosis I-H)
  Maroteaux-Lamy syndrome (mucopolysaccharidosis VI)*
  Trisomy 13

*Personal observation.

enth month. The angle recess does not become fully opened until sometime during the first year after birth.

Two hypotheses have been proposed to explain the disappearance of mesoderm and the consequent formation of the anterior chamber [1, 2, 28, 37]. The earlier idea was that the mesoderm disappears by means of atrophy and absorption. The more recent concept is that the mesoderm is pulled apart passively as a result of different growth rates of the anterior tissues. Both mechanisms may operate to some extent.

POSTERIOR EMBRYOTOXON

Posterior embryotoxon is an exaggeration of the normal anterior border ring of Schwalbe (Schwalbe's ring). This structure is a collagenous band that encircles the periphery of the cornea on its posterior surface [16]. The collagen fibers of Schwalbe's ring course circumferentially (parallel to the limbus), whereas the fibers elsewhere in the cornea run radially. Schwalbe's ring is bounded anteriorly by the termination of Descemet's membrane and posteriorly by the trabecular meshwork. Gonioscopically, it is seen just above the meshwork and is then referred to as Schwalbe's line. It may be flat and indistinct, or elevated and ridgelike.

In most persons, Schwalbe's ring is not visible biomicroscopically because it lies behind the opaque portion of the limbus; but it is sufficiently promi-

nent and anteriorly displaced as to be visible in 15 to 30 percent of normal eyes. If it can be seen by external examination, it is referred to as posterior embryotoxon. It appears clinically as an arcuate or scalloped translucent membrane on the posterior surface of the cornea just inside the limbus (Fig. 10-4). It is usually seen in the horizontal meridian, nasally and temporally, but may encircle the entire cornea.

Posterior embryotoxon is inherited as a dominant trait. The eye is usually otherwise normal unless Axenfeld's anomaly or syndrome (discussed below) is present. Cornea plana, corectopia, and aniridia have also been present from time to time.

Even a Schwalbe's ring that is not anteriorly displaced may be visible without gonioscopy if there is a sectoral deficiency of the normal extension of sclera into the superficial tissues of the limbus. This extremely rare anomaly is called the *partial limbal coloboma of Ascher* and exposes Schwalbe's ring and the meshwork to direct view [11].

PROMINENT IRIS PROCESSES

Although prominent iris processes are not corneal anomalies, they should be mentioned because they are part of the spectrum of mesodermal dysgenesis and because it is necessary to determine their relationship to the peripheral cornea in order to evaluate their pathologic significance [51].

It is normal for some slender processes (usually fewer than 100) to extend from the peripheral iris to the scleral roll (also known as the scleral spur) at the posterior edge of the trabecular meshwork or, occa-

TABLE 10-4. *Comparative Features of Anterior Keratoconus, Posterior Keratoconus, and Keratoglobus*

Feature	Anterior Keratoconus	Generalized Posterior Keratoconus	Circumscribed Posterior Keratoconus	Keratoglobus
Frequency	Most common	Least common	Third most common	Second most common
Heredity	Uncertain	None	Usually none	Uncertain
Sex predilection	Slightly more females	All females	Mostly females	Uncertain
Laterality	Usually bilateral	Usually unilateral	Usually unilateral	Bilateral
Progression	Yes	No	No	Yes
Decreased acuity	Yes	Rarely	Sometimes	Yes
Corneal clouding	Sometimes	Seldom	Usually	Seldom
Anterior curve	Increased, distorted	Normal	Normal or distorted	Increased, distorted
Posterior curve	Increased	Increased	Increased locally	Increased
Corneal thinning	Central	Central	Variable	Peripheral
Acute hydrops	Occasionally	No	Seldom	Seldom

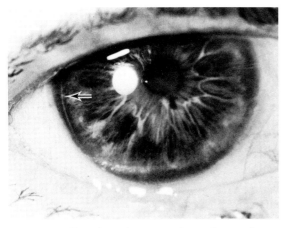

FIGURE 10-4. *Posterior embryotoxon. A prominent and anteriorly displaced anterior border ring of Schwalbe is visible just inside the limbus* (arrow).

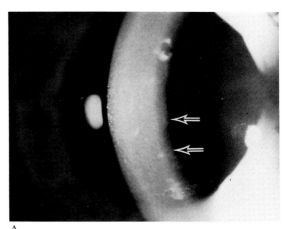

A

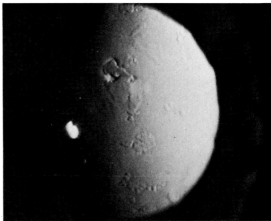

B

FIGURE 10-5. *A. Posterior polymorphous dystrophy. A prominent vesicular lesion, convex toward the stroma and surrounded by an opaque halo, is seen in the upper portion of the slitlamp beam at the level of Descemet's membrane. Similar, but smaller, bleblike lesions are also present* (arrows), *and there is a nondescript deep opacity near the inferior edge of the pupil. B. Posterior polymorphous dystrophy. Sinuous and geographic opacities are evident at the level of Descemet's membrane by retroillumination.*

sionally, even to the central portion of the meshwork itself. Extensions to or beyond Schwalbe's ring are abnormal and are referred to as prominent iris processes. Abnormal processes are often more numerous, in addition to being more prominent and anteriorly displaced, than are normal processes.

Prominent iris processes can occur with any of the other manifestations of mesodermal dysgenesis. They are also seen in many cases of primary congenital glaucoma and in several systemic disorders that are associated with congenital glaucoma: phakomatosis; homocystinuria; rubella; and Marfan's, Lowe's, Pierre Robin, Hallermann-Streiff, Rubenstein-Taybi, and Turner's syndromes [51].

MESODERMAL DYSGENESIS OF THE IRIS
In addition to prominent iris processes, mesodermal dysgenesis may be associated with congenital peripheral anterior synechiae and a variety of abnormalities of the iris itself, including atrophy of the iris stroma, corectopia, and pseudopolycoria.

POSTERIOR POLYMORPHOUS DYSTROPHY
Posterior polymorphous dystrophy (Fig. 10-5) may be classified either as a dystrophy or as a congenital anomaly. Its histopathologic features suggest a relationship to mesodermal dysgenesis, and it not infrequently occurs with other forms of mesodermal dysgenesis [22, 23, 64]. This entity is described in detail in Chapter 9.

CONGENITAL CORNEA GUTTATA
Cornea guttata can occur rarely as a congenital anomaly. It is sometimes familial. A dominant pedigree with associated anterior polar cataract has been

described, suggesting an abnormality in the anterior segment mesoderm that helps to separate the lens from the surface ectoderm at about the sixth to eighth week of embryonic life [10]. Congenital cornea guttata is also described in Chapter 9.

CIRCUMSCRIBED POSTERIOR KERATOCONUS
Circumscribed posterior keratoconus is characterized by the presence of a localized, craterlike defect (convex toward the stroma) in the posterior surface of the cornea (Fig. 10-6) [23, 56–58, 62, 67]. Contrary to former belief, Descemet's membrane and en-

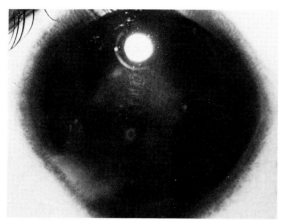

FIGURE 10-6. *Circumscribed posterior keratoconus. A localized crater, convex toward the stroma, is present in the posterior cornea. The area is hazy, and small stromal opacities overlie the defect.*

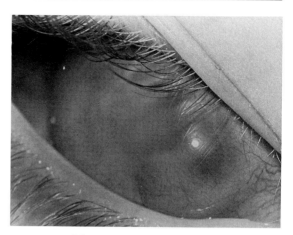

FIGURE 10-7. *Sclerocornea. Scleralization is virtually complete, but the central cornea is slightly less affected, as is typical. The cornea is vascularized by extensions of normal epibulbar vessels, without evidence of inflammation.*

dothelium are usually present in the area of the defect, although the collagen of Descemet's membrane may be abnormal in structure and configuration [23, 56–58, 67]. More than one pit may be present. The overlying stroma often has nonspecific opacities. Most cases are in females and are unilateral.

Circumscribed posterior keratoconus is mainly sporadic, although familial examples have occurred. It is probably the result of excessive absorption or cleavage of mesoderm in the area of involvement, perhaps secondary to some problem with separation of the lens vesicle. Some cases show evidence of being related to intrauterine inflammation: corneal infiltrates and vascularization, keratic precipitates, anterior synechiae, and uveitis; these cases do often have defects in Descemet's membrane and endothelium and are sometimes referred to as *von Hippel's posterior* (or *internal*) *corneal ulcer*.

The characteristics of circumscribed posterior keratoconus, as compared with generalized posterior keratoconus, anterior keratoconus, and keratoglobus, are summarized in Table 10-4. Associated ocular and systemic abnormalities are listed in Table 10-5 [23].

SCLEROCORNEA

Sclerocornea is an abnormality in which the second mesodermal wave forms tissue resembling sclera instead of clear corneal stroma (Fig. 10-7) [17, 29, 33]. The scleralization may be only peripheral or virtually complete. Even when it is complete, the central cornea is apt to be slightly less opaque than the

TABLE 10-5. *Abnormalities Associated with Circumscribed Posterior Keratoconus*

Ocular
Fleischer ring
Aniridia
Mesodermal dysgenesis
Anterior lenticonus
Systemic
Hypertelorism
Poorly developed nasal bridge
Brachydactyly
Bull neck
Mental retardation
Growth retardation

periphery. Affected areas have fine, superficial vessels that are direct extensions of normal scleral, episcleral, and conjunctival vessels. Sclerocornea is usually bilateral [29].

Histopathologic studies reveal elastic fibers and collagen fibers of increased and variable diameters in the anterior corneal stroma. The deeper collagen fibers have smaller diameters than do the more anterior ones, as is typical of sclera; the reverse is true of normal cornea [33].

About 50 percent of cases of sclerocornea are sporadic, and the remainder can be dominant or recessive [29]. The dominant forms are less severe than the recessive ones [48]. There is no sex predilection. The most common associated finding is cornea plana. Other ocular and systemic associations are given in Table 10-6 [15, 21, 29, 41, 48].

AXENFELD'S ANOMALY AND SYNDROME

Axenfeld's *anomaly* is the combination of posterior embryotoxon with prominent iris processes. The *syndrome* is the same plus glaucoma [28, 62]. Both the anomaly and the syndrome are dominantly inherited. Hypertelorism is occasionally present.

RIEGER'S ANOMALY AND SYNDROME

Rieger's anomaly (iridocorneal mesodermal, or mesoectodermal, dysgenesis) consists of posterior embryotoxon, atrophy of the iris stroma, and prominent iris processes (Fig. 10-8) [1, 28, 62]. Peripheral anterior synechiae, corectopia, and pseudopolycoria are often present also, as is glaucoma in 50 to 60 percent of cases.

In *Rieger's syndrome*, dental, cranial, facial, or skeletal abnormalities are also present. Some patients are mentally retarded.

Rieger's anomaly and syndrome are usually dominant but are occasionally sporadic. One case showed a presumptive isochromosome of the long arm of chromosome 6 [54], and another had a pericentric inversion of chromosome 6 [25].

GONIODYSGENESIS WITH GLAUCOMA

Goniodysgenesis with glaucoma is probably just a minor form of Rieger's anomaly, lacking only posterior embryotoxon [26, 62]. Transmission is dominant.

TABLE 10-6. *Abnormalities Associated with Sclerocornea*

Ocular
  High refractive errors
  Blue sclera
  Cornea plana
  Horizontally oval cornea
  Aniridia
  Mesodermal dysgenesis
  Uveal and retinal coloboma
  Cataract
  Open-angle glaucoma
  Angle-closure glaucoma
  Pseudoptosis
  Microphthalmos
Systemic
  Anomalies of skull and facial bones
  Deformities of the external ear
  Deafness
  Polydactyly
  Cerebellar dysfunction
  Testicular abnormalities
  Hereditary osteo-onychodysplasia
  Osteogenesis imperfecta
  Others (numerous and variable)

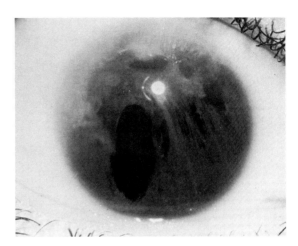

FIGURE 10-8. *Rieger's anomaly. Posterior embryotoxon, peripheral anterior synechiae, corectopia, atrophy of the iris stroma (producing pseudopolycoria), prominent iris processes, and glaucoma are present.*

IRIDOGONIODYSGENESIS WITH CATARACT

Iridogoniodysgenesis with cataract differs from Rieger's anomaly in that cataract is present, posterior embryotoxon is absent, and the heredity is autosomal recessive [26, 62]. Iridogoniodysgenesis is not associated with systemic abnormalities, but Conradi's syndrome (congenital stippled epiphyses) sometimes manifests other forms of mesodermal dysgenesis in association with cataract.

PETERS' ANOMALY

In the *mesodermal form* of Peters' anomaly, the central cornea has a congenital leukoma with strands of iris adherent to it (see Fig. 10-3) [1, 11, 28, 37, 52, 56–58, 62]. The adhesions usually, but not invariably, arise from the iris collarette and represent persisting remnants of the pupillary membrane. The lens, which is ectodermal in origin, is clear in the classic and purely mesodermal form of the anomaly. It is most often sporadic but may be transmitted recessively or as an irregularly dominant trait [52]. Approximately 80 percent of cases are bilateral, and about half include glaucoma [52]. Mesodermal Peters' anomaly is caused by incomplete absorption or cleavage of the mesoderm that is associated with the central portions of the iris, anterior chamber, and cornea. Descemet's membrane and endothelium are generally absent at the site of the leukoma, as is true also of the other two forms of the anomaly that are discussed below.

The *ectodermal form* is the result of faulty separation of the lens vesicle from surface ectoderm (Fig.

10-9). In addition to the features of the mesodermal type, anterior cataract (polar, subcapsular, or reduplication) is present.

The *inflammatory form* follows intrauterine inflammation and so is nonhereditary. The inflammation can interfere with ectodermal or mesodermal development or both. There is no definitive way to make the diagnosis, although signs of inflammation may still be present after birth, and the iris adhesions are extensive and do not arise only from the vicinity of the collarette. Cases of inflammatory Peters' anomaly nearly always fulfill the criteria for use of the term *von Hippel's posterior corneal ulcer*, namely, inflammatory signs in association with congenital defects of Descemet's membrane and endothelium. We have already seen that some examples of circumscribed posterior keratoconus have these same features and so may also be referred to as cases of von Hippel's ulcer; in fact, there seems to be little, if any, difference between the inflammatory form of Peters' anomaly and the inflammatory form of circumscribed posterior keratoconus.

OTHER COMBINED FORMS OF MESODERMAL DYSGENESIS

Although the foregoing disorders are the most frequently encountered combined forms of mesodermal dysgenesis, it is worth reemphasizing that any combination of features is possible. This is illustrated well by the family reported by Grayson in which some members had all of the following findings: cornea guttata, posterior polymorphous dystrophy, posterior embryotoxon, circumscribed posterior keratoconus, iris atrophy, peripheral anterior synechiae, prominent iris processes, and glaucoma [22]. These patients also developed corneal edema and fibrocalcific band keratopathy.

CONGENITAL MASS LESIONS OF THE CORNEA

METAPLASIAS

A metaplasia is a transformation of tissue from one type to another, usually in response to exposure, inflammation, or trauma [11, 69]. As mentioned earlier, the cornea can undergo metaplasia to skin (dermoid transformation) in the conditions of keratectasia, corneal staphyloma, and true cryptophthalmos. The metaplasia is at times of such proportions as to produce an apparent tumor of the cornea.

If the metaplasia is strictly ectodermal, the corneal epithelium is replaced by tissue resembling epidermis, sometimes with related derivatives such as hairs and glandular structures being present. Me-

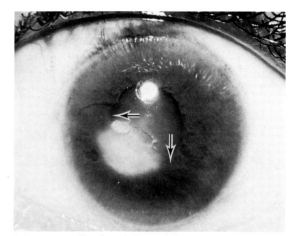

FIGURE 10-9. *Ectodermal form of Peters' anomaly. Corneal leukoma with adherent strands of iris (arrows). Anterior polar and subcapsular cataracts are also present, indicating faulty separation of the lens vesicle from surface ectoderm.*

sodermal metaplasia brings about the appearance in subepithelial stroma of the fibrofatty elements of dermis, and sometimes cartilage or bone. When the metaplasia consists primarily of a hypertrophic overgrowth of fibrous tissue, the term *corneal keloid* may be used [44].

CHORISTOMAS

A choristoma is a mass of tissue that has been displaced during prenatal development from its normal position to a location where it would not normally be found [69].

CORNEAL, LIMBAL, AND EPIBULBAR DERMOIDS

Corneal, limbal, and epibulbar dermoids consist of masses of tissue that were destined to become skin but were displaced to the surface of the eye [11, 69]. They can also occur in the orbit.

Choristomatous dermoids contain ectodermal elements (keratinizing epithelium, hair, sebaceous and sudoriferous glands, nerve, smooth muscle, and, rarely, teeth) and mesodermal derivatives (fibrous tissue, fat, blood vessels, and cartilage) in various combinations. They are called lipodermoids if fatty tissue predominates.

Clinically, an epibulbar dermoid is usually a round or ovoid, yellowish white, domelike mass (Fig. 10-10). Occasionally, a dermoid may be rather diffuse or may encircle the limbus or peripheral cornea. Hairs often protrude from the lesion. The surface may be pearly or clear and glistening, depending on the presence or absence of epithelial keratinization. The most common location is at the inferotemporal limbus, but dermoids can occur anywhere on the surface of the eye. The central cornea

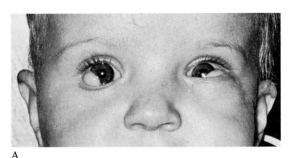

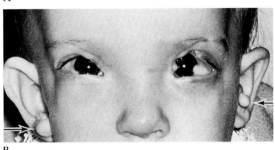

FIGURE 10-10. *A. Bilateral limbal dermoids of Goldenhar's syndrome. Note also that the left ear is malformed. B. Goldenhar's syndrome with bilateral limbal and epibulbar dermoids, colobomas of the upper eyelids, and preauricular appendages* (arrows).

can be affected, although some of these lesions are probably the result of dermoid transformation (metaplastic dermoids) rather than being choristomatous malformations. The second most common site for a dermoid is the superotemporal orbit. Dermoids usually exhibit little or no growth but do enlarge occasionally, especially at the time of puberty [5]. They do not become malignant.

A limbal or corneal dermoid can cause decreased visual acuity by covering the visual axis or by causing astigmatism. An arcuate deposition of lipid often develops along the central (corneal) edge of a limbal dermoid and is another possible source of decreased vision. The lipid sometimes increases as long as the dermoid is present [5].

Limbal dermoids always involve some of the corneal stroma and can even extend into the anterior chamber. Any attempt at excision must be limited merely to shaving away the elevated portion of the lesion, unless one is willing to undertake a corneoscleral graft, which would rarely, if ever, be indicated. It is important to explain to the parents, or to the patient who is old enough to understand, that the shaving procedure can only eliminate the elevation and that the corneal opacity will remain. The surgery is not without some difficulty and risk. The cornea may be thin in the area of the dermoid, and perforation is possible. I have observed that if the

dermoid covers the anterior portion of the sclera, the underlying extraocular muscles and their insertions may be anomalous and that they may inadvertently be transected if the surgeon is not careful.

Perhaps 30 percent of patients who have epibulbar dermoids have other abnormalities [5]. These most often consist of some or all of the features of *Goldenhar's syndrome* (oculoauriculovertebral dysplasia; Fig. 10-10) [4–6, 18, 19]. Goldenhar's syndrome is the result of maldevelopment of the first and second branchial arches, which give rise to the maxilla, mandible, malar bone, auricle, and structures of the upper neck. The syndrome comprises a triad of findings: epibulbar (usually limbal) dermoid(s), abnormalities of the ear such as auricular appendages or pretragal fistulas, and anomalies of the vertebral column. Other abnormalities that sometimes occur are listed in Table 10-7 [4–6, 18, 19].

The cause of Goldenhar's syndrome is unknown. It is nearly always sporadic and nonhereditary, although familial examples have been reported twice [36, 53]. Most isolated epibulbar dermoids are also sporadic, but bilateral corneal dermoids can be hereditary, and dermoids that encircle the limbus (ring dermoid syndrome) can be dominantly transmitted [27, 42].

Epibulbar dermoids are occasionally associated with systemic disorders other than Goldenhar's syndrome (Table 10-8) [5, 19].

ABNORMALITIES OF TRANSPARENCY

In a heterogeneous group of disorders, the clarity of the cornea is disturbed, but the cornea is not grossly malformed. Loss of transparency can be caused by edema, trauma, inflammation, biochemical depositions, or drying, as well as by any of the various mechanisms that have already been discussed. Many of these problems are not truly congenital anomalies and so will be mentioned only briefly.

EDEMA

CONGENITAL HEREDITARY ENDOTHELIAL DYSTROPHY

Congenital hereditary endothelial dystrophy (CHED) is characterized by the presence, at birth or soon thereafter, of bilateral corneal edema that is often slightly worse centrally and that is not associated with vascularization or inflammation [32, 35, 43, 45, 64]. Epithelial edema is not prominent, but the stroma may be swollen to 2 or 3 times its normal thickness. Descemet's membrane, when visible, is seen to be thick and opaque, but guttate changes are not present. Intraocular pressures are normal. The corneas are not enlarged.

Two types of CHED having different modes of transmission are recognized [32, 45, 63, 64]. The recessive form is more common, and is usually more severe, than the dominant form. In the recessive disease, the corneas are cloudy at birth, and nystagmus is common. The condition is essentially nonprogressive and is asymptomatic except for severely decreased vision. Deafness is sometimes present; otherwise, there are no related systemic abnormalities [24, 64].

Corneal edema in dominant CHED may not become apparent until sometime during the first or second year after birth [32, 63, 64]. Nystagmus is

TABLE 10-7. *Abnormalities Associated with Goldenhar's Syndrome**

Ocular
  Coloboma of upper eyelid
  Uveal coloboma
  Aniridia
  Miliary retinal aneurysms
  Duane's retraction strabismus syndrome
  Lacrimal stenosis
  Microphthalmos
Systemic
  Mandibular and malar hypoplasia
  Other facial and oral abnormalities
  Cardiac abnormalities
  Renal abnormalities
  Gastrointestinal abnormalities
  Genitourinary abnormalities
  Mental retardation

*In addition to the basic triad of epibulbar dermoid(s), anomalies of the ear, and anomalies of the vertebral column.

TABLE 10-8. *Systemic Malformation Syndromes Sometimes Associated with Epibulbar Dermoids*

Branchial arch syndromes
  Goldenhar's syndrome (oculoauriculovertebral
    dysplasia)
  Franceschetti (or Treacher Collins) syndrome
    (mandibulofacial dysostosis)
Congenital neurocutaneous syndromes
  Bloch-Sulzberger syndrome (incontinentia
    pigmenti)
  Encephalocraniocutaneous lipomatosis
  Linear sebaceous nevus syndrome
Chromosomal abnormalities
  Cri du chat syndrome (deletion of short arm of
    chromosome 5)

absent. The edema is likely to progress slowly, and some patients develop pain, photophobia, and tearing.

Histopathologically, the anterior ("banded") portion of Descemet's membrane is normal, but the posterior nonbanded layer (which is formed later during development) is abnormal and consists of a variably thickened, or occasionally thinned, layer of aberrant collagen [3, 34, 35, 64]. Guttate excrescences do not form. Endothelial cells are absent or atrophic. The primary abnormality is presumed to be with the endothelial cells and must manifest itself during or after the fifth month of gestation, at which time the endothelial cells begin to form the posterior nonbanded portion of Descemet's membrane.

Asymptomatic relatives of patients with CHED may show corneal changes resembling posterior polymorphous dystrophy [38]. An attempt should be made to identify such persons because their children seem to have a greater risk of having CHED. (See Chapter 9 for additional comments.)

BIRTH TRAUMA
Mild trauma during birth can damage the corneal epithelium. More severe injury, usually from forceps, can produce ruptures in Descemet's membrane and the endothelium. These ruptures tend to be linear and seem to occur more often in the left eye (when related to the use of forceps) because babies most commonly present in the left-occiput-anterior position; in such a case, the tears would run in an inferonasal-superotemporal axis. As healing ensues, a ridge of hypertrophic Descemet's membrane develops along the line of rupture. The edema may or may not clear and can recur later in life.

PRIMARY OR SECONDARY CONGENITAL GLAUCOMA
Congenital glaucoma of any cause can produce corneal edema. The cornea enlarges, which causes ruptures of Descemet's membrane and endothelium (Haab's striae) and still more edema [51].

CONGENITAL HEREDITARY STROMAL DYSTROPHY
Congenital hereditary stromal dystrophy (CHSD) is a rare, dominant condition in which the superficial corneal stroma of both eyes has an ill-defined, feathery cloudiness [66]. The haze is more prominent centrally and fades peripherally. There is no edema. CHSD is nonprogressive, but the opacity can be sufficiently dense as to cause substantial loss of vision. Searching nystagmus is usually present. The stromal collagen fibers are abnormal in form, size, and distribution. (See also Chapter 9.)

KERATITIS

RUBELLA

Rarely, rubella produces keratitis in the form of disciform stromal edema. It more often causes a cloudy cornea by virtue of its association with congenital glaucoma.

SYPHILIS

Luetic interstitial keratitis may occasionally be present at birth, although it characteristically appears during the first or second decade of life, as does the associated deafness.

MISCELLANEOUS INFECTIONS

Many other infectious agents, including gonococcus, staphylococcus, and influenza virus (among others) can cause intrauterine keratitis. If the process is active, the presentation is with inflammatory signs in the cornea; if not, leukoma, keratectasia, or congenital anterior staphyloma may be seen.

DEPOSITIONS

ARCUS JUVENILIS

Arcus juvenilis, a deposition of lipid in the peripheral cornea (also known as *anterior embryotoxon*), is the same as corneal arcus (arcus senilis; see Chapter 9), except that the congenital variety is more often unilateral and sectoral in its distribution (Fig. 10-11) [13, 40]. The anomaly is of unknown etiology. When truly congenital, it is not related to elevated serum cholesterol. However, the patient with juvenile arcus is often not seen until sometime after infancy, and it is then uncertain whether the finding was present at birth. In such a case, the serum cholesterol should be checked because it can be elevated (and associated with premature atherosclerosis) in some cases of developmental juvenile arcus. Arcus juvenilis is sometimes found in association with megalocornea, aniridia, blue sclera and osteogenesis imperfecta; hereditary nephritis and nerve deafness (Alport's syndrome); or corneal inflammation or malformation of any cause.

OTHER DEPOSITIONS

Biochemical deposits can appear in the cornea early in life as a manifestation of any of several systemic diseases, but most of these deposits are not clinically apparent at birth. These diseases are listed in Table 10-9.

NEUROTROPHIC CHANGES AND DRYING OF THE CORNEA

The cornea may become dry soon after birth because of decreased corneal sensation, as happens

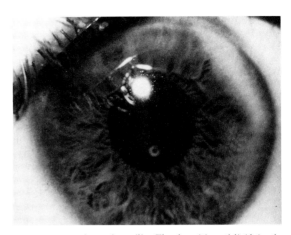

FIGURE 10-11. *Arcus juvenilis. The deposition of lipid in the corneal stroma resembles that of corneal arcus (arcus senilis) but is more likely to be unilateral and sectoral in its distribution.*

TABLE 10-9. *Systemic Diseases That Cause Corneal Opacities Early in Life**

Biochemical deposits
  Cystinosis
  Fabry's disease (angiokeratoma corporis diffusum)
  Mucopolysaccharidosis
  Mucolipidosis
  Tyrosinemia
  Tangier disease (high-density alpha-lipoprotein deficiency)
  Familial plasma lecithin-cholesterol acyltransferase deficiency
  Refsum's syndrome (heredopathia atactica polyneuritiformis)
  Schnyder's crystalline corneal dystrophy
Nonspecific (usually patchy or spotty) opacities
  Trisomy 13
  Trisomy 18
  Turner's syndrome (ovarian dysgenesis, XO karyotype)
  Phenylketonuria
  Chédiak-Higashi syndrome
  Genodermatoses

*Most of these opacities are not clinically apparent at birth.

with the Riley-Day syndrome (familial dysautonomia) or with isolated congenital dysfunction of the trigeminal nerve. Other causes of drying include congenital deficiency of tears (which may be idiopathic or may occur as another manifestation of the Riley-Day syndrome) and exposure from lagophthalmos.

KERATOPLASTY IN INFANTS

Specific therapy is not available for most congenital anomalies of the cornea, so the ophthalmologist must decide whether to attempt corneal transplantation. In general, the prognosis is poor. Apparently pleasing results have been reported from time to time, but little information is available concerning risks and long-term benefits [7, 8, 50, 52, 61, 68]. The difficulties of follow-up care are formidable, and problems related to the presence of associated abnormalities of the eye are often insurmountable.

Most authorities believe that corneal grafting in infancy is seldom indicated if the fellow eye is normal. Even if clarity of the graft is attained, amblyopia is likely to persist because of the presence of astigmatism and other refractive problems. On the other hand, keratoplasty is justifiable in some cases of severe bilateral involvement. Any improvement in such a desperate situation might be worthwhile, but it is important to evaluate the possible visual benefits in relation to the risks of anesthesia. The parents' attitudes, reliability, and expectations must also be taken into consideration. All concerned should realize that there is frequently little realistic chance of success, although the slight possibility of a rewarding result makes the endeavor worthwhile in selected cases.

REFERENCES

1. Alkemade, P. P. H. *Dysgenesis Mesodermalis of the Iris and Cornea: A Study of Rieger's Syndrome and Peters' Anomaly.* Assen, Netherlands: Thomas and Royal van Gorcum, 1969.
2. Allen, L., Burian, H. M., and Braley, A. E. New concept of development of anterior chamber angle. *Arch. Ophthalmol.* 53:783, 1955.
3. Antine, B. Histology of congenital hereditary corneal dystrophy. *Am. J. Ophthalmol.* 69:964, 1970.
4. Baum, J. L., and Feingold, M. Ocular aspects of Goldenhar's syndrome. *Am. J. Ophthalmol.* 75:250, 1973.
5. Benjamin, S. N., and Allen, H. F. Classification for limbal dermoid choristomas and branchial arch anomalies: Presentation of an unusual case. *Arch. Ophthalmol.* 87:305, 1972.
6. Bergsma, D. (Ed.). *Birth Defects: Atlas and Compendium.* Baltimore: Williams & Wilkins, 1973.
7. Brown, S. I. Corneal transplantation in the anterior chamber cleavage syndrome. *Am. J. Ophthalmol.* 70:942, 1970.
8. Brown, S. I. Corneal transplantation of the infant cornea. *Trans. Am. Acad. Opthalmol. Otolaryngol.* 78:461, 1974.
9. Codère, F., Brownstein, S., and Chen, M. F. Cryptophthalmos syndrome with bilateral renal agenesis. *Am. J. Ophthalmol.* 91:737, 1981.
10. Dohlman, C. H. Familial congenital cornea guttata in association with anterior polar cataract. *Acta Ophthalmol.* (Copenh.) 29:445, 1951.
11. Duke-Elder, S. Normal and Abnormal Development: Congenital Deformities. In S. Duke-Elder (Ed.), *System of Ophthalmology*, Vol. 3, Pt. 2. St. Louis: Mosby, 1964.
12. Duke-Elder, S., and Cook, C. Normal and Abnormal Development: Embryology. In S. Duke-Elder (Ed.), *System of Ophthalmology*, Vol. 3, Pt. 1. St. Louis: Mosby, 1963.
13. Duke-Elder, S., and Leigh, A. G. Diseases of the Outer Eye: Cornea and Sclera. In S. Duke-Elder (Ed.), *System of Ophthalmology*, Vol. 8, Pt. 2. St. Louis: Mosby, 1965.
14. Erikkson, A. W., Lehmann, W., and Forsius, H. Congenital cornea plana in Finland. *Clin. Genet.* 4:301, 1973.
15. Fenske, H. D., and Spitalny, L. A. Hereditary osteo-onychodysplasia. *Am. J. Ophthalmol.* 70:604, 1970.
16. Fine, B. S., and Yanoff, M. *Ocular Histology: A Text and Atlas* (2nd ed.). Hagerstown, Md.: Harper & Row, 1979.
17. Friedman, A. H., et al. Sclero-cornea and defective mesodermal migration. *Br. J. Ophthalmol.* 59:683, 1975.
18. Geeraets, W. J. *Ocular Syndromes* (3rd ed.). Philadelphia: Lea & Febiger, 1976.
19. Gellis, S. S., and Feingold, M. *Atlas of Mental Retardation Syndromes: Visual Diagnosis of Facies and Physical Findings.* Washington, D.C.: U.S. Government Printing Office, 1968.
20. Goldhammer, Y., and Smith, J. L. Cryptophthalmos syndrome with basal encephaloceles. *Am. J. Ophthalmol.* 80:146, 1975.
21. Goldstein, J. E., and Cogan, D. G. Sclerocornea and associated congenital anomalies. *Arch. Ophthalmol.* 67:99, 1962.
22. Grayson, M. The nature of hereditary deep polymorphous dystrophy of the cornea: Its association with iris and anterior chamber dysgenesis. *Trans. Am. Ophthalmol. Soc.* 72:516, 1974.
23. Grayson, M. *Diseases of the Cornea.* St. Louis: Mosby, 1979.
24. Harboyan, G., et al. Congenital corneal dystrophy: Progressive sensorineural deafness in a family. *Arch. Ophthalmol.* 85:27, 1971.
25. Heinemann, M., Breg, R., and Cotlier, E. Rieger's syndrome with pericentric inversion of chromosome 6. *Br. J. Ophthalmol.* 63:40, 1979.
26. Henkind, P., and Friedman, A. H. Iridogoniodysgenesis with cataract. *Am. J. Ophthalmol.* 72:949, 1971.
27. Henkind, P., et al. Bilateral corneal dermoids. *Am. J. Ophthalmol.* 76:972, 1973.

28. Henkind, P., Siegel, I., and Carr, R. E. Mesodermal dysgenesis of the anterior segment: Rieger's anomaly. *Arch. Ophthalmol.* 73:810, 1965.

29. Howard, R. O., and Abrahams, I. W. Sclerocornea. *Am. J. Ophthalmol.* 71:1254, 1971.

30. Ide, C. H., and Wollschlaeger, P. B. Multiple congenital abnormalities associated with cryptophthalmia. *Arch. Ophthalmol.* 81:638, 1969.

31. Jacobs, H. B. Posterior conical cornea. *Br. J. Ophthalmol.* 41:31, 1957.

32. Judisch, G. F., and Maumenee, I. H. Clinical differentiation of recessive congenital hereditary endothelial dystrophy and dominant congenital hereditary endothelial dystrophy. *Am. J. Ophthalmol.* 85:606, 1978.

33. Kanai, A., et al. The fine structure of sclerocornea. *Invest. Ophthalmol.* 10:687, 1971.

34. Kenyon, K. R., and Maumenee, A. E. The histological and ultrastructural pathology of congenital hereditary corneal dystrophy: A case report. *Invest. Ophthalmol.* 7:475, 1968.

35. Kenyon, K. R., and Maumenee, A. E. Further studies of congenital hereditary endothelial dystrophy of the cornea. *Am. J. Ophthalmol.* 76:419, 1973.

36. Krause, U. The syndrome of Goldenhar affecting two siblings. *Acta Ophthalmol.* 48:494, 1970.

37. Laibson, P. R., and Waring, G. O. Diseases of the Cornea. In R. D. Harley (Ed.), *Pediatric Ophthalmology*. Philadelphia: Saunders, 1975.

38. Levenson, J. E., Chandler, J. W., and Kaufman, H. E. Affected asymptomatic relatives in congenital hereditary endothelial dystrophy. *Am. J. Ophthalmol.* 76:967, 1973.

39. Malbran, E., and Dodds, R. Megalocornea and its relation to congenital glaucoma. *Am. J. Ophthalmol.* 49:908, 1960.

40. Mann, I. *Developmental Abnormalities of the Eye.* London: Cambridge University Press, 1937.

41. March, W. F., and Chalkley, T. H. F. Sclerocornea associated with Dandy-Walker cyst. *Am. J. Ophthalmol.* 78:54, 1974.

42. Mattos, J., Contreras, F., and O'Donnell, F. E., Jr. Ring dermoid syndrome. A new syndrome of autosomal dominantly inherited, bilateral, annular limbal dermoids with corneal and conjunctival extension. *Arch. Ophthalmol.* 98:1059, 1980.

43. Maumenee, A. E. Congenital hereditary corneal dystrophy. *Am. J. Ophthalmol.* 50:1114, 1960.

44. O'Grady, R. B., and Kirk, H. Q. Corneal keloids. *Am. J. Ophthalmol.* 73:206, 1972.

45. Pearce, W. G., Tripathi, R. C., and Morgan, G. Congenital endothelial corneal dystrophy: Clinical, pathological and genetic study. *Br. J. Ophthalmol.* 53:477, 1969.

46. Reese, A. B., and Ellsworth, R. M. The anterior chamber cleavage syndrome. *Arch. Ophthalmol.* 75:307, 1966.

47. Reinecke, R. D. Cryptophthalmos. *Arch. Ophthalmol.* 85:376, 1971.

48. Rodrigues, M. M., Calhoun, J., and Weinreb, S. Sclerocornea with an unbalanced translocation (17 p, 10 q). *Am. J. Ophthalmol.* 78:49, 1974.

49. Ross, J. V. M. Keratoconus posticus generalis. *Am. J. Ophthalmol.* 33:801, 1950.

50. Schanzlin, D. J., Goldberg, D. B., and Brown, S. I. Transplantation of congenitally opaque corneas. *Ophthalmology* 87:1253, 1980.

51. Shaffer, R. N., and Weiss, D. I. *Congenital and Pediatric Glaucomas*. St. Louis: Mosby, 1970.

52. Stone, D. L., et al. Congenital central corneal leukoma (Peters' anomaly). *Am. J. Ophthalmol.* 81:173, 1976.

53. Summitt, R. L. Familial Goldenhar syndrome. *Birth Defects* 5:106, 1969.

54. Tabbara, K. F., Khouri, F. P., and der Kaloustian, V. M. Rieger's syndrome with chromosomal anomaly (report of a case). *Can. J. Ophthalmol.* 8:488, 1973.

55. Thomas, C., Cordier, J., and Reny, A. Les manifestations ophthalmologiques du syndrome de Turner. *Arch. Ophtalmol.* (Paris) 29:565, 1969.

56. Townsend, W. M. Congenital corneal leukomas: I. Central defect in Descemet's membrane. *Am. J. Ophthalmol.* 77:80, 1974.

57. Townsend, W. M., Font, R. L., and Zimmerman, L. E. Congenital corneal leukomas: II. Histopathologic findings in 19 eyes with central defect in Descemet's membrane. *Am. J. Ophthalmol.* 77:192, 1974.

58. Townsend, W. M., Font, R. L., and Zimmerman, L. E. Congenital corneal leukomas: III. Histopathologic findings in 13 eyes with noncentral defect in Descemet's membrane. *Am. J. Ophthalmol.* 77:400, 1974.

59. Vail, D. T., Jr. Adult hereditary anterior megalophthalmos sine glaucoma: A definite disease entity. With special reference to the extraction of cataract. *Arch. Ophthalmol.* 6:39, 1931.

60. Waardenburg, P. J., Franceschetti, A., and Klein, D. *Genetics and Ophthalmology*. Assen, Netherlands: Royal van Gorcum, 1961. Vol. I, Chap. 8.

61. Waring, G. O., III, and Laibson, P. R. Keratoplasty in infants and children. *Trans. Am. Acad. Ophthalmol. Otolaryngol.* 83:283, 1977.

62. Waring, G. O., III, Rodrigues, M. M., and Laibson, P. R. Anterior-chamber cleavage syndrome: A stepladder classification. *Surv. Ophthalmol.* 20:3, 1975.

63. Waring, G. O., III, Rodrigues, M. M., and Laibson, P. R.   Corneal dystrophies: I. Dystrophies of the Bowman's layer, epithelium and stroma. *Surv. Ophthalmol.* 23:71, 1978.

64. Waring, G. O., III, Rodrigues, M. M., and Laibson, P. R.   Corneal dystrophies: II. Endothelial dystrophies. *Surv. Ophthalmol.* 23:147, 1978.

65. Wilkins, L.   *The Diagnosis and Treatment of Endocrine Disorders in Childhood and Adolescence.* Springfield, Ill.: Thomas, 1950.

66. Witschel, H., et al.   Congenital hereditary stromal dystrophy of the cornea. *Arch. Ophthalmol.* 96:1043, 1978.

67. Wolter, J. R., and Haney, W. P.   Histopathology of keratoconus posticus circumscriptus. *Arch. Ophthalmol.* 69:357, 1963.

68. Wood, T. O., and Kaufman, H. E.   Penetrating keratoplasty in an infant with sclerocornea. *Am. J. Ophthalmol.* 70:609, 1970.

69. Yanoff, M., and Fine, B. S.   *Ocular Pathology: A Text and Atlas.* Hagerstown, Md.: Harper & Row, 1975.

70. Young, A. I.   Megalocornea and mosaic dystrophy in identical twins. *Am. J. Ophthalmol.* 66:734, 1968.

11. METABOLIC DISEASES

Mitchell H. Friedlaender

PROTEIN

PORPHYRIA

The term *porphyria* embraces a group of diseases, each with characteristic and unusual features, that have in common the excessive excretion of one or more fluorescent pigments known as porphyrins. Porphyria can be divided into two general groups: *erythropoietic porphyria*, in which excessive quantities of porphyrins accumulate in red blood cells, and *hepatic porphyria*, in which porphyrins accumulate in the liver. The latter may be subdivided into at least four different types: acute intermittent porphyria, porphyria variegata, porphyria cutanea tarda, and hereditary coproporphyria. Although there is some overlap between the erythropoietic and hepatic groups, specific inherited enzymatic defects have been identified in at least three of the porphyrias (erythropoietic uroporphyria, acute intermittent porphyria, and porphyria cutanea tarda). The enzymatic defects are present in many tissues; however, the resulting metabolic derangements are most prominent in either the liver or erythroid tissue.

CLINICAL FEATURES

GENERAL

Erythropoietic porphyria may be divided into two types: erythropoietic uroporphyria and erythropoietic protoporphyria. Erythropoietic uroporphyria is a very rare disorder inherited as a recessive mendelian trait. The disease becomes manifest within a few days of birth and is due to the excessive deposition of porphyrins in the tissues, leading to pronounced photosensitization. Blisters occur on the skin surfaces exposed to light, especially the face and the hands. With time, scarring and mutilation occur, with loss of fingers and facial tissues. Skin not exposed to light remains unaffected. Red discoloration of the teeth may be seen grossly or with a Wood's light. Uroporphyrin I, derived from bone marrow normoblasts, is excreted in the urine, which appears pink or red. The disease is slowly progressive, and death generally results from infection or hemolytic anemia.

Erythropoietic protoporphyria is a more common, autosomal dominant disease. It becomes manifest in childhood and is characterized by skin photosensitivity with intense itching, edema, and erythema of the exposed skin. Protoporphyrins are increased in normoblasts and erythrocytes and in the plasma. They are also excreted in large amounts in the feces. The disease is usually benign, consisting of chronic skin changes on the hands and face and sometimes a mild hemolytic anemia.

Acute intermittent porphyria is a rare disease inherited as a mendelian dominant trait. It is rare before the age of 15 and after age 60. It is characterized clinically by (1) periodic attacks of intensive colic, usually accompanied by nausea and vomiting; (2) severe constipation; (3) neurotic or even psychotic behavior; and (4) neuromuscular disturbances. Increased quantities of porphyrin are found in the liver and excreted in the urine. On standing in sunlight, the urine turns a burgundy color or black. The inherited metabolic defect is a partial deficiency of the enzyme uroporphyrinogen I synthetase. The course of the disease is extremely variable; however, recurrent abdominal crises may occur for many years, and the mortality is high.

Porphyria variegata is a non-sex-linked mendelian dominant condition characterized by cutaneous lesions or attacks of colic. Coproporphyrins and protoporphyrins are excreted in the feces in large amounts. The skin is unusually sensitive to light and blisters and abrades easily. Jaundice, colic, and psychosis may occur during acute attacks. Between attacks, there may be no symptoms.

Porphyria cutanea tarda (Fig. 11-1) is the most common form of porphyria and is characterized by photosensitive dermatitis, hyperpigmentation of the skin, liver disease, and hypertrichosis. The skin is sensitive to light and trauma, and blisters, ulcers, and scars may occur on areas exposed to light. Uroporphyrin I is synthesized excessively by the liver and excreted in the urine. The disease is inherited as an autosomal dominant trait and is due to a partial deficiency of the enzyme uroporphyrinogen decarboxylase. Porphyria cutanea tarda may remain latent for several years only to be precipitated by alcoholic cirrhosis or exposure to drugs or toxins.

Hereditary coproporphyria is an autosomal dominant disease characterized by increased excretion of coproporphyrin in the urine and feces. Acute attacks may be precipitated by ingestion of barbiturates and other drugs. Symptoms consist of psychiatric crises and skin abnormalities.

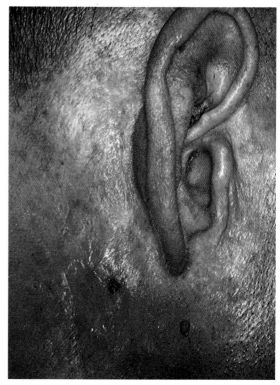

FIGURE 11-1. *Porphyria cutanea tarda. (Courtesy P. Thygeson, M.D.)*

OCULAR

The ocular findings in coproporphyria are variable and may affect all tissues of the eye. The eyebrows may be thinned or thickened and may meet in the midline [2]. Bullous lesions of the eyelids may be followed by pigmentation and scarring. Blisters may develop on the exposed area of the conjunctiva, resulting in symblepharon and shrinkage of the conjunctival sac. Lacrimation, photophobia, and blepharospasm are common features [87]. The conjunctiva becomes infiltrated by chronic inflammatory cells and forms adhesions to the underlying sclera.

Corneal complications are the result of cicatricial ectropion or vesiculation of the cornea. Vesicles occur in exposed areas of the cornea and heal forming nebulae or leukomas. Occasionally, the vesicles may lead to perforation [87]. The cornea may be thin peripherally, contain numerous crystals in Bowman's layer, and have deep stromal lamellar opacification [12]. Lesions resembling phlyctenules may precede corneal ulceration. Exposure keratitis and corneal opacification may result from severe ectropion.

Scleral involvement in porphyria is often described as scleromalacia perforans [12]. Punched-out scleral ulcers may occur between the limbus and the lateral rectus insertion, and these ulcers may sometimes extend over the limbus onto the cornea. A brawny scleritis is sometimes seen, and red fluorescence has been observed in the sclera, vitreous, and retina. The tissue damage that is seen is probably the result of oxidative or fluorochemical reactions.

Ophthalmoscopic changes include brown cotton-wool patches of edema. After 3 weeks these become dense, black globular patches. Retinal hemorrhages and discrete anular choroidal lesions are sometimes observed [12]. Atrophy of the ganglion cell and nerve fiber layer of the retina has also been described [108]. Optic atrophy has recently been reported [16].

DIFFERENTIAL DIAGNOSIS
The conjunctival changes of porphyria must be differentiated from those of cicatricial pemphigoid. The scleral and corneal changes must be distinguished from keratomalacia associated with vitamin A deficiency and peripheral corneal degenerations associated with local and systemic immunologic diseases. The retinal and choroidal lesions of porphyria can be confused with various types of uveitis. The systemic features of porphyria, the excretion of porphyrins, and the fluorescence of skin and ocular tissues will help in making a definitive diagnosis.

TREATMENT
If ultraviolet exposure causes damage, sunlight should be avoided. Beta carotene 30 mg orally per day may be of value in reducing dermal photosensitivity to sunlight. Splenectomy and phlebotomy to remove the excess iron load from the liver are effective treatments for certain kinds of porphyria. For acute attacks, a liberal intake of glucose orally or intravenously is the most effective treatment. Supportive therapy, including analgesics, fluids, and respiratory support is also important for acute attacks.

Treatment of ocular lesions begins with proper medical management of systemic porphyria. Protection from the sun and abstention from alcohol seem to be helpful. Corticosteroids have been recommended for the brawny scleritis of porphyria [12], but surgical treatment with scleral grafting may be necessary.

GOUT
Primary gout comprises a group of inborn metabolic disorders leading to hyperuricemia, recurrent attacks of arthritis, and tophaceous deposits of

sodium urate. Secondary gout is an acquired form of the disease in which hyperuricemia occurs. Gout affects 0.3 percent of the population in Europe and the United States and 10 percent of the adult male Maori population in New Zealand. Although usually considered a disease of the middle and upper social classes, gout affects all nationalities and income groups. Over 90 percent of gout is found among adult men but 3 to 7 percent may occur in postmenopausal women. Secondary gout constitutes 5 to 10 percent of all cases and usually is a complication of myeloproliferative disorders or hypertensive cardiovascular disease.

PATHOGENESIS
Uric acid is formed by oxidation of purine bases, which may be of dietary or biosynthetic origin. Two-thirds of these bases are excreted in the urine, and one-third is excreted in the bile, gastric, and intestinal secretions where they are destroyed by colonic bacteria. In gout, there are abnormalities of endogenous purine production and of uric acid excretion. In certain patients, purine biosynthesis is increased owing to the excess availability of key substrates, enzymatic activity, and inadequate feedback controls. Multiple enzyme abnormalities and renal tubular abnormalities would, however, be necessary to explain all cases of gout.

PATHOLOGIC CHANGES
The pathognomonic lesion of gout is the tophus, a uric acid deposit surrounded by inflammatory cells and a foreign-body reaction. Urate crystals are brilliantly anisotropic when viewed with polarized light under the microscope. Urate deposits accumulate in cartilage, epiphyseal bone, prearticular structures, and the kidneys. Tophi may accumulate in the ear, tendons, skin, nose, large vessels, myocardium, vocal cords, arytenoid cartilages, cornea, sclera, and tarsal plates of the eyelid. Destructive changes occur in the tissues because of these deposits. Sodium urate crystals may also be deposited in the kidney and produce serious interstitial inflammatory changes.

CLINICAL FEATURES
GENERAL
The natural history of gout consists of three phases: asymptomatic hyperuricemia, acute gouty arthritis, and chronic gouty arthritis. Fifty percent of initial acute attacks involve the great toe (podagra), and 90 percent of gouty patients experience podagra dur-

ing the course of their disease. The instep, ankle, heel, knee, and wrist are other common sites of involvement. In general, the more distal locations of the lower extremities are typically affected. Attacks may be precipitated by many kinds of stress. Dietary, physical, and emotional factors have also been implicated. Chronic gouty arthritis is associated with a progressive inability to dispose of urate and deposition of urate crystals in the cartilage, synovial membranes, tendons, and soft tissues. Tophaceous deposits may produce irregular swelling over the joints or the helix of the ear. Eventually, destruction of the joints ensues. The incidence of permanent joint change is considerably less now that drugs are available to control uric acid levels.

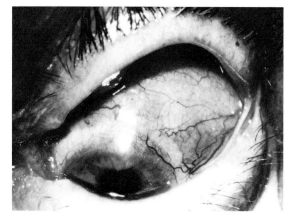

FIGURE 11-2. *Gouty scleritis. (Courtesy G. Smolin, M.D.)*

OCULAR

Acute ocular inflammation in gout is characterized by marked hyperemia and scanty discharge. This has been referred to by Hutchinson as the "hot eye of gout" [43]. The conjunctival vessels are dilated and tortuous, and the patient experiences a burning, hot, prickly sensation. Conjunctival tophi have also been reported [66]. The inflammation is episodic and associated with acute attacks of gouty arthritis. Scleritis (Fig. 11-2) and episcleritis can be associated with gout, and urate crystals occasionally are found in these tissues [66]. Acute iritis lasting about 10 days has also been reported [66]. The cornea can be affected, perhaps because of its avascularity and peripheral location [23]. Monosodium urate crystals may be deposited in the superficial stroma and epithelium of both the conjunctiva and cornea (Fig. 11-3) [89]. Corneal scraping reveals urates that can be demonstrated by colorimetry and spectrophotometry [23]. Urate crystals occur within the nuclei of the corneal epithelial cells [89]. The crystals are needlelike and demonstrate negative birefringence. Band keratopathy has also been described in gout [23]; it may be impossible to distinguish this condition from calcific band keratopathy by slit lamp examination.

DIFFERENTIAL DIAGNOSIS

Ocular gout should be distinguished from keratitis urica [107], a localized dystrophic disease of the cornea having an uncertain cause but unassociated with gout. Uric acid levels, a history of typical attacks of gouty arthritis, and the presence of tophi will help in making a correct diagnosis. In the absence of the characteristic features of gout, corneal urate deposits must be differentiated from the deposits of other metabolic corneal diseases as well

as certain drug depositions. The arthritis of rheumatoid disease, acute rheumatic fever, and osteoarthritis should be distinguished from gouty arthritis.

TREATMENT

Treatment of gouty arthritis is aimed at terminating the acute attack and preventing new recurrences, as well as preventing and reversing uric acid deposition in the joints and kidneys. Colchicine, indomethacin, and phenylbutazone are effective in treating the acute gouty arthritis attack. Hydrocortisone may be injected intraarticularly for prompt relief of pain. Drugs that lower the serum level of uric acid include probenecid, salicylates, and allopurinol. Allopurinol is a potent inhibitor of xanthinoxidase. In selected patients, surgical removal of urate deposits may be necessary. Tophaceous deposits can also be surgically removed from the conjunctiva. Superficial keratectomy may be necessary to remove the urate band keratopathy [23]. Purified uricase may supplement the scraping of the superficial deposits.

CYSTINOSIS

Cystinosis (Lignac-Fanconi syndrome) is a rare genetic disorder of cystine storage. No consistent enzymatic abnormality has been found to date. The disease is transmitted as an autosomal recessive trait. Cystine is found in lipid-storing membranes of circulating leukocytes, fibroblasts, and macrophages, probably within lysosomes [82]. Cystinosis usually occurs in childhood in association with Fanconi's syndrome. *Fanconi's syndrome* is a descriptive term for a group of physiologic abnormalities that include proximal renal tubular dysfunction, notably glucosuria, generalized aminoaciduria, phosphaturia, and renal tubular acidosis. Occasionally, ocular and systemic cystine

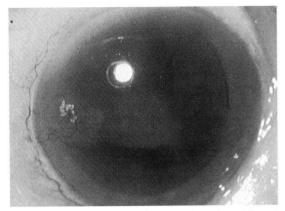

FIGURE 11-3. *Urate crystals in the cornea of a patient with gout. (Courtesy D. D. Donaldson, M.D.)*

storage occurs in the adult in the absence of renal disease.

PATHOGENESIS
Cystinosis results from the intracellular deposition of crystalline cystine in the reticuloendothelial cells of the bone marrow, liver, spleen, lymphatic system, and kidney.

CLINICAL FEATURES

GENERAL
Cystine storage disease with Fanconi's syndrome is a severe disorder usually leading to death by the age of 10. Severe rickets with stunting of growth and failure to thrive are evident in the first few months of life. Secondary hyperparathyroidism, glucosuria, and urinary loss of potassium and amino acids are characteristic features. Pyelonephritis is frequent and may contribute to renal failure.

OCULAR
Cystinosis rarely occurs in the adult in the absence of renal disease. In such cases, cystine crystals may be deposited in the cornea (Fig. 11-4) and conjunctiva as the only manifestation of adult cystinosis. These crystals, which are glistening, polychromatic, and needlelike to rectangular, are distributed throughout the anterior stroma with a slight predilection for the periphery. They appear as early as 6 months of age and can cause intense photophobia. Crystals may be found throughout the entire thickness of the cornea (Fig. 11-5) [112]; if they are extensive, visual acuity may be reduced. Intracellular crystals have been demonstrated within corneal stromal cells as well as cells of the iris, ciliary body, choroid, and retinal pigment epithelium [54, 82, 112]. Retinopathy associated with extensive degeneration and loss of the pigment epithelium has also

been described [109]. These peripheral fundus abnormalities may precede the corneal deposits and prove helpful in making an early diagnosis of cystinosis. Macular alterations, characterized by scintillating, crystalline-appearing structures in the fundus, may represent cystine crystals in the choroid or pigment epithelium [78, 82]. Recently, retinoschisis and retinal detachment have been reported in conjunction with adult cystinosis [19].

DIFFERENTIAL DIAGNOSIS
Cystinosis must be differentiated from other types of corneal depositions, including the paraproteinemias. Conjunctival biopsy is a useful technique in which cystine can be extracted and analyzed by column chromatography [110]. In addition, the characteristic retinal lesions may be very useful in making a proper diagnosis [86].

Cystinosis is sometimes classified as juvenile, adolescent, and adult. The juvenile form is usually associated with severe renal disease; the adult form appears to have only ocular manifestations since the renal disease is usually minimal. The adolescent form appears to be intermediate between the juvenile and adult forms. In the adolescent form, corneal crystals and nephropathy may be present, but retinopathy is absent [114].

TREATMENT
Attempts at treating cystinosis have been disappointing in the absence of information about the disease's exact biochemical defect. Dietary restriction has not been successful, since cystine is synthesized from the essential amino acid methionine. Renal transplantation has been carried out successfully in a number of patients. Potassium replacement to reverse chronic acidosis and vitamin D therapy to promote normal calcification of bone are important. Despite treatment, early death from uremia usually occurs in the juvenile form. The adult form of the disease is benign and requires no treatment.

ALKAPTONURIA
Alkaptonuria is a rare hereditary error of metabolism. It is due to an absence of the enzyme homogentisic acid oxidase, which results in an accumulation of homogentisic acid, a normal intermediary in the metabolism of phenylalanine and tyrosine, in the urine and other tissues including the eye. Oxidation of homogentisic acid produces a form of degenerative arthritis and a dark pigmentary change in connective tissues known as ochronosis.

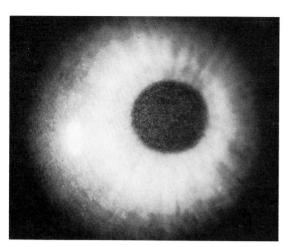

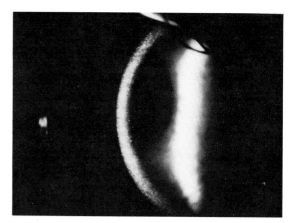

FIGURE 11-5. *Slit lamp photo of cystine crystals throughout entire thickness of the cornea. (Courtesy J. Krachmer, M.D., and D. Meisler, M.D.)*

FIGURE 11-4. *Cystine crystals in the cornea of a patient with cystinosis. (Courtesy J. Krachmer, M.D., and D. Meisler, M.D.)*

CLINICAL FEATURES

GENERAL

The first description of alkaptonuria was by Garrod in 1902 [31]. He recognized that the disease might be transmitted as a single recessive mendelian trait and that homogentisic acid arose in the normal course of tyrosine metabolism. The frequency of the disease is about 1 in 200,000 births. In the infant, darkening of the urine on a wet diaper may be the first sign. Alkaptonuria is a benign disorder until middle life when degenerative joint changes begin to take place in the majority of cases. The large joints and the spine are severely affected with pain, stiffness, and inflammation. Small joints tend to be spared. Ochronotic pigmentation of the ear, nose, and sclera are often seen. Internal structures such as the costochondral junctions, joints, and ligaments have also been noted to have ochronotic pigmentation. A diagnosis is usually made on the basis of the triad of arthritis, ochronotic pigmentation, and urine that darkens on the addition of a strong alkali.

OCULAR

Ocular pigmentation is found in the interpalpebral area at the insertion of the recti muscles (Fig. 11-6) [91]. In addition, a more diffuse pigmentation may also be found in the conjunctiva and cornea. The pigment may be gray to bluish black but microscopically appears ochre. Corneal pigment is located in the deep epithelium and in Bowman's layer. Pigmentation of the tarsal plates and lids may also be seen.

TREATMENT

Attempts to treat alkaptonuria with vitamins and cortisone have been successful [58]. Dietary restriction of phenylalanine and tyrosine is not practical except for brief periods and may be dangerous. Enzyme replacement is also not practical at present.

AMYLOIDOSIS

Amyloid is an eosinophilic hyaline material that has a striking affinity for dyes such as Congo red. Amyloid can be deposited in various tissues of the body including the eye as part of a localized or systemic disease. A specialized form of amyloid deposition in the cornea is seen in lattice corneal dystrophy. (See Chapter 9.) Amyloid is not a homogeneous substance but consists of at least two different substances. Type A amyloid (also known as AA) is a nonimmunoglobulin protein of unknown origin. It has a molecular weight of approximately 8000 and may be formed by proteolytic digestion of an unidentified protein precursor. Type B amyloid has been shown by amino acid sequence analysis to be identical to a fragment of the light chain of immunoglobulin. The amino acid sequence is most compatible with the variable region of light chain. Amyloid deposits are associated with a structural protein known also as P or AP [93]. Amyloidosis is sometimes classified as primary or secondary. Either type A or type B amyloid can occur in both forms. Amyloidosis may also be defined as systemic or localized. A third type of amyloid, known as type C, may be seen adjacent to tumors of neuroectodermal origin and in aging.

PATHOGENESIS

Several mechanisms may account for the deposition of amyloid in the tissues of the body, especially in

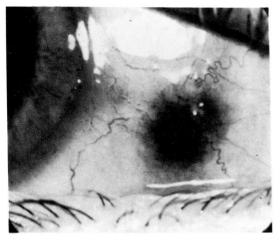

FIGURE 11-6. *Ocular pigmentation in alkaptonuria. (Courtesy G. Smolin, M.D.)*

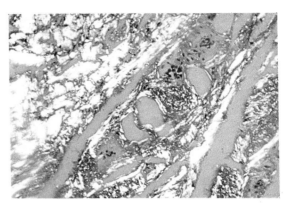

FIGURE 11-7. *Amyloid deposit stained with Congo red and viewed with polarized light. (Courtesy L. Schwartz, M.D.)*

the case of protein B: (1) catabolism by macrophages of deposited antigen-antibody complexes, (2) de novo synthesis of whole immunoglobulins or light chains with reduced solubility, (3) genetic deletions in the light chain gene producing an anomalous protein of reduced solubility, or (4) separate synthesis of discrete regions of light chain. Other types of amyloid may be formed by complexing precursors of polypeptide hormones. The reason for amyloid deposition is unknown. It may be a disorder of protein metabolism, an abnormality of the reticuloendothelial system, the result of chronic immunologic stimulation, a disorder of delayed hypersensitivity, or a combination of these defects [85].

PATHOLOGIC CHANGES

Homogeneous amyloid consists of characteristic long fibrils, which measure 80 Å. It is not known whether these fibrils are synthesized as such or if they are the result of degradation of intact protein molecules. Clinically suspected amyloidosis must be confirmed by biopsy of appropriate tissues. Amyloid stains with H&E. It is PAS-positive and stains mahogany brown with iodine, changing to blue with the addition of sulfuric acid. Amyloid stains brown with Congo red and exhibits dichroism and birefringence with polarized light (Fig. 11-7). Amyloid fluoresces yellow green with thioflavine T.

CLINICAL FEATURES

GENERAL

Many classifications of amyloidosis exist. The simplest and most widely used one is based on the four major categories described by Reiman and colleagues [79]: (1) Primary amyloidosis occurs in the absence of a preexisting disease. Almost any mesenchymal tissue, including the heart, can be involved. Bence Jones protein may be present in the urine. (2) Secondary amyloidosis usually follows chronic diseases such as neoplasms, infections, or connective tissues disorders, especially rheumatoid arthritis. The kidney, liver, spleen, and intestine are often affected. Bence Jones protein is usually absent. Amyloidosis associated with multiple myeloma and other plasma cell dyscrasias is characterized by homogeneous proteins in the serum and urine. Amyloid deposits have also been found in small amounts in postmortem examinations of various tissues. (3) Tumor-forming amyloid is an isolated mass of amyloid that appears in the skin, eye, or urinary tract. (4) Familial types of amyloidosis affect different organ systems and have different patterns of inheritance. The most common is associated with familial Mediterranean fever, seen mostly in Sephardic Jews.

Virtually any organ system can be affected in amyloidosis. Kidney involvement is potentially the most serious manifestation of the disease and is usually the main cause of death. Renal involvement is the preponderant manifestation in secondary amyloidosis, in amyloidosis accompanying familial Mediterranean fever, in multiple myeloma, and in approximately half the patients with primary amyloidosis. Cardiac deposition of amyloid may be asymptomatic but on occasion leads to congestive heart failure. This pattern may occur in primary amyloidosis or in amyloidosis associated with multiple myeloma and familial Mediterranean fever. Amyloid may be deposited in any portion of the gastrointestinal tract, from the tongue to the anus.

Tongue involvement is more commonly seen in the primary form of amyloidosis. Gastrointestinal symptoms include obstruction, ulceration, malabsorption, hemorrhage, and protein loss. Diagnosis can sometimes be made on biopsy of the rectum, conjunctiva, or gingivae. Amyloid infiltration may also be seen in nearly every other tissue of the body. Involvement is often limited to the walls of small blood vessels, and clinical manifestations may be absent.

OCULAR

The skin of the eyelid is a frequent site of amyloid deposition. Small papules with a waxy, yellowish appearance are typical. Conjunctival amyloid nodules, although rarely seen, may follow various forms of conjunctivitis, including trachoma. Occasionally, large tumorlike conjunctival nodules may be seen in the absence of any apparent predisposing condition [7].

Amyloid may be deposited in the cornea as the result of preexisting chronic inflammation. Amyloid has been demonstrated in the corneal epithelium of a patient with retrolental fibroplasia [94]. It has also been detected in the corneas in 7 unsuspected cases of amyloidosis showing corneal scarring and opacification [65]. Corneal involvement is characterized by the presence of cobblestone masses (Fig. 11-8) of yellowish pink material, which stain bright salmon pink with 0.2% Congo red [76]. A gelatinous or droplike change in the cornea has been described in primary corneal amyloidosis, especially in Japan [30, 55, 70, 105]. Familial amyloidosis of the cornea has also been described [95] and may be associated with cataracts (which do not contain amyloid). Lattice dystrophy of the cornea is considered a localized form of amyloidosis [9, 67]. Recently, type A amyloid has been identified in the cornea of a patient with lattice corneal dystrophy [69].

Amyloid may be deposited in the iris secondary to chronic infection [77], or it may be found in the vitreous where it has a characteristic glass-wool appearance. Most patients with vitreous amyloid have familial amyloidosis, although some have no family history of the disease. Vitreous opacities can be unilateral or bilateral. They may be in contact with the posterior lens surface. Pupillary abnormalities are not uncommon in familial amyloidosis. The irides may show segmented paralysis [104], pupillary dissociation [57], inequality [22], or heterochromia [1]. Scalloped pupils are a characteristic feature of familial amyloidosis and may be a helpful clue in making a correct diagnosis [1, 60]. This pupillary abnormal-

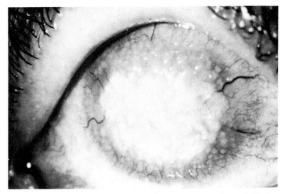

FIGURE 11-8. *Cobblestone mass in localized corneal amyloidosis.*

ity may be due to infiltration of the sphincter of nonadjacent ciliary nerves with amyloid.

Orbital involvement may be seen in amyloidosis and may lead to proptosis [56, 83]. Lacrimal gland and extraocular muscle involvement have also been described [56].

TREATMENT

In amyloidosis associated with plasma cell tumors, treatment is directed at the tumor; however, regression of the amyloid lesions may be slow or imperceptible. Primary amyloidosis should not be treated with antitumor chemotherapy unless definite evidence of a neoplasm is found [26]. Treatment of an infection or an inflammatory process may cause mobilization of systemic amyloid. Colchicine may abort the febrile episodes of familial Mediterranean fever, a disease often accompanied by amyloidosis. This drug can also prevent the development of amyloidosis in mice [48] and may be useful in far advanced human cases. Various other agents including steroids, ascorbic acid, and immunosuppressive agents have also been tried without clear-cut benefit.

The vitreous deposits associated with amyloidosis may be removed by vitrectomy [47]; however, redeposition tends to occur. Corneal transplantation may be necessary in advanced lattice corneal dystrophy or for the localized form of corneal amyloidosis.

LIPID

MUCOLIPIDOSES

The mucolipidoses are inherited metabolic diseases characterized by abnormal accumulation of acid mucopolysaccharides, sphingolipids, and glycolipids. Corneal opacities as well as psychomotor retardation and other systemic abnormalities are associated with this group of diseases.

GENERAL

In mucolipidosis I, physical growth is normal in the first years of life but slows after the age of 10. Hepatosplenomegaly and hernias are sometimes seen. Mental development is slow and patients usually have a moderate degree of mental retardation. The disease is recessively inherited but the specific enzymatic defect is unknown.

Mucolipidosis II is also recessively inherited and is characterized by severe growth and psychomotor retardation, hepatomegaly, gargoylelike facies, severe growth and psychomotor retardation, and thickened skin. The disease is also known as I-cell disease because of the cytoplasmic inclusions in fibroblasts and macrophages of affected persons [17]. One also sees gingival hypoplasia, frequent hernias, and a marked tendency toward infections. This entity, like other mucolipidoses, may be a type of lysosomal enzyme defect [62]. Acid mucopolysaccharides and glycolipids are stored in excess, and a deficiency of the enzyme beta-galactosidase seems to exist.

Mucolipidosis III, also known as pseudo-Hurler polydystrophy, is a recessively inherited disease in which acid mucopolysaccharides, sphingolipids, and glycolipids accumulate. The enzymatic defect is unknown. Musculoskeletal abnormalities including small stature, short neck, scoliosis, hip dysplasia, and restricted joint mobility are seen. Moderate mental retardation is present, and gargoylelike facies sometimes appear. Neither hepatosplenomegaly, severe psychomotor retardation, nor excessive secretion of mucopolysaccharides in the urine occur in this entity.

Mucolipidosis IV is probably a recessive disorder with an unknown enzymatic defect. Mucopolysaccharides presumably accumulate in excess. This condition affects mainly Ashkenazi Jews. It is characterized clinically by corneal clouding and profound psychomotor retardation but no skeletal or facial deformity, organomegaly, gross neurologic abnormalities, or mucopolysacchariduria. The specific enzyme defect remains unknown.

OCULAR

In mucolipidosis I, corneal opacities are rarely seen, but when they occur, they are associated with a cherry red spot [61]. Mucolipidosis II may be associated with bilateral corneal haziness, early cortical cataracts, and bilateral prominence of the eyes [8, 53, 61]. Glaucoma, megalocornea, optic atrophy, absent retinal blood vessels, and severe retinal degeneration have also been described [71]. Mucolipidosis III can be associated with fine corneal opacities, pre-

sumably abnormal storage material around stromal keratocytes [74]. Severe corneal clouding may be seen at birth or early infancy in mucolipidosis IV [51, 68]. The severe and early corneal involvement distinguishes type IV from the other mucolipidoses. Light microscopy reveals swollen corneal epithelial cells containing foamy cytoplasm and vacuolated keratocytes. Extensive vacuolization of the conjunctival epithelium is also seen.

FABRY'S DISEASE

Fabry's disease is a sphingolipidosis caused by a deficiency of ceramide trihexosidase and the accumulation of ceramide trihexoside in the tissues. The disease is sometimes known as angiokeratoma corporis diffusum, but since it is a multisystem disease, the term *Fabry's disease* is preferred. The disease is transmitted as an X-linked recessive trait, and the hemizygous male is the most seriously affected. Female carriers may be asymptomatic or exhibit mild symptoms. The skin is affected with clusters of punctate lesions that vary from purple to maroon to brownish but have a very characteristic distribution over the genitalia and lumbosacral area. The genitourinary system, the central nervous system, the musculoskeletal system, and the cardiovascular system may all be involved. Common neurologic changes include hemiplegia, aphasia, cerebellar disorders, and strokes. Pain in the fingers and toes is common.

Ocular findings are frequent and quite characteristic. The most typical ocular feature is a fine, whorl-like superficial corneal opacity (Fig. 11-9). This corneal change can be found in both the affected male patient and in the female carrier. It resembles the corneal opacities found after administration of chloroquine and amiodarone. Corneal opacities have been seen as early as 6 months of age and are presumably caused by the accumulation of sphingolipids in the corneal epithelium [25, 92, 106]. Visual acuity is generally unaffected.

Other ocular alterations include dilatation and tortuosity of the conjunctival vessels, sometimes associated with aneurysms. Periorbital and retinal edema, optic atrophy and papilledema, and dilatation and tortuosity of the retinal vessels may be present. Spokelike posterior sutural cataracts consisting of 9 to 12 spokes are seen in 50 percent of patients.

The visual prognosis in Fabry's disease is excellent, although severe visual loss caused by central retinal artery occlusion has been reported [88]. No satisfactory treatment has been reported for the systemic disease. It is compatible with long life; however, some deaths related to cardiovascular, renal, and gastrointestinal complications occur in middle adult life [46].

HYPERLIPOPROTEINEMIAS

Five types of hyperlipoproteinemias have been distinguished by Fredrickson, Levy, and Lees [27]. Type I hyperlipoproteinemia is characterized clinically by hepatosplenomegaly, eruptive xanthomas, fat intolerance, and episodes of abdominal pain. Ocular findings include lipemia retinalis and palpebral eruptive xanthomas [102]. Lipid keratopathy is occasionally seen, but corneal arcus usually does not occur.

Type II hyperlipoproteinemia is common and is associated with high levels of beta-lipoprotein and cholesterol with normal triglyceride levels. The disease is inherited as a mendelian dominant trait, but homozygous persons have a more severe expression of the disease. Patients exhibit xanthomatous lesions of the tendonous areas and coronary artery disease. Ocular findings include cornal arcus, xanthelasma, conjunctival xanthomas, and lipid keratopathy.

Type III hyperlipoproteinemia is a rare disorder transmitted as an autosomal recessive trait. Triglycerides, cholesterol, and beta-lipoproteins are elevated. Tuberous xanthomas on the hands and tendons are characteristic. There is a high incidence of peripheral vascular and coronary artery disease as well as diabetes. Ocular findings include xanthelasma, lipemia retinalis, and corneal arcus.

Type IV hyperlipoproteinemia is associated with increased prebetalipoproteins (very low-density lipoproteins), elevated serum triglycerides, and normal or slightly elevated cholesterol. Diabetes and hyperuricemia may also be present. Clinically, this condition is characterized by eruptive xanthomas, peripheral vascular disease, coronary artery disease, gout, diabetes, and abdominal pain. Ocular findings include xanthelasma, corneal arcus, and lipemia retinalis.

Type V hyperlipoproteinemia is marked by an increase in both chylomicrons and prebetalipoproteins with corresponding elevation of serum triglycerides and cholesterol. Abdominal pain, xanthomas, and hepatosplenomegaly may occur in the second or third decade of life. Peripheral vascular disease and coronary artery disease are not important features of this syndrome. Ocular findings include lipemia retinalis and palpebral xanthomas.

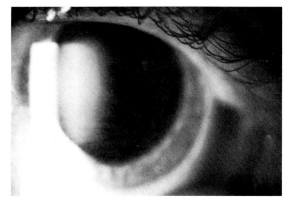

FIGURE 11-9. *Fabry's disease. (Courtesy I. Schwab, M.D.)*

FAMILIAL PLASMA CHOLESTEROL ESTER DEFICIENCY

Familial plasma cholesterol ester deficiency (lecithin cholesterol acyltransferase [LCAT] deficiency) is characterized by a marked reduction of plasma cholesterol esters and lysolecithin, and an increase in the level of unesterified cholesterol, triglycerides, and phospholipids. The deficiency of LCAT prevents the maintenance of a normal balance between cholesterol and cholesterol esters in cell membranes [33]. The cornea shows a nebulous cloudiness and a pronounced anular opacity near the limbus. The opacity, found in the stroma, is composed of innumerable tiny dots and resembles a corneal arcus, but the peripheral border is not as sharply demarcated. It is believed that the corneal opacity is due to lipid deposits as a consequence of abnormal plasma lipid and glycoprotein deposition. Occasionally, crystals appear near Descemet's membrane peripheral to the opacity.

TANGIER DISEASE

Tangier disease is an autosomal recessive disease associated with the complete absence of plasma high-density alpha-lipoproteins. Corneal involvement consists of stromal clouding caused by deposition of cholesterol esters [42] and many small dots in the posterior stroma, sometimes in a whorllike distribution. A haze in the peripheral horizontal meridian may be seen, but no arcus is present.

CARBOHYDRATE

MUCOPOLYSACCHARIDOSES

Mucopolysaccharide storage diseases (Table 11-1) are inborn errors of metabolism characterized by excessive storage of mucopolysaccharides and defective processes of degradation owing to deficiencies of lysosomal acid hydrolases. The normal cornea contains 4 to 4.5 percent mucopolysaccharides, of which 50 percent are keratan sulfate, 25 percent chondroitin, and 25 percent chondroitin 4-sulfate [15]. In the mucopolysaccharidoses, excess dermatan and keratan sulfate appear in the cornea, and heparan sulfate accumulates in the retina and central nervous system.

HURLER'S SYNDROME

Hurler's syndrome (mucopolysaccharidosis I) is characterized by moderate dwarfism, grotesque facial appearance (Fig. 11-10), protuberant abdomen, joint contractures, and mental retardation. A large head, hypertelorism, and thick lips with a large tongue and hypertrophic gums are generally seen. The bridge of the nose is depressed, and the chest is usually enlarged with marked flaring of the lower ribs. A prominent gibbus is present in a large percentage of patients. The hands are broad, the fingers short and stubby. There may be contractures of the hips and other joints. The spleen and liver are generally enlarged, and hernias are common. The skin is usually thickened, and there may be nodules over the scapular region. Hirsutism is often present. Deafness is frequent, but the cause is unclear. Respiratory disease results in deformity of the nasal and facial bones. Heart damage may be due to specific valvular lesions. Coronary artery and myocardial disease also occurs. Neurologic findings are

variable, but spasticity and mental retardation have frequently been reported.

Corneal clouding is a prominent feature of the disease (Fig. 11-11) [63] and helps to differentiate it from Hunter's syndrome. The opacities are located first in the anterior stroma and consist of fine gray punctate opacities. Later, the posterior stroma and endothelium become involved. Histologically, grossly ballooned macrophages are found in the cornea [52]. Pigmentary retinopathy and optic atrophy are also commonly seen [32].

SCHEIE'S SYNDROME

Scheie's syndrome (mucopolysaccharidosis I-S) is a variant of Hurler's syndrome and has the same enzymatic defect, a deficiency of alpha-L-iduronidase. Increased amounts of dermatan sulfate and heparan sulfate are excreted in the urine [45]. Originally described by Scheie and associates [84], this syndrome is characterized by corneal clouding early in life caused by an accumulation of acid mucopolysaccharides. Scheie's syndrome does not have the typical features of Hurler's syndrome except for the clawhand deformity and bony changes in the feet. Physical growth is in the normal range, and mental impairment is minimal or absent [64]. The gar-

TABLE 11-1. *Ocular Manifestations of Mucopolysaccharidoses*

Mucopolysaccharidosis	Enzyme Deficiency	Corneal Clouding	RPE Degeneration	Optic Atrophy
Hurler (I-H)	α-L-iduronidase	+	+	+
Scheie (I-S)	α-L-iduronidase (partial)	+	+	+
Hurler-Scheie compound (I-H/S)	α-L-iduronidase (partial)	+	+	+
Hunter A (IIA) (severe phenotype)	Iduronate sulfatase	−	+	+
Hunter B (IIB) (mild phenotype)	Iduronate sulfatase	+	+	+
Sanfilippo A (IIIA)	Heparan sulfate sulfamidase	−	+	+
Sanfilippo B (IIIB)	N-acetyl-α-D-glucosaminidase	−	+	+
Morquio (IV)	N-acetyl-galactosamine sulfatase	+	−	+
Maroteaux-Lamy A (VIA) (severe phenotype)	Arylsulfatase B	+	−	+
Maroteaux-Lamy B (VIB) (mild phenotype)	Arylsulfatase B	+	−	−
Macular corneal dystrophy (Groenouw type II)	?	+	−	−

RPE = retinal pigment epithelium; CRS = cherry red spot or grayness; + = present; − = absent; ± = variable.
SOURCE. Modified from K. R. Kenyon, Lysosomal Disorders Affecting the Ocular Anterior Segment. In D. H. Nicholson (Ed.), *Ocular Pathology Update.* New York: Masson Publishing USA, Inc., 1980.

goylelike facial appearance does not occur. However, the mouth is broad, and an atypical facial appearance has been noted. Hepatomegaly, usually without splenomegaly; aortic regurgitation with diastolic murmurs; stiff joints; and carpal tunnel syndrome have all been reported.

The most prominent ocular feature in Scheie's syndrome is a corneal haze that is often present at birth and very slowly progressive. The cornea appears thickened and somewhat edematous. The cloudiness is more marked in the corneal periphery. Corneal transplantation may be necessary later in life; however, transplants may do poorly over a period of time [96]. Other ocular findings include pigmentary disease of the retina and optic nerve atrophy. Acute glaucoma has been reported [75], but the cause is unclear. It may be due to a narrow angle or possibly a thickening of the anterior ocular structures caused by abnormal acid mucopolysaccharide storage. A thickening and decrease in the elasticity of the conjunctiva has also been observed. Mucopolysaccharide deposits are found in the keratocytes, and vacuoles or pleomorphic inclusions are found with electron microscopy [98, 100]. The disease is inherited as an autosomal recessive trait.

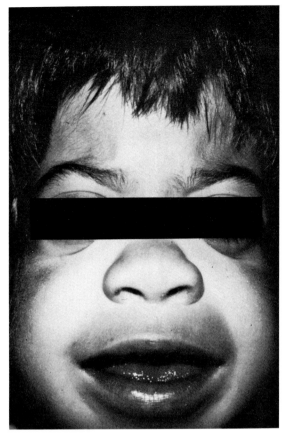

FIGURE 11-10. *Hurler syndrome.*

HUNTER'S SYNDROME

Hunter's syndrome (mucopolysaccharidosis II) has clinical and biochemical features similar to those of Hurler's syndrome except Hunter's syndrome is less severe. Again, there is a failure to degrade dermatan sulfate and heparan sulfate. Lysosomal storage of these polymers leads to numerous clinical problems including skeletal abnormalities, limitation of joint motion, hepatomegaly, deafness, and cardiovascular disease [20, 63]. The gross facial features are similar to those in Hurler's syndrome, and patients suffer from dwarfism, noisy breathing, hernias, and skin changes. Mental retardation is less severe than in Hurler's syndrome, and lumbar gibbus does not usually occur. Deafness, however, is a common feature of Hunter's syndrome. Patients usually die in their 20s and 30s because of cardiac involvement with congestive heart failure. Although Hunter's syndrome is similar to Hurler's syndrome clinically and biochemically, the two diseases are genetically distinct. Hunter's syndrome is inherited as an X-linked recessive trait, whereas Hurler's syndrome is autosomal recessive. Hunter's syndrome is also seen more frequently than is Hurler's syndrome.

Corneal clouding is generally considered to be ab-

sent in Hunter's syndrome, although exceptions have been recorded [101]. Pathologic studies have also demonstrated the accumulation of mucopolysaccharides in the cornea and other ocular tissues [34, 99]. Two forms of Hunter syndrome are said to exist. In the mild form, corneal opacities occur later in life but are mild compared with those of other mucopolysaccharidoses. In the severe form, subclinical corneal clouding can be demonstrated histochemically. Thus, although the presence of corneal clouding has been used to distinguish Hurler's syndrome from Hunter's syndrome, this distinction is not always a reliable one. Some Hurler's patients have clear corneas up to 14 years of age [29]; some Hunter's patients have clear corneas until late in life. Retinal pigmentary changes and optic atrophy have been noted in Hunter's syndrome, and the sclera and cilia may also be affected [34, 99].

SANFILIPPO'S SYNDROME

Sanfilippo's syndrome (mucopolysaccharidosis III) is an autosomal recessive disease in which patients

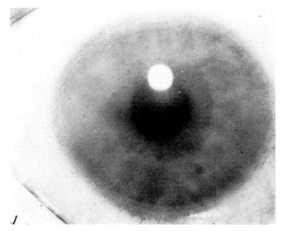

FIGURE 11-11. *Corneal clouding in Hurler's syndrome. (Courtesy G. Smolin, M.D.)*

excrete only heparan sulfate. It is seen less frequently than the Hurler or Hunter variants. It is characterized by severe mental retardation but fewer craniofacial changes than in Hurler's. Dwarfism is not a prominent feature. Joint movements are restricted, and neurologic symptoms including seizures and athetosis are quite prominent. Death usually occurs by age 14. Corneal cloudiness does not occur in Sanfilippo's syndrome. Retinal pigmentary degeneration and optic atrophy have been observed.

MORQUIO'S SYNDROME

Morquio's syndrome (mucopolysaccharidosis IV) is inherited as an autosomal recessive trait and is associated with the accumulation of keratan sulfate in the tissues. The cartilaginous and bony structures are primarily affected. These patients have a dwarf appearance, knock knees, barrel chest with pigeon breast, short neck, and generalized osteoporosis. The facial appearance is characteristic, with a broad mouth, short nose, widely spaced teeth with defective enamel, and a prominent maxilla. Hepatosplenomegaly, deafness, and metachromatic granulation of leukocytes has also been noted. Intelligence is normal, but neurologic symptoms may result from deformity of the spine, and cardiac complications may result from malformation of the chest. Corneal clouding can occur but may not be grossly evident until after 10 years of age. Cloudiness may consist of a mild stromal haze, or it may be severe [103]. Retinopathy and optic nerve changes are not present.

MAROTEAUX-LAMY SYNDROME

Maroteaux-Lamy syndrome (mucopolysaccharidosis VI) is an autosomal recessive disease in which

dermatan sulfate accumulates in the tissues. Skeletal changes are a prominent feature of this syndrome. Lumbar kyphosis, protrusion of the sternum, and genu valgum are found. The facial appearance is abnormal, but not as striking as in Hurler's syndrome. Intellectual function is normal. Corneal opacities occur in all cases (Fig. 11-12), but slit lamp examination may be necessary to see them [35]. Hydrocephalus, papilledema, and optic atrophy may also be seen [35]. The cornea shows an accumulation of lipidlike material in addition to glycosaminoglycans [97]. This suggests a relationship of Maroteaux-Lamy syndrome to the mucolipidoses.

BETA-GLUCURONIDASE DEFICIENCY

Beta-glucuronidase deficiency (mucopolysaccharidosis VII) is an autosomal recessive trait in which dermatan sulfate accumulates in the tissues. Skeletal dysplasia, hepatosplenomegaly, and mental retardation are known to occur, but no ocular complications have been reported [90].

GLUCOSE 6-PHOSPHATASE DEFICIENCY

Glucose 6-phosphatase deficiency (von Gierke's disease) is characterized by enlargement of the liver and kidneys and bouts of severe hypoglycemia. It is transmitted as an autosomal recessive characteristic and is due to the loss of activity of a single tissue enzyme, glucose 6-phosphatase. Clinically, the disease is characterized by slow development, a fat face and neck, and a markedly distended abdomen containing a huge liver. Xanthomas with prominent lipemia are characteristic. Seizures and vomiting also occur. The cornea may show a faint brown peripheral clouding, and discrete yellow perimacular lesions have also been observed. Although no treatment exists for this disease, early diagnosis and recognition has led to an increased life expectancy.

MINERALS

CALCIUM

Calcium deposition can occur in the cornea under a wide variety of circumstances ranging from local ocular inflammation to widespread systemic metabolic abnormalities. The most frequent pattern of corneal calcification is band keratopathy (Figs. 11-13 and 11-14). However, diffuse corneal calcification, sometimes accompanied by conjunctival calcification, is known to occur [14].

Band keratopathy begins in the peripheral cornea in the exposed areas. A clear interval is usually

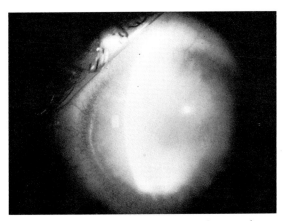

FIGURE 11-12. *Corneal clouding in Maroteaux-Lamy syndrome. (Courtesy J. Krachmer, M.D.)*

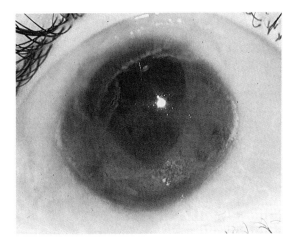

FIGURE 11-13. *Band keratopathy.*

present between the band and the limbus. If severe, the deposit may extend across the visual axis. In many cases, the band simply remains in the periphery. Tiny Swiss-cheese-like holes are usually present in the deposit. These are thought to be located in areas where corneal nerves penetrate Bowman's layer.

Histologically, the calcium is deposited in and around Bowman's layer. The early histologic change consists of a basophilic stippling of the epithelial basement membrane followed by deposition and fragmentation within Bowman's layer.

When calcific deposits in the cornea impair visual acuity, they can be removed by a variety of methods [111]. (See Chapter 9.)

HYPERPARATHYROIDISM
Corneal calcification has been studied extensively in both primary and secondary hyperparathyroidism [4, 44]. Calcium, in the form of hydroxyapatite crystals, is found intracellularly in both the conjunctiva and the cornea. In other cases of band keratopathy, calcium spherules and conglomerates are usually found extracellularly. It has been suggested that parathyroid hormone may have an effect on the intracellular deposition of calcium [4].

HYPOPHOSPHATASIA
Hypophosphatasia is a rare familial disease characterized clinically by multiple skeletal abnormalities, pathologic fractures of long bones, malformation of the skull and orbits, early loss of teeth, failure to thrive, and often early death caused by nephrocalcinosis and the other sequelae of hypercalcemia [10]. Band keratopathy and conjunctival calcifi-

cation have been noted in this syndrome and may be associated with blue sclera, harlequin orbits, pathologic lid retraction, papilledema, and increased intracranial pressure [10].

DIETARY CAUSES
Excessive vitamin D intake in a range of 100,000 to 500,000 IU daily may lead to band keratopathy and nephrocalcinosis in a few months to a few years [13]. Excessive ingestion of antacids, a condition known as the milk-alkali syndrome, has been associated with similar changes.

RENAL FAILURE
Patients with renal failure may demonstrate uremia, hypercalcemia, and band keratopathy. In some cases, renal damage may result from high calcium and alkali intake. Red eyes and conjunctival irritation are sometimes associated with renal failure [5, 6]. The conjunctival injection and granular appearance of the conjunctiva is due to a deposition of microcrystals of calcium phosphate salts in the conjunctiva and cornea. Over 80 percent of severely uremic patients will have corneal and conjunctival calcific deposits. Most of these patients are asymptomatic, and chronic hemodialysis does not seem to have any influence on the deposits [40]. Typical conjunctival and corneal changes associated with chronic renal failure consist of diffuse opacification of the peripheral limbal area and the interpalpebral zone [18]. Such deposits may regress after kidney transplantation.

NEOPLASTIC AND INFLAMMATORY DISEASES
Diffuse or bandlike calcific changes may be associated with sarcoidosis [14] and with various malignancies with and without bone metastases. Multiple

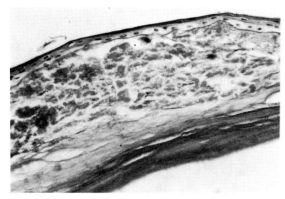

FIGURE 11-14. *Calcium deposition in Bowman's layer in band keratopathy. (× 80)*

myeloma and Paget's disease of bone may also lead to band keratopathy.

CORNEAL SCARS
Band keratopathy is frequently associated with chronic ocular inflammation such as trachoma and interstitial keratitis [28]. The severity of the band reflects the duration of the inflammation.

IRIDOCYCLITIS
Band keratopathy is a well-known complication of chronic iridocyclitis, especially cases occurring in children. The exact mechanism for this deposition is unknown. It has been suggested that gaseous exchange at the surface of the exposed cornea with loss of carbon dioxide and a localized elevation of pH may be an important factor [73]. Experimental band keratopathy can regularly be induced in rabbits with immunogenic uveitis that have been given systemic calciferol [21]. Lid closure may prevent the development of these calcific deposits.

DRY EYE SYNDROMES
Rapid development of band keratopathy has been reported in dry eye patients with corneal inflammation who use artificial tears frequently [59]. Whether this corneal change is due to some component of the artificial tears or another mechanism is still unclear. (See Chapter 7.)

MERCURIAL COMPOUNDS
Atypical band keratopathy has been reported in glaucoma patients using pilocarpine with the preservative phenylmercuric nitrate [49, 50]. The reason for this deposition is unclear, and this preservative is no longer used in eyedrops.

COPPER
Copper deposition in the eye may be the result of metabolic diseases or intraocular foreign bodies

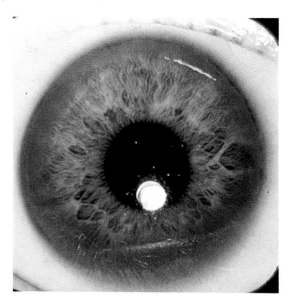

FIGURE 11-15. *Kayser-Fleischer ring in Wilson's disease. (Courtesy G. Smolin, M.D.)*

composed of copper or copper alloys. Hepatolenticular degeneration or Wilson's disease is a deficiency of the copper-binding serum protein ceruloplasmin. This condition is characterized by deposition of free copper in nearly all the body's tissues, especially the liver, basal ganglia of the brain, kidney, and cornea. Patients with Wilson's disease have ataxia, hepatosplenomegaly, cirrhosis of the liver, and progressive neurologic impairment. The disease is inherited as an autosomal recessive trait. Copper excretion is high, but serum copper is low since it is deposited in tissues. The most characteristic ocular feature of Wilson's disease is the Kayser-Fleischer ring in the peripheral cornea (Fig. 11-15). This ring is a deposition of copper 1 to 3 mm in width in the peripheral cornea. It is green, blue, red, yellow brown, or a mixture of any of these colors. There is no lucid interval unless an anterior embryotoxon is present. The ring is at the level of Descemet's membrane. It may be absent below the age of 10, and it may also disappear upon treatment with chelating agents and restricted copper intake. Anterior subcapsular cataracts, sometimes called sunflower cataracts, may be part of the ocular picture of Wilson's disease.

Copper may also be deposited in the cornea in primary biliary cirrhosis, progressive intrahepatic cholestasis of childhood, and chronic active hepatitis [24].

Intraocular foreign bodies of pure copper produce

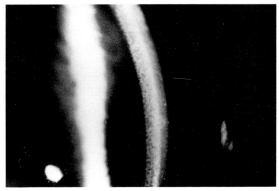

FIGURE 11-17. *Slit lamp photo of silver deposition in the cornea. (Courtesy J. Krachmer, M.D.)*

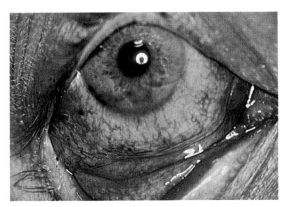

FIGURE 11-16. *Silver deposition in the conjunctiva and cornea. (Courtesy G. Smolin, M.D.)*

a marked suppurative reaction and loss of the eye. Copper alloys containing less than 85 percent copper result in less severe reactions [72, 81]. Intraocular copper produces a blue green discoloration between the endothelium and Descemet's membrane, especially in the peripheral cornea. The iris, vitreous, and lens may also be affected. If electroretinographic changes develop, the copper foreign body should be removed and medical treatment with a chelating agent instituted. Penicillamine 250 mg can be taken orally four times per day for extended periods.

GOLD

Intramuscular gold therapy has been used in the treatment of rheumatoid arthritis and other collagen vascular diseases. The exact therapeutic mode of action is uncertain; however, gold may be capable of inhibiting lysosomal hydrolases. With continued therapy, gold is deposited in various tissues including the kidney, liver, spleen, and eye [11].

Two forms of gold deposition have been reported in the cornea. Corneal chrysiasis consists of numerous, minute, yellowish brown to violet, glistening deposits that are distributed irregularly throughout the cornea at various depths [11, 36, 41]. Sometimes the deposits are described as dustlike and are gold to purple violet in color [80]. Deposits may be seen in the deep stroma or in the epithelium [11]. Occasionally, a vortex distribution can be seen. Most patients receiving an excess of 1500 mg of gold or 25 mg per week for 6 months will demonstrate corneal chrysiasis. Other ocular features include deposition of gold in bulbar conjunctiva and anterior lens capsule. Dermatitis and stomatitis are signs of gold toxicity. Ocular chrysiasis does not usually produce any symptoms, and visual acuity is not ordinarily impaired. A second form of ocular disease caused by gold is a possibly allergic response consisting of marginal ulceration and keratitis [37]. Painful, white, crescent-shaped ulcers bordering the limbus are seen. Distinct, flat, white, superficial opacities have also been noted.

Corneal gold deposition is not necessarily an indication for discontinuing gold therapy. Deposits tend to resolve when gold treatment is stopped and penicillamine appears to be effective for the toxic reactions.

SILVER

Silver deposition in the cornea, conjunctiva, and lens has been observed during the use of topical silver preparations, such as mild silver protein (Argyrol), and after industrial exposure to organic silver salts. Argyrosis is rare today, although a number of cases have been reported [3, 38, 39, 113].

The conjunctiva develops a slate gray appearance (Fig. 11-16). The nasal portion where the tear pool accumulates may be nearly black. The cornea may contain fine, blue gray, green, or gold deposits (Fig. 11-17). These are found in the deep stroma and in Descemet's membrane, especially inferiorly. Electron microscopic examination has shown that minute silver deposits are located intracellularly in the connective tissue of the conjunctiva and extracellularly in Descemet's membrane [39]. Ocular argyrosis produces only cosmetic changes; it does not impair vision. The skin and the eyelids may develop a slate gray hue. Argyrosis of the nasolacrimal sac has been reported [113], and iridescent cataracts have been described as well [3]. Severe silver nitrate injury to the cornea has been reported after use of the concentrated applicator sticks [38]. Obviously, these applicators should not be used around the eye.

REFERENCES

1. Andrade, C. A peculiar form of peripheral neuropathy: Familial atypical generalized amyloidosis with special involvement of peripheral nerves. *Brain* 75:408, 1952.

2. Barnes, H. D., and Boshof, F. P. A. Ocular lesions in patients with porphyria. *Arch. Ophthalmol.* 48:567, 1952.

3. Bartlett, R. E. Generalized argyrosis with lens involvement. *Am. J. Ophthalmol.* 38:402, 1954.

4. Berkow, J. W., Fine, B. S., and Zimmerman, L. E. Unusual ocular calcification in hyperparathyroidism. *Am. J. Ophthalmol.* 66:812, 1968.

5. Berlyne, G. M. Microcrystalline conjunctival calcification in renal failure. *Lancet* 2:366, 1968.

6. Berlyne, G. M., and Shaw, A. B. Red eyes in renal failure. *Lancet* 1:4, 1967.

7. Blodi, F. C., and Apple, D. J. Localized conjunctival amyloidosis. *Am. J. Ophthalmol.* 88:346, 1979.

8. Borit, A., Sugarman, G. I., and Spencer, W. H. Ocular involvement in I-cell disease (mucolipidosis II): Light and electron microscopic findings. *Albrecht Von Graefes Arch. Klin. Ophthalmol.* 198:25, 1976.

9. Boysen, G., et al. Familial amyloidosis with cranial neuropathy and corneal lattice dystrophy. *J. Neurol. Neurosurg. Psychiatry* 42:1020, 1979.

10. Brenner, R. L., et al. Eye signs of hypophosphatasia. *Arch. Ophthalmol.* 81:614, 1969.

11. Bron, A. J., McLendon, B. F., and Camp, A. V. Epithelial deposition of gold in the cornea in patients receiving systemic therapy. *Am. J. Ophthalmol.* 88:354, 1979.

12. Chumbley, L. C. Scleral involvement in symptomatic porphyria. *Am. J. Ophthalmol.* 84:729, 1977.

13. Cogan, D. G., Albright, F., and Bartter, F. C. Hypercalcemia and band keratopathy. *Arch. Ophthalmol.* 40:624, 1948.

14. Cogan, D. G., and Henneman, P. H. Diffuse calcification of the cornea in hypercalcemia. *N. Engl. J. Med.* 257:451, 1957.

15. Cotlier, E. The Cornea. In R. H. Moses (Ed.), *Adler's Physiology of the Eye*. St. Louis: Mosby, 1966.

16. DeFrancisco, M., Savino, P. J., and Schatz, N. J. Optic atrophy in acute intermittent porphyria. *Am. J. Ophthalmol.* 87:221, 1979.

17. DeMars, R., and Leroy, J. G. The remarkable cells cultured from a human with Hurler's syndrome. *In Vitro* 2:107, 1967.

18. Demco, T. A., McCormick, A. G., and Richard, J. S. F. Conjunctival and corneal changes in chronic renal failure. *Can. J. Ophthalmol.* 9:208, 1974.

19. Dodd, M. J., Pusin, S. M., and Green, W. R. Adult cystinosis. *Arch. Ophthalmol.* 96:1054, 1978.

20. Dorfman, A., and Matalon, R. The Mucopolysaccharidoses. In J. B. Stanbury, J. B. Wyngaarden, and D. S. Fredrickson (Eds.), *The Metabolic Basis of Inherited Disease* (3rd ed.). New York: McGraw-Hill, 1972.

21. Doughman, D. J., et al. Experimental band keratopathy. *Arch. Ophthalmol.* 81:264, 1969.

22. Falls, H. F., et al. Ocular manifestations of hereditary primary systemic amyloidosis. *Arch. Ophthalmol.* 54:660, 1955.

23. Fishman, R. S., and Sunderman, F. W. Band keratopathy in gout. *Arch. Ophthalmol.* 75:367, 1966.

24. Fleming, C. R., et al. Pigmented corneal rings in non-Wilsonian liver disease. *Ann. Intern. Med.* 86:285, 1977.

25. Francois, J., Hanssens, M., and Teuchy, H. Corneal ultrastructural changes in Fabry's disease. *Ophthalmologica* 176:313, 1978.

26. Franklin, E. D. Amyloidosis. *Bull. Rheum. Dis.* 26:832, 1976.

27. Fredrickson, D. S., Levy, R. I., and Lees, F. S. Fat transport in lipoproteins—An integrated approach to mechanisms and disorders. *N. Engl. J. Med.* 276:34, 94, 148, 215, 273, 1967.

28. Friedlaender, M. H., and Smolin, G. Corneal degenerations. *Ann. Ophthalmol.* 11:1485, 1974.

29. Gardner, R. J. M., and Hay, J. R. Hurler's syndrome with clear corneas. *Lancet* 2:845, 1974.

30. Garner, A. Amyloidosis of the cornea. *Br. J. Ophthalmol.* 53:73, 1969.

31. Garrod, A. E. The incidence of alkaptonuria: A study in chemical individuality. *Lancet* 2:1616, 1902.

32. Gills, P. J., et al. Electroretinography and fundus oculi findings in Hurler's disease and allied mucopolysaccharidoses. *Arch. Ophthalmol.* 74:596, 1965.

33. Gjone, E., and Bergaust, B. Corneal opacity in familial plasma cholesterol ester deficiency. *Acta Ophthalmol.* (Copenh.) 47:222, 1969.

34. Goldberg, M. F., and Duke, J. R. Ocular histopathology in Hunter's syndrome. *Arch. Ophthalmol.* (Copenh.) 77:503, 1967.

35. Goldberg, M. F., Scott, C. I., and McKusick, V. A. Hydrocephalus and papilledema in the Maroteaux-Lamy syndrome (mucopolysaccharidosis type VI). *Am. J. Ophthalmol.* 69:969, 1970.

36. Gottlieb, N. L., and Major, J. C. Ocular chrysiasis correlated with gold concentrations in the crystalline lens during chrysotherapy. *Arthritis Rheum.* 21:704, 1978.

37. Grant, W. M. *Toxicology of the Eye.* Springfield, Ill.: Thomas, 1974. Pp. 530–533.

38. Grayson, M., and Pieroni, D. Severe silver nitrate injury to the eye. *Am. J. Ophthalmol.* 70:227, 1970.

39. Hanna, C., Fraunfelder, F. T., and Sanchez, J. Ultrastructural study of argyrosis of the cornea and conjunctiva. *Arch. Ophthalmol.* 92:18, 1974.

40. Harris, L. S., et al. Conjunctival and corneal calcific deposits in uremic patients. *Am. J. Ophthalmol.* 72:130, 1971.

41. Hashimoto, A., et al. Corneal chrysiasis. A clinical study in rheumatoid arthritis patients receiving gold therapy. *Arthritis Rheum.* 15:309, 1972.

42. Hoffman, H., II., and Fredrickson, D. S. Tangier disease (familial high-density lipoprotein deficiency): Clinical and genetic features in two adults. *Am. J. Ophthalmol.* 39:582, 1965.

43. Hutchinson, J. The relation of certain diseases of the eye to gout. *Br. Med. J.* 2:995, 1884.

44. Jensen, O. A. Ocular calcifications in primary hyperparathyroidism. *Acta Ophthalmol.* (Copenh.) 53:173, 1975.

45. Kajii, T., et al. Hurler/Scheie genetic compound (mucopolysaccharidosis IH/IS) in Japanese brothers. *Clin. Genet.* 6:394, 1974.

46. Karr, W. J., Jr. Fabry's disease (angiokeratoma corporis diffusum universale). *Am. J. Med.* 27:829, 1959.

47. Kasner, D., et al. Surgical treatment of amyloidosis of the vitreous. *Trans. Am. Acad. Ophthalmol. Otolaryngol.* 72:410, 1968.

48. Kedar, I., et al. Colchicine inhibition of casein induced amyloidosis in mice. *Isr. J. Med. Sci.* 10:787, 1974.

49. Kennedy, R. E., Roca, P. D., and Landers, P. H. Atypical band keratopathy in glaucomatous patients. *Am. J. Ophthalmol.* 72:917, 1972.

50. Kennedy, R. E., Roca, P. D., and Platt, D. S. Further observations on atypical band keratopathy in glaucoma patients. *Trans. Am. Ophthalmol. Soc.* 72:107, 1974.

51. Kenyon, K. R., et al. Mucolipidosis IV: Histopathology of conjunctiva, cornea, and skin. *Arch. Ophthalmol.* 97:1106, 1979.

52. Kenyon, K. R., et al. The systemic mucopolysaccharidoses. *Am. J. Ophthalmol.* 73:811, 1972.

53. Kenyon, K. R., and Sensenbrenner, J. A. Mucolipidosis II (I-cell disease): Ultrastructural observation of conjunctiva and skin. *Invest. Ophthalmol.* 10:555, 1971.

54. Kenyon, K. R., and Sensenbrenner, J. A.

55. Kirk, H. Q., et al. Primary familial amyloidosis of the cornea. *Trans. Am. Acad. Ophthalmol. Otolaryngol.* 77:411, 1973.

56. Knowles, D. M., et al. Amyloidosis of the orbit and adnexa. *Surv. Ophthalmol.* 19:367, 1975.

57. Konigstein, H., and Spiegel, E. A. Muskelatrophie bei Amyloidose. *Neurol. Psychiatr.* (Bucur) 88:220, 1924.

58. La Du, B. N. Alkaptonuria. In J. B. Stanbury, J. B. Wyngaarden, and D. S. Fredrickson (Eds.), *The Metabolic Basis of Inherited Disease* (3rd ed.). New York: McGraw-Hill, 1972. Pp. 308–324.

59. Lemp, M. A., and Ralph, R. A. Rapid development of band keratopathy in dry eyes. *Am. J. Ophthalmol.* 83:657, 1977.

60. Lessell, S., et al. Scalloped pupils in familial amyloidosis. *N. Engl. J. Med.* 293:914, 1975.

61. Libert, J., et al. Ocular findings in I-cell disease (mucolipidosis type II). *Am. J. Ophthalmol.* 83:617, 1977.

62. Lightbody, J., et al. I-cell disease: Multiple lysosomal-enzyme defect. *Lancet* 1:451, 1971.

63. McKusick, V. A. *Heritable Disorders of Connective Tissue* (3rd ed.). St. Louis: Mosby, 1966.

64. McKusick, V. A., et al. The genetic mucopolysaccharidoses. *Medicine* (Baltimore) 44:445, 1965.

65. McPherson, S. D., Kiffney, T. G., Jr., and Freed, C. C. Corneal amyloidosis. *Am. J. Ophthalmol.* 62:1025, 1966.

66. McWilliams, J. R. Ocular findings in gout. *Am. J. Ophthalmol.* 35:1778, 1952.

67. Meretoja, J. Comparative histopathological and clinical findings in eyes with lattice corneal dystrophy of two types. *Ophthalmologica* 165:15, 1972.

68. Merin, S., et al. The cornea in mucolipidosis IV. *J. Pediatr. Ophthalmol.* 13:289, 1976.

69. Mondino, B. J., et al. Protein AA and lattice corneal dystrophy. *Am. J. Ophthalmol.* 89:377, 1980.

70. Nagataki, S., Tanishima, T., and Sakimoto, T. A case of primary gelatinous drop–like corneal dystrophy. *Jpn. J. Ophthalmol.* 16:107, 1972.

71. Newell, F. W., Matalon, R., and Meyer, S. A new mucolipidosis with psychomotor retardation, corneal clouding, and retinal degeneration. *Am. J. Ophthalmol.* 80:440, 1975.

72. Oae, N. A., Tso, M. O. M., and Rosenthal, A. R. Chalcosis in the human eye: A clinicopathologic study. *Arch. Ophthalmol.* 94:1379, 1976.

Electron microscopy of cornea and conjunctiva in childhood cystinosis. *Am. J. Ophthalmol.* 78:68, 1974.

73. O'Connor, G. R. Calcific band keratopathy. *Trans. Am. Ophthalmol. Soc.* 70:58, 1972.

74. Quigley, H. A., and Goldberg, M. F. Conjunctival ultrastructure in mucolipidosis III (pseudo-Hurler polydystrophy). *Invest. Ophthalmol.* 10:568, 1971.

75. Quigley, H. A., Maumenee, A. E., and Stark, W. J. Acute glaucoma in systemic mucopolysaccharidosis I-S. *Am. J. Ophthalmol.* 80:70, 1975.

76. Ramsey, M. S., Fine, B. S., and Cohen, S. W. Localized corneal amyloidosis. *Am. J. Ophthalmol.* 73:560, 1972.

77. Ratnaker, K. S., and Mohan, M. Amyloidosis of the iris. *Can. J. Ophthalmol.* 89:377, 1980.

78. Read, J., et al. Nephropathic cystinosis. *Am. J. Ophthalmol.* 76:791, 1973.

79. Reimann, H. A., Koucky, R. F., and Eklund, C. M. Primary amyloidosis limited to tissue of mesodermal origin. *Am. J. Pathol.* 11:977, 1935.

80. Roberts, W. H., and Wolter, J. R. Ocular chrysiasis. *Arch. Ophthalmol.* 56:48, 1956.

81. Rosenthal, A. R., Appleton, B., and Hopkins, J. L. Intraocular copper foreign bodies. *Am. J. Ophthalmol.* 78:671, 1974.

82. Sanderson, P. O., et al. Cystinosis: A clinical, histopathologic and ultrastructural study. *Arch. Ophthalmol.* 91:270, 1974.

83. Sarino, P. J., Schatz, N. J., and Rodrigues, M. M. Orbital amyloidosis. *Can. J. Ophthalmol.* 11:252, 1976.

84. Scheie, H. G., Hambrick, G. W., Jr., and Barness, L. A. A newly recognized forme fruste of Hurler's disease (gargoylism). *Am. J. Ophthalmol.* 53:753, 1962.

85. Scheinberg, M. A., and Cathcart, E. S. Casein-induced experimental amyloidosis: III. Responses to mitogens, allogeneic cells and graft versus host reactions in the murine model. *Immunology* 27:953, 1974.

86. Schneider, J. A., Wong, V., and Seegmiller, J. E. The early diagnosis of cystinosis. *J. Pediatr.* 74:114, 1969.

87. Sevel, D., and Burger, D. Ocular involvement in cutaneous porphyrias. *Arch. Ophthalmol.* 85:580, 1971.

88. Sher, N. A., Letson, R. D., and Desnick, R. J. The ocular manifestations in Fabry's disease. *Arch. Ophthalmol.* 97:671, 1979.

89. Slansky, H. H., and Kuwabara, T. Intranuclear urate crystals ·in corneal epithelium. *Arch. Ophthalmol.* 80:338, 1969.

90. Sly, W. S., et al. β-glucuronidase deficiency: Report of clinical, radiologic, and biochemical features of a new mucopolysaccharidosis. *J. Pediatr.* 82:249, 1973.

91. Smith, J. W. Ochronosis of the sclera and cornea complicating alkaptonuria: Review of the literature and report of four cases. *JAMA* 120:1282, 1942.

92. Spaeth, G. L., and Frost, P. Fabry's disease. *Arch. Ophthalmol.* 74:760, 1965.

93. Spark, E. D., et al. The identification of amyloid P-component (protein AP) in normal cultured human fibroblasts. *Lab. Invest.* 38:556, 1978.

94. Stafford, W. R., and Fine, B. S. Amyloidosis of the cornea: Report of a case without conjunctival involvement. *Arch. Ophthalmol.* 75:53, 1966.

95. Stock, E. L., and Kielar, R. Primary familial amyloidosis of the cornea. *Am. J. Ophthalmol.* 82:266, 1976.

96. Sugar, J. Corneal manifestations of the systemic mucopolysaccharidoses. *Am. Ophthalmol.* 11:531, 1979.

97. Süveges, I. Histological and ultrastructural studies of the cornea in Maroteaux-Lamy syndrome. *Albrecht Von Graefes Arch. Klin. Exp. Ophthalmol.* 212:29, 1979.

98. Tabone, E., et al. Ultrastructural aspects of corneal fibrous tissue in Scheie syndrome. *Virchows Arch.* [*Cell Pathol.*] 27:63, 1978.

99. Topping, T. M., et al. Ultrastructural ocular pathology of Hunter's syndrome. *Arch. Ophthalmol.* 86:164, 1971.

100. Tremblay, M., Dube, I., and Gagne, R. Alterations de la cornée dans la maladie de Scheie. *J. Fr. Ophtalmol.* 2:193, 1979.

101. Van Pelt, J. F., and Huizinga, J. Some observations on the genetics of gargoylism. *Acta Genet.* 12:1, 1962.

102. Vinger, P. F., and Sachs, B. A. Ocular manifestations of hyperlipoproteinemia. *Am. J. Ophthalmol.* 70:563, 1970.

103. Von Noorden, G. K., Zellweger, H., and Ponseti, I. V. Ocular findings in Morquio-Ullrich's disease. *Arch. Ophthalmol.* 64:137, 1960.

104. Walsh, F. B., and Hoyt, W. F. *Clinical Neuro-ophthalmology* (3rd ed.). Baltimore: Williams & Wilkins, 1969. P. 811.

105. Weber, F. L., and Babel, J. Gelatinous drop–like dystrophy. *Arch. Ophthalmol.* 98:144, 1980.

106. Weingeist, T. A., and Blodi, F. D. Fabry's disease: Ocular findings in a female carrier. *Arch. Ophthalmol.* 85:169, 1971.

107. Weve, H. J. M. *Uric Acid Keratitis and Other Ocular Findings in Gout.* Rotterdam: W. J. Van Hengel, 1924.

108. Wolter, J. R., Clark, R. L., and Kallet, H. A. Ocular involvement in acute intermittent porphyria. *Am. J. Ophthalmol.* 74:666, 1972.

109. Wong, V. G., Lietman, P. E., and Seegmiller, J. E. Alterations of pigment epithelium in cystinosis. *Arch. Ophthalmol.* 77:361, 1967.

110. Wong, V. G., Schulman, J. D., and Seegmiller, J. E. Conjunctival biopsy for the biochemical diagnosis of cystinosis. *Am. J. Ophthalmol.* 70:278, 1970.

111. Wood, T. O., and Walker, G. G. Treatment of band keratopathy. *Am. J. Ophthalmol.* 80:553, 1975.

112. Yamamoto, G. K., et al. Long-term ocular changes in cystinosis: Observations in renal transplant recipients. *J. Pediatr. Ophthalmol.* 16:21, 1979.

113. Yanoff, M., and Scheie, H. G. Argyrosis of the conjunctiva and lacrimal sac. *Arch. Ophthalmol.* 72:57, 1964.

114. Zimmerman, T. J., Hood, I., and Gasset, A. F. "Adolescent" cystinosis. *Arch. Ophthalmol.* 92:265, 1974.

12. CORNEAL TUMORS

Devron H. Char

This chapter reviews the diagnosis and management of acquired benign and malignant corneal mass lesions. Primary tumors of the cornea are extraordinarily rare; most benign or potentially malignant corneal masses occur as a result of conjunctival or limbal tumors that secondarily involve the corneal epithelium or stroma. Congenital corneal tumors are discussed in Chapter 10. In order of frequency, the most common acquired masses at the limbus are pterygium, pseudopterygium, papilloma, and conjunctival melanoma. Other tumors can rarely involve the limbus or the cornea. These include epithelial cysts, pyogenic granuloma, keratocanthoma, adenoma, fibroma, fibrochondroma, fibrous histiocytoma, angioma, lymphangioma, alveolar endothelioma, neurolemmoma, malignant schwannoma, mycosis fungoides, juvenile xanthogranuloma, leukemia, dermoid, episcleral osseous choristoma, ectopic lacrimal tissue, lipoma, amyloid, blue nevus, and nevi [5, 11–13, 16, 21, 26, 35, 38, 55]. There are no pathognomonic findings with these rare tumors; with the exception of neurofibroma in conjunction with von Recklinghausen's disease or metastatic corneal tumors, the clinical history and appearance are not helpful in distinguishing these tumors from more common causes of corneal mass lesions.

BENIGN CORNEAL TUMORS

PTERYGIUM

PATHOGENESIS
The cause of pterygia is unclear. Epidemiologically, these lesions occur most frequently in populations living near the equator [41]. The common denominator appears to be exposure to ultraviolet radiation; however, other environmental factors such as heat, dry atmosphere, high winds, and abundant dust may also be important inciting factors [10].

Supported in part by a grant from That Man May See and NIH grants EY01441, EY01759, and EY03675. Dr. Char is a recipient of a NIH Research Career Development Award (K04 EY00117).

Although environmental factors play an important role in causing pterygia, the pathophysiologic mechanisms in their development remain unclear. Trantas and Barraquer suggested that conjunctival degenerative changes cause an uneven tear film at the limbus and peripheral cornea; corneal dellen develop, and the inflamed conjunctival tissues secondarily cover this "injured" corneal area [2, 52]. Pterygia occur much more commonly in the nasal than the temporal portion of the conjunctiva, and this is consistent with the above hypothesis.

CLINICAL FEATURES

Pterygia usually involve the nasal portion of the bulbar conjunctiva in the interpalpebral fissure. They consist of thickened, inflamed, fibrovascular conjunctival tissue that involves the limbus and may extend onto the cornea.

A fully developed pterygium almost never involves more than one-half of the cornea (Fig. 12-1). These lesions have a triangular, blunt apex, and usually there are small irregular opacities at the level of Bowman's membrane. Immediately anterior to these opacities is Stocker's line, which probably results from hemosiderin deposition [49]. When a pterygium is active, growing, and inflamed, the tissue is red and fibrovascular; as the pterygium becomes inactive, vascularity diminishes and the redness disappears.

PATHOLOGIC FINDINGS

Histologically, pterygia have changes consistent with solar elastosis. Collagen is degenerated; the fibers are hypertrophic and hyalinized and may have some granular basophilic degenerative material [18].

DIFFERENTIAL DIAGNOSIS

A number of other lesions can simulate pterygia, and pterygia can occasionally simulate a conjunctival malignancy. Any peripheral corneal inflammation, infection, or dystrophy can cause a superficial overgrowth of conjunctival tissue. These pseudopterygia usually occur in areas other than the interpalpebral fissure, and there is a history of peripheral corneal disease. Both pterygia and pinguecula can have a leukoplakic appearance; occasionally, conjunctival carcinoma develops in the area of a pterygium (Fig. 12-2).

TREATMENT

Therapeutic intervention (surgery, chemotherapy, or irradiation) in the management of pterygia

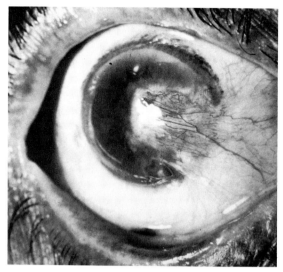

FIGURE 12-1. *A pterygium.*

should be judicious; there is a 30 to 50 percent incidence of recurrence, depending on environmental factors [10, 41]. Lesions that present only a marginal cosmetic problem can often be managed with the use of sunglasses to diminish ultraviolet exposure and prevent further progression over the corneal surface. Relative indications for surgery include periodic inflammation, cosmetic defect, persistent vascularity, and documented growth. Absolute indications include visual disability because of either opacification of the central cornea or major irregular astigmatism and the development of diplopia caused by traction by the pterygium.

A myriad of surgical techniques have been proposed for the management of pterygia [10]. These include, among others, the bare sclera technique, excision with simple closure of the wound, excision with repair using a movable conjunctival flap, graft of free conjunctiva, mucous membrane graft, skin graft, or other transplantation procedures in which the head of the pterygium is dissected off the cornea and moved elsewhere.

I have used a graded approach to the management of pterygia. In patients who are constantly exposed to environmental factors, small pterygia (with less than 1–2 mm of cornea involved) are treated with sunglasses; the cosmetic removal of such lesions if the patient is constantly in the sunlight usually results in a recurrence. Patients with progressively growing pterygia and those with either threatened vision or diplopia are treated with a simple excision of the pterygia using the operating microscope. The corneal surface from which the pterygium is removed is "polished" with a diamond

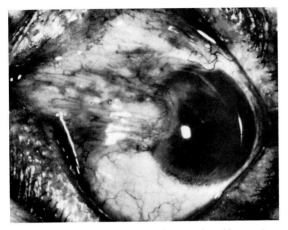

FIGURE 12-2. *Carcinoma in situ in the area of an old pterygium.*

burr or a scalpel to provide a more even surface for the tear film. In addition, the sclera adjacent to the corneal defect is scraped, and all of the vessels are gently cauterized to diminish the vascularity in the area. A bare scleral zone is created at the limbus and beyond by recessing the conjunctiva 2 to 3 mm and tacking it in this position with 8-0 nylon sutures. Careful attention to a smooth residual surface and the absence of vessels decreases the likelihood of a recurrence after surgery. Patients are given topical steroids and topical triethylenethiophosphoramide (Thiotepa 1:2000) every 6 hours for 6 weeks. Triethylenethiophosphoramide is unstable and must be refrigerated and replaced weekly. The patients are examined weekly to determine if they are steroid responders. Triethylenethiophosphoramide is an excellent adjunct in the management of pterygia; however, especially in dark-skinned patients, there is a major risk of skin depigmentation. I have not observed any of the hematologic complications that can occur when this agent is used parenterally. Patients are advised to avoid excess sun exposure and use sunglasses after removal of their pterygia.

Patients referred with a recurrent pterygium are managed differently, depending on the number of recurrences and their current environmental status. In a patient who has had only one recurrence, the above surgical technique is used plus beta radiation with 2000 to 4000 rads from strontium 90 applicators. I usually use 3 applications of 1000 rads per session. Steroid and triethylenethiophosphoramide drops are instituted after irradiation. The recurrence rate after surgery and irradiation is reported to be between 5 and 16 percent [8].

In patients who have had multiple recurrent pterygia unresponsive to the above techniques, I have attempted to remove the pterygia using a lamellar keratectomy and then covered the corneal

and scleral defect with a corneal-scleral lamellar graft. Although donor tissue obtained from the central cornea will usually remain clear over the central portion of the recipient bed and become opaque over the sclera, I have obtained a better cosmetic result when corneal and scleral lamellar donor material is obtained to match the ratio of corneal and scleral defect created during the removal of the pterygium [40]. This graft should be sutured with either interrupted or running 10-0 nylon sutures and both triethylenethiophosphoramide and topical steroids used as described. I believe this technique offers the best cosmetic result and the lowest incidence of recurrence for refractory pterygia.

PAPILLOMAS

CLINICAL FEATURES
Conjunctival papillomas have a predilection for the limbus, caruncle, and lid margin (Fig. 12-3) [11]. The majority of papillomas are caused by viruses; these papillomas usually occur as multiple lesions in young people. Conjunctival carcinoma can simulate a papilloma; carcinoma usually occurs as a single conjunctival lesion in older patients. Clinical differentiation between viral and nonviral papillomas can be difficult [54]. In contradistinction to noninfectious papillomas, viral papillomas are often pedunculated, have a smooth surface, are multiple or bilateral, are transmissible, and may have associated epithelial keratitis. Noninfectious papillomas are unilateral, single, and often either sessile or diffuse and have an irregular surface with corneal involvement only by direct extension. A papilloma occurring at the limbus can spread onto the cornea as a reddish gray elevated lesion.

PATHOLOGIC FINDINGS
Histologically, papillomas consist of a central core of connective tissue covered by proliferating stratified epithelium. It can sometimes be difficult to distinguish between a viral and a malignant papilloma on histologic examination; occasionally, sufficient fibrous tissue is present to simulate a fibroma [17]. Papillomas almost always remain superficial and do not invade the corneal stroma.

TREATMENT
In viral papillomas, a period of observation of at least 6 months is indicated before intervention; often these lesions will spontaneously involute. The usual treatment of solitary conjunctival papillomas involving the limbus is surgical. When the cornea is

involved, the lesion may be shaved off because there is usually an easily defined surgical plane between the lesion and the cornea at or above Bowman's membrane; a lamellar keratoplasty is usually not necessary. Viral lesions have a tendency to be multiple and to recur. In some cases, surgical excision with cautery of the base is not sufficient to destroy the tumor. Although radiation therapy has been advocated by some authors, complications including corneal vascularization and opacification limit its use as a treatment of this benign disease [4, 9, 27]. Cryosurgery has been used successfully by some investigators to treat viral and malignant papillomas [3, 17]. In resistant cases, topical chemotherapeutic drugs or immunostimulants (dinitrochlorobenzene) may be a useful adjunct. The management of conjunctival carcinoma, which may present as a papilloma clinically, is covered in a subsequent section of this chapter.

MALIGNANT CORNEAL TUMORS

Corneal melanomas and carcinomas almost always occur as a result of contiguous spread from a limbal or bulbar conjunctival neoplasm [7]. Although rare cases of allegedly primary corneal melanomas have been reported, almost all malignant tumors involving the cornea arise from conjunctival elements that either are present at the limbus or migrate onto the cornea as a result of inflammation and secondary pseudopterygium formation [39]. As a general rule, almost all neoplasms involve only the superficial corneal layers; it is distinctly unusual for either a melanoma or a squamous cell carcinoma to invade either the corneal stroma or the intraocular structures.

CORNEAL MELANOMA

Corneal melanomas are rare; although a few case reports exist, most oncologists believe that melanomas of the cornea develop either as a result of contiguous spread from a conjunctival melanoma or as a result of malignant degeneration of melanocytes that have migrated onto the corneal surface from the limbus. Conjunctival melanomas account for approximately 2 percent of eye malignancies [46]. The rarity of both conjunctival and corneal melanomas has resulted in insufficient data on which to base definitive statements on the cause, pathogenesis, or management of pigmented conjunctival and corneal neoplasms [7].

PATHOGENESIS
Probably about one-half of conjunctival melanomas arise de novo; the other half arise equally from nevi

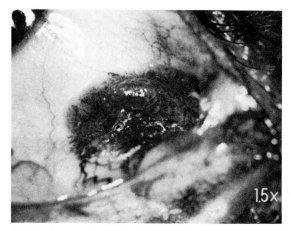

FIGURE 12-3. *Conjunctival papilloma.*

or as a result of malignant degeneration of acquired melanosis [22, 24, 30, 47]. Epidemiologic studies of cutaneous melanomas show that sun exposure plays an important role in their development; similar studies in ocular melanomas have not conclusively demonstrated the importance of ultraviolet radiation in their pathogenesis [46].

CLINICAL FEATURES
The vast majority of corneal melanomas occur either as a single large tumor at the limbus (Fig. 12-4) or as a diffuse superficial lesion secondary to malignant degeneration of acquired melanosis. The latter type occurs either as a fungating mass or as a thin sheet of melanocytic tissue across the superficial cornea (Fig. 12-5). In a patient with a pigmented corneal mass lesion, conjunctival scrapings or biopsy or both should yield a definitive diagnosis.

DIFFERENTIAL DIAGNOSIS
Most of the lesions that can simulate a conjunctival melanoma elsewhere in the bulbar conjunctiva do not present diagnostic difficulties at the limbus. Melanosis oculi, oculodermal melanocytosis, argyrosis, trachoma, exposure to toxins (radiation or arsenic), or certain systemic conditions (pregnancy or Addison's disease) usually do not simulate a corneal or limbal melanoma. Occasionally, exposure to manganese or epinephrine or corneal tattooing either after foreign-body injury or to camouflage a corneal scar may mimic a pigmented corneal neoplasm [36]. Conjunctival nevi or blue nevus at the limbus can also mimic a corneal melanoma; nevi often have microcysts visible on slit lamp biomicroscopy, whereas melanomas never do. Acquired melanosis may also involve the limbus and may be difficult to differentiate from a melanoma. Patients develop acquired epithelial melanosis insidiously

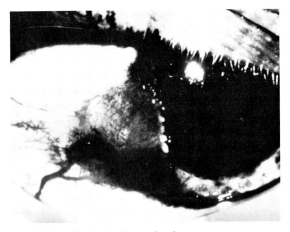

FIGURE 12-4. *Conjunctival-corneal melanoma.*

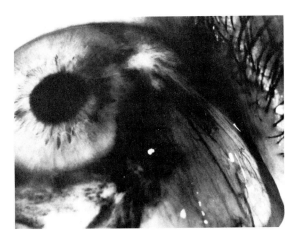

FIGURE 12-5. *Malignant degeneration of acquired melanosis.*

during middle age; approximately 17 percent of cases undergo malignant degeneration [43]. The clinical course of acquired melanosis is extraordinarily varied. Areas of conjunctival and limbal pigmentation can disappear, new areas can crop up, and other areas may develop a malignant degeneration. Since approximately 17 percent of patients with acquired melanosis develop frank melanoma, frequent careful serial examinations should be performed [56]. Although some authors believe that early histologic changes are quite useful prognostically, this hypothesis has not been proved [22]. In patients who develop new vessels, discrete tumor thickening, inflammation, or the spread of diffuse disconnected pigment, a biopsy should be performed.

TREATMENT

The relative rarity of conjunctival and especially corneal melanomas precludes definitive management guidelines. Conjunctival melanoma usually occurs in later life; rarely, it develops in patients in their late teens. A biopsy should be done of suspicious lesions; this does not adversely affect prognosis. At present, there are no statistically significant data, even in the relatively more common conjunctival melanomas, that demonstrate the superiority of any type of therapeutic modality in the management of these lesions. Most patients with conjunctival melanomas less than 1.5 mm thick do well regardless of the type of therapy employed [47].

I have treated conjunctival and corneal melanomas as follows: In any suspicious pigmented lesion, I attempt an excisional biopsy; if the margins are free of tumor, no further therapy is undertaken. If I am unable to remove the entire tumor with adequate margins, I treat the area of microscopic tumor extension with either beta radiation using approxi-

mately 6000 to 10,000 rads over a 5-week course or double–freeze-thaw cryotherapy [23]. The use of beta radiation has the lowest incidence of x-ray complications; however, marked morbidity can occur, especially in corneal lesions. The complication rate with irradiation of conjunctival melanomas has been reported to be between 5 and 12 percent [28, 29, 33, 51]. If there is obvious tumor present or multiple areas of involvement of both the cornea and bulbar conjunctiva, orthovoltage radiation or more extensive beta radiation is probably indicated.

In acquired melanosis with malignant degeneration, there can often be areas of melanoma involving the limbus with a thin spread of tumor onto the corneal surface. Usually the corneal portion can be peeled off the cornea using a microsurgical dissection technique. In such cases, I have not performed a lamellar keratoplasty but have instead simply excised the area and treated the superficial cornea with cryotherapy.

In bulky melanomas occurring at the limbus, gonioscopy and examination of the posterior pole should be performed. Gow and Spencer have observed patients in whom corneal-conjunctival melanomas had entered the anterior chamber and even diffusely involved the posterior choroid [15]. In patients with lesions such as shown in Figure 12-6, an excision of the tumor with a lamellar keratoplasty and partial thickness scleral dissection should be performed.

I have not used radiation as a primary means of therapy in corneal-conjunctival melanomas except in patients with diffuse malignant degeneration of acquired conjunctival melanosis. Similarly, my experience with cryotherapy in the management of conjunctival and corneal melanomas is limited. At

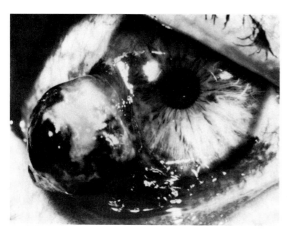

FIGURE 12-6. *Large conjunctival-corneal melanoma. This tumor eventually involved the entire uveal tract.*

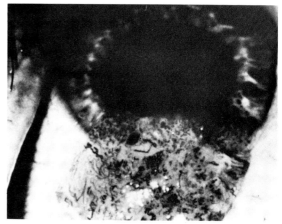

FIGURE 12-7. *Conjunctival carcinoma with typical gelatinous strawberry fronds.*

present, I have chosen to use cryotherapy only as an adjunct to surgery to treat a margin around an area of excised melanoma.

The role of exenteration in the management of conjunctival and corneal melanoma is unclear. Some authors have questioned the efficacy of this technique in prolonging survival in any patient, especially those with large conjunctival melanomas. I have been inclined to use this technique in patients with tumors invading the orbital or intraocular structures or with a large recurrence after surgery and irradiation. The effect of exenteration on the natural history and prognosis of conjunctival melanomas is unclear. Conjunctival melanoma can metastasize to local lymph nodes, bone, liver, and brain [15, 44]. Before a mutilating procedure such as an exenteration, a thorough physical examination, body and brain computed tomographic studies, bone survey, and blood tests for liver involvement (lactate dehydrogenase) should be performed. In patients with diffuse conjunctival melanoma, enucleation is not a reasonable therapeutic option since the entire conjunctiva is at risk for the development of further tumors.

The prognosis in conjunctival melanoma is generally favorable. Patients with malignant degeneration of acquired melanosis have a slightly worse prognosis that those with localized conjunctival tumors [25, 32, 44]. The combined 5-year mortality of all types of conjunctival melanomas is approximately 22 percent. Patients with diffuse melanoma secondary to acquired melanosis have a five-year mortality between 20 and 30 percent. Those with localized tumors have a 17 percent five-year mortality.

SQUAMOUS CELL CARCINOMA OF THE CONJUNCTIVA

The nomenclature regarding conjunctival tumors is confusing. *Bowen's disease, dyskeratosis,* and *leukoplakia* have been used interchangeably to denote carcinoma in situ (intraepithelial epitheliomas). *Bowen's disease* is not applicable to conjunctival tumors; patients with Bowen's disease have a significant incidence of visceral malignancies, and this has not been observed in patients with squamous cell carcinoma of the conjunctiva [34]. *Leukoplakia* denotes a white plaque of the conjunctiva; these are also frequently observed in nonmalignant lesions. Pizzarello and Jakobiec have suggested *conjunctival intraepithelial neoplasia* to substitute for these other terms [42]; given the previous confusion, this change in nomenclature may prove beneficial. Squamous cell carcinoma of the conjunctiva with secondary involvement of the cornea is the most frequent nonpigmented malignant conjunctival and corneal tumor.

CLINICAL FEATURES

Advanced conjunctival squamous cell carcinomas at the limbus have an almost pathognomonic appearance (Fig. 12-7). These lesions appear gelatinous with strawberrylike fronds of blood vessels on their surface.

Conjunctival carcinomas commonly develop in the limbal area in the interpalpebral fissure. Older patients are typically affected; the majority of patients are over age 60 when they develop either conjunctival intraepithelial neoplasia or frank conjunctival carcinoma. In any patient with a chronic

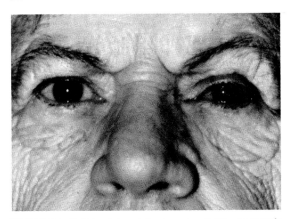

FIGURE 12-8. *Unilateral chronic keratoconjunctivitis-masquerade syndrome (squamous cell carcinoma of the conjunctiva).*

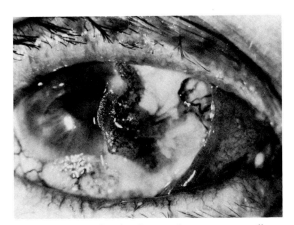

FIGURE 12-9. *Corneal perforation secondary to squamous cell carcinoma of the conjunctiva.*

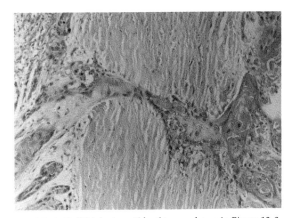

FIGURE 12-10. *Histologic section of tumor shown in Figure 12-9.*

unilateral keratoconjunctivitis refractory to therapy (Fig. 12-8), a conjunctival carcinoma should be suspected. Conjunctival scrapings in the area of the lesions will often demonstrate the presence of bizarre cells with large clumped nuclei, which is highly suggestive of malignancy [48]. Often the lesions will stain with rose bengal, although this staining pattern may be nonspecific [53].

PATHOLOGIC FINDINGS
Histologically, squamous cell carcinoma involving the conjunctiva and the cornea appears quite malignant; metastatic disease as a result of either conjunctival intraepithelial neoplasia or frank squamous cell carcinoma is very rare. In the American literature, there are only 3 reported cases of tumor-related deaths from these entities, and in only 1 has metastatic death been documented by postmortem examination [1, 6, 19, 20].

TREATMENT
The treatment of conjunctival and corneal squamous cell carcinoma is predicated on two factors: These tumors have very little metastatic potential, and they have a high rate of recurrence if they are incompletely excised.

The treatment of conjunctival and corneal intraepithelial neoplasia or frank malignancy is with an excisional biopsy. Lesions that involve the cornea secondary to pagetoid spread can usually be excised under the microscope without the need for a lamellar keratoplasty [14]. Suspicious residual areas of superficial corneal tumors are treated with single-freeze cryotherapy without thermocouple monitoring. Frozen section control should be used in the surgical removal of limbal tumors since the recurrence rate in incompletely excised conjunctival car-

cinomas approaches 35 percent [6, 20, 45]. In patients treated by local excision obtaining tumor-free margins, the recurrence rate is less than 5 percent. In lesions that cannot be adequately excised in the cornea or in which the borders of the surgical resection are not free of tumor, either beta radiation or cryotherapy is a reasonable adjunct.

Before surgical resection of conjunctival carcinoma involving either the limbus or the cornea, a gonioscopic examination should be performed. Four cases in which there was either microscopic or frank invasion of the eye secondary to the conjunctival corneal tumor have been reported [31, 37, 50]. Figure 12-9 shows a spontaneous corneal perforation secondary to a squamous cell carcinoma. A histologic section of this lesion is shown in Figure 12-10.

Enucleation or exenteration is almost never indicated for squamous cell carcinoma involving the conjunctiva or the cornea. The indication for these procedures is limited to tumor involving the intraocular structures or the orbit, which is quite rare.

REFERENCES

1. Ash, J. E., and Wilder, H. C. Epithelial tumors of the limbus. *Am. J. Ophthalmol.* 25:926, 1942.
2. Barraquer, J. I. Etiologia y patogenia del pterigiom y de las excavaciones de la cornea de Fuchs. *Arch. Soc. Am. Oftal. Optom.* 5:45, 1964.
3. Beard, C. B. Cryosurgery in the Treatment of Eyelid Tumors. In A. Hornblass (Ed.), *Tumors of the Ocular Adnexa and Orbit.* St. Louis: Mosby, 1979. Pp. 147–152.
4. Bell, L. G. Conjunctival papillomata. *Trans. Ophthalmol. Soc. N.Z.* 14:46, 1962.
5. Boudet, C., et al. Naevus bleu à localisation limbique: Évolution anatomique et attitude therapeutique. *Bull. Soc. Ophtalmol. Fr.* 77:867, 1977.
6. Carroll, J. M., and Kuwabara, T. A classification of limbal epitheliomas. *Arch. Ophthalmol.* 73:545, 1965.
7. Char, D. H. The management of lid and conjunctival malignancies. *Surv. Ophthalmol.* 14:679, 1980.
8. Cooper, J. S. Postoperative irradiation of pterygia: Ten more years of experience. *Radiology* 128:753, 1978.
9. Doherty, W. B. Ocular papilloma. *Am. J. Ophthalmol.* 15:1016, 1932.
10. Duke-Elder, S. Diseases of the Outer Eye. In S. Duke-Elder (Ed.), *System of Ophthalmology.* St. Louis: Mosby, 1965. Vol. 8, Pt. 1, pp. 573–585.
11. Duke-Elder, S. Diseases of the Outer Eye. In S. Duke-Elder (Ed.), *System of Ophthalmology.* St. Louis: Mosby, 1965. Vol. 8, Pt. 1, pp. 1137–1242.
12. Emamy, H., and Ahmadian, H. Limbal dermoid with ectopic brain tissue. *Arch. Ophthalmol.* 95:2201, 1977.
13. Faludi, J. E., Kenyon, K., and Green, W. R. Fibrous histiocytoma of the corneoscleral limbus. *Am. J. Ophthalmol.* 80:619, 1975.
14. Freedman, J., and Rohm, G. Surgical management and histopathology of invasive tumours of the cornea. *Br. J. Ophthalmol.* 63:632, 1979.
15. Gow, J. A., and Spencer, W. H. Intraocular extension of an epibulbar malignant melanoma. *Arch. Ophthalmol.* 90:57, 1973.
16. Grayson, M. *Disease of the Cornea.* St. Louis: Mosby, 1979. Pp. 501–513.
17. Harkey, M. E., and Metz, H. S. Cryotherapy of the conjunctival papillomata. *Am. J. Ophthalmol.* 66:872, 1968.
18. Hogan, M. J., and Zimmerman, L. E. *Ophthalmic Pathology: An Atlas and Textbook* (2nd ed.). Philadelphia: Saunders, 1962. Pp. 253–254.
19. Iliff, W. J., Marback, R., and Green, W. R. Invasive squamous cell carcinoma of the conjunctiva. *Arch. Ophthalmol.* 93:119, 1975.
20. Irvine, A. R., Jr. Dyskeratotic epibulbar tumors. *Trans. Am. Ophthalmol. Soc.* 61:243, 1963.
21. Jakobiec, F. A. Fibrous histiocytoma of the corneoscleral limbus. *Am. J. Ophthalmol.* 78:700, 1974.
22. Jakobiec, F. A. Conjunctival melanoma: Unfinished business. *Arch. Ophthalmol.* 98:1378, 1980.
23. Jakobiec, F. A., et al. Combined surgery and cryotherapy for diffuse melanoma of the conjunctiva. *Arch. Ophthalmol.* 98:1390, 1980.
24. Jay, B. A follow-up study of limbal melanomata. *Proc. R. Soc. Med.* 57:497, 1964.
25. Jay, B. Naevi and melanomata of the conjunctiva. *Br. J. Ophthalmol.* 49:169, 1965.
26. Kessing, S. V. Ectopic lacrimal gland tissue at the corneal limbus (glands of Manz). *Acta Ophthalmol.* (Copenh.) 46:398, 1966.
27. Koellner, S. Epithelial new formation at the corneal limbus which recurred for five years and was finally cured with mesothorium. *Arch. Ophthalmol.* 46:130, 1917.
28. Lederman, M. Radiotherapy of malignant melanomata of the eye. *Br. J. Radiol.* 34:21, 1961.
29. Lederman, M. Discussion of Pigmented Tumors of the Conjunctiva. In M. Boniuk (Ed.), *Ocular and Adnexal Tumors.* St. Louis: Mosby, 1964. Pp. 24–48.
30. Lewis, P. M., and Zimmerman, L. E. Delayed recurrences of malignant melanomas of the bulbar conjunctiva. *Am. J. Ophthalmol.* 45:536, 1958.
31. Li, W. W., Pettit, T. H., and Zakka, K. A. Intraocular invasion by papillary squamous cell carcinoma of the conjunctiva. *Am. J. Ophthalmol.* 90:697, 1980.
32. Liesegang, T. J., and Campbell, R. J. Mayo Clinic experience with conjunctival melanomas. *Arch. Ophthalmol.* 98:1385, 1980.
33. Lommatzsch, P. K. Beta-ray treatment of malignant epibulbar melanoma. *Albrecht Von Graefes Arch. Klin. Exp. Ophthalmol.* 29:111, 1978.
34. McGavic, J. S. Intraepithelial epithelioma of the cornea and conjunctiva (Bowen's disease). *Am. J. Ophthalmol.* 25:167, 1942.
35. Minckler, D. Pyogenic granuloma of the cornea simulating squamous cell carcinoma. *Arch. Ophthalmol.* 97:516, 1979.
36. Nicholson, D. H. Epibulbar Tumors. In *Ocular Pathology Update.* New York: Masson, 1980. Pp. 253–259.
37. Nicholson, D. H., and Herschler, J. Intraocu-

lar extension of squamous cell carcinoma of the conjunctiva. *Arch. Ophthalmol.* 95:843, 1977.

38. Nicolitz, E. Kaposi's sarcoma of the conjunctiva. *Ann. Ophthalmol.* 13:205, 1981.

39. Niedobitek, F. Der melanotische Tumor der Kornea. *Klin. Monatsbl. Augenheilkd.* 144:540, 1964.

40. Paton, D. Pterygia management based upon a theory of pathogenesis. *Trans. Am. Acad. Ophthalmol. Otolaryngol.* 79:603, 1975.

41. Pico, G. Pterygium: Current Concept of Etiology and Management. In J. H. King, Jr., and J. W. McTigue (Eds.), *First World Congress on the Cornea.* London: Butterworths, 1965. Pp. 280–291.

42. Pizzarello, L. D., and Jakobiec, F. A. Bowen's Disease of the Conjunctiva: A Misnomer. In F. A. Jakobiec (Ed.), *Ocular and Adnexal Tumors.* Birmingham, Ala.: Aesculapius, 1978. Pp. 553–571.

43. Reese, A. B. Precancerous and cancerous melanosis. *Am. J. Ophthalmol.* 61:1272, 1966.

44. Reese, A. B. *Tumors of the Eye* (3rd ed.). Hagerstown, Md.: Harper & Row, 1976. P. 257.

45. Sanders, N., and Bedotto, C. Recurrent carcinoma in situ of the conjunctiva and cornea (Bowen's disease). *Am. J. Ophthalmol.* 74:688, 1972.

46. Scotto, J., Fraumeni, J. F., and Lee, J. A. H. Melanomas of the eye and other noncutaneous sites: Epidemiologic aspects. *J. Natl. Cancer Inst.* 56:489, 1976.

47. Silvers, D. N., et al. Melanoma of the Conjunctiva: A Clinical Pathologic Study. In F. A. Jakobiec (Ed.), *Ocular and Adnexal Tumors.* Birmingham, Ala.: Aesculapius, 1978. Pp. 585–599.

48. Spinak, N., and Friedman, A. H. Squamous cell carcinoma of the conjunctiva: Value of exfoliative cytology and diagnosis. *Surv. Ophthalmol.* 21:351, 1977.

49. Stocker, F. W. Eine pigmentierte Hornhautlinie beim Pterygium. *Klin. Monatsbl. Augenheilkd.* 102:384, 1939.

50. Stokes, J. J. Intraocular extension of epibulbar squamous cell carcinoma of the limbus. *Trans. Am. Acad. Ophthalmol. Otolaryngol.* 59:143, 1955.

51. Ten Napel, J. A. Conjunctival melanoma: A retrospective study. *Ophthalmology* (Rochester) 42:321, 1977.

52. Trantas, N. G. Sur une nouvelle keratopathie par déshydration locale. *Bull. Mem. Soc. Fr. Ophtalmol.* 42:401, 1955.

53. Wilson, F. M., II. Rose bengal staining of epibulbar squamous neoplasms. *Ophthalmic Surg.* 7:21, 1976.

54. Wilson, F. M., II, and Ostler, H. B. Conjunctival papillomas in siblings. *Am. J. Ophthalmol.* 77:103, 1974.

55. Wolter, J. R., Leenhouts, T. M., and Hendrix, R. C. Corneal involvement in mycosis fungoides. *Am. J. Ophthalmol.* 55:317, 1963.

56. Zimmerman, L. E. Criteria for management of melanosis. *Arch. Ophthalmol.* 76:307, 1966.

13. DIETARY DEFICIENCY

Richard A. Thoft

In most developed countries, dietary deficiencies only rarely produce clinical disease, but they are an important factor in the production of systemic and ocular disease in much of the world. By far the most common ocular problems are those related to vitamin A deficiency and associated protein-energy malnutrition. Only recently have reliable estimates of the magnitude of nutritional eye disease in certain populations become available [40]; these indicate wide variability in the prevalence of ocular manifestations. Nevertheless, hundreds of thousands of preschool children may be afflicted each year with potentially blinding disease as a result of poor nutrition.

This chapter is designed to acquaint ophthalmologists with the most important nutritional ocular disease, that associated with vitamin A deficiency. A review of all the details of vitamin A absorption, transport, and cellular function is beyond the scope of this chapter, but a brief discussion is included. The conventional classification of xerophthalmia and keratomalacia is included, with illustrations of some of the more common clinical manifestations. Finally, therapy for and prevention of nutritional eye disease are discussed.

TYPES OF MALNUTRITION

Two categories of malnutrition in children have been associated with specific clinical syndromes. These are marasmus, a generalized protein-energy deficiency, and kwashiorkor, which is associated primarily with protein deficiency. Both of these clinical entities are seen most frequently in the age group from weaning to 6 years of age. One or the other of these types of malnutrition is almost always associated with the ocular findings of vitamin A deficiency in children.

MARASMUS

If competition for food within the family group or widespread famine leads to chronic deficiency of all food categories, the result is marasmus, a dramatic manifestation of starvation in young children. As shown in Figure 13-1A, children so afflicted are small and poorly developed. There is failure to develop body fat, wastage of muscle, decreased muscle tone, loss of skin elasticity, and mental dullness. There is little animation, with weak cries and little response to stimulation. The eyes are staring, with a low blink rate.

The prognosis for children with marasmus is poor. Even if the deficiency is relieved in a hospital setting, when the child returns to the home the same factors that led to starvation in the first place are still at work. It has been estimated that, in some areas, at least 40 percent of children who are treated for marasmus will ultimately die of starvation. Such children are also at high risk for the development of specific deficiency states, such as vitamin A deficiency. Moreover, additional stresses such as infection impose further burdens on their already depleted reserves, making such children very vulnerable to serious complications from otherwise routine childhood diseases such as measles.

KWASHIORKOR
Kwashiorkor is caused by weaning the infant to a diet high in carbohydrate and low in protein. Many of the manifestations are related to inadequate protein synthesis from insufficient supplies of essential amino acids. Characteristic of the child with kwashiorkor is massive edema of the abdomen and extremities with wastage of the normal musculature (Fig. 13-1B). The pattern of starvation takes weeks to months to develop and may be present in various degrees of severity. Changes in the color and texture of the hair are common, with a loss of the usual pigmentation and a coarsening of the strands. Depigmentation of the skin is also seen, with patches of normal skin adjacent to the involved areas.

The edema is a result of inadequate serum protein synthesis, leading to failure to maintain the usual intravascular volume. Such defects in protein synthesis may have a direct effect on the transport of nutrients such as vitamin A that are carried on protein carriers.

NONSPECIFIC PROTEIN-ENERGY MALNUTRITION
The above descriptions indicate the broad spectrum of findings in malnutrition in children; however, inadequate diets for children and adults may not lead to specific clinical syndromes. Such nutritional deficiency may be considered under the more general grouping of protein-energy malnutrition, with the implication that replacement therapy should encompass a wide variety of nutrients [19].

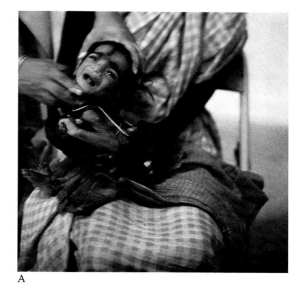

A

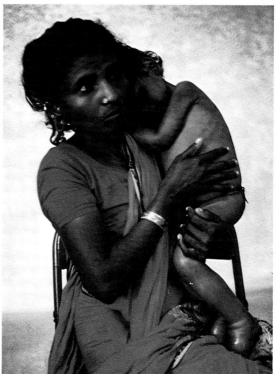

B

FIGURE 13-1. *A. Marasmus. This disease is caused by a chronic deficiency of all food categories. B. Kwashiorkor. The manifestations of this clinical entity are due largely to protein deficiency. Characteristic features are massive edema of the abdomen and extremities, concurrent with muscle wastage.*

Although children, with the high energy demands that growth imposes, are particularly vulnerable to dietary deficiencies, adults may also show a number of general systemic abnormalities associated with protein-energy malnutrition. The organs and physiologic functions most vulnerable are those in which cells are constantly turning over and being replaced. These include the skin and mucous membranes, hematopoietic tissue, and the gastrointestinal tract. Intestinal changes further reduce absorption, compounding the inadequate intake with malabsorption.

Vitamin A deficiency, although frequently associated with more generalized protein-energy malnutrition, is a serious ophthalmic problem in much of the world today. The next two sections will, therefore, be devoted to a review of the metabolism of this compound and to a description of the ocular abnormalities believed to be caused by vitamin A deficiency.

VITAMIN A METABOLISM

SOURCES AND ABSORPTION

The major sources of vitamin A for humans are beta carotene from plants and vitamin A itself derived from animal tissue (Fig. 13-2). The beta carotene must be hydrolyzed, either as a consequence of or immediately after absorption, into two molecules of retinaldehyde that are subsequently reduced to vitamin A alcohol (retinol). Preformed vitamin A from animal tissue usually exists in the form of the al-

cohol or the alcohol esterified with a long-chain fatty acid (retinyl ester, frequently palmitate ester [Fig. 13-2]). These esters are hydrolyzed in the gut but are promptly re-esterified once they are in the cells of the gastrointestinal tract (Fig. 13-3).

TRANSPORT

After absorption from the gut, vitamin A molecules are then transported (probably as esters) in the chylomicra of lymph and blood to the liver, where absorption into the hepatic cells probably involves ester hydrolysis.

Storage in the liver is usually in the form of the retinyl ester. The level of vitamin A storage in the liver depends, of course, on the dietary history, the demand for vitamin A, and the integrity of the transport mechanism of vitamin A out of the liver to the peripheral tissues.

Vitamin A is transported in plasma from the liver to other tissues as the alcohol (retinol) bound to a specific transport protein, retinol-binding protein (RBP). RBP, which is produced by the liver itself, interacts with plasma prealbumin so that it is a com-

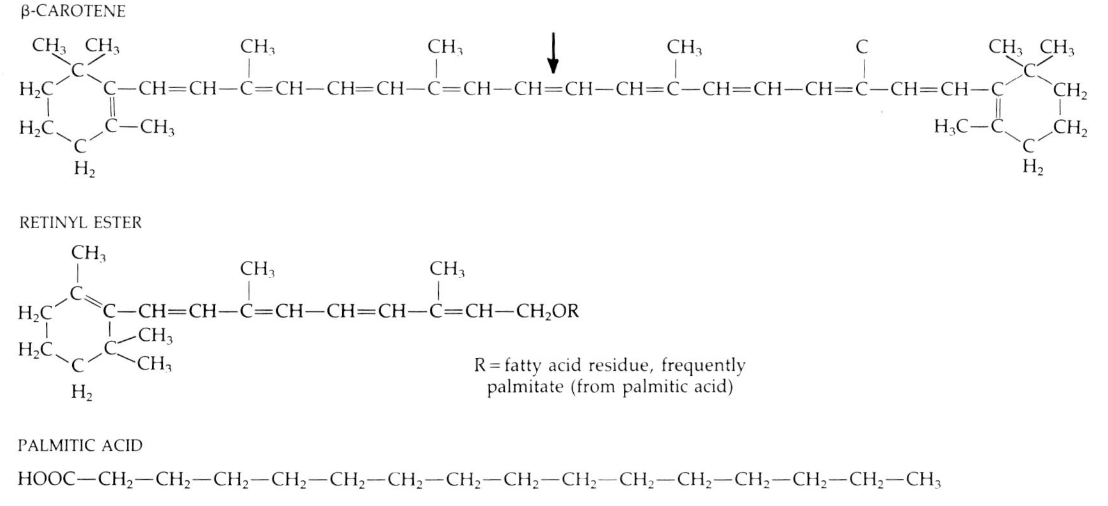

FIGURE 13-2. Chemical formulae of the major forms of vitamin A. Arrow indicates cleavage point of beta carotene. (See also Figure 13-3.)

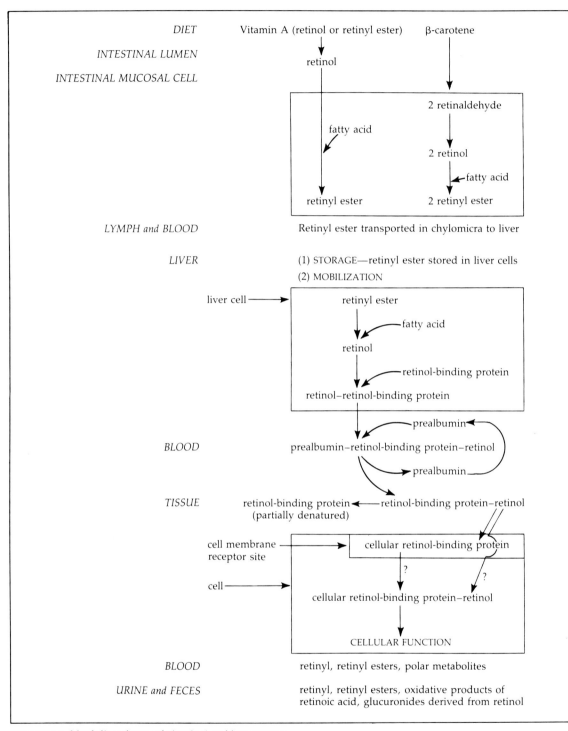

DIET   Vitamin A (retinol or retinyl ester)   β-carotene

INTESTINAL LUMEN   retinol

INTESTINAL MUCOSAL CELL

2 retinaldehyde

fatty acid

2 retinol

fatty acid

retinyl ester   2 retinyl ester

LYMPH and BLOOD   Retinyl ester transported in chylomicra to liver

LIVER   (1) STORAGE—retinyl ester stored in liver cells
(2) MOBILIZATION

liver cell ⟶ retinyl ester

fatty acid

retinol

retinol-binding protein

retinol–retinol-binding protein

BLOOD   prealbumin

prealbumin–retinol-binding protein–retinol

prealbumin

TISSUE   retinol-binding protein ⟵ retinol-binding protein–retinol
(partially denatured)

cell membrane
receptor site ⟶ cellular retinol-binding protein

cell ⟶ ?

cellular retinol-binding protein–retinol   ?

CELLULAR FUNCTION

BLOOD   retinyl, retinyl esters, polar metabolites

URINE and FECES   retinyl, retinyl esters, oxidative products of
retinoic acid, glucuronides derived from retinol

FIGURE 13-3. *Metabolic pathways of vitamin A and beta-carotene.*

plex of these three molecules bound together that circulates in the blood. The usual level of RBP in plasma is about 40 to 50 µg per milliliter, with prealbumin at 200 to 300 µg per milliliter. In normal subjects, the level of circulating retinol (in whatever form) is over 20 µg/100 ml [25]. Secretion of RBP from the liver is inhibited in vitamin A deficiency. Conversely, RBP is necessary for adequate retinol release by the liver, so that regulation of RBP is as important as that of vitamin A itself in ensuring adequate levels of the vitamin are available to peripheral tissues. Accumulation of unbound RBP occurs in the liver during deficiency states, with release when vitamin A is again available [6, 24, 29, 30, 47, 50, 51].

ACTION IN PERIPHERAL TISSUES

Figure 13-3 sketches what are believed to be the main metabolic pathways for vitamin A in peripheral tissues, but much of this is still very speculative.

In contrast to the visual cycle, where the fundamental role played by vitamin A is well understood [7], there is little information regarding the specific action of vitamin A in the maintenance of conjunctival and corneal integrity. Several morphologic studies of ocular surface epithelium in vitamin A–deficient animals have shown increased thickening and keratinization of these tissues, with loss of conjunctival goblet cells and loss of the cell surface microplicae [4, 5, 14, 20, 21, 48]. Even before frank xerophthalmia is present, certain morphologic changes, e.g., loss of goblet cells, increased density of keratofilaments, and large numbers of exfoliating cells, can be seen in corneal epithelium of vitamin A–deficient rats [5].

Only a few pieces of information are available regarding the penetration of vitamin A into ocular surface cells. At the level of individual corneal epithelial cells, binding sites for retinol complexed with serum RBP have been described [24, 50, 51]. Corneal epithelial cells accumulate retinol from RBP. Retinoic acid binding has not, however, been demonstrated specifically for corneal epithelium but may be present in conjunctiva [50].

Once the vitamin A molecules are in the cells, very little is known of how they act in metabolic processes. Vitamin A does play a role in glycoprotein synthesis in cornea as it does in other tissues. It stimulates incorporation of glucose and glucosamine into some glycoproteins of corneal epithelium [11, 15–17] while decreasing synthesis of other glycoproteins. How interference with glycoprotein synthesis is related to the ocular surface epithelial cell abnormalities seen in vitamin A deficiency has not yet been determined [18].

Another feature of cellular activity that appears to be mediated by vitamin A is the differentiation of ocular surface epithelium. In animals, in the absence of vitamin A, conjunctiva loses its goblet cells and begins to keratinize [4, 5, 14, 20, 48]. In addition, the differentiation of epithelial tissue in vitro is influenced by the vitamin A content of the medium. Vitamin A favors the production of mucus-producing cells in some tissues (e.g., skin, esophagus); in others (e.g., trachea) vitamin A inhibits the differentiation of goblet cells [1, 2, 8, 9]. Recently, retinoic acid was found to increase the rate of corneal epithelial healing in nondeficient rabbits [31], although such therapy in humans may not be useful because of the high doses used [33].

DEFICIENCY IN PERIPHERAL TISSUE

There are a number of causes that can result in inadequate supplies of vitamin A to peripheral tissue. The first is an actual dietary deficiency of the vitamin, seen most commonly in diets deficient in animal sources (meat, milk) and vegetables. The second factor is inadequate synthesis and release of the RBP, prealbumin, or both necessary for the transport of vitamin A. For example, even in the presence of adequate vitamin A, severe protein deficiency would be expected to lead to inadequate synthesis of RBP or prealbumin. A third cause, theoretically possible, would be the lack of specific enzymes required for any of the steps involving retinol, from absorption through epithelial cell metabolism.

CLINICAL ASPECTS OF VITAMIN A DEFICIENCY AND ASSOCIATED NUTRITIONAL EYE DISEASE

As the preceding discussion indicates, it is nearly impossible in most cases to separate various vitamin deficiencies from the larger picture of protein-energy malnutrition. Nevertheless, by convention there are a number of clinical manifestations that are ascribed primarily to vitamin A deficiency. Most of these can be reproduced in animal studies [21], which lends further credence to the pivotal role played by vitamin A deficiency in their development. *Xerophthalmia* is the term used to describe these changes in the ocular surface. This condition has been seen in experimental studies of vitamin A–deficient animals and has been reversed by topical vitamin A [21, 22]. *Keratomalacia*, a term best reserved for actual dissolution of the cornea, has not been produced in animals, except when additional trauma or infection is superimposed on the underlying xerophthalmia [27, 52].

The first classification of ocular changes in vitamin A deficiency to gain general acceptance was that proposed by ten Doeschate [46]. Her initial scheme was later expanded to include night blindness and the more severe corneal changes. The descriptions given here for the various stages are only minimally modified from those presented in the World Health Organization Technical Report No. 590, which resulted from a joint WHO–United States Agency for International Development meeting held in Jakarta in 1974 [49].

Classification	Primary Signs
X1A	Conjunctival xerosis
X1B	Bitot's spot with conjunctival xerosis
X2	Corneal xerosis
X3A	Corneal ulceration with xerosis
X3B	Keratomalacia
XN	Night blindness
XF	Xerophthalmic fundus
XS	Corneal scars

OCULAR MANIFESTATIONS OF VITAMIN A DEFICIENCY

X1A—CONJUNCTIVAL XEROSIS

The conjunctival changes characteristic of vitamin A deficiency are usually confined to the bulbar region. Features include dryness, lack of wettability, loss of transparency, thickening, wrinkling, and pigmentation. Overdiagnosis of conjunctival xerosis is a common error and makes this a relatively "soft" sign of vitamin A deficiency. The variability from one observer to the next makes it very difficult to standardize the use of xerosis as a criterion of the presence of nutritional eye disease. In many studies in the past, this unreliable sign has been used either alone or with biochemical or dietary data to support the contention that xerophthalmia and, by association, vitamin A deficiency, are present in a population. When such prevalence surveys have been used as a basis for dietary supplementation programs, subsequent analysis of the population's response to vitamin supplementation has been hard to interpret.

X1B—BITOT'S SPOT WITH CONJUNCTIVAL XEROSIS

A Bitot's spot is a small, light gray plaque with a foamy surface (Fig. 13-4A). Histologically, Bitot's spots show inflammatory infiltration of the sub-epithelial tissue. The conjunctival epithelium is keratinized and shows acanthotic thickening and loss of goblet cells [38]. The foamy appearance is due to accumulation of bacteria and mucus on the surface of the lesion. The spot is invariably on the bulbar conjunctiva, usually temporal to the limbus, and is frequently bilateral.

Bitot's spots with underlying conjunctival xerosis have been shown to be responsive to systemic vitamin A, promptly reversing to a more normal conjunctival appearance [37]. Such a prompt response long before the general nutritional status has shown much change is good evidence for the role of vitamin A deficiency per se in the production of this ocular mucous membrane lesion.

Although a Bitot's spot accompanied by conjunctival xerosis in a child under 6 is taken as a "hard" sign of vitamin A deficiency, serious eye disease caused by vitamin A deficiency may develop and progress to keratomalacia and blindness without a Bitot's spot having developed. Thus, the disease does not necessarily evolve through a series of clinical stages—X1A to X1B to X2 to X3A—but may manifest any one of the stages alone. Of course, evolution of the disease has not been observed in humans since therapeutic intervention with vitamin A is possible. In animal deficiency, Bitot's spots are not seen, even though corneal xerosis and clouding are prominent [20, 21, 48].

X2—CORNEAL XEROSIS

Corneal xerosis, a roughened, lusterless corneal appearance, is usually seen in association with conjunctival xerosis and may or may not represent a more severe or advanced stage of epithelial involvement (Fig. 13-4B). The appearance is keratinization, stromal edema, and superficial punctate keratitis visible with biomicroscopy [36]. There is a lack of wettability of the cornea, even in the presence of an apparently normal tear supply. The tear film breakup time is much reduced as a consequence of this surface change, which leads to desiccation of the corneal epithelial cells. It is important to note that the early tear breakup is secondary to surface irregularity and need not indicate an abnormality in the composition of the tears themselves, although there may be decreased tearing. To date, no information regarding the composition of the tear film in vitamin A deficiency is available. However, because of the possible role of vitamin A in the normal differentiation of the conjunctiva and in the maintenance of the usual percentage of goblet cells, abnormalities in tear film mucin content might certainly be expected in deficiency states.

Corneal xerosis is rapidly reversed in both hu-

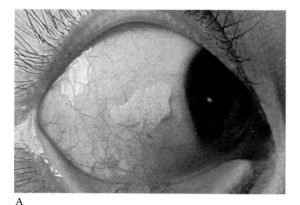

A

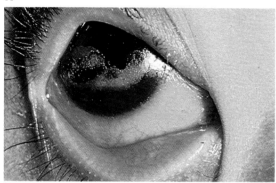

B

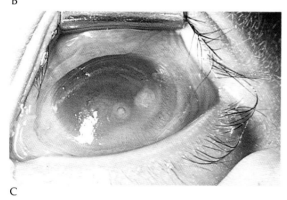

C

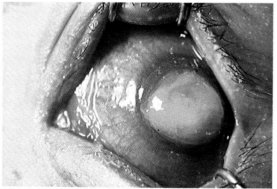

D

mans and animals by vitamin A supplements, with no permanent damage to the corneal surface or to the conjunctiva [35].

X3A—CORNEAL ULCERATION WITH XEROSIS

Dissolution of corneal stroma indicates that more than just the ocular surface is involved in the process (Fig. 13-4C). It is still not certain to what extent ulceration of the cornea (not just epithelial loss) can be caused by pure vitamin A deficiency. Clinically, such stromal loss is found frequently but not always in association with marked protein-energy malnutrition. It is certain that epithelial loss in other conditions does not always lead to stromal ulceration, so that it seems possible that the stroma is, in some way, particularly vulnerable in these patients. In experimental animals, stromal ulceration in animals with severe vitamin A deficiency is rare, but trauma can precipitate ulceration [27], which suggests again the susceptibility of the stroma to dissolution when the epithelium is damaged. The finding of severe stromal edema in animals may reflect the tendency for corneal swelling seen in nonprimate species when the epithelial barrier is lost.

Only recently have studies been directed toward the ulcerative process in vitamin A deficiency in animals [27]. There is some evidence that vitamin A supplementation can reduce collagenase production by thermally burned vitamin A–deficient rats [23], but there has been no correlation of that with clinical ulceration. Isolated vitamin A therapy does appear to reverse ulceration of the corneal stroma in humans [34]. The role of inflammatory cells, proteolytic enzymes, and the composition and structure of the corneal collagen itself will have to be evaluated before the best immediate treatment for acute stromal ulceration can be determined. Local

FIGURE 13-4. *A. Bitot's spot, a foamy light gray area of conjunctiva frequently found in vitamin A deficiency in humans. (From A. Sommer* Nutritional Blindness and Keratomalacia. *Oxford: Oxford University Press, 1982.) B. Corneal xerosis. Keratinization and superficial punctate keratitis are characteristic of epithelial involvement in nutritional disease. (From A. Sommer Field guide to the detection and control of xerophthalmia. Geneva: World Health Organization, 1978.) C. Corneal ulceration with xerosis. (From A. Sommer and S. Tjakrasudjatma, Corneal xerophthalmia and keratomalacia. Arch. Ophthalmol. 100:404, 1982. Copyright 1982, American Medical Association.) D. Keratomalacia. Rapid melting of cornea accompanies advanced starvation in children. (From A. Sommer* Nutritional Blindness and Keratomalacia. *Oxford: Oxford University Press, 1982.)*

infection does not appear to play an important precipitating role [34].

X3B—KERATOMALACIA

An extreme form of corneal dissolution is that seen in advanced starvation in very young children (Fig. 13-4D). The cornea melts away in part or entirely, seemingly overnight. There is subsequent extrusion or prolapse of intraocular contents, with blindness as the end result. The inflammatory response is minimal, appearing more like that of the central ulceration in rheumatoid arthritis than that seen in active herpes simplex. The role of local and systemic infection in the production of keratomalacia is not clear. Local bacterial infection may be important in hastening the ulceration of an already compromised cornea. Systemic infection with measles, parasites, and other agents also seems to throw children with precarious nutritional balance into outright ocular manifestations of vitamin A deficiency.

SECONDARY SIGNS OF VITAMIN A DEFICIENCY

XN—NIGHT BLINDNESS

Retinal function depends upon adequate sources of vitamin A for the visual cycle. Night blindness has been produced in volunteers subjected to a diet deficient in vitamin A [13] and is thought to be an early sign of vitamin A deficiency. Although sophisticated electrical and psychophysical tests can detect changes in rod function long before subjects complain of night blindness, such diagnostic maneuvers are not practical for surveying the status of vitamin A in large populations. As a symptom, however, night blindness can suggest that vitamin A may not be in adequate supply in the local diet, and in at least some cultures it has proved a sensitive and specific screening tool [34, 39].

XF—XEROPHTHALMIC FUNDUS

Although rarely sought and observed, a characteristic appearance of the fundus associated with chronic night blindness has been reported [12]. These whitish yellow changes in the pigment epithelium appear to be window defects on fluorescein angiography and may correspond to areas of temporary visual field loss [43]. Both eyes are said to be affected, although not necessarily to the same degree. There has been no attempt to use fundus changes as either a survey parameter or for assessing the severity of vitamin A deficiency in individual cases.

XS—CORNEAL SCARS

By a process of exclusion it seems reasonable to attribute otherwise nonspecific scars to nutritional deficiencies in appropriate populations. The clinical picture is that of a healed ulcer in a child known to have had an episode of severe malnutrition. If other diseases (measles, bacterial infection, herpes simplex, trachoma, trauma) have been ruled out, the scar may be due to vitamin A deficiency. The danger in such diagnosis by exclusion is apparent.

NUTRITIONAL EYE DISEASE IN DEVELOPED COUNTRIES

In adults, protein-energy malnutrition can be a manifestation of decreased dietary intake or reduced absorption. In developed countries, the most common forms of dietary deficiencies seen are those in alcoholism, malabsorption, and self-imposed bizarre diets.

Malnutrition is a problem frequently associated with alcoholism. Usually, deficiencies of specific vitamins such as folic acid, thiamine, niacin, and vitamin B_6 are found, leading to a variety of clinical signs. The fatty liver of alcoholism is morphologically indistinguishable from that seen in childhood protein-energy malnutrition. Although it has been suggested that the liver damage may be the result of nutritional deficiencies seen when much of the dietary intake is confined to alcohol, there also appear to be direct hepatotoxic effects of ethanol. In addition to the possible lack of nutrients in the alcoholic's diet, the altered hepatic metabolism in the alcoholic influences the uptake and storage of nutrients and may interfere with the synthesis of carrier proteins [10, 26].

Descriptions of possible nutritional eye disease in seemingly well nourished populations have been limited to case reports with a variety of dietary and pathologic observations, as well as documentation of response to therapy [3, 28, 45]. One report describes 2 cases of ocular abnormalities in alcoholic patients [45]; vitamin A levels were abnormally low in both cases. An important observation was made regarding the conjunctiva in these cases. Initially, biopsy specimens of conjunctival tissue showed virtually no goblet cells although the specimens were taken from the inferonasal location, the area with the highest proportion of goblet cells under normal circumstances. In addition, there were loss of nuclei and keratinization of the superficial cells, which was viewed as epidermalization. After 3 weeks of vitamin A therapy coupled with improvement in the general nutritional status, the biopsy specimen in the one case that could be followed showed a restoration of the normal cuboidal basal cells, with loss of most of the superficial keratinization and reappearance of a few goblet cells. After 6 weeks of nutritional therapy, the conjunctival biopsy specimen was essentially normal. In addition to these histologic changes, the blood levels of vitamin A in this patient promptly rose into the normal range. The clinical appearance changed dramatically also, from an irregular surface of both the conjunctiva and cornea to the normal lustrous appearance. It is notable that there was no demonstrable deficiency of aqueous tears, as judged by normal Schirmer test values in both patients.

Another series of two patients highlights the difficulty in separating specific vitamin deficiencies from generalized starvation [3]. In two cachectic hospitalized patients, ocular signs consistent with stage X2 (corneal xerosis) were observed. In these cases, serum protein levels were quite abnormal, evidenced by very low albumin and globulin. Vitamin A levels, which were not below 40 μg per milliliter, were normal, however. Such cases suggest that nutritional eye disease may exist in the absence of vitamin A deficiency.

TREATMENT OF VITAMIN A DEFICIENCY

In the presence of conjunctival or corneal xerosis (X1A, X2) or more advanced corneal disease (X3A, X3B) with or without possible concurrent infection, therapy with vitamin A should be instituted. Ideally, serum should be drawn for serum protein and vitamin A levels to confirm the clinical diagnosis. In virtually all cases, the malnutrition is more general, either as a result of the loss of appetite customarily found with vitamin A deficiency or as part of the overall dietary deficiency.

Vitamin A supplementation can be oral or parenteral or both; oral dosage has been found as effective as parenteral [41]. The initial dose is 200,000 IU of vitamin A in oil, orally, or, if judged necessary, 200,000 IU of water soluble vitamin A intramuscularly. The next day, an additional 200,000 IU of vitamin A should be given. A week or two later, or at discharge, the oral 200,000 IU dose should be repeated. For children under 1 year, half of these doses should be given [53]. Larger doses of vitamin A are not necessary or desirable, particularly on a chronic basis, since vitamin A toxicity must be avoided. In persons with severe protein deficiency, it is probably useful to repeat massive doses every 2 weeks until protein status returns to normal.

In the presence of normal interstitial absorption, no more than 195 IU/kg body weight in children to 36 IU/kg body weight in adults must be supplied daily to maintain adequate stores of the vitamin after the initial deficiency is eliminated. Since liver stores generally last 6 months after a massive dose, daily supplementation is not necessary even in populations very deficient in vitamin A.

PREVENTION OF NUTRITIONAL EYE DISEASE

Recently, sophisticated field survey techniques have been used to evaluate the prevalence of vitamin A–related ocular findings in populations of preschool children [32, 34, 44]. Such surveys have directed national and world attention to the problems of how best to achieve adequate nutrition in developing nations. Although the best method would be the provision of adequate quantities of all the essential foodstuffs, the magnitude and difficulty of such a solution has led to the proposal that vitamin A supplementation per se might be effective in reducing the prevalence of blinding disease.

A variety of techniques have been suggested to achieve vitamin A supplementation, including fortification of diets, periodic dosing, and nutritional education and rehabilitation. Fortification usually depends on adding small quantities of vitamin A to everyday foods such as sugar or monosodium glutamate. Periodic dosing with vitamin A in oil has been carried out in large populations, without clear-cut evidence of its effectiveness. Reeducation of parents in areas where leafy vegetables are plentiful is another way to alter the dietary intake of vitamin A. The efficacy of each of these methods awaits convincing demonstration, however. Until all children can receive adequate protein, calories, and vitamins as part of their regular diet, the search will continue for useful methods of supplementation.

ACKNOWLEDGMENT
I am grateful to Alfred Sommer, M.D., for his review of this chapter, as well as for the color photographs in Figure 13-4.

REFERENCES
1. Aydelotte, M. V. The effects of vitamin A and citral on epithelial differentiation *in vitro*: I. The chick tracheal epithelium. *Acta Embryol. Morphol. Exp.* 11:279, 1963.
2. Aydelotte, M. V. The effects of vitamin A and citral on epithelial differentiation *in vitro*: II. The chick esophageal and corneal epithelia and epidermis. *Acta Embryol. Morphol. Exp.* 11:621, 1963.
3. Baum, J., and Rao, G. Keratomalacia in the

cachectic hospitalized patient. *Am. J. Ophthalmol.* 82:435, 1976.

4. Beitch, I. The induction of keratinization in the corneal epithelium. *Invest. Ophthalmol.* 9:827, 1970.

5. Carter-Dawson, L., et al. Early corneal changes in vitamin A–deficient rats. *Exp. Eye Res.* 30:261, 1980.

6. Chytil, F., and Ong, D. E. Cellular retinol and retinoic acid–binding proteins in vitamin A action. *Fed. Proc.* 38:2510, 1980.

7. Duke-Elder, S. The Physiology of the Eye and of Vision. In S. Duke-Elder (Ed.), *System of Ophthalmology*. St. Louis: Mosby, 1968. Vol. 4, p. 469.

8. Elias, P. M., and Friend, D. S. Vitamin A–induced mucus metaplasia. *J. Cell Biol.* 68:173, 1976.

9. Fell, H. B. The effect of excess vitamin A on cultures of embryonic chicken skin implanted at different stages of differentiation. *Proc. R. Soc. Lond.* [Biol.] 146:246, 1957.

10. Halsted, C. H. Nutritional Implications of Alcohol. In *Present Knowledge in Nutrition* (4th ed., Nutrition Reviews Series). Washington, D.C.: Nutrition Foundation, 1976.

11. Hassell, J. R., Newsome, D. A., and DeLuca, L. Increased biosynthesis of specific glycoconjugates in rat corneal epithelium following treatment with vitamin A. *Invest. Ophthalmol. Vis. Sci.* 19:642, 1980.

12. Hing, T. K. Fundus changes in hypovitaminosis A. *Ophthalmologica* 137:81, 1959.

13. Hume, E. M., and Krebs, H. A. Vitamin A requirement of human adults: An experimental study of vitamin A deprivation in man (Medical Research Council Special Report Series No. 264). London: Her Majesty's Stationery Office, 1949.

14. Jayaraj, A. P., Leela, R., and Rama Rao, P. B. Studies on cornea and conjunctiva mucus metaplasia in vitamin A deficient rats. *Exp. Eye Res.* 12:1, 1971.

15. Kim, Y-C. L., Wang, E., and Wolf, G. Vitamin A and the nucleic acids and proteins of rat corneal epithelium. *Nutr. Rep. Int.* 11:93, 1975.

16. Kim, Y-C. L., and Wolf, G. Vitamin A deficiency and the glycoproteins of rat corneal epithelium. *J. Nutr.* 104:710, 1974.

17. Kiorpes, T. C., Kim, Y-C. L., and Wolf, G. Stimulation of the synthesis of specific glycoproteins in corneal epithelium by vitamin A. *Exp. Eye Res.* 28:23, 1979.

18. Kiorpes, T. C., et al. α_2-macroglobulin in vitamin A–deficient children. *Am. J. Clin. Nutr.* 32:1842, 1979.

19. Milner, R. D. G. Protein-Calorie Malnutrition.

In *Present Knowledge in Nutrition* (4th ed., Nutrition Reviews Series). Washington, D.C.: Nutrition Foundation, 1976.

20. Pfister, R. R., and Renner, M. E. The corneal and conjunctival surface in vitamin A deficiency: A scanning electron microscope study. *Invest. Ophthalmol. Vis. Sci.* 17:874, 1978.

21. Pirie, A. Xerophthalmia. *Invest. Ophthalmol.* 15:417, 1976.

22. Pirie, A. Effects of locally applied retinoic acid on corneal xerophthalmia in the rat. *Exp. Eye Res.* 25:297, 1977.

23. Pirie, A., Werb, A., and Burleigh, M. C. Collagenase and other proteinases in the cornea of retinol-deficient rats. *Br. J. Nutr.* 34:297, 1975.

24. Rask, L., et al. Vitamin A supply of the cornea. *Exp. Eye Res.* 31:201, 1980.

25. Report of the International Vitamin A Consultative Group (IVACG). Washington, D.C.: Nutrition Foundation, 1976. P. III-5.

26. Sebrell, W. H. Malnutrition. In J. F. Moxey-Rosenau and P. F. Sartwell (Eds.), *Preventive Medicine and Public Health.* New York: Appleton-Century-Crofts, 1973.

27. Seng, W. L., et al. The effect of thermal burns on the release of collagenase from corneas of vitamin A–deficient rats. *Invest. Ophthalmol. Vis. Sci.* 19:1461, 1980.

28. Smith, R., Farrell, T., and Bailey, T. A. Keratomalacia. *Surv. Ophthalmol.* 20:213, 1975.

29. Smith, F. R., and Goodman, D. S. Vitamin A metabolism and transport. In *Present Knowledge in Nutrition* (4th ed., Nutrition Reviews Series). Washington, D.C.: Nutrition Foundation, 1976.

30. Smith, F. R., et al. Serum vitamin A, retinol-binding protein and prealbumin concentrations in protein-calorie malnutrition: I. A. Functional defect in retinol release. *Am. J. Clin. Nutr.* 26:973, 1973.

31. Smolin, G., and Okumoto, M. Vitamin A acid and corneal epithelial wound healing. *Ann. Ophthalmol.* 13:563, 1981.

32. Sommer, A. Field guide to the detection and control of xerophthalmia. Geneva: World Health Organization, 1978.

33. Sommer, A. Vitamin A treatment for herpes keratitis. *Arch. Ophthalmol.* 98:1656, 1980.

34. Sommer, A. *Nutritional Blindness: Xerophthalmia and Keratomalacia.* New York; London: Oxford University Press, 1982.

35. Sommer, A., and Emran, N. Topical retinoic acid in the treatment of corneal xerophthalmia. *Am. J. Ophthalmol.* 86:615, 1978.

36. Sommer, A., Emran, N., and Tamba, T. Vitamin A–responsive punctate keratopathy in xerophthalmia. *Am. J. Ophthalmol.* 87:330, 1979.

37. Sommer, A., Emran, N., and Tjakrasudjatma, S. Clinical characteristics of vitamin A–re-

sponsive and nonresponsive Bitot's spots. *Am. J. Ophthalmol.* 90:160, 1980.

38. Sommer, A., Green, R., and Kenyon, K. R. Clinical histopathologic correlations of vitamin A responsive and nonresponsive Bitot's spots. *Arch. Ophthalmol.* In press.

39. Sommer, A., et al. History of night blindness: A simple tool for xerophthalmia screening. *Am. J. Clin. Nutr.* 33:887, 1980.

40. Sommer, A., et al. Incidence, prevalence and scale of blinding malnutrition. *Lancet* 1:1407, 1981.

41. Sommer, A., et al. Oral vs. intramuscular vitamin A in the treatment of xerophthalmia. *Lancet* 1:557, 1980.

42. Sommer, A., and Tjakrasudjatma, S. Corneal xerophthalmia and keratomalacia. *Arch. Ophthalmol.* 100:404, 1982.

43. Sommer, A., et al. Vitamin A–responsive panocular xerophthalmia in a healthy adult. *Arch. Ophthalmol.* 96:1630, 1978.

44. Sommer, A., et al. Xerophthalmia Determinants and Control. In K. Shimieu and J. A. Oosterhuis (Eds.), *XXIII Concilium Ophthalmologicum.* Amsterdam: Excerpta Medica, 1978. P. 1615.

45. Sullivan, W. R., McCulley, J. P., and Dohlman, C. H. Return of goblet cells after vitamin A therapy in xerosis of the conjunctiva. *Am. J. Ophthalmol.* 75:720, 1973.

46. ten Doeschate, J. Causes of blindness in and around Surabaya, East Java, Indonesia. University of Indonesia (Jakarta) Ph.D. Thesis, 1968.

47. Underwood, B. A., Loerch, J. D., and Lewis, K. C. Effects of dietary vitamin A deficiency, retinoic acid and protein quantity and quality on serially obtained plasma and liver levels of vitamin A in rats. *J. Nutr.* 109:796, 1979.

48. Van Horn, D. L., et al. Xerophthalmia in vitamin A–deficient rabbits: Clinical and ultrastructural alterations in the cornea. *Invest. Ophthalmol. Vis. Sci.* 9:1067, 1980.

49. Vitamin A Deficiency and Xerophthalmia (Technical Report No. 590). Geneva: World Health Organization, 1976.

50. Wiggert, B., et al. Vitamin A receptors: Retinoic acid binding in ocular tissues. *Biochem. J.* 169:87, 1978.

51. Wiggert, B., et al. Retinol receptors in corneal epithelium, stroma and endothelium. *Biochim. Biophys. Acta* 491:104, 1977.

52. Wolbach, S. B., and Howe, P. R. Tissue changes following deprivation of fat soluble vitamin A. *J. Exp. Med.* 42:753, 1925.

53. Xerophthalmia Club Bulletin, No. 23, August, 1981.

14. CORNEAL INJURIES

Trauma

Robert G. Webster, Jr.

DIAGNOSIS

The circumstances of the occurrence of an injury to the eye are very important and should be elicited in great detail. The cornea may be compromised by blunt trauma, penetrating injury, or a perforating foreign body. The possibility of bacterial or fungal contamination or inoculation should be explored, even to the point of culturing for the offending agent. If a high-speed missile has entered the eye, careful description by the patient of his or her exact activity at the moment of impact will often give the ophthalmologist a good idea of the character of the missile. With metallic intraocular foreign bodies it is particularly important to identify the substance, both to estimate its possible toxicity to the eye and to determine if it is magnetic.

The preinjury status of the eye should be recorded in order to determine realistic goals of therapy. The history should include note of prior eye surgery or injury and subsequent visual function, the presence of amblyopia, and possible family history of eye disease.

Examination should include measurement of visual acuity; check of papillary responses; slit lamp examination for epithelial defects, concussion corneal edema, and foreign body; extent of any laceration; and integrity of the anterior and posterior segment structures. The examination should be done as early as possible, since findings may later be obscured by hyphema, hypopyon, or membranes. Appropriate studies (x-ray, ultrasound, and other studies that do not threaten the integrity of the globe) for possible foreign bodies may be crucial. Fluorescein staining may help verify epithelial defects. In cases of uncertainty about anterior segment perforation, Seidel's test is useful after an initial white light examination (Fig. 14-1). The fellow eye should be examined to determine its function, anatomic integrity, and possible involvement in the trauma.

A lacerated globe may produce nausea, particularly in children. Vomiting should be pharmacologically suppressed as necessary, with due consideration for possibly imminent general anesthesia.

TREATMENT TECHNIQUES

GENERAL

Many kinds of surface and superficial corneal injuries are treated by nonsurgical techniques. If the globe is not perforated, only topical antibiotic treatment is necessary to accompany other therapy. If surgical repair is to be performed, appropriate preoperative measures should be taken, including questioning about any known drug allergies, tetanus prophylaxis, the signing of operative permits covering all possible procedures, and selection of anesthesia. General anesthesia is mandatory in children and uncooperative adults and is often preferable to retrobulbar anesthesia in the presence of open or gaping ocular wounds. If the globe is perforated or ruptured, systemic and probably topical antibiotics are indicated postoperatively and possibly preoperatively, depending on the likelihood of contamination.

In the operating room, careful thought should be given to the materials, equipment, and techniques that might be needed during the procedure. For example, if one is removing a foreign body that is imbedded only in or through the cornea of a phakic patient, one would not have to ask that the vitrectomy instruments be available; if the cornea is lacerated with a dislocated or lacerated lens, one must be prepared to deal with lens material and vitreous presenting during the course of the repair. Depending on the nature and degree of anterior segment disorganization, one may decide to approach repair in a one-step or a multistep procedure. One may do a simple initial corneal repair, and then at some later date do an anterior segment reconstruction involving synechialysis, iridoplasty, and possible lensectomy and penetrating keratoplasty. If the corneal wound is complex, one may elect to close it primarily and at the same time create a well-ordered limbal incision to give one safer access to the anterior segment for possible removal of foreign body or reconstruction at that time [5]. In the case of a lacerated globe in an infant, young child, or adult of advanced age, one might prefer, after primary repair, to affix a Flieringa ring to the

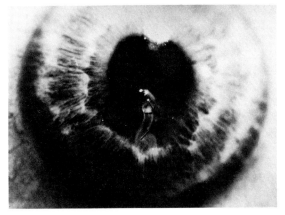

FIGURE 14-1. *Positive result of Seidel's test in inadequately closed corneal wound.*

globe before attempting any further procedure that involves a major aperture in the globe.

In acute injuries, cultures are usually indicated. If the corneal trauma is nonperforating, the most important culture is of the foreign body, if one is present, and of corneal scrapings from the wound, but lid and conjunctival cultures should also be done. These are usually inoculated into aerobic and anaerobic nutrient broth, blood and chocolate culture media, and Sabouraud agar. Gram and Giemsa stains of corneal wound scrapings are also often helpful. If the anterior chamber has been entered, its contents should also be inoculated in a similar array of media. Again, lid and conjunctival cultures should be done.

An operating microscope and microsurgical instruments should be available, and sutures should be selected. Suture choice will vary somewhat, depending on the habits of the individual surgeon, but corneal and limbal defects are usually best closed with 10-0 monofilament nylon. Consideration should be given to the possible need for diathermy, cryotherapy, and a cryoextractor. Surgical adhesives (isobutyl cyanoacrylate) and a therapeutic soft contact lens should be available.

Unless there is total disorganization of the globe, primary repair rather than enucleation should always be attempted. Salvage is often accomplished even in severe injuries. The surgeon may then safely observe the eye for approximately 10 days to 2 weeks before major risk of sympathetic ophthalmia develops. In fact, a greater waiting period might be observed, since in the last two decades sympathetic ophthalmia seems to have decreased in frequency and severity, possibly because of steroid therapy [8]. The effort to save with vitrectomy eyes that otherwise would be lost may possibly increase the risk of sympathetic ophthalmia [7].

OBSERVATION, PATCHING

Observation with or without patching is usually the only treatment needed for blunt trauma to or abrasion of the cornea. In an otherwise healthy eye, the epithelium rapidly slides to cover denuded areas. Topical antibiotics may be used prophylactically. If gram-negative bacterial contamination is suspected, an aminoglycoside ointment may be applied twice daily while a pressure patch is maintained for the period required for re-epithelialization. If there is minimal suspicion of a virulent organism contaminating the abraded cornea, erythromycin or sulfacetamide ointment may be used once daily while the pressure patch is maintained. In the case of a generally compromised epithelium, e.g., the diabetic cornea, one may cover for most gram-negative possibilities with chloramphenicol ointment, which is far less toxic to the healing epithelium than are the aminoglycosides. Other good broad-spectrum antibiotic ointments are a chloramphenicol-polymyxin combination (Chloromyxin) and a polymyxin B-bacitracin-neomycin combination (Neosporin). Neomycin-containing medicaments should be used with the knowledge that approximately 5 percent of the population is hypersensitive to this antibiotic. Topical steroids, usually in suspension or solution form, may be indicated for postinjury anterior uveitis. The physician will usually give a moderately long-acting cycloplegic once daily during the healing phase for patient comfort. For simple corneal abrasions, often neither antibiotic nor steroid is necessary, but many practitioners are in the habit of prescribing an antibiotic ointment four times per day until the epithelial defect is healed.

For small epithelial defects, the patching time is usually 24 to 48 hours for full recovery. For larger geographic epithelial defects, the patching time may be longer. In recalcitrant epithelial defects caused by metabolic problems, neurotrophic influences, or associated keratitis, one may have to patch for several days or resort to a therapeutic soft contact lens for an extended period. The fact that topical corticosteroids inhibit healing to some extent should be remembered if they are used. They may be titrated for maximal antiinflammatory benefit and minimal inhibition of repair.

Partial-thickness stromal lacerations and even some small, self-sealed full-thickness perforations and lacerations can also be treated nonsurgically. The physician will usually employ a moderately long-acting cycloplegic at least once daily and a topical antibiotic chosen by criteria analogous to those above. To promote healing, the eye in these cases can be patched or bandaged with a therapeutic soft contact lens. Some perforating injuries are closed from the time of injury, and some that leak initially close within a few hours owing to stromal swelling around the injury site. Epithelial ingrowth rarely occurs in these injuries. In my opinion, small full-thickness lacerations and perforations that are self-sealing and do not show aqueous leakage with Valsalva maneuver can be treated with observation rather than immediate suturing. An injury with spontaneous aqueous leakage should have prompt surgical repair, since development of a chronic corneal fistula can be a perplexing corneal and anterior segment problem. Some small leaking corneal defects, especially if far off the visual axis, may be approached with surgical adhesive. See the discussions of general treatment techniques (above) and surgical adhesive (below).

REMOVAL OF FOREIGN BODIES

Surface and superficial stromal foreign bodies are usually easily removed in the office. An ophthalmic topical anesthetic is given every minute for two or three doses. With the patient settled at the slit lamp, a fine needle (usually 20 gauge or smaller), affixed to a small syringe for firm and steady control by the surgeon, can be used to tease the foreign material from the cornea. Surrounding rust may be removed with a hand-held motorized burr, and traumatized epithelium peripheral to the injury site should be gently scraped away with a sharp or semisharp spatulated instrument. Children, patients with several corneal bodies at various stromal depths, or patients whose anterior chambers may collapse during the removal procedure should be hospitalized for general anesthesia and removal of as much of the foreign substance as possible with the aid of an operating microscope. In most cases, a corneal foreign body should be removed along the path of its entrance. If the foreign material is particularly friable or noncohesive, it may be necessary to cut perpendicularly through the cornea directly down to the foreign substance, which may then be scraped or irrigated away.

Multiple foreign bodies, if inert, may be left in place after one has removed those immediately adjacent to Bowman's membrane (Fig. 14-2). Occasionally, the deeper foreign bodies will work their way anteriorly and ultimately extrude through the epithelium, but this is unusual. Deeply imbedded foreign bodies should be treated as indicated by the ophthalmologist's knowledge of the nature of the foreign body and his observation of its behavior and the reaction of the involved cornea. Some substances, such as glass, sand, and certain minerals,

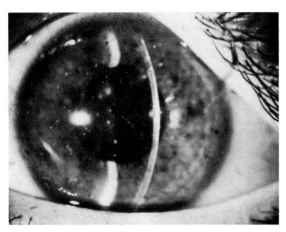

FIGURE 14-2. *Multiple stromal corneal foreign bodies, primarily sand, caused by bomb explosion, shown 4 years after injury. Vision, 20/30.*

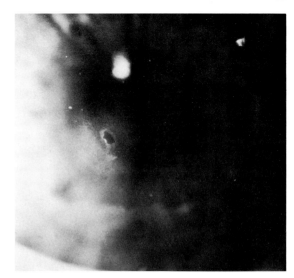

FIGURE 14-3. *Early siderosis surrounding metallic intracorneal foreign body.*

are well tolerated, and may remain within the stroma for long periods without reaction. Other substances, including many metals, vegetable substances, and insect parts, are poorly tolerated, and can lead to surrounding edema, inflammatory reaction, opacification secondary to ion deposition (Fig. 14-3), vascularization, and stromal necrosis. These foreign bodies should be removed promptly for many reasons: They are easier to see before the onset of surrounding reaction, early removal may prevent permanent visual loss secondary to stromal response, and the tissue heals better before the onset of marked stromal inflammation. The operating microscope and microsurgical instruments have made possible the successful removal of very fine particles.

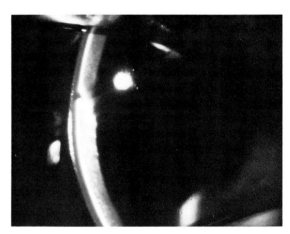

FIGURE 14-4. *Therapeutic soft contact lens placed over corneal laceration to restore anterior chamber until it can be surgically repaired.*

THERAPEUTIC SOFT CONTACT LENSES

Soft contact lenses have become an important therapeutic device in the treatment of a wide range of corneal diseases (see Chapter 17). In corneal trauma, they can be of assistance in many ways. Large abrasions may heal more rapidly and with increased patient comfort beneath a soft contact lens. For recurrent erosions, this device has become the treatment of choice (see Complications below). Some corneal perforations will seal permanently after buttressing with a soft contact lens. Application of a soft lens over a perforation or laceration often will restore the anterior chamber until needed surgery can be performed (Fig. 14-4). One of the most helpful uses of the device is its application over sutures or adhesive, allowing the patient more

comfort and ensuring cooperation (especially in children) and compliance. The soft contact lens applied over a sutured or glued cornea is truly therapeutic in that it decreases mucus pickup by these foreign bodies and minimizes reactive edema and vascularization.

APPOSITIONAL SUTURING

Before primary closure of a corneoscleral laceration can be accomplished, prolapse of any intraocular contents through the wound must be dealt with. If lens material or fibrin is extruding, it can be irrigated from the wound with balanced salt solution (BSS) or swept from the wound with a cellulose sponge. Particular care must be taken, if there is any chance that the fibrinous material is enmeshed in vitreous, that minimal traction be put on the vitreous before severing it flush with the wound and attempting to manipulate the remaining tuft from the wound back fully inside the eye. If prolapsed iris has been exposed less than a few hours and appears "clean," it may be gently reposited with an iris spatula. If prolapsed iris appears contaminated or has been exposed for more than a few hours, it should be excised and the edges of the iris massaged back through the wound into the anterior chamber. Prolapsed ciliary body should be reposited with rare exceptions. If not already done, one may at this time attempt at least partially to reform the anterior chamber with either a viscoelastic substance, for example, sodium hyaluronate (Healon), or BSS or air. Penetrating or partially penetrating transsceral diathermy can be applied to portions of the injured ciliary body.

If iris or vitreous adhesions persist after reformation of the anterior chamber, one may substitute air for a portion of the sodium hyaluronate or BSS and then sweep through the air-filled portion of the anterior chamber via a limbal stab incision remote from the wound. Sodium hyaluronate or BSS can then be resubstituted for air. Use of sodium hyaluronate in this fashion is probably the best way to maintain the anterior chamber during primary repair of a corneal laceration since it minimizes peripheral anterior synechiae and leaks out through wounds much more slowly than does BSS. When all the maneuvers of the primary repair are complete, the material that has filled the chamber up to that point should be exchanged for BSS.

Microscopes, microsurgical instruments, and fine sutures have improved techniques for, and results of, repair of corneal injuries and have made direct appositional suturing the treatment of choice for this entity. Direct appositional suturing allows the most uniform approximation of corneal tissue, can be modified as needed, allows satisfactory healing, and permits removal of separate sutures as healing and vascularization progress.

In my opinion, corneal defects requiring surgery are best closed with interrupted fine nylon sutures (Fig. 14-5). Corneal tissue can be closed with 8-0 or 9-0 silk, but 9-0 or 10-0 nylon is preferable. In addition to causing minimal tissue reaction, fine nylon sutures expand with tissue swelling and contract with resolution and are very comfortable for the patient. Absorbable sutures (variable absorption time, relatively inflammatory) should not be used in corneal tissue, with the exception of stab incision closures at the limbus in children. They may be used at the limbus if covered by a conjunctival flap.

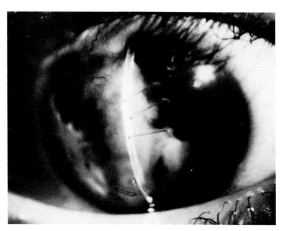

FIGURE 14-5. *Closure of laceration with 10-0 nylon sutures.*

Several microsurgical needles with a swaged-on suture are marketed for use in corneal surgery. The choice of a particular needle is left to the preference of the individual surgeon; those with the sharpest point and finest wire diameter seem most effective.

Suturing techniques are adequately described in surgical textbooks, and only brief comment is needed here. An attempt should be made to make suture bites about three-quarters depth, and bites should be longer in edematous tissue than in nonedematous tissue. Full-thickness sutures are occasionally helpful, but generally are not indicated. For stellate lacerations, a purse-string suture may be advantageous. Particular care should be taken in the optical axis to approximate tissue carefully and to place the minimum number of sutures. Corneal tissue should never be excised unless mandatory, because this brings increased difficulty in wound closure, marked tissue distortion and thus astigmatism, and more frequent wound disruption. Patch grafts, whether lamellar or full-thickness, can be laid in as needed.

Corneal trauma is frequently accompanied by anterior and posterior segment injuries, including hyphema, iris prolapse or laceration, lens disruption and dislocation, and vitreous incarceration. Although the course of action that may seem easiest is simple corneal repair, leaving other problems for later surgery, there is ample evidence that undertaking repair of associated anterior segment problems at the time of primary repair offers many advantages: Intraocular inflammation is reduced, the endothelium is protected from contact with various structures, synechiae can be prevented, glaucoma is reduced, secondary membranes are not as readily formed, further surgery may be obviated, and visualization of the posterior segment is made possible. Mechanical microsurgical instrumentation has made intraocular repair possible, and a surgeon caring for corneal wounds should not hesitate to undertake simultaneous anterior segment repair.

If a definite lens rupture greater than approximately 2 mm exists, and cortical material has begun to flocculate, as complete a lens extraction as possible should be done at the time of the primary repair. If the original corneal wound involves large loss of corneal substance, the lens aspiration or extraction may be accomplished through that site. Otherwise, the usual approach is to perform a limbal incision after primary repair of the corneal wound and carry out any needed lensectomy or vitrectomy through the limbal wound. The limbal wound is then closed in a routine fashion.

SURGICAL ADHESIVE

During the last 10 years, the use of surgical adhesive has become an important closure technique in corneal disease [1, 4]. Its use in trauma, however, is limited because of the effectiveness of appositional suturing. For a stellate laceration in which suturing does not achieve tight closure, adhesive applied over the sutures may be an important adjunct. A rare linear perforation, and traumatic rupture of thinned cornea (e.g., in Terrien's dystrophy), may be better closed with adhesive than with sutures. The main use of tissue adhesive in trauma, however, is as the primary bonding agent in the case of a leaking punctate perforation or leaking or "large" descemetocele and in cases in which focal infection follows laceration or perforation. Many infected, necrotic perforations have been successfully closed with adhesive when suturing was impossible, allowing healing beneath the adhesive and eliminating the need for more imposing surgery in the face of corneal infection.

One technique of surgical adhesive application to a corneal perforation or laceration is summarized as follows: The patient is best positioned supine. The surface to be bonded is meticulously cleaned of any debris, including vitreous, lens material, or iris pigment. Any epithelium covering the precisely outlined corneal surface to be bonded is removed. This is most conveniently accomplished with a No. 64 or 69 Beaver blade (Rudolph Beaver, Inc., Belmont, Mass.). This bared surface is then meticulously dried. Drying is most conveniently achieved with

successively applied cellulose sponges. If the area to be bonded is continually moistened by aqueous leaking through the adjacent wound, the anterior chamber may be gently massaged with the blunt, rounded instrument to "milk" some aqueous from the anterior chamber. Thus, when one next dries the wound, aqueous does not immediately leak onto the area to be bonded. Such anterior chamber massage of the globe is carried out only, of course, if there are no contraindications.

Surgical adhesive equipment includes a supply of thin polyethylene discs ranging in size from 2 to 4 mm and stored in any convenient antiseptic solution, a small smooth forceps of the surgeon's choice to retrieve a disc from the antiseptic solution, a blunt-end sterile applicator stick (conveniently the back end of a sterile cotton-tip applicator), ophthalmic topical anesthetic (if the procedure is done in the office and not under general anesthesia), a pair of surgeon's magnifying loupes, and a tube of sterile ointment.

Once these articles are assembled and the patient is supine, the most efficient approach is to have an assistant apply a small amount of ointment to the flat end of the applicator stick, affix the appropriate-size disc to this sticky flat surface, and then apply a minuscule drop of the fluid surgical adhesive to the center of the polyethylene disc. These maneuvers can be performed while the surgeon is de-epithelializing and drying the cornea. Once the corneal surface is prepared, the assistant quickly hands the glue-loaded disc on the stick held upright to the surgeon and assumes responsibility for holding open the patient's lids (if they are not maintained by a lid retractor). The surgeon then quickly inverts the glue applicator and accurately applies it to the corneal wound with mild pressure. This maneuver will transform the tissue adhesive into a flat confluent disc beneath the polyethylene disc. While the surgeon maintains slight pressure with the applicator stick on the polyethylene disc, the assistant drops several drops of BSS or topical anesthetic onto the perimeter of the polyethylene disc in order to polymerize any remaining fluid adhesive. This accomplished, the surgeon withdraws the applicator stick, leaving the polyethylene disc and a disc of now-solidified tissue glue beneath it straddling the wound. If the proper amount of adhesive monomer is originally applied to the polyethylene disc, the polymerized glue will not extend more than several tenths of a millimeter from the edge of the disc in any meridian.

If the anterior chamber was shallow before gluing, it is then observed for spontaneous deepening. Otherwise, the wound can be checked for aqueous

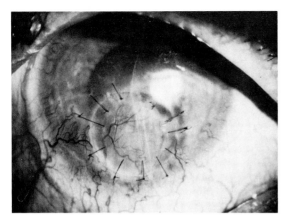

FIGURE 14-6. *Lamellar inlay graft, attached with interrupted 10-0 nylon sutures.*

leakage by carefully drying it with a cellulose sponge, as one typically does in the testing of any corneal wound closure, or by using Seidel's test. If the anterior chamber does not notably deepen within several minutes, or if the wound is evidently insecure, e.g., leaks visibly, the glue chip is removed. This is done by gently rotating it in the corneal plane to break its inadequate bond to the subjacent tissue and then gently lifting the chip away from the cornea. Pulling the partially bonded plaque off without first freeing its adhesions risks removing some corneal substance with it. The application procedure is then repeated in detail. Once hermetic wound closure is achieved and any other primary surgery is completed, a bandage soft contact lens is applied to the eye to minimize lid irritation by the glue and glue disturbance by lid motion.

"BLOWOUT" PATCH, LAMELLAR KERATOPLASTY, PENETRATING KERATOPLASTY

Although "blowout" patch, lamellar keratoplasty, and penetrating keratoplasty are frequently used in corneal disease, they are seldom indicated as a primary procedure in corneal trauma. When a large amount of corneal tissue is lost in the injury, donor tissue can be placed in a fashioned lamellar or full-thickness bed, with appositional or overlying support [2, 10]. Also, when trauma causes penetration or rupture of previously degenerated or thinned tissue, lamellar keratoplasty may be more effective than attempted primary closure (Fig. 14-6). Penetrating and lamellar keratoplasty are, of course, frequently used secondarily after trauma to eliminate scarring in the optical axis. These cases, particularly in young people, do not have the good prognosis for long-term graft clarity seen in some other conditions. This is thought to be due to corneal vascularization, inflammation, and associated anterior seg-

ment disorders secondary to trauma. Chapter 15 contains details regarding keratoplasty.

CONJUNCTIVAL FLAP

In the past, a conjunctival flap was frequently used alone or in association with other closure methods for the treatment of corneal perforations or lacerations. With modern surgical techniques and therapeutic substances and devices, a conjunctival flap is usually not the appropriate primary therapy for trauma. If there is leakage after suturing, a flap will seldom stop it. Placing a flap makes it difficult if not impossible to observe the healing process or the leakage site. Both the optical and cosmetic results of a conjunctival flap are poor. For all of these reasons, serious consideration should be given to all other modes of therapy before resorting to a conjunctival flap in this context.

COMPLICATIONS

RECURRENT EROSION

Recurrent corneal epithelial erosions may occur after disruption of basal cell adherence by hemidesmosomes to the basement membrane [3, 6]. Recurrent erosions are usually due to poor or delayed hemidesmosome reformation, which may result from local causes, e.g., diffuse mechanical or microbiologic injury to basement membrane or a primary basement membrane dystrophy, or from systemic causes, e.g., diabetes mellitus, severe malnutrition, and other systemic metabolic derangements.

Treatment may include lightly scraping loose epithelial flaps from the basement membrane to form a clean basal surface onto which adjacent epithelium may slide and bond. The involved eye may be pressure patched for a few days, with application once or twice daily of topical antibiotic selected according to the criteria in Observation, Patching above. After the initial period of pressure patching during which, one hopes, a major part of the healing occurs, one may discontinue the patch and switch to an emollient or antibiotic ointment as the case requires, applied 4 to 5 times daily. One may use in combination with the antibiotic ointment a hyperosmotic ointment, e.g., 5% sodium chloride ointment. An intermediate-acting cycloplegic should be used approximately once daily from the onset of the recurrent erosion for patient comfort. If these simple measures have failed after several days' trial, long-term bandage soft contact lenses seem to be the best treatment. Chapter 17 has more details regarding this entity.

FISTULA FORMATION

In my experience, chronic fistula formation after trauma is not only a very difficult problem to cure, but also is a major threat to the health of the eye. A fistula can lead to anterior chamber epithelialization, corneal infection, and endophthalmitis. Surgical closure is difficult, and tissue adhesive tamponade is often the best approach. If the fistula has been present for some time, closure often causes a severe and recalcitrant secondary glaucoma, even though no anatomic problem is seen in the angle structures. All of these possible problems lead to the recommendation of very aggressive early treatment of post-traumatic corneal fistulas.

INFECTION

Infection can occur after superficial or penetrating corneal injury. Its occurrence depends both on the offending agent and on the time between trauma and therapy. Infection is rare after superficial injury, particularly so after the common industrial occurrence of a metallic foreign body imbedded in the corneal surface, but these should probably be treated with broad-spectrum topical antibiotics until the epithelial defect is closed. Herpes simplex is frequently reported as a sequela of minor surface injury but probably is primary rather than secondary in many cases. Fungus infection can occur after surface injury with vegetable matter, leading to the recommendation of judicious postinjury steroid administration, removal of all foreign material, and surveillance for several weeks.

Topical antibiotics are usually sufficient therapy in surface and anterior penetrating injuries, and relatively clean penetrating injuries can be treated with topical and subconjunctival antibiotics. If the offending agent in a penetrating injury is suspected of carrying major bacterial contamination (i.e., in farmyard or pasture injuries), if the injury occurred more than 24 hours before treatment, or if purulence is obvious, pretreatment cultures are mandatory, and these cases should probably be treated as presumed endophthalmitis during early care. Bacterial Diseases in Chapter 5 has more details on this subject.

ULCERATION

Delayed epithelial healing and sterile superficial stromal ulceration have occurred in the past after repair of corneal injuries. This probably was due to surface irregularity, suture trauma to the surface, irregular tear film in the repair area with dellen formation, and antibiotic epithelial toxicity. Fortunately, the new refined sutures that become covered with epithelium and our current knowledge of antibiotic toxicity, surfacing and lubricating agents, and adjunctive devices such as the therapeutic soft contact lens have diminished this complication. If a sterile ulcer becomes infected, the treatment approach may be as discussed above under Infection.

ANTERIOR AND POSTERIOR SEGMENT COMPLICATIONS

Many complications can occur after major corneal trauma. Retained lens material can result in ocular inflammation, pupillary membranes, and secondary glaucoma, as well as formation of a "secondary cataract." Vitreous loss attendant upon corneal laceration may cause a higher incidence of epithelial or stromal fibrous downgrowth, iris prolapse, uveitis, glaucoma, retinal detachment, cystoid macular edema, vitreous opacities, vitreous contraction bands, pupillary membrane, endophthalmitis, and optic neuritis. Vitreous incarceration is probably the single most likely cause of ocular morbidity after vitreous loss. It may be better to excise anterior vitreous once it has been disturbed than to allow it to cause these potentially disastrous changes. It is interesting to note that recent research seems to indicate that vitreous hemorrhage followed by condensation, traction, and detachment may be better treated 1 to 2 weeks after primary repair of the injured eye [9].

Expulsive subchoroidal hemorrhage is a rare but dramatic and disastrous complication that may occur whenever the eye is traumatically or surgically opened. If it occurs during the course of closure of a complicated corneal wound, the wound can be tamponaded with a soft contact lens and digital pressure. If this does not relieve the expulsive process and if the wound cannot be closed by progressively tightening strong sutures (e.g., 7-0 or 6-0 silk), an immediate posterior sclerotomy, as first recommended by Verhoeff [11], is the procedure of choice. When the pressure of the hemorrhage is released, the wound may be surgically closable. If the wound cannot be closed by progressively tightening several strong sutures, partial anterior vitrectomy may be required finally to secure the wound. In this instance, particular care should be taken not to excise any anteriorly presenting retina.

Simple choroidal detachment may be due to the primary ocular insult or to persistent hypotony.

After scleral laceration, bleeding may occur from episcleral vessels, from a lacerated ciliary body, or from abnormal iris vascularization if any part of the eye is opened. Intraocular or extraocular bleeding or both may limit the view of the surgical field. If left in a disorganized eye, blood may organize pathologically. Bloodstaining of the cornea occurs if there is repeated intraocular bleeding and if the intraocular pressure is elevated. Endothelial trauma may predispose to corneal bloodstaining without elevated intraocular pressure.

Bullous keratopathy may occur from concussion endotheliopathy, traumatic or surgical endothelial damage, or attrition of endothelium by persistent glaucoma or uveitis. The incidence of late wound dehiscence may be increased by the use of topical or systemic corticosteroids to suppress intraocular inflammation. To promote wound healing, the patient, particularly if elderly or alcoholic, should be encouraged to have a balanced diet. Use of a high-quality multivitamin can do no harm and may do much good in the postoperative (stressed) patient.

Postinjury early endophthalmitis is usually septic and bacterial in origin but may be sterile. Endophthalmitis occurring several days to several weeks after surgery may be due to a wound leak and therefore either bacterial or fungal. Endophthalmitis occurring approximately 2 weeks or later after surgery in the absence of wound leak or filtering bleb may be fungal.

Chronic uveitis is often highly resistant to treatment in a severely traumatized eye. It may lead to anterior and posterior synechiae.

Further anterior and posterior segment complications of corneal trauma include the following: Commotio retinae is often attendant on major ocular trauma. Cystoid macular edema may result from the initial ocular shock, vitritis, simple aphakia, or aphakia with recurrent uveitis. Macular hole most often results from direct ocular trauma, although it may occur as a degenerative condition in cystoid macular edema. Rubeosis iridis may occur from severe ocular trauma alone, from severe anterior segment disorganization, or as a result of retinal ischemia, as may occur with optic nerve avulsion.

REFERENCES

1. Boruchoff, S. A., et al. Clinical applications of adhesives in corneal surgery. *Trans. Am. Acad. Ophthalmol. Otolaryngol.* 73:499, 1969.
2. Dohlman, C. H., Boruchoff, S. A., and Sullivan, G. L. A technique for the repair of perforated corneal ulcers. *Arch. Ophthalmol.* 77:519, 1967.
3. Goldman, J. M., Dohlman, C. H., and Kravitt, B. A. The basement membranes of the human cornea in recurrent epithelial erosion syndrome. *Trans. Am. Acad. Ophthalmol. Otolaryngol.* 73:471, 1969.
4. Hyndiuk, R. A., Hull, D. S., and Kinyoun, J. L. Free tissue patch and cyanoacrylate in corneal perforations. *Ophthalmic Surg.* 5:50, 1974.
5. Keates, R. H., and Lichtenstein, S. B. The management of anterior segment trauma with multiple small incisions. *Ophthalmology* (Rochester) 87:887, 1980.
6. Khodadoust, A. A., et al. Adhesion of regenerating corneal epithelium: The role of the basement membrane. *Am. J. Ophthalmol.* 65:339, 1968.
7. Lewis, M. L., Gass, D. M., and Spencer, W. H. Sympathetic uveitis after trauma and vitrectomy. *Arch. Ophthalmol.* 96:263, 1978.
8. Liddy, B. S., and Stuart, J. Sympathetic ophthalmia in Canada. *Can. J. Ophthalmol.* 7:157, 1972.
9. Ryan, S. J., and Allen, A. W. Pars plana vitrectomy in ocular trauma. *Am. J. Ophthalmol.* 88:483, 1979.
10. Troutman, R. C. *Microsurgery of the Anterior Segment of the Eye.* St. Louis: Mosby, 1974. Vol. 1, pp. 281–285.
11. Verhoeff, F. H. Scleral punctures for expulsive choroidal hemorrhage following sclerotomy—scleral rupture for postoperative separation of the choroid. *Ophthalmol. Res.* 24:55, 1915.

segments below.

Chemical Injuries

James P. McCulley

In most cases, chemical injuries of the eye are relatively minor and are easily treated. Occasionally, alkaline and acidic substances may cause severe ocular damage and permanent loss of vision, but usually they result in only minor tissue damage and rarely lead to permanent visual loss [43]. Because severe ocular injuries caused by chemicals are uncommon, it appears that they have received unjustified and disproportionate attention in the literature, but such attention is deserved, not only because severe chemical injuries are usually bilateral and often occur in young people, but also because the basic tissue responses to these injuries have been the focus of a great deal of experimental work aimed at understanding corneal ulceration and healing (see Chapter 2, Morphology and Pathologic Responses of the Cornea to Disease).

Since more is known about alkali injuries of the eye than about other chemical injuries, and much of this information can be applied to other types of chemical injuries, especially those caused by acids, alkali injuries are covered in depth in this chapter, and ocular acid burns are discussed in less detail. Other types of chemical injuries of the eye are usually less severe than alkali and acid injuries, and little has been written about them. The reader is referred to Grant's *Toxicology of the Eye* for a detailed discussion of the adverse ocular effects of petroleum products, other organic chemicals, and common household products such as detergents and cleaning agents [43].

ALKALI INJURIES

ALKALIES THAT CAUSE OCULAR INJURY

AMMONIA

Ammonia (NH_3) is encountered as a fertilizer and a refrigerant as well as in the manufacturing of other chemicals. The most common form is household ammonia, a 7% solution used as a cleaning agent [79]. Ammonia fumes stimulate the eye to secrete tears, which tends to dilute the chemical, reducing its potential for major ocular damage. However, the gas is soluble in water and tears, and, with prolonged exposure to the eye, ammonia gas forms ammonium hydroxide (NH_4OH), which does cause major ocular damage. Because ammonia is also highly soluble in lipid, it rapidly penetrates the eye, causing severe corneal injury, frequently accompanied by iris and lens damage. Penetration of the

eye by ammonia occurs in less than a minute, making the injury very difficult to ameliorate by subsequent irrigation.

LYE

Lye (i.e., sodium hydroxide, NaOH, caustic soda, sodium hydrate) penetrates the eye nearly as fast as does ammonium hydroxide. Lye burns occur most often as a result of getting solid sodium hydroxide (used as a drain cleaner) into the eye. These burns rank second in severity to those produced by ammonium hydroxide.

OTHER HYDROXIDES

Potassium hydroxide (KOH, caustic potash) and magnesium hydroxide [$Mg(OH)_2$] are encountered infrequently as causes of chemical injuries of the eye. Potassium hydroxide penetrates the eye only slightly less rapidly than does sodium hydroxide and cause injuries of similar severity. Magnesium hydroxide is found in sparklers and flares, and the combination of thermal injury and chemical injury accounts for the fact that the ocular injury associated with these devices is more severe than injuries that occur as a result of heat alone [45].

LIME

Lime [$Ca(OH)_2$, fresh lime, quicklime ($CaO + H_2O = Ca(OH)_2$, calcium hydrate, slaked lime, hydrated lime, plaster, mortar, cement, whitewash] is one of the more commonly encountered substances producing ocular burns. It penetrates the eye relatively poorly because it reacts with the epithelial cell membrane, forming calcium soaps that precipitate and hinder further penetration. Therefore, the injuries are less severe; however, calcium hydroxide does cause corneal opacity that is visible before the opacities seen as a result of ammonium or sodium hydroxide [44].

TOXIC EFFECTS

pH CHANGES

The mechanism of tissue damage is the same for all alkaline substances and is caused by changes in pH produced by the hydroxyl ion. Alkalies produce a high pH in the tissue water, which saponifies the fatty components of the cell membrane, leading to cell disruption. The variation in the severity of injury from one substance to another resides in the particular alkali's cation, which determines the penetrability of the individual molecules. At high pH, cations bind to collagen and glycosaminoglycans by reacting with carboxyl groups [44]. Since the corneal stroma is made up primarily of extracellular collagen, this change in pH causes hydration (swelling) of the individual collagen fibrils and results in thickening and shortening of the fibrils. However, no visible changes in the collagen molecules themselves can be detected by electron microscopy [46].

The alkali does appear to make the collagen more susceptible to enzymatic degradation. It has been postulated that this susceptibility is caused by the hydroxyl ion hydrolyzing the protective interfibrillar glycosaminoglycans, thus leaving the collagen "naked" and less resistant to enzymatic degradation [26, 40].

Increased aqueous pH correlates with increasing tissue damage, with serious, irreversible damage occurring at approximately pH 11.5. An increase in aqueous pH occurs within seconds of exposure to ammonium hydroxide; the aqueous pH change after sodium hydroxide exposure occurs a little more slowly, peaking between 3 to 5 minutes after exposure [71]. The pH returns to normal for all alkalies within ½ to 3 hours, with or without external irrigation [69].

If the alkaline substances penetrate to the ciliary body, changes in addition to pH elevation occur in the aqueous humor [26]. Both aqueous glucose [70] and ascorbate levels are decreased. This ascorbate deficiency may be the cause of subsequent reduced collagen synthesis [26, 58].

ULCERATION

Alkali burns commonly cause stromal ulceration. Ulceration is secondary to the initial effects of the chemical on the tissues, usually occurring approximately 2 to 3 weeks after the alkali burn as a result of accelerated proteolytic processes coupled with inadequate collagen synthesis.

PROTEOLYTIC EFFECTS

Several enzymes found in the chemically injured cornea account for the ulcerative process, including acid glycosidases [25], elastase, cathepsin G, and collagenolytic enzymes [19, 20, 22, 52, 78], one of which is true mammalian collagenase [8, 33, 41]. These enzymes have been found in both polymorphonuclear cells and epithelial cells in the ulcerating stroma, implying synthesis of at least some of the enzymes by these cells. As discussed in Chapter 2, after chemical injury it is thought that polymorphonuclear leukocytes are attracted to the region of tissue damage, infiltrating the stroma [53]. Although the normal cornea contains no latent or active collagenase [9, 41], 9 hours after an alkali burn to the cornea such enzymatic activity can be detected [10, 71]. The peak of collagenase activity does not occur until 14 to 21 days after the burn, however [8, 9].

The corneal epithelium has also been shown to produce a true collagenase after chemical injury [17, 71]. However, the epithelium probably plays a

greater role in the modulation of collagenase production by polymorphonuclear leukocytes [56] than it does in contributing to ulceration of the corneal stroma [53]. In addition to these two cell types, corneal stromal fibroblasts have also been shown to produce collagenase, although the role of such collagenase in ulceration after injury has not been delineated [48, 65].

When the cornea has re-epithelialized, or when the corneal stroma becomes totally vascularized, corneal ulceration ceases. Epithelial healing blocks the penetration of polymorphonuclear leukocytes into the corneal stroma from the tear film and also seems to inactivate the synthesis of collagenase by the white blood cells present in the stroma. Blood vessel growth into the stroma supplies nutrient precursors for protein and proteoglycan synthesis, which is accomplished by fibroblasts that migrate into the stroma some weeks after the injury.

COLLAGEN SYNTHESIS DEFECTS

Not only is collagen breakdown after alkali burns instrumental in the ulcerative process, but so also are defects in collagen synthesis. It has been noted that, in the reparative stages after severe ocular alkali burns, localized scorbutus can be seen in the cornea [40, 58, 72]. Aqueous humor ascorbate levels are greatly decreased after severe alkali burns. The ciliary body normally concentrates ascorbate in the aqueous humor to a level approximately 20-fold that in plasma. If the ciliary body is damaged, this concentrating ability appears to be compromised or lost. Ascorbate is required for the conversion of proline and lysine to hydroxyproline and hydroxylysine, respectively; these are necessary steps in the synthesis of mature collagens (c.f. Physiology of the Cornea: Metabolism and Biochemistry in Chapter 1). Ascorbate is also necessary for the conversion of monocytes to fibroblasts and in the formation of normal rough endoplasmic reticulum. Ascorbate also plays a role important in the synthesis of glycosaminoglycans.

It was found that if the aqueous humor ascorbate was greater than 15 mg/100 ml, no ulceration occurred in the rabbit [72]. By giving systemic or local ascorbate to increase the ascorbate level above 15 mg/100 ml, no ulceration occurred in an experimental alkali injury.

CLINICAL FEATURES

CLASSIFICATION OF SEVERITY

An ideal classification or grading system for ocular alkali burns does not exist because of the complex-

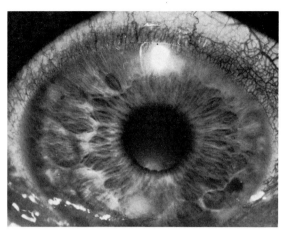

FIGURE 14-7. *Grade I alkali injury with minimal damage to corneal epithelium and associated conjunctival hyperemia. Iris details easily seen through a relatively clear cornea. This eye recovered in 10 days with return of vision to 20/20.*

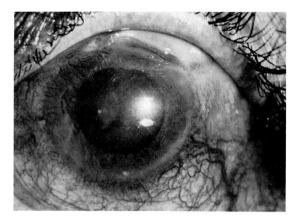

FIGURE 14-8. *Grade II alkali injury with moderate epithelial damage and associated stromal edema resulting in minimal blurring of iris detail. Minimal conjunctival ischemia present from 12 to 3 o'clock at the limbus. The eye recovered totally within 3 weeks.*

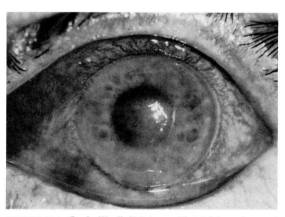

FIGURE 14-9. *Grade III alkali injury with total loss of corneal epithelium and marked stromal edema blurring but not obscuring the iris detail. The pupil is dilated, and the border can be seen between 8 and 2 o'clock. Conjunctival ischemia is present from 4 to 8 o'clock in the perilimbal region. The eye recovered after 2 months of therapy; however, residual minimal diffuse stromal scarring and vascularization decreased the visual acuity to 20/70.*

ities and variables associated with these injuries. However, the classification proposed by Hughes [49, 50] and modified by Ballen [4] and Roper-Hall [74] is useful in providing a guide to prognosis and treatment. The classification divides the injuries into four groups as follows:

Grade I
    Good prognosis
    Corneal epithelial damage (Fig. 14-7)
    No ischemia
Grade II
    Good prognosis
    Cornea hazy but iris details seen (Fig. 14-8)
    Ischemia at less than one-third of the limbus
Grade III
    Guarded prognosis
    Total loss of corneal epithelium
    Stromal haze blurring iris details (Fig. 14-9)
    Ischemia at one-third to one-half of limbus
Grade IV
    Poor prognosis
    Cornea opaque, obscuring view of iris or pupil
    Ischemia at more than one-half of the limbus
      (Fig. 14-10)

As is evident from the grading system, clinical prognosis is related to the area of chemical exposure as well as its depth of penetration. Determinants of the area of exposure are the extent of corneal epithelial loss and the degree of conjunctival involvement. The depth of penetration is determined not only by the degree of scleral injury initially, but also by the

subsequent development of hypotony or cataracts. Other factors that govern the severity of the injury include the quantity of chemical exposure, the hydroxyl ion concentration (pH) of the solution, the nature of the associated cation (which affects penetrability, and, in the case of ammonia, directly reacts with tissue), and the duration of exposure to the chemical.

EVALUATION OF TISSUE INJURY

ACUTE CHANGES (IMMEDIATE TO 1 WEEK AFTER INJURY)

Acute ocular chemical injury causes destruction of cellular membranes and some or all of the following structures, depending on the depth of the penetration: the corneal and conjunctival epithelium,

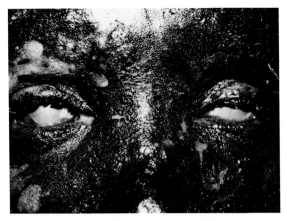

FIGURE 14-10. *Grade IV alkali injury with total corneal opacification blurring pupil and iris detail. Ischemia is present 360 degrees around the limbus. After 6 months of therapy, the corneas were severely scarred and vascularized bilaterally; however, the visual acuity in a dark room was 20/80 OD and 20/200 OS.*

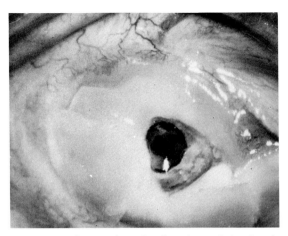

FIGURE 14-11. *Large pericentral perforated corneal ulcer 6 weeks after a neglected grade IV alkali injury. Note surrounding necrotic tissue and absence of vascularization.*

keratocytes, corneal nerves, endothelium of the cornea and blood vessels, cellular and vascular components of iris and ciliary body, and lens epithelium. Even if the deeper ocular structures such as the lens, ciliary body, and iris are spared, penetration of the cornea by the chemical leads to epithelial defects, stromal clouding, perilimbal necrosis, and hemorrhage. The damage to the corneal endothelium and deeper structures may not be apparent immediately, since they may be obscured by the anterior stromal clouding [2].

In the first few hours after alkali burns, the intraocular pressure may be increased in a bimodal fashion, although the pressure is occasionally normal [27, 67, 68, 80]. The initial increase appears to be due to collagen fibril hydration, which results in longitudinal shortening of the collagen fibers, compression of the globe, and distortion of the filtration angle. Within a few hours, a second increase in pressure may occur as a result of obstruction of the outflow channels by increased episcleral venous pressure, as well as accumulation of inflammatory debris within the trabecular meshwork. Prostaglandin released from the iris and other ocular structures may contribute to the second phase of increased intraocular pressure also [67, 69]. Once these two early phases of elevation of intraocular pressure have passed, the pressure may fluctuate from glaucoma to hypotony for several days, depending on the balance between decreased aqueous humor production and decreased outflow.

EARLY REPARATIVE PHASE (1–3 WEEKS)
After the first week, the conjunctival and corneal epithelia begin to regenerate and, in all but the most

severe injuries, completely cover the ocular surfaces during the early reparative phase [50]. Ingrowth of vessels and invasion of the corneal stroma by inflammatory cells parallel the epithelial regrowth.

Corneal opacity begins to clear and, in mild to moderate cases, may completely resolve during this period. However, if corneal ulceration ensues, it typically begins 2 to 3 weeks after the injury and may subsequently become a serious problem.

LATE REPARATIVE PHASE AND SEQUELAE (3 WEEKS TO SEVERAL MONTHS)
The onset of stromal ulceration depends on the balance between collagen synthesis and collagen degradation in the cornea during the late reparative phase. Such ulceration can cause irregularities of the surface with the production of severe astigmatism and poor vision. However, the most serious consequence of ulceration is descemetocele formation or even perforation, both of which threaten the integrity of the globe [50] (Fig. 14-11). If perforation can be avoided in this interval, the eye will heal, although frequently with severe vascularization and scarring. In the final stages of healing after moderately severe injuries, a fibrovascular pannus may overgrow the cornea. Corneal vascularization often occurs after severe alkali burns and often progresses until the entire cornea is vascularized. In very severe injuries, total corneal vascularization is desirable in a sense, since the cornea is not apt to perforate in areas where it is vascularized [16].

If the alkali has destroyed the corneal endothelium, retrocorneal, iridic, and ciliary body fibrous membranes may develop in the late reparative stage [60]. With severe injuries, permanent loss of corneal innervation with resultant neurotrophic keratitis may occur in the late reparative phase. Thus, in addition to permanent ocular surface abnormalities, the loss of corneal innervation contributes to the poor prognosis for corneal transplantation in these patients.

Loss of the accessory lacrimal glands or scarring of the ductule openings of the major lacrimal gland may result in tear deficiency. However, tear deficiency is less common after alkali injury than is copious tear secretion. Nevertheless, the tear film may be unstable as the result of a mucin-deficient state produced as a consequence of a diffuse loss of goblet cells [57]. Tear film abnormalities are one of the more common and important sequelae of all but mild alkali burns and lead to epithelial abnormalities manifested by epithelial cell damage and keratinization.

Intraocular pressure in the late phase after alkali burn may range from a state of hypotony to glaucoma. Fibrosis of the ciliary body may occur after severe injuries, resulting in hypotony and subsequent phthisis bulbi. With less severe injuries or injuries affecting the outflow channels more than the ciliary body, severe secondary glaucoma may develop. Fibrous proliferation in the anterior chamber angle, extensive peripheral anterior synechiae obstructing the trabecular meshwork, or increased episcleral venous pressure may contribute to the secondary glaucoma.

The development of symblepharon after alkali burns is variable, depending on the extent of conjunctival necrosis. If the palpebral and bulbar conjunctival regions are both injured, the two opposing surfaces may fuse during the healing process, leading to shortening of the fornix. Contracture of the subepithelial tissues leads to progressive symblepharon formation, producing lid abnormalities manifested as entropion and trichiasis. This may cause exposure of the globe and mechanical irritation, resulting in further damage to the ocular surface.

TREATMENT

Regeneration of intact epithelial covering of the ocular surface, general support of the reparative process, control of the acute inflammatory reaction, and avoidance of complications are the primary goals of therapy. Specific therapeutic measures vary, however, depending on the severity of the alkali burn. Dividing treatment into four phases—

immediate, early, and intermediate treatment, and rehabilitation—is helpful in discussing these therapeutic variations. For mild to moderate alkali burns, treatment can be accomplished on an outpatient basis, but patients with more severe burns require hospitalization and observation for 1 to 2 weeks.

IMMEDIATE TREATMENT

Immediate treatment of ocular alkali burns consists of irrigation with any nontoxic liquid. The nature of the irrigant, provided it is nontoxic, is less important than the speed with which is it begun. Water, ionic solutions, and buffered solutions have all proved to be equally effective. However, acidic irrigating solutions to neutralize the alkali are risky and are not recommended. The implantation of a T tube or the use of an irrigating scleral lens has been recommended as a method of irrigation by Morgan [61]. However, these methods have not proved to be superior to simply retracting the lids and using IV tubing connected to the irrigating solution under manual control.

Although it may be helpful to determine the pH in the inferior cul-de-sac by using litmus paper before irrigation, in no circumstances should irrigation be greatly delayed to accomplish this. However, determination of pH and its return to neutrality may be used to monitor the effectiveness of irrigation in some cases.

On the principle that it is better to irrigate too much rather than too little, irrigation for 30 minutes has come to serve as the standard approach [79]. In addition to adequate cleansing of the eye, one must be certain that the pH is not abnormal because of slow release of the chemical from retained particulate matter. In some cases, even prolonged irrigation will not bring the pH to normal, and thus it is essential to examine the superior and inferior cul-de-sacs carefully for particles. If examination, done by double everting the upper lid, reveals chemical imbedded in the tissue, a 0.01- to 0.05-M solution of sodium EDTA, should be used as an irrigant [44]. If this also fails to remove all of the remaining material, a cotton-tip applicator soaked in sodium EDTA should be used.

Although paracentesis alone or in combination with irrigation of the anterior chamber with buffered solutions, e.g., phosphate buffer, has been advocated [6, 69], efficacy has not been proved. Therefore, I advise against this procedure because of the inherent risks.

EARLY (ACUTE PHASE) TREATMENT

After immediate irrigation of the eye, the next phase of treatment is directed toward making the patient comfortable, preventing infection, reducing ocular inflammation, and preventing stromal loss. In mild injuries, application of a topical antibiotic, a mydriatic-cycloplegic, and a pressure patch are all that may be necessary for treatment. In more severe injuries, other therapeutic modalities including topical steroids, collagenase inhibitors, and therapeutic soft contact lenses may be necessary.

ANTIBIOTICS, CYCLOPLEGICS, AND ACUTE GLAUCOMA THERAPY

Antibiotics should be given routinely to prevent infection. Chloramphenicol drops (0.5% 3 times daily) or gentamicin drops (0.3% 3 times daily) provide broad-spectrum prophylaxis against a variety of gram-negative and gram-positive bacteria. Because of the decreased resistance of the injured tissue, it is also advisable to include prophylaxis against normally nonpathogenic bacteria such as *Staphylococcus epidermidis*. This can be achieved by using bacitracin ointment 3 times daily.

Mydriatics and cycloplegics (10% phenylephrine and 2% atropine 3 times daily) should be given to prevent the development of posterior synechiae and to alleviate ciliary spasm and its attendant discomfort. If the intraocular pressure is elevated or if it is not possible to measure it, treatment with carbonic anhydrase inhibitors (acetazolamide 250 mg PO 4 times daily) or topical timolol maleate (0.5% twice daily) should be instituted.

TOPICAL STEROIDS

Because inflammatory cells produce proteolytic enzymes that are responsible for corneal ulceration, the use of topical steroids to decrease inflammation of the eye is indicated in severe injury. The drug of choice is 1% prednisolone or 0.1% dexamethasone applied topically several times a day for the first 10 days. This regimen has proved to be safe and is effective in reducing post-traumatic iritis and inflammation.

Contradictory data exist as to whether steroids inhibit or potentiate the effects of tissue collagenase [21, 48, 55]. Nevertheless, most clinicians feel that stromal ulceration is accelerated by the use of steroids once it has begun. This adverse effect generally occurs only if the administration is continued longer than the first 10 days after the injury. A study in rabbits supports this observation, showing no deleterious effect from the use of topical steroids during the first week after alkali burns [32]. In humans, also, topical steroids may be administered for the first 10 days after alkali burn even if the epithelium is not intact. However, if after 10 days corneal re-epithelialization has not occurred, the steroid dosage must be tapered rapidly and discontinued within 1 or 2 days, since at this point the risk

of potentiating ulceration by promoting collagen breakdown outweighs the potential antiinflammatory benefits. On the other hand, if the epithelium is intact after 10 days of steroid therapy, steroids can be safely continued for weeks and months. However, there are no clinical studies that prove that such steroid usage reduces the eventual scarring and vascularization that occur with healing.

COLLAGENASE INHIBITORS

Collagenase can be assayed within 9 hours after an acute alkali burn; however, the basement membrane does not break down until approximately 7 days after injury, and stromal ulceration usually begins 2 to 3 weeks after injury. Therefore, the use of collagenase inhibitors may be delayed until there is evidence of collagen breakdown at 7 to 14 days.

Several different substances including 0.2-M sodium EDTA (Na$_4$EDTA) [18], 0.2-M calcium EDTA (CaNa$_2$EDTA) [18, 51, 77], 0.2-M cysteine [12, 15, 18, 76], 0.1-M penicillamine [35], and 10 to 20% acetylcysteine (Mucomyst) [76], have been found to inhibit collagenase. The in vivo effect of most of these substances is quite weak. Some of them are relatively toxic and are therefore not suitable inhibitors for clinical use. The only inhibitor that is clinically available at present is 10 to 20% acetylcysteine. It may be given every 2 hours while the patient is awake. It has been shown in animals to be an effective irreversible inhibitor of collagenase [76]. It chelates divalent ions and disrupts disulfide bonds. It is a relatively unstable solution but can be kept in the refrigerator and used for approximately 1 week. Acetylcysteine also has a powerful, disagreeable odor that patients find objectionable.

Other inhibitors of collagenase occur naturally in serum. These include alpha-1-macroglobulin, alpha-2-macroglobulin, and beta-1-globulin. These have been shown to be effective natural inhibitors in the rabbit, and alpha-2-macroglobulin and beta-1-globulin have been shown to be effective inhibitors in humans. The inability to obtain these materials in pure form has made their use in prevention of stromal ulceration impossible.

Another approach to collagenase inhibition is to interfere with the synthesis of the enzyme itself. A 0.5% suspension of medroxyprogesterone (Provera) in 1% aqueous methylcellulose used twice daily has been shown to inhibit the production of collagenase in rabbits [64]. This compound has the added advantage of decreasing the inflammatory response. Although it has been used in isolated cases in which perforation seemed inevitable, its use in the treatment of alkali burns on a routine basis is not yet established.

SOFT CONTACT LENSES

In patients in whom inadequate epithelial healing becomes evident, soft contact lenses have proved to be of great benefit in many instances. It is best to fit the soft contact lens as soon as possible after the acute injury, since its use may facilitate adhesion of the regenerating epithelial edge. The usual antibiotic, cycloplegic, and antiglaucomatous drops can be used with the lens in place.

After fitting the lens, evaluation of its effectiveness in promoting epithelial healing and integrity may be difficult to accomplish. In general, however, the lens can be taken off briefly, and fluorescein can be used to determine the size of the residual defect. In general, the therapeutic soft lens must be left in place for at least 6 to 8 weeks after the epithelium has healed to ensure adequate adhesion between the epithelium and its underlying substrate.

OTHER THERAPY

In the early phase, various forms of treatment including the subconjunctival injections of serum or blood, topical vasodilators, lamellar keratoplasty, mucous membrane grafts [3, 5, 28], and artificial epithelium (glued-on contact lenses) have been recommended but have fallen into disuse. However, ascorbate supplement may prove to be a therapeutic benefit when the aqueous humor ascorbate level is decreased after a chemical injury. The beneficial effect of ascorbate has not been established in humans, but trials are in progress using oral ascorbate, 2 gm 4 times daily, and a topical 10% solution of ascorbate in artificial tears, given hourly 14 times each day. Based on animal experiments, if the aqueous humor ascorbate level is maintained at 15 mg/100 ml or higher, it is likely that the cornea will not ulcerate [72]. However, supplemental ascorbate has been shown to have an adverse effect with increased resultant stromal ulceration in conditions in which there is no loss of ciliary body concentrating ability [34]. It is therefore important not to generalize this proposed use of ascorbate from alkali burns, in which the aqueous humor level of ascorbate is probably low, to other ulcerating conditions in which it is entirely normal.

Subconjunctival injection of 0.75 ml heparin (750 U) mixed with 0.2 ml lidocaine hydrochloride 2% and 0.35 ml NaCl given every other day has been reported to reduce stromal ulceration [1]. It is re-ported that the therapeutic effect may not be obvious for several weeks, and this lack of clear relationship to the therapy has led to skepticism about the effectiveness of conjunctival heparin in inhibiting stromal ulceration in alkali burns.

The most prominent conjunctival complication of alkali burn is symblepharon formation. This gradual loss of fornix depth, with adhesion between the bulbar and palpebral conjunctiva, can be minimized by the use of scleral lenses or symblepharon rings, which keep the raw tarsal and bulbar surfaces from coming into apposition with one another. A simple, effective means of decreasing symblepharon formation is lysis of the symblepharons daily with an ointment-coated glass rod.

INTERMEDIATE TREATMENT

The characteristics of the alkali burn and the response to early treatment will determine treatment from 3 to 4 weeks after injury until the eye has stabilized. Appropriate measures that have been instituted earlier, such as antibiotics, cycloplegic-mydriatics, and antiglaucoma therapy, should be continued.

The persistence of epithelial defects and associated stromal ulceration are the major problems during this period. Epithelial healing may be abetted by refitting therapeutic soft contact lenses at frequent intervals. If this fails, topical echothiophate iodide (Phospholine Iodide) can be given in an attempt to stimulate epithelial mitosis by increasing the acetylcholine concentration available to the epithelium [24]. Echothiophate iodide inhibits acetylcholine esterase, which leads to an elevation of the acetylcholine level in the epithelium. It is thought that the increased level acetylcholine in turn increases the level of intracellular guanosine 3',5'-cyclic phosphate, which stimulates cellular mitosis [24].

Mucomimetic tears may be given to help stabilize the tear film in more severe injuries. Even with their use, there may be continued signs of epithelial breakdown even if a gross epithelial defect does not occur. If exposure secondary to poor lid function is considered to be a serious problem, a tarsorrhaphy should be considered. Scarring of the lids may also lead to trichiasis, with mechanical abrasion of the globe. In most cases, the continued use of a soft contact lens will eliminate this potential cause of epithelial loss.

A conjunctival flap should be considered if continued stromal ulceration occurs despite all measures taken. However, the flap should not be done until the conjunctiva itself is repopulated, which can take 3 to 6 weeks (see Chapter 16, Conjunctival Surgery for Corneal Disease). If the conjunctiva has been so severely injured that it does not appear to

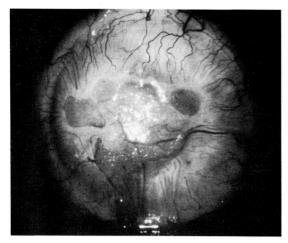

FIGURE 14-12. *Scarred vascularized cornea 6 months after grade IV alkali injury. Note areas of faceting centrally, secondary to recurrent erosions with resultant ulceration.*

be mobile enough to cover the cornea, a 0.4-mm-thick mucous membrane graft from the mouth can be transplanted to the corneal surface. Mucous membrane grafts are effective in halting stromal ulceration, but they do not restore the normal anatomy of the surface of the eye [3, 28]. They have their greatest utility in restoration of the depth of the fornix after symblepharon formation.

If corneal perforation occurs, and the site of perforation is relatively small, one may consider the use of a tissue adhesive such as cyanoacrylate [83] or a patch graft [30] to seal the perforation.

REHABILITATION
After the eye is totally healed and inflammation has subsided, the potential for useful vision in the eye can be assessed. In the case of serious injury, anterior segment scarring and vascularization may be severe enough to interfere with examination of the posterior pole by conventional funduscopy (Fig. 14-12). Nevertheless, the gross visual response to light can be determined, and ultrasonography can be used to check the position of the lens and to ascertain that the retina is not detached.

The surgical procedures that have been found useful for rehabilitation of the chemically injured eye include conjunctival transplantation, penetrating keratoplasty, and keratoprosthesis.

CONJUNCTIVAL TRANSPLANTATION
As described in detail in Chapter 16, Conjunctival Surgery for Corneal Disease, transplantation of conjunctiva obtained from the other eye can be used in unilateral injuries [81]. The procedure has been shown to be effective in rehabilitation of the ocular

surface [81] and in selected circumstances may prove to benefit the vision as well. Whether or not this procedure is useful before keratoplasty to provide a stable epithelium is not yet known.

PENETRATING KERATOPLASTY
In patients with chemical injury of the eye, there are a number of complications that threaten the success of the corneal grafting [13, 14]. These include lid scarring and distortion, trichiasis, symblepharon formation, long-standing glaucoma, anterior chamber fibrosis with membrane formation, and retinal detachment. In addition, poor postoperative compliance with medical recommendations has proved to be a major problem in many cases and occasionally thwarts otherwise potentially successful surgical outcomes [54].

Because of the complications, a penetrating keratoplasty should be delayed for at least 1 year from the time the eye is healed and inflammation has resolved. This gives the tissue time to resume structural and biochemical normalcy.

In all cases, stromal and epithelial wound healing represent major postoperative problems. This occurs despite the fact that most surgeons leave the donor epithelium in place to avoid immediate postoperative epithelial defects. Eventually, the donor epithelium appears to be replaced by host epithelium, which does not seem to re-epithelialize the donor stroma in a normal fashion. It has been demonstrated in animals that conversion of conjunctival epithelium to morphologically and biochemically normal corneal epithelium is a slow and incomplete process [38, 82]. This lack of conversion into corneal epithelium may account for the delayed epithelial defects that are so characteristic of penetrating keratoplasty in chemical injury.

The technical details of keratoplasty in chemical injury are similar to those described for other diseases in Therapeutic Keratoplasty in Chapter 15. Postoperatively, it is essential to suppress inflammation with the vigorous use of topical steroids. Soft contact lenses are also necessary to assist in the maintenance of an intact corneal epithelium. Mucomimetic artificial tears may be effective in helping to maintain a normal corneal epithelium. The possibility of developing glaucoma should be carefully monitored, and increased pressure should be controlled if it develops.

KERATOPROSTHESIS
Many severe chemical injuries leave the patient blind. Repeated attempts at keratoplasty may be

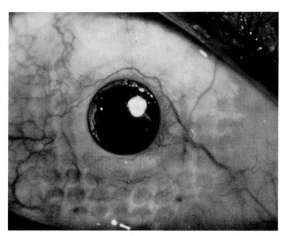

FIGURE 14-13. *Nut-and-bolt keratoprosthesis 2 years after alkali injury. Visual acuity is hand motions only because of severe glaucomatous damage.*

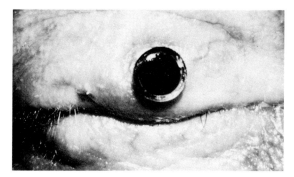

FIGURE 14-14. *Through-and-through keratoprosthesis 1 year after severe alkali injury. Vision fluctuated between 20/20 and 20/40 for 2 years but subsequently deteriorated because of an irreparable retinal detachment.*

made but are usually unsuccessful because of immunologic rejection. In such patients, keratoprosthesis may offer the only means for at least temporary visual improvement. Such procedures are outlined in Therapeutic Keratoplasty in Chapter 15.

A nut-and-bolt or collar-button prosthesis is generally not successful because of melting and extrusion [23, 31, 39] (Fig. 14-13). However, through-and-through prostheses, with the optical post extending through the upper lid, have had limited success [23, 73] (Fig. 14-14). The major complications associated with all types of keratoprostheses include extrusion, retroprosthetic membrane, glaucoma, retinal detachment, and infection.

ACID INJURIES

Ocular acid injuries occur only slightly less frequently than do injuries produced by alkaline substances [74]. However, with the exception of isolated case reports, little has appeared in the literature about acid injuries. Fortunately, most acid injuries are mild because the exposure is to weak acids or diluted strong acids. However, severe injuries do occur and are most commonly associated with exposure to heavy metal acid such as chromic acid or mineral acids such as sulfuric, sulfurous, or hydrofluoric acid. These acids tend to produce more severe injuries for reasons that will be discussed below. The clinical appearance and subsequent evolution of all severe ocular acid injuries are similar, regardless of which acid was responsible. For the most part, the approach to managing acid injuries of the eyes is similar to that for managing alkaline injuries, and therefore on the following pages emphasis is placed on areas in which the management of acid injuries is different.

CLINICALLY IMPORTANT ACIDS

SULFURIC ACID
The most commonly encountered acid causing ocular injury is sulfuric acid (H_2SO_4), which is a widely used industrial chemical as well as the acid used in batteries. Concentrated sulfuric acid has a great avidity for water. The reaction produced from the combination of sulfuric acid with the water contained in the corneal tissue is accompanied by the release of heat, resulting in tissue charring. Sulfuric acid produces injuries ranging from mild to very severe: Highly concentrated sulfuric acid causes severe ocular injuries; mild injury similar to injuries caused by hydrochloric acid results from a lower concentration of sulfuric acid.

Battery acid injuries are increasing in frequency [47]. The majority are minor; however, severe injuries with loss of vision or loss of the globe do occur. Most of the injuries, especially the more severe ones, occur as the result of battery explosions. Hydrogen and oxygen are produced by electrolysis when sulfuric acid combines with water in the battery. This gaseous mixture explodes on contact with flame. Matches or cigarette lighters used as illumination sources or sparks produced by jumper cables are the most common modes of ignition. Injuries that result from battery explosions commonly are combinations of acid burn and contusion from particulate matter but may also show laceration or intraocular foreign-body penetration.

SULFUROUS ACID
Sulfur dioxide (SO_2), which forms sulfurous acid (H_2SO_3) when it combines with water in corneal tissue, may be encountered as sulfurous anhydride or

sulfurous oxide, which is used as a fruit and vegetable preservative, bleach, or refrigerant. When used as a refrigerant, it is mixed with oil. If this combination gets into the eye, contact is prolonged because of the hydrocarbon present, with more severe tissue damage as a result. However, because SO_2 is volatile and tends to evaporate from its oily carrier, ocular and tissue damage do not occur unless a direct jet of the gas or liquid and oil hits the skin or eye.

Sulfur dioxide damages the corneal nerves, resulting in anesthesia and little discomfort. Initially, visual acuity is not severely affected but it worsens greatly over hours to days as the ocular signs worsen.

Sulfur dioxide's freezing effect on the tissue does not produce the injury [42]. Rather, the damage is caused by the sulfurous acid itself, which denatures protein and inactivates numerous enzymes, causing the destruction of the corneal tissue. Because of its high lipid and water solubility, sulfurous acid penetrates the tissues easily.

HYDROFLUORIC ACID
Hydrofluoric acid (HF, hydrogen fluoride) is a weak inorganic acid but a strong solvent. In industry, it is found either in its pure form (in solutions ranging from 0.5% to 70% in strength) or mixed with other agents such as nitric acid, ammonium difluoride, and acetic acid. It breaks down the molecular structure of most substances; however, it does not affect polyethylene or polypropylene. Rubber can withstand hydrofluoric acid for limited periods.

Hydrofluoric acid is used in etching and polishing glass and silicone and in frosting glass. It is also used in the pickling or chemical milling of metals, as well as in the refining of uranium, tantalum, and beryllium. It is also used in the alkylation of high-octane gasoline, the production of elemental and inorganic fluoride, and the preparation of organic fluorocarbons. Its most frequent use is in the expanding semiconductor business, in which it is used in the production of silicone products.

Much has been written on skin burns caused by hydrofluoric acid; however, the literature is sparse relative to ocular injuries. A rabbit model was developed to evaluate ocular hydrofluoric acid burns [63], and it was found that hydrofluoric acid produces a severe injury because of its high degree of activity in dissolving cellular membranes. In addition, the low molecular weight and small size of hydrofluoric acid molecule allow it to penetrate the tissues readily.

OTHER ACIDS
Chromic acid is a strong caustic derived from chromic oxide and chromium trioxide (Cr_2O_3). Rare cases of severe ocular injury have occurred after direct instillation of the liquid in the eye. However, ocular injuries caused by chromic acid are more often associated with exposure to droplets of the acid in the chrome-plating industry, resulting in chronic conjunctival inflammation and a brown discoloration of the epithelium in the interpalpebral fissure.

Hydrochloric acid is commonly used as 32 to 38% solution. The hydrogen chloride gas is irritating to the eye, producing protective tearing and thus preventing severe ocular damage. On the other hand, at high concentrations and with prolonged exposure, liquid hydrochloric acid may produce severe ocular damage.

Burns produced by nitric acid (HNO_3) are similar to those produced by hydrochloric acid, except that the epithelial opacity produced by nitric acid is yellowish rather than white as it is in the other acid burns.

Acetic acid (CH_3COOH), a relatively weak inorganic acid, is also known as ethanoic acid, ethylic acid, methane carboxylic acid, vinegar acid, and glacial acetic acid. The various forms of acetic acid, especially vinegar acid, which is only 4 to 10% acetic acid, typically produce only minor ocular damage, unless exposure is prolonged. Exposure to a greater than 10% solution is required to produce a severe injury unless the time of exposure is exceedingly long. "Essence of vinegar" is 80% acetic acid and may produce severe damage. Glacial acetic acid is the most concentrated form of acetic acid (90%) and may also produce severe ocular injury.

TOXIC EFFECTS
All acids coagulate and precipitate protein, causing tissue destruction. The degree of protein precipitation and denaturation depends upon the protein affinity of the particular acid's anion [37]. Therefore, both the pH change caused by the hydrogen ion and the adverse effect on the tissue proteins caused by the ionic portion of the acid contribute to tissue destruction. However, because tissue proteins in turn have a buffering effect on the action of the acid, most acid burns are limited and localized [36]. Coagulated epithelial cells also serve as a relative barrier to deep and extensive penetration of acid.

Acids react with collagen, resulting in a shortening of collagen fibers, which causes a rapid increase in intraocular pressure [27, 66]. Acids have a variable effect on corneal glycosaminoglycans as measured by the effect on stromal swelling pressure [42] and changes in metachromatic staining [37, 63, 75]. The stromal turbidity seen after acid burns is probably not caused by changes in collagen but rather by precipitation of the extracellular glycosaminoglycans [59].

Changes in the aqueous humor after exposure to acid have been less thoroughly examined than aqueous humor changes after alkaline injuries. However, aqueous humor pH has been found to be decreased 15 minutes after exposure to hydrochloric acid [66]. Aqueous humor protein content and prostaglandin activity have been found to be elevated during the first several hours after exposure to hydrochloric acid [66].

Proteolytic enzyme activity after acid burns has not been evaluated. However, it can be surmised that when ulceration occurs the same kind of endogenous proteolytic enzymes that are present after alkali burns are present. Ulceration has been found to be rare after hydrofluoric acid burns, unless divalent ions from some other chemical mixed with the acid are present. In cases in which hydrofluoric acid is combined with another chemical, the ulcerative process becomes prominent [62].

A defect in collagen synthesis has not been established after alkali burns. However, after severe burns with ciliary body damage it has been demonstrated that aqueous humor and corneal ascorbate are decreased and that a localized scorbutic state, similar to that found after severe alkali burns, exists [58, 72].

CLINICAL FEATURES

CLASSIFICATION OF SEVERITY

A classification system has not been proposed specifically for acid burns. However, the Roper-Hall [74] and Ballen [4] modification of the Hughes [49, 50] scheme for alkali burns (see page 424) can also be used to classify acid burns. As in the case of alkali burns, an acid injury has a bad prognosis if there is evidence that the acid has penetrated the tissue, e.g., complete corneal anesthesia, conjunctival and episcleral ischemia, severe iritis, and lens opacification.

In general, however, acids produce less severe injuries than do alkalies. This is attributed to the fact that the acid coagulates the epithelial surface, forming a relative barrier to penetration of the acid, and that the corneal stroma has a buffering effect on acid solutions with a pH less than 4 (Fig. 14-15) [36]. Exceptions to this include sulfuric acid, which has a tissue-charring effect related to its avidity for water; sulfurous acid, which is water and lipid soluble; and hydrofluoric acid, which penetrates well and the fluoride ion of which produces associated tissue damage [63].

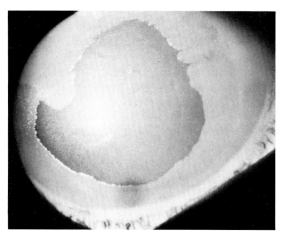

FIGURE 14-15. *Whitish coagulated epithelium overlying edematous opaque stroma after a moderately severe sulfuric acid injury. Central epithelium has sloughed; however, the peripheral white, coagulated epithelium persisted for 1 week before sloughing. The eye ultimately scarred and vascularized with best visual acuity of 20/60 in a darkened room.*

After exposure to any acid, the amount of tissue damage depends on the pH, quantity, and concentration of the acid, and the time of exposure. Other individual biochemical characteristics such as lipid solubility [42] and protein affinity [37] also affect the severity of the injury. Fumes containing hydrogen ions and droplets of acidic solutions cause minor injury, with the more severe injuries occurring from direct splashes of acidic chemicals onto the ocular surface.

TREATMENT

Treatment of acid burns, as with alkali burns, must be adjusted to the severity of the injury. The primary goals are the restoration of an intact epithelial covering of the ocular surface, control of the acute inflammatory process, the support of the reparative process, and the avoidance of complications.

Acid burn therapy is similar to that for alkali burns of similar severity. As a general rule, the majority of acid burns are mild and do not require the extensive treatment necessary for alkali burns, which are usually more severe. However, although severe acid burns are uncommon, they do occur and must be treated in a manner similar to that for severe alkali burns. In the following discussion of specific treatment, therapeutic measures for acid burns are detailed only if they vary from treatment of comparably severe alkali burns.

IMMEDIATE (EMERGENCY) TREATMENT

The most important consideration is the speed with which irrigation begins. It is inadvisable to attempt to neutralize the acid solution either with alkali or a buffer solution. Saline or water are acceptable for irrigation; however, if both are equally available, it is preferable to use normal saline to avoid damage caused by the hypotonicity of water alone. If saline is not immediately available, the damage caused by water is minimal and may be more than balanced by the beneficial effect of rapid irrigation.

The inferior cul-de-sac pH should be measured before beginning irrigation. A shorter period is required for the pH to return to normal after acid burns than after alkali burns. However, irrigation for 20 to 30 minutes as a starting point is not excessive. After 20 to 30 minutes of irrigation and a delay of approximately 5 minutes to allow for equilibration, the cul-de-sac pH should be remeasured and irrigation continued only if the pH is still abnormally low.

Although 0.03% benzalkonium chloride has been recommended as an irrigant for ocular hydrofluoric acid burn [29], it has been found to cause additional ocular damage and has no beneficial therapeutic effect [62]. Therefore, this solution should not be used. It has also been suggested that various substances used to treat hydrofluoric acid burns of the skin could be used to treat hydrofluoric acid ocular burns, but all have proved to be toxic or simply ineffective. Pastes of 25 to 50% magnesium sulfate or magnesium oxide have been recommended but were found to be too toxic for use in the eye [62]. Isotonic calcium chloride, calcium gluconate, or 0.2% benzethonium (Hyamine) irrigation has also been found to be toxic to the normal eye and to produce an additive toxic effect with hydrofluoric acid [62]. Injection of 10% calcium chloride, calcium gluconate, or isotonic lanthanum chloride subconjunctivally has been found to be very toxic to the normal as well as hydrofluoric acid–burned eye [62]. Injection of isotonic magnesium chloride subconjunctivally has been found to have no therapeutic benefit [62].

Apart from the suggested alterations in irrigating solutions mentioned above, there are no specific immediate or ongoing therapeutic measures for the treatment of acid burns that differ from those for alkali burns. Since the usual acid burn is less severe than an alkali burn, the severe complications of delayed epithelial healing, stromal ulceration, perforation, and secondary glaucoma are less likely to occur, making these injuries less ominous than those caused by alkali.

REFERENCES
1. Aronson, S. B., et al. Pathogenetic approach to therapy of peripheral corneal inflammatory disease. *Am. J. Ophthalmol.* 70:65, 1970.
2. Awan, K. J. Delayed cataract formation after alkali burn. *Can. J. Ophthalmol.* 10:423, 1975.
3. Ballen, P. H. Mucous membrane grafts in chemical (lye) burns. *Am. J. Ophthalmol.* 55:302, 1963.
4. Ballen, P. H. Treatment of chemical burns of the eye. *Eye Ear Nose Throat Mon.* 43:57, 1964.
5. Bennett, J. E. The management of total xerophthalmia. *Arch. Ophthalmol.* 81:667, 1969.
6. Bennett, T. O., Peyman, G. A., and Rutgard, J. Intracameral phosphate buffer in alkali burns. *Can. J. Ophthalmol.* 13:93, 1978.
7. Berman, M. B., et al. Corneal ulceration and the serum antiproteases: I. α-1-antitrypsin. *Invest. Ophthalmol.* 12:759, 1973.
8. Berman, M. B., et al. Characterization of collagenolytic activity in the ulcerating cornea. *Exp. Eye Res.* 11:255, 1971.
9. Berman, M. B., Leary, R., and Gage, J. Latent collagenase in the ulcerating rabbit cornea. *Exp. Eye Res.* 25:435, 1977.
10. Berman, M. B., Leary, R., and Gage, J. Evidence for a role of the plasminogen activator–plasmin system in corneal ulceration. *Invest. Ophthalmol. Vis. Sci.* 19:1204, 1980.
11. Berman, M. B., and Manage, R. Corneal collagenase—evidence for a zinc metaboenzyme. *Ann. Ophthalmol.* 5:1193, 1973.
12. Brown, S. I., Akiya, S., and Weller, C. A. Prevention of the ulcers of the alkali-burned cornea: Preliminary studies with collagenase inhibitors. *Arch. Ophthalmol.* 82:95, 1969.
13. Brown, S. I., Bloomfield, S. E., and Pearce, D. B. A follow-up report on transplantation of the alkali-burned cornea. *Am. J. Ophthalmol.* 77:538, 1974.
14. Brown, S. I., Tragakis, M. P., and Pearce, D. B. Corneal transplantation for severe alkali burns. *Trans. Am. Acad. Ophthalmol. Otolaryngol.* 76:1266, 1972.
15. Brown, S. I., Tragakis, M. P., and Pearce, D. B. Treatment of the alkali-burned cornea. *Am. J. Ophthalmol.* 74:316, 1972.
16. Brown, S. I., Wassermann, H. E., and Dunn, M. W. Alkali burns of the cornea. *Arch. Ophthalmol.* 82:91, 1969.
17. Brown, S. I., and Weller, C. A. Cell origin of collagenase in normal and wounded corneas. *Arch. Ophthalmol.* 83:74, 1970.
18. Brown, S. I., and Weller, C. A. Collagenase inhibitors in prevention of ulcers of alkali-burned cornea. *Arch. Ophthalmol.* 83:352, 1970.
19. Brown, S. I., and Weller, C. A. The pathogenesis and treatment of collagenase-induced diseases of the cornea. *Trans. Am. Acad. Ophthalmol. Otolaryngol.* 74:375, 1970.
20. Brown, S. I., Weller, C. A., and Akiya, S. Pathogenesis of ulcers of the alkali-burned cornea. *Arch. Ophthalmol.* 83:205, 1970.
21. Brown, S. I., Weller, C. A., and Vidrich, A. M.

Effect of corticosteroids on corneal collagenase of rabbits. *Am. J. Ophthalmol.* 70:744, 1970.

22. Brown, S. I., Weller, C. A., and Wassermann, H. E. Collagenolytic activity of alkali-burned corneas. *Arch. Ophthalmol.* 81:370, 1969.

23. Cardona, H., and DeVoe, A. G. Prosthokeratoplasty. *Trans. Am. Acad. Ophthalmol. Otolaryngol.* 83:OP271, 1977.

24. Cavanagh, H. D. Herpetic ocular disease: Therapy of persistent epithelial defects. *Int. Ophthalmol. Clin.* 15(4):67, 1975.

25. Cejkova, J., et al. Alkali burns of the rabbit cornea: I. A histochemical study of β-glucuronidase, β-galactosidase and N-acetyl-β-D-glucosaminidase. *Histochemistry* 45:65, 1975.

26. Cejkova, J., et al. Alkali burns of the rabbit cornea: II. A histochemical study of glycosaminoglycans. *Histochemistry* 45:71, 1975.

27. Chiang, T. S., Moorman, L. R., and Thomas, R. P. Ocular hypertensive response following acid and alkali burns in rabbits. *Invest. Ophthalmol.* 10:270, 1971.

28. Denig, R. G. Transplantation of mucous membrane of mouth for various diseases and burns of the cornea. *N.Y. Med. J.* 57:1074, 1918.

29. de Treville, R. T. P. Hydrofluoric acid burns management (Medical Series Bulletin No. 17-70). Industrial Hygiene Foundation of America, Washington, D.C., 1970.

30. Dohlman, C. H., Boruchoff, S. A., and Sullivan, G. L. A technique for the repair of perforated corneal ulcers. *Arch. Ophthalmol.* 77:519, 1967.

31. Dohlman, C. H., Schneider, H. A., and Doane, M. G. Prosthokeratoplasty. *Am. J. Ophthalmol.* 77:694, 1974.

32. Donshik, P. C., et al. Effect of topical corticosteroids on ulceration in alkali-burned corneas. *Arch. Ophthalmol.* 96:2117, 1978.

33. Eisen, A. Z., Jeffrey, J. J., and Gross, J. Human skin collagenase: Isolation and mechanism of attack on the collagen molecule. *Biochim. Biophys. Acta* 151:637, 1968.

34. Foster, C. S., et al. Ascorbate therapy for experimental corneal burns. *Invest. Ophthalmol. Vis. Sci.* 19(ARVO Suppl.):227, 1980.

35. Francois, J., et al. Collagenase inhibitors (penicillamine). *Ann. Ophthalmol.* 5:391, 1973.

36. Friedenwald, J. S., Hughes, W. F., Jr., and Herrmann, H. Acid-base tolerance of the cornea. *Arch. Ophthalmol.* 31:279, 1944.

37. Friedenwald, J. S., Hughes, W. F., Jr., and Herrmann, H. Acid burns of the eye. *Arch. Ophthalmol.* 35:98, 1946.

38. Friend, J., and Thoft, R. A. Functional competence of regenerating ocular surface epithelium. *Invest. Ophthalmol. Vis. Sci.* 17:134, 1978.

39. Girard, L. J., et al. Keratoprosthesis: A 12-year follow-up. *Trans. Am. Acad. Ophthalmol. Otolaryngol.* 83:OP252, 1977.

40. Gnadinger, M. C., et al. The role of collagenase in the alkali-burned cornea. *Am. J. Ophthalmol.* 68:478, 1969.

41. Gordon, J. M., Bauer, E. A., and Eisen, A. Z. Collagenase in human cornea: Immunologic localization. *Arch. Ophthalmol.* 98:341, 1980.

42. Grant, W. M. Ocular injury due to sulfur dioxide: II. Experimental study and comparison with ocular effects of freezing. *Arch. Ophthalmol.* 38:762, 1947.

43. Grant, W. M. *Toxicology of the Eye* (2nd ed.). Springfield, Ill.: Thomas, 1974.

44. Grant, W. M., and Kern, H. L. Action of alkalies on the corneal stroma. *Arch. Ophthalmol.* 54:931, 1955.

45. Harris, L. S., Cohn, K., and Galin, M. A. Alkali injury from fireworks. *Ann. Ophthalmol.* 3:849, 1971.

46. Henriquez, A. S., Pihlaja, D. J., and Dohlman, C. H. Surface ultrastructure in alkali-burned rabbit corneas. *Am. J. Ophthalmol.* 81:324, 1976.

47. Holekamp, T. I. R., and Becker, B. Ocular injuries from automobile batteries. *Trans. Am. Acad. Ophthalmol. Otolaryngol.* 83:805, 1977.

48. Hook, R. M., Hook, C. W., and Brown, S. I. Fibroblast collagenase: Partial purification and characterization. *Invest. Ophthalmol.* 12:771, 1973.

49. Hughes, W. F., Jr. Alkali burns of the eye: I. Review of the literature and summary of present knowledge. *Arch. Ophthalmol.* 35:423, 1946.

50. Hughes, W. F., Jr. Alkali burns of the eye: II. Clinical and pathologic course. *Arch. Ophthalmol.* 36:189, 1946.

51. Itoi, M., et al. Prévention d'ulcères du stroma de la cornée grâce a l'utilisation d'un sel de calcium d'E.D.T.A. *Arch. Ophtalmol.* (Paris) 29:389, 1969.

52. Itoi, M., et al. Collagenase in the cornea. *Exp. Eye Res.* 8:369, 1969.

53. Kenyon, K. R., et al. Prevention of stromal ulceration in the alkali-burned rabbit cornea by glued-on contact lens: Evidence for the role of polymorphonuclear leukocytes in collagen degradation. *Invest. Ophthalmol. Vis. Sci.* 18:570, 1979.

54. Klein, R., and Lobes, L. A., Jr. Ocular alkali burns in a large urban area. *Ann. Ophthalmol.* 8:1185, 1976.

55. Koob, T. J., Jeffrey, J. J., and Eisen, A. Z. Regulation of human skin collagenase activity by hydrocortisone and dexamethasone in organ culture. *Biochem. Biophys. Res. Commun.* 61:1083, 1974.

56. Lazarus, G. S., et al. Human granulocyte collagenase. *Science* 159:1483, 1968.

57. Lemp, M. A. Cornea and sclera. *Arch. Ophthalmol.* 92:158, 1974.

58. Levinson, R. A., Paterson, C. A., and Pfister, R. R. Ascorbic acid prevents corneal ulceration and perforation following experimental alkali burns. *Invest. Ophthalmol.* 15:986, 1976.

59. Lewin, L., and Guillery, H. *Die Wurkurgen von Arznermitteln und Giften auf des Auge* (2nd ed.). Berlin: August Huishwald, 1913.

60. Matsuda, H., and Smelser, G. K. Endothelial cells in alkali-burned corneas. *Arch. Ophthalmol.* 89:402, 1973.

61. Morgan, L. B. A new drug delivery system for the eye. *Indus. Med.* 40:11, 1971.

62. McCulley, J. P., Pettit, M., and Lauber, S. Treatment of experimental ocular hydrofluoric acid burns. *Invest. Ophthalmol. Vis. Sci.* 19(ARVO Suppl.):228, 1980.

63. McCulley, J. P., Whiting, D. W., and Lauber, S. Experimental ocular hydrofluoric acid burns. *Invest. Ophthalmol. Vis. Sci.* 18(ARVO Suppl.):195, 1979.

64. Newsome, D. A., and Gross, J. Prevention by medroxyprogesterone of perforation in the alkali-burned rabbit cornea: Inhibition of collagenolytic activity. *Invest. Ophthalmol. Vis. Sci.* 16:21, 1977.

65. Newsome, D. A., and Gross, J. Regulation of corneal collagenase production: Stimulation of serially passaged stromal cells by blood mononuclear cells. *Cell* 16:895, 1979.

66. Paterson, C. A., et al. The ocular hypertensive response following experimental acid burns in the rabbit eye. *Invest. Ophthalmol. Vis. Sci.* 18:67, 1979.

67. Paterson, C. A., and Pfister, R. R. Ocular hypertensive response to alkali burns in the monkey. *Exp. Eye Res.* 17:449, 1973.

68. Paterson, C. A., and Pfister, R. R. Intraocular pressure changes after alkali burns. *Arch. Ophthalmol.* 91:211, 1974.

69. Paterson, C. A., Pfister, R. R., and Levinson, R. A. Aqueous humor pH changes after experimental alkali burns. *Am. J. Ophthalmol.* 79:414, 1975.

70. Pfister, R. R., Friend, J., and Dohlman, C. H. The anterior segments of rabbits after alkali burns. *Arch. Ophthalmol.* 86:189, 1971.

71. Pfister, R. R., et al. Collagenase activity of intact corneal epithelium in peripheral alkali burns. *Arch. Ophthalmol.* 86:308, 1971.

72. Pfister, R. R., and Paterson, C. A. Additional clinical and morphological observations on the favorable effect of ascorbate in experimental ocular alkali burns. *Invest. Ophthalmol. Vis. Sci.* 16:478, 1977.

73. Rao, G. N., Blatt, H. L., and Aquavella, J. V. Results of keratoprosthesis. *Am. J. Ophthalmol.* 88:190, 1979.

74. Roper-Hall, M. J. Thermal and chemical burns. *Trans. Ophthalmol. Soc. U.K.* 85:631, 1965.

75. Schultz, G., Henkind, P., and Gross, E. M. Acid burns of the eye. *Am. J. Ophthalmol.* 66:654, 1968.

76. Slansky, H. H., et al. Cysteine and acetylcysteine in the prevention of corneal ulcerations. *Ann. Ophthalmol.* 2:488, 1970.

77. Slansky, H. H., Dohlman, C. H., and Berman, M. B. Prevention of corneal ulcers. *Trans. Am. Acad. Ophthalmol. Otolaryngol.* 75:1208, 1971.

78. Slansky, H. H., Freeman, M. I., and Itoi, M. Collagenolytic activity in bovine corneal epithelium. *Arch. Ophthalmol.* 80:496, 1968.

79. Stanley, J. A. Strong alkali burns of the eye. *N. Engl. J. Med.* 273:1265, 1965.

80. Stein, M. R., Naidoff, M. A., and Dawson, C. R. Intraocular pressure response to experimental alkali burns. *Am. J. Ophthalmol.* 75:99, 1973.

81. Thoft, R. A. Conjunctival transplantation. *Arch. Ophthalmol.* 95:1425, 1977.

82. Thoft, R. A., and Friend, J. Biochemical transformation of regenerating ocular surface epithelium. *Invest. Ophthalmol. Vis. Sci.* 16:14, 1977.

83. Webster, R. G., Jr., et al. The use of adhesives for the closure of perforations: A report of two cases. *Arch. Ophthalmol.* 80:705, 1968.

15. KERATOPLASTY

Therapeutic Keratoplasty

S. Arthur Boruchoff

Therapeutic keratoplasty is an operation in which diseased corneal tissue is removed and replaced by donor corneal material or, in the case of keratoprosthesis, some other substitute material. The procedure is performed either to provide structural support for the cornea (tectonic keratoplasty) or to improve vision.

From a historic point of view, the concept of corneal transplantation is about 150 years old, but the modern era in clinical keratoplasty can be dated from pioneer surgeons such as von Hippel [23], who advocated lamellar keratoplasty in Germany in the latter part of the nineteenth century. In Prague, Elschnig [9] emphasized the use of penetrating keratoplasty soon after 1910. Tudor-Thomas [21] popularized keratoplasty in Great Britain two decades later. The procedures initially described by these authors have been refined by contributions by many other surgeons in the United States and other countries.

The modern era of keratoplasty began in 1952, when Stocker [18] first reported successful keratoplasty for the treatment of corneal edema. The success was in large part due to the use of topical steroids, coupled with the availability of fine sutures and needles. Whereas only 25 or 30 years ago, keratoplasty was still a medical rarity, now it is estimated that approximately ten thousand corneal transplants are performed each year in the United States alone.

Not only has the success of keratoplasty broadened its application to a greater number of diseases; increasing numbers of patients are afflicted with abnormalities that can be treated by corneal transplantation. The increasing longevity of the population alone is responsible for much of the increase in the number of cases of corneal edema ophthalmologists are seeing. In addition, other commonly performed operative procedures such as cataract extraction and intraocular lens implantation are associated with additional endothelial cell loss, which may lead to corneal edema later in the patient's life.

Even today, however, certain conditions can only rarely be improved by keratoplasty. These include primary ocular surface diseases such as cicatricial pemphigoid and Stevens-Johnson syndrome, severe keratitis sicca, chemical burns, and other forms of trauma that severely damage the ocular surface.

Keratoplasty can be done to replace only a part of the corneal thickness (lamellar keratoplasty) or the full thickness (penetrating keratoplasty). Depending on the location of the corneal abnormality, it may be sufficient to replace just the anterior layers with a lamellar keratoplasty. When the endothelium is involved, however, replacement of corneal tissue must include the endothelial layer, and thus a penetrating keratoplasty must be performed. The failure of both types of keratoplasty is likely in a number of severe anterior segment diseases and injuries, and such failure has prompted the development of a technique that depends on the implantation of an inert optical prosthesis, fabricated from plastic (keratoprosthesis). The indications, techniques, care, and complications associated with these three procedures—lamellar keratoplasty, penetrating keratoplasty, and keratoprosthesis—are discussed in this section.

LAMELLAR KERATOPLASTY

Lamellar keratoplasty is defined as removal and replacement of less than the total thickness of the cornea. As a rule, lamellar grafts tend to be relatively large (greater than 8 mm in diameter), and they replace tissue removed by deep stromal dissection but leave behind some stroma, Descemet's membrane, and the endothelium.

INDICATIONS

Lamellar keratoplasty is indicated for those corneal conditions in which the pathologic changes are limited to anterior stromal and surface irregularities but in which the endothelium is healthy. Lamellar keratoplasty is most useful for superficial scars or surface irregularities caused by stromal or surface disease and may be highly useful if most of the abnormal tissue can be excised, leaving behind a healthy stromal bed free of vessels. It is never indicated for disease secondary to endothelial dysfunction. In addition, the dry eye syndromes, ocular surface diseases, severe conjunctival scarring after inflammation or injury, and the aftereffects of

chemical or radiation burns of the anterior segment all carry with them a dire prognosis for lamellar keratoplasty, since epithelial healing is so poor in such conditions. Tear quantity, tear function, and the ability to resurface the cornea may also be compromised in the presence of major lid abnormalities, since notches of the lids and malposition or incomplete lid closure may all produce localized or generalized areas of inadequate corneal epithelial wetting.

Although popular in France, where 75 percent of grafts have been reported to be clear with improvement in vision [14], in the experience of most surgeons lamellar keratoplasty does not yield visual results comparable to those attained with penetrating keratoplasty. This fact alone limits the indications for lamellar keratoplasty. In general, the procedure is used primarily to strengthen and thicken the corneal substance in anticipation of a subsequent penetrating keratoplasty. Examples of such conditions include markedly thin corneas in keratoconus or extensive loss of stromal tissue after inflammatory disease.

DONOR MATERIAL

Since the primary goal of lamellar keratoplasty is to provide a normal stromal matrix, none of the cell types (epithelial, stromal, endothelial) need be viable. Re-epithelialization of the graft occurs from the host's peripheral cornea in a few days; repopulation of the stroma, which occurs in a few weeks, is by keratocytes derived from the host. These factors permit considerable latitude in the choice of donor material and the method of its interim storage. For example, none of the special criteria important in ensuring the viability of the endothelium for penetrating keratoplasty, such as age of the donor, interval of time from death to use, or method of preservation, are important. Obviously, however, the same safeguards taken to ensure "clean" or uncontaminated donor material should be observed in lamellar keratoplasty. In addition, the use of whole eyes is helpful, since it is very difficult to do a lamellar dissection on only the isolated corneal-scleral preparation.

SURGICAL PROCEDURE

Lamellar keratoplasty is extraocular in the sense that the anterior chamber is not entered. Inadvertent movement or straining on the part of the patient are less likely to affect the outcome of the procedure, permitting more flexibility in the type of anesthesia chosen. Control of intraocular pressure by the use of osmotic agents is also of little importance to the success of the procedure.

The actual technique involves three separate activities: preparation of the host stromal bed, preparation of the donor material, and suturing of the donor material to the host stromal bed [5].

PREPARATION OF THE HOST STROMAL BED
Since the exact extent of the surgery cannot be predicted in most cases until the pathologic material is actually dissected free, it is obvious that the lamellar bed should be prepared first so that the donor len-

ticule can be chosen accordingly. After the usual preparation and draping for ophthalmic surgery, a trephine of adequate size is chosen (Fig. 15-1A). In most lamellar keratoplasties, the size is 8 mm or larger and may even extend virtually to the limbus.

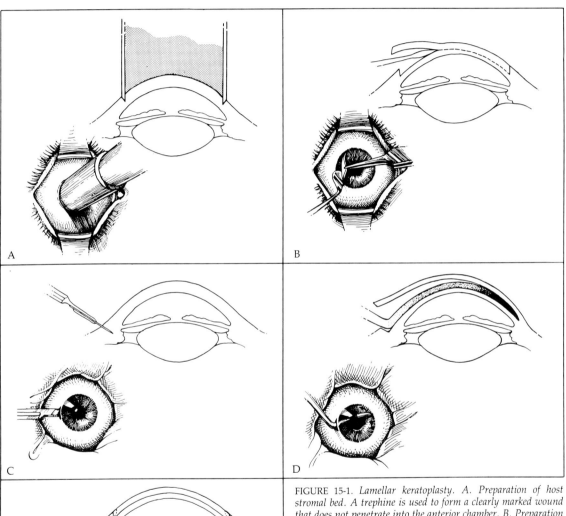

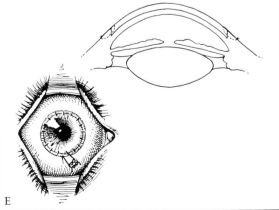

FIGURE 15-1. *Lamellar keratoplasty. A. Preparation of host stromal bed. A trephine is used to form a clearly marked wound that does not penetrate into the anterior chamber. B. Preparation of stromal bed. A knife or corneal splitter is used to dissect off the lamellar tissue. C. Preparation of donor material. A sharp incision is made at the limbus of the donor cornea at a depth corresponding to the depth of the host bed previously prepared. D. Preparation of donor material. A fine spatula with a curved blade is introduced through the incision and is used to separate the cornea into anterior and posterior parts. The central anterior portion corresponding in size to the stromal bed is cut out with a trephine and removed. E. Suturing donor tissue in place. Approximately 16 sutures are used to secure the graft. The sutures are placed nearly full-thickness depth in the donor lamellar disc. (From G. Spaeth (Ed.),* Ophthalmic Surgery. *Philadelphia: Saunders, 1982.)*

The trephine is set for partial penetration of the host tissue (e.g., 0.4 mm), pressed against the host, and rotated to form a partially penetrating, clearly marked wound. After checking to see that the incision is well marked in all areas, the central lamellar tissue is grasped with a fine forceps and elevated. A suitable knife blade, e.g., Bard-Parker No. 15 (Becton, Dickinson & Co., Rutherford, N.J.), Beaver No. 64 (Rudolph Beaver, Inc., Belmont, Mass.), or a Desmarre's scarifier, is then used to dissect off the lamellar tissue in the plane established by the depth of the cut (Fig. 15-1B). Care should be taken to make the bed as smooth as possible; this is best performed by cutting the fine fibers horizontally while pressing downward with the blade of the knife against the deep host tissues. At the end of this dissection, it is useful to undermine the remaining peripheral cornea for approximately ½ mm to create a lip of tissue to facilitate subsequent suturing.

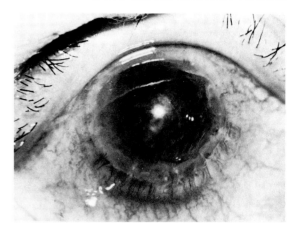

FIGURE 15-2. *Haze at the interface resulting in poor vision is one of the major complications of lamellar keratoplasty. (From G. Spaeth (Ed.),* Ophthalmic Surgery. *Philadelphia: Saunders, 1982.)*

PREPARATION OF THE DONOR MATERIAL
Attention is then directed to the donor material, which should be at room temperature. If the tissue is fresh, the epithelium may be removed if it is not thought to be necessary for subsequent surface healing. Frozen tissue should have the epithelium removed, since it is nonviable. At the limbus, a sharp incision is made (Fig. 15-1C) to correspond to the depth of the host bed previously dissected. A fine spatula with a curved blade (e.g., Martinez dissecting spatula) is then introduced into the incision and turned parallel to the plane of the cornea (Fig. 15-1D). Using a sweeping motion, a clean dissection of the donor tissue is carried out across the dome of the cornea to the limbus in all directions, separating the donor tissue into a superficial layer corresponding to the depth of the previously dissected bed and leaving beneath it the remaining corneal tissue. A trephine corresponding to the size of the lamellar host dissection is then chosen, applied to the donor material, and rotated so that the dissected disc of tissue is removed by the trephine.

SUTURING
The dissected donor tissue is then placed in the host bed and sutured in place (Fig. 15-1E). As a rule, interrupted sutures are used, and either 9-0 silk or 10-0 nylon or Prolene (Ethicon, Inc., Somerville, N.J.) may be used. The sutures go deep into the donor tissue, exiting at the base of the vertical edge, crossing into the vertical edge of the host. Approximately 16 sutures are employed, and the knots are pulled toward the limbus. Since such sutures are usually removed in 10 to 20 days, the knots are not buried. Usually the exposed knots are felt by the patient and may cause some tissue irritation, but the irritation has the beneficial effect of earlier healing and permits earlier suture removal.

POSTOPERATIVE CARE
Postoperative care involves use of appropriate quantities of topical antibiotics and corticosteroids during the several weeks the sutures are left in place.

Since there has been no entry into the anterior chamber, marked inflammation is not usually encountered. However, topical corticosteroids (e.g., 0.1% dexamethasone 5–10 times daily for 1 week) may be useful in preventing recrudescence of stromal inflammatory disease if such inflammation was part of the original disease. The sutures are removed when they become loose, when vessels bridge the wound from host to donor, or when healing is apparent. It is probably wise to remove sutures in two stages. A typical regimen is to remove every other stitch in 10 to 14 days and the remaining sutures a week or so later.

COMPLICATIONS
Since the surgery does not usually involve penetration into the eye, most complications are not serious. Premature loosening of sutures, ingrowth of vessels, infection, or later appearance of the original disease may all occur. Perhaps the major complication is the inherent relatively poor visual result in most cases of lamellar keratoplasty because of haze at the interface (Fig. 15-2).

PENETRATING KERATOPLASTY

Penetrating keratoplasty is essential if the primary defect is in the endothelium or if the stroma is deeply ulcerated or perforated. Many surgeons favor a penetrating keratoplasty even if the endothelial layer itself is not diseased, since the visual results appear to be better than with lamellar procedures. This point of view is reflected in the current practice of United States surgeons, in which well over 90 percent of keratoplasties are penetrating. Because of entry into the anterior chamber, however, additional considerations enter into the performance of the technique itself, as well as the management of postoperative complications.

INDICATIONS

The indications for penetrating keratoplasty include cases in which tissue strengthening is the primary goal (tectonic) and cases in which increased visual acuity is the immediate goal. Tectonic penetrating keratoplasty is indicated for those situations in which lamellar keratoplasty would not be expected to alleviate the situation because of inadequate peripheral or central host corneal thickness. For example, deep ulcerations with an active diffuse stromal involvement, corneal perforations, marked variation in the thickness of the stroma, or an ongoing diffuse inflammatory process in which medical measures have failed to halt stromal loss might all be indications for tectonic penetrating keratoplasty.

The major indication for penetrating keratoplasty, however, is restoration of optical clarity. Among the clinical situations encountered are the following: (1) irregularity of the corneal surface (e.g., epithelial edema or scarring seen in some epithelial dystrophies); (2) abnormal corneal contour (e.g., keratoconus or healed stromal ulceration); (3) opacification of the stroma (as the end result of a wide variety of inflammatory or degenerative conditions); and (4) thickening of the stroma secondary to edema, with concurrent epithelial edema. However, the surgeon should have exhausted all medical measures (antibiotics, antiinflammatory agents, hypertonic agents) and should have attempted visual correction by optical means (e.g., contact lenses) before embarking on penetrating keratoplasty.

Needless to say, the surgeon must be convinced that the patient will benefit from a keratoplasty if it is done. Consideration of the vision in the other eye and the needs of the patient as defined by age, occupation, and activity must be taken into account. In addition, there must be reasonable expectation that the visual potential of the macula and retina is sufficient to warrant the operation.

There are conditions in the cornea itself that may limit the usefulness of keratoplasty. Diffuse and deep stromal vascularization, particularly if the vessels are numerous and active, produces a stromal bed that is inhospitable for a penetrating graft because of the likelihood of immunologic graft reaction. Although minor degrees of vascularization are not important, the more diffuse and active the vessels in the stroma, the more likely that, sooner or later, the graft will be involved in and succumb to a graft rejection.

The activity of the disease (e.g., active melting, progressive vascularization, marked edema) also affects the prognosis. Superimposing the trauma of keratoplasty upon preexistent inflammation, such as that found in herpetic keratouveitis, further jeopardizes the graft endothelium. In addition, the donor tissue may be subject to the same factors that cause inflammation and stromal loss in the host tissue. For these reasons, most surgeons prefer to do keratoplasty in the inactive stage of inflammatory disease, if possible.

As in the case of lamellar keratoplasty, the dry eye syndromes, ocular surface diseases, and chemical or radiation burns of the anterior segment all represent relative contraindications to penetrating keratoplasty, since epithelial healing from the peripheral host epithelial cells may be inadequate. Likewise, pronounced lid abnormalities and aberrations of the lashes may jeopardize the success of penetrating keratoplasty.

Abnormal intraocular pressure may also be associated with graft failure. In particular, abnormally low tensions may be further aggravated by partial vitrectomy, whch is frequently performed in aphakic keratoplasty. Although high pressure itself can usually be controlled postoperatively by a combination of medical and surgical means, preoperative glaucoma is frequently made worse by partial loss of the filtration angle. The chronic use of steroids after keratoplasty may induce yet another type of glaucoma.

DONOR MATERIAL

In contrast to lamellar keratoplasty, in penetrating keratoplasty it is essential that the donor cornea have a viable endothelial layer. A variety of methods ranging from cold storage at 4°C or storage in nutrient medium [10] to cryopreservation [6] have been developed to ensure such viability. In most developed nations, the local need for corneal tissue exceeds the supply, so that there need not be banking of tissue for any length of time. Even in such countries, however, local lack of donor corneal tissue may require transportation over considerable distances, making effective storage for several days mandatory. In most cases, storage in nutrient medium (McCarey-Kaufman [10]) has been found to preserve endothelial viability for several days, facilitating distribution of the tissue.

The endothelial layer is acknowledged to be of fundamental importance, but controversy exists about the desirability or need for viable epithelial and stromal cells. In most cases, these layers are probably also viable if the endothelial layer is; however, the role of such donor cells in the outcome of the transplant is not yet known. In ocular surface disorders, it seems desirable to transplant healthy epithelial cells [20]. At the same time, however, it can be argued that transplantation of such cells increases the risk of immunologic rejection by the host [17].

There are other factors that bear on the decision about the suitability of donor tissue for transplantation. The Eye Bank Association of America, in conjunction with the American Academy of Ophthalmology, has an ongoing committee that periodically reviews available data, makes suggestions, and sets criteria for donor tissue selection and eye banking in the United States. Their most recent criteria are reproduced in Table 15-1.

Because immunologic graft reaction occurs so often in highly vascularized corneas, it has been suggested by some that the corneal donor should be chosen on the basis of compatible tissue antigens. The human leukocyte antigen (HLA) system is a major histocompatibility system in humans, and matching the donor to the recipient has proved beneficial in renal transplantation in siblings [12]. Given the impossible task of HLA matching for corneal transplantation, Stark has suggested that serologic cross-match testing of serum from the prospective recipient against lymphocytes of the donor may disclose the presence of specific recipient presensitization against one or more HLA antigens of the donor [17]. Even though such a test is likely to detect only recipient humoral antibodies to the donor, such testing is thought to reduce the possibility of cell-mediated incompatibility also. Although such lymphocyte-serum cross matching is available only on an experimental basis at present, prospective studies currently underway may indicate the desirability of this technique for selecting donor corneas for heavily vascularized corneal recipients.

PREOPERATIVE EVALUATION

A complete preoperative ocular evaluation should be done and a course of action planned before ad-

mission of the patient to the hospital, since keratoplasty is often done with little advance notice, depending upon the availability of donor tissue. A general medical evaluation to assess the anesthesia risks is useful with particular attention to the possible desirability of general anesthesia. Since adequate visualization of the interior of the eye is frequently not possible in patients with corneal disease, ultrasonography and electrophysiologic testing may be helpful in planning the extent of surgery. Preexisting inflammation should be controlled as well as possible, and preliminary treatment with topical steroids for a day or so before surgery often improves the outcome if the eye is inflamed. Preexistent glaucoma should be treated, with adequate pressure control attained before keratoplasty, particularly since keratoplasty may aggravate glaucoma.

SURGICAL PROCEDURE

KERATOPLASTY TECHNIQUE

The size of the graft is usually determined at the time of surgery. As a generalization, grafts performed for endothelial dysfunction should be as large as feasible, usually 8.0 to 8.5 mm in diameter. A graft larger than 8.5 mm is frequently accompanied by extensive synechiae and subsequent glaucoma; grafts much smaller than 6.5 mm are frequently inadequate because of central optical distortion. The donor trephine is often 0.5 mm larger than the trephine used for the host, although this is not mandatory.

The donor button is usually prepared from the cornea and its scleral rim, which has been removed from the refrigerated donor eye at the time of operation or earlier, with subsequent storage in McCarey-Kaufman (M-K) medium. A trephine is applied from the endothelial surface with uniform pressure to penetrate through to the epithelial surface (Fig. 15-3A). It is useful to place a single-armed suture of 9-0 or 10-0 silk or nylon through the cut edge of the button at this stage to facilitate later handling of the tissue. With the suture in place, the button is set aside, endothelial side up, on an appropriate storage material, care being taken to keep the endothelial side thoroughly moistened with M-K medium or balanced salt solution. If a whole eye is available at the time of operation, the epithelium may be left on or removed by scraping, depending on the relative merits of keeping the epithelial layer.

The next step in the procedure is the excision of the diseased corneal tissue. A trephine of appropriate size is chosen, the blade is exposed to approximately 0.3 or 0.4 mm, and this blade is then pressed against the eye and rotated in a uniform manner, making a partial penetration of the cornea (Fig. 15-

TABLE 15-1. *Criteria for Donor Material for Corneal Transplants*

I. Cases in which donor tissue may present a health-threatening condition for the recipient or may be contraindicated because of endothelial dysfunction:
 A. Death of unknown cause
 B. Jakob-Creutzfeldt disease
 C. Subacute sclerosing panencephalitis
 D. Congenital rubella
 E. Progressive multifocal leukoencephalopathy
 F. Reye's syndrome
 G. Subacute encephalitis, cytomegalovirus brain infection
 H. Septicemia
 I. Hepatitis
 J. Rabies
 K. Intrinsic eye disease (retinoblastoma, conjunctivitis, iritis, glaucoma, corneal disease, malignant tumors of the anterior segment)
 L. Blast-form leukemia
 M. Hodgkin's disease
 N. Lymphosarcoma

II. Cases in which donor tissue may require caution in use:
 A. Multiple sclerosis
 B. Parkinson's disease
 C. Amyotrophic lateral sclerosis
 D. Jaundice (rule out infectious hepatitis)
 E. Chronic lymphocytic leukemia
 F. Diabetes
 G. Surgically induced eye abnormality, e.g., aphakia
 H. Syphilis

III. Age of donor:
 The lower limit is full-term birth. There is no absolute upper limit. It is recognized, however, that endothelial abnormalities increase and cell density decreases with age.
 The interval between donor death and enucleation should be as short as possible. Cooling the body and/or placing ice packs over the closed lids is helpful.

IV. Corneal retrieval procedures:
 The enucleation should be performed by sterile technique, following which the globe should be irrigated with sterile solution and placed in a sterile glass container, which is then put into a shipping container. The contents should be kept as cold (not freezing) as possible.
 At the Eye Bank, the whole eye should be vigorously irrigated with sterile saline and immersed for five minutes in Neosporin solution.
 The Eye Bank should report the following information to the surgeon:
 A. Gross appearance (e.g., presence of gross scars) of the eye
 B. Microscopic appearance of the eye, including
  1. State of the epithelium
  2. Gross thickness of the stroma
  3. Presence of folds in deep layers
  4. Presence of guttata (if possible)

V. Methods of preservation of donor material:
 A. The whole eye is placed in a closed, sterile moist chamber, cooled to 4°C. Eyes so prepared need not necessarily pass through an Eye Bank.
 B. The cornea with a rim of sclera is excised, using sterile technique, and placed into a sterile solution consisting of tissue culture medium (TC 199), dextran, and antibiotics (M-K [McCarey-Kaufman] technique).
 C. Cryo-preserved tissue is still available in some Eye Banks. It requires meticulously careful preserving and thawing.
 D. Organ-cultured tissue is a technique available in only a few centers and not generally available to the surgeon.
 E. Tissue stored in glycerin or frozen at −80°C is useful for lamellar grafts and, rarely, as an emergency patch-graft for a perforation.

VI. Time interval between death and surgery:
 A. Whole or refrigerated eyes may be used up to 48 hours after the death of the donor. Surgery is advisable as soon as possible.
 B. Tissue preserved by the McCarey-Kaufman technique may be used up to 4 days after the death of the donor.
 C. Cryopreserved tissue may be used up to at least 1 year after the death of the donor.

VII. Responsibility of surgeon and eye bank:
 The decision to accept a given donor rests with the operating surgeon. The Eye Bank's responsibility lies in furnishing as full and accurate data as possible to the surgeon, including
 A. Age of donor
 B. Cause of death
 C. Associated diseases
 D. Time of death
 E. Time of enucleation
 F. Method of preservation

VIII. Miscellaneous:
 Pre-operative cultures are left to the discretion of the individual Eye Bank.
 The surgeon can also take cultures.
 Emergency situations may arise where it is necessary to use donor tissue that does not meet all the criteria mentioned above. In such cases the urgency of the situation must be balanced against the overall quality of the donor.

SOURCE: Standards Committee, Eye Bank Association of America, 1981.

3B). The anterior chamber is then entered by cutting with a sharp knife such as a Haab or Super Blade (Superblade, Inc., Ft. Lauderdale, Fl.). Once the chamber has been entered, scissors are introduced to complete the excision (Fig. 15-3C). It is my preference to bevel the posterior part of the cornea, leaving behind an edge of posterior host stroma that effectively exerts a gasketlike pressure, assuring firm apposition of the posterior aspect of the donor and the host (Fig. 15-3C). The bed is carefully inspected, and any adventitious tissue is removed. In addition, other procedures such as lysis of synechiae, vitrectomy, or cataract extraction can now be performed (see Concurrent Surgical Procedures, below).

The donor button is then placed in the host bed with the previously placed suture positioned at 12 o'clock. This suture is tied. Most surgeons prefer to place additional interrupted sutures at 3, 6, and 9 o'clock. The final suturing may be done either with interrupted sutures or a running suture. Interrupted sutures are probably the sutures of choice if there are vessels, areas of inflammation, or irregularity of the host bed. In the presence of such conditions the healing is likely to be uneven and more rapid in some areas than others, and therefore the more controlled suture removal possible with interrupted sutures is desirable. Regardless of the type of suturing, there should be four to five sutures per quadrant, halfway through the thickness of the cornea, approximately ¾ mm into the donor and extended into the host almost to the limbus (Fig. 15-3D).

After suturing, all the sutures or suture loops should have approximately equal tension. The knots of the running or interrupted sutures can be buried, which increases patient comfort. If the ends

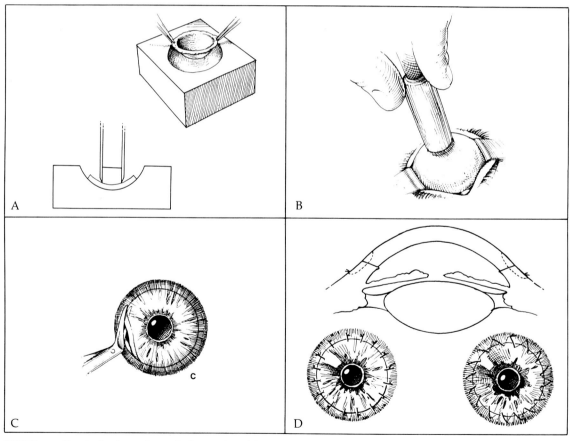

FIGURE 15-3. *Penetrating keratoplasty. A. Preparation of donor material. A corneal-scleral ring is removed from the donor eye and placed epithelial side down in a holder. The corneal button is cut out using a trephine. B. Preparation of host. A trephine is used to make a partial penetration, and a knife is used to enter the anterior chamber. C. Preparation of host. Excision of the host corneal button is completed using scissors. D. The donor button is sutured in place using either interrupted sutures or a running suture. (From G. Spaeth (Ed.),* Ophthalmic Surgery. *Philadelphia, Saunders, 1982.)*

are left exposed, the discomfort can usually be managed by the application of a soft contact lens. At the end of the procedure, the anterior chamber should be reformed. Particular attention should be paid to the depth of the periphery of the chamber as well as of the center. This is particularly important in inflammatory conditions such as herpes simplex, in which the tendency for iris to adhere to the back of the wound should be recognized. Reinflation of the chamber is most easily performed by instilling saline from a 2-ml glass syringe through a bent blunt 30-gauge needle directly into the anterior chamber between adjacent wound suture loops. Sodium hyaluronate (Healon) may be useful in establishing the chamber and in keeping the iris away from the wound [11, 13].

CONCURRENT SURGICAL PROCEDURES

CATARACT EXTRACTION

If it is obvious that a lens opacity that would prevent restoration of vision even with a clear cornea is present, cataract extraction is usually indicated. Other indications are a very shallow anterior chamber with a severe lens opacity, and even only moderate lens opacity if the other eye is already aphakic. For this procedure, a soft eye is particularly helpful, and intravenous mannitol and general anesthesia are useful in achieving that end. A Flieringa ring to stabilize the anterior segment is also helpful in facilitating accurate suture placement. Either intracapsular or extracapsular extraction can be performed, in conformity with the usual indications for one or the other procedure. An iridectomy is indicated in combined keratoplasty–cataract extraction procedures, even though this is not routinely done for the usual phakic keratoplasty patient.

VITRECTOMY

Prognosis for aphakic grafts is virtually the same as for phakic grafts if the vitreous is handled appropriately. In the phakic patient, or after lens extraction in a combined procedure, if the vitreous face is unbroken and does not protrude, it is prudent to leave the vitreous undisturbed. If, on the other hand, there is loose vitreous in the anterior chamber, or if vitreous protrudes beyond the wound margins, vitreous should be removed so that when the Flieringa ring is elevated, the vitreous face falls well back of the iris plane. Vitreous may be removed either by one of the vitreous cutting and suction instruments or with Weck Cell sponges (Edward Weck & Co., Inc., Research Triangle Park, N.C.). Either method is effective. The evacuation of fluid vitreous through the pars plana before opening the cornea is advocated by some surgeons. If massive vitreous organization or extensive vitreous hemorrhage is known to exist before the keratoplasty, it is also possible to perform an open-sky vitrectomy. It is perhaps best for the patient and most reassuring to the surgeons if a corneal surgeon and a retina-vitreous surgeon join together in such an effort.

ANTERIOR SEGMENT RECONSTRUCTION

In addition to cataract removal and handling of the vitreous, it is also possible to combine keratoplasty with suturing of iris colobomas in case of a full iridectomy or with lysis of synechiae with no increase in operative complications.

POSTOPERATIVE CARE

Antibiotics (e.g., 0.5% chloramphenicol) are instilled routinely three times a day for several days and are then used less frequently. Inflamed eyes or eyes that have had extensive surgery previously usually benefit from frequent instillation of corticosteroids—up to 1 drop per hour of 0.1% dexamethasone for several days. Gradually the steroids can be reduced as the inflammation within the eye diminishes. Systemic steroids are usually not necessary but may be advisable if marked uveitis is seen despite the use of topical steroids.

Elevation of pressure is found so frequently after penetrating keratoplasty that its presence should always be expected, and routine measures should be taken to avoid it. Vigorous dilation of the pupil is essential in cases with aphakia, since pupillary block can occur even in the absence of an intact vitreous face. In addition to potential pupillary block, inflammatory blockage of the filtration angle is another compelling reason to use high doses of corticosteroids topically. Even with such measures, pressures may rise to levels that lead to patient discomfort, making the temporary use of osmotic agents advisable. With such measures, pressure elevation rarely lasts for more than a few days.

COMPLICATIONS

It is convenient to divide the complications of penetrating keratoplasty into three categories: those that occur during the operation, those that occur in the immediate postoperative period, and those that occur weeks or months after surgery.

INTRAOPERATIVE COMPLICATIONS

For the most part, intraoperative complications are technical. Meticulous technique will prevent poor excision of the donor button, trauma to the underlying lens or iris by inadvertent contact of trephine or scissors, or the leaving behind of strands of vitreous or remnants of Descemet's membrane. Modern instrumentation such as bipolar endocoagulators permits treatment of complications such as intraocular bleeding from the wound edge or iris.

COMPLICATIONS IN THE IMMEDIATE
POSTOPERATIVE PERIOD

Wound leak, pupillary block, synechiae formation, wound ulceration, and failure of re-epithelialization are the most common problems seen in the immediate postoperative period. A wound leak leading to a shallow or flat anterior chamber may become apparent either at the time of surgery or in the immediate postoperative period. Pupillary block may also cause a flat anterior chamber, so that leakage from the wound must be evaluated. Bathing the surface with concentrated 2% fluorescein solution (Seidel's test) may point to an unsuspected area of wound leakage (Fig. 15-4). Although the intraocular pressure is likely to be low in the presence of a wound leak, it may be normal or high if a pupillary block accompanies the leak. Not infrequently, a pressure bandage over the eye is all that is necessary to reappose the wound and seal a wound leak. A contact lens may accomplish the same effect. If a small wound leak persists for more than 2 days, or if there is a major wound dehiscence, resuturing in the operating room is always indicated.

Iris prolapse accompanying a wound leak also requires surgical repair. If at all possible, retention of the iris is desirable to provide a normal pupil, reducing the glare that accompanies iridectomy. If the iris prolapse is relatively small and recent and if the iris appears to be reasonably healthy rather than macerated, reposition of the iris is feasible. It may be necessary to remove one or two extra sutures and reposit the iris while breaking any pupillary block. If, on the other hand, the iris appears to be macerated or devitalized or if the iris prolapse is of long duration, excision is preferable.

A shallow anterior chamber, particularly if the pupil is not well dilated, should raise the possibility of pupillary block, irrespective of whether the intraocular pressure is elevated, normal, or even low. Vigorous dilation with 1% cyclopentolate and 5% phenylephrine frequently produces dramatic and rapid restoration of the chamber depth. One should always keep in mind the possibility that choroidal detachment is present and is either leading to or perpetuating a shallow anterior chamber. Ultrasonography is helpful in making this diagnosis if observation is not possible with an indirect ophthalmo-

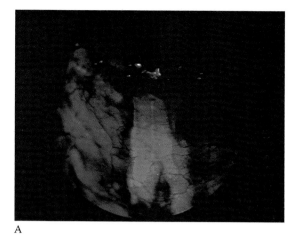

A

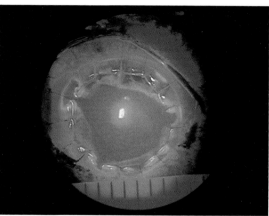

B

FIGURE 15-4. *Complications of penetrating keratoplasty. A. Seidel's test is used to demonstrate an area of wound leakage. If a wound leak is present, fluorescein applied to the eye is diluted by the aqueous in the area of the leak. B. Inadequate surface healing may result in persistent epithelial defect, especially if the surrounding host epithelium is diseased.*

scope. Watchful waiting is a reasonable course to follow for several days, but operative drainage of the fluid may be necessary if the angle appears to be anatomically compromised for more than several days.

Synechiae of iris to the graft border of some degree are not rare, and they do not per se lead to complications if small and not progressive. However, extensive synechiae to the wound are undesirable because of the likelihood of subsequent glaucoma (Fig. 15-5). Vigorous movement of the pupil can sometimes break early synechiae. Entering the chamber to sweep minor synechiae may lead to more serious problems than the synechiae themselves.

Wound ulceration is uncommon immediately after keratoplasty but can be present after grafting in those conditions in which ulceration is prominent,

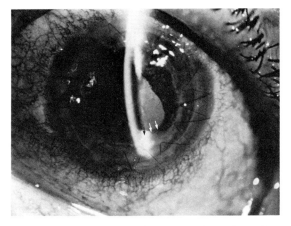

FIGURE 15-5. *Complications of penetrating keratoplasty. Synechiae (arrows) are potentially dangerous since glaucoma may ensue.*

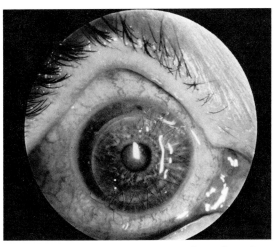

FIGURE 15-6. *Complications of penetrating keratoplasty. Loose sutures may result in wound separation and loss of the anterior chamber.*

e.g., herpes simplex and ocular surface diseases. Ulceration is best avoided by good wound apposition, moderate topical corticosteroid use, and facilitation of epithelial healing.

Epithelial healing is best achieved by retaining the donor epithelium on the donor graft and by the use of soft contact lenses to reduce traumatic loss of epithelial cells. Even with these measures, however, epithelial failure may occur later in the postoperative period.

COMPLICATIONS IN THE LATE POSTOPERATIVE PERIOD

Complications that occur several weeks or longer after surgery are most frequently related to wound healing, either stromal or epithelial. Wound separation is a frequent complication of premature loosening of sutures. The loosening of one interrupted suture is often not serious, but if one loop of a running suture should loosen, frequently loops on either side of it will loosen as a consequence, and therefore a relatively large area of wound may be permitted to separate (Fig. 15-6). The use of interrupted sutures in cases in which wound healing may be abnormal prevents this complication. Minor surface dehiscences with no tendency for wound separation and loss of the anterior chamber are best left alone. However, if the chamber is lost and does not reform rapidly with the use of pressure patching, soft contact lenses, or the application of cyanoacrylate adhesive, surgical repair becomes mandatory.

In the avascular graft, wound healing is slow, particularly if a nylon suture with buried knots is employed. Interrupted sutures, particularly if the knots are exposed, lead to earlier wound healing. Wounds are frequently not truly secure for a year or longer in the avascular graft, and the patient should be warned that the wound is *never* so strong as the surrounding tissue and is the most vulnerable area of the eye should blunt trauma occur. For this reason, sutures are frequently left in place for a year or longer under ordinary circumstances before being removed. However, sutures should be removed as soon as the wound appears fully healed as manifested by a strong gray scar at the wound margin or if vessels come up to and branch out along the wound margin. Postoperative infection or suture abscess is more likely to occur if the suture is left in place after the wound is well healed, since the suture frequently loosens at that time and may prove a nidus for infection. Fortunately, postoperative infection is rare, but it should always be considered if the eye becomes inflamed and irritated and intraocular inflammation is present.

The other major late postoperative problem is inadequate surface healing. Obviously this complication is more likely to occur if surrounding host epithelium is diseased as in chemical burns or the dry eye syndromes. Herpetic patients also frequently have wound surface problems, quite apart from the possibility of recurrent viral disease in the epithelium. If the epithelium is slow to reestablish itself, simply keeping the eyelids taped closed to prevent their rubbing the corneal surface may prove helpful. Soft contact lenses play a similar role, but the risk of a superinfection, particularly in the compromised eye, may be aggravated by soft contact lenses. The longer a persistent defect is present, the more likely it is that the surface will be irregular, with compromise of vision.

CORNEAL GRAFT FAILURE

Corneal grafts may lose their transparency for a variety of reasons. It is important to differentiate between *graft failure,* a general term for a hazy or opacified graft, and *graft rejection,* a term that refers to a specific immunopathophysiologic process.

GRAFT FAILURE

The common denominator of graft failure is a lack of clarity of the graft. While technical problems are an infrequent cause of graft failure, many of the complications of surgery may lead to surface irregularity or loss of stromal transparency.

Graft failure can occur at any time after keratoplasty. In the immediate postoperative period, graft failure is often due to some defect in the donor material itself. Despite biomicroscopy, specular microscopy, and strict adherence to the standards of use of donor material, adequate functioning of the donor material is not assured. If there is faulty donor endothelium, from the first postoperative day the graft will appear unduly thickened, with characteristic deep folds in the posterior limiting layers of the cornea (Fig. 15-7). Although this is sometimes reversible, it is undoubtedly a serious portent, and if it persists for several weeks without clearing, the graft must be considered irreversibly damaged. High doses of topical steroids (0.1% dexamethasone drops hourly for several days) should be immediately instituted and lower doses continued for several weeks, although the fate of the graft has been sealed if the edema persists for 4 to 6 weeks. It is reasonable to expect that intraoperative factors, such as trauma, that may not have come to the attention of the surgeon may also play a role in this *primary donor failure.*

In the immediate postoperative period, adventitious tissue adhering to the graft may also cause endothelial failure. Prolonged flat chamber causing the iris to rub on the endothelium, massive protrusion of vitreous causing its adherence to endothelium, or other mechanical causes of graft failure such as intraoperative trauma or excessive irrigation during surgery may all contribute to endothelial dysfunction and corneal edema. For this reason, intensive postoperative topical steroids (0.1% dexamethasone every other hour) to minimize postoperative inflammation are a useful adjunct to surgery even in atraumatic surgery.

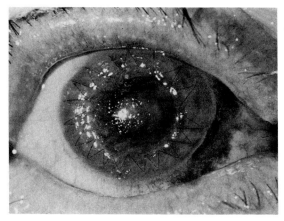

FIGURE 15-7. *Primary graft failure is caused by faulty donor endothelium and is apparent within hours after keratoplasty.*

Although it has not been demonstrated that increased intraocular pressure has an adverse effect on the survival of the endothelial cells, the wound integrity and the optic nerve may both suffer if glaucoma develops. Therefore, intraocular pressure should be carefully monitored postoperatively, timolol and carbonic anhydrase inhibitors should be given, and all medications used preoperatively for preexistent glaucoma should be reinstituted. Filtration surgery for postkeratoplasty glaucoma is usually not successful, but cyclocryotherapy may be done; it offers the best chance of controlling increased postoperative intraocular pressure that does not yield to medication. Movement of the pupil with cycloplegics to prevent pupillary block and vitreous entrapment against the endothelium is also important in preventing glaucoma.

In the late postoperative period, even in "uncomplicated" surgery, some grafts will fail. In some cases, this is undoubtedly due to the natural attrition of endothelial cells that occurs with age, particularly when one realizes that the trauma of the surgery itself may already have led to the loss of some endothelial cells. Postoperative inflammation may also contribute to the attrition of some endothelial cells.

GRAFT REJECTION

The term *graft rejection* deserves special consideration. The term is used to define a specific process in which a clear graft, having been established for at least several weeks (usually longer), suddenly succumbs to graft edema in conjunction with inflammatory signs. This process is immunologically mediated and is independent of any of the types of graft failure mentioned above. Although the most common type of rejection is associated with en-

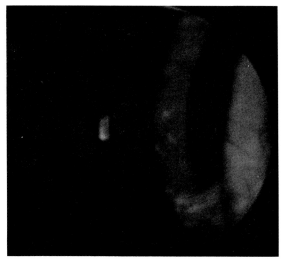

FIGURE 15-8. *Corneal graft rejection. Epithelial rejection may be manifested by subepithelial deposits similar to those seen in epidemic keratoconjunctivitis.*

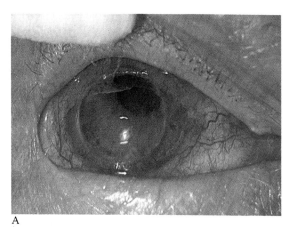

A

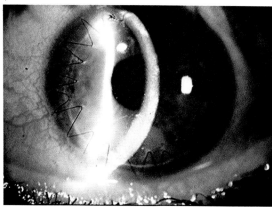

B

FIGURE 15-9. *A. Corneal endothelial graft rejection. This immunologic phenomenon occurs 1 month or more after surgery. It is characterized by graft edema in conjunction with inflammatory signs. B. Classic endothelial graft rejection causes endothelial dysfunction resulting in corneal edema. The "rejection line" of keratitic precipitates on the endothelium may be a late manifestation of the immunologic process destroying the endothelium.*

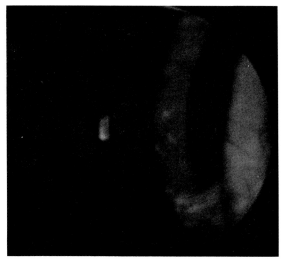

dothelial dysfunction, it has been suggested that epithelial rejection may be seen as well.

In cases of immunologic graft rejection, the precise role of donor and recipient HLA antigens is not fully known. Some authors have found a correlation between the number of matching donor and recipient antigens and the graft results in high risk cases of transplantation [4, 22], but other studies have not shown a similar correlation [3]. In renal transplantation [1], the importance of HLA-DR matching has been demonstrated, adding support to the idea that such matching or its lack may have an effect on the outcome of corneal grafting in vascular corneas.

Epithelial rejection is manifested in one of two ways. The first form is the development of an irregularly elevated line on the epithelium that moves rapidly across the cornea, disappearing with or without steroid treatment in a few days. The second form of epithelial rejection is the presence of round subepithelial deposits, similar in appearance to those found in the end stages of epidemic keratoconjunctivitis. These lesions change their location and configuration as time goes on and disappear after several weeks [2] (Fig. 15-8). Both of these reactions respond to steroids, but even without treatment they do not per se cause major visual problems, although the patient is aware of irritation in many cases.

The classic endothelial rejection causes endothelial dysfunction, which leads to corneal edema. Edema usually occurs in one of two locations. It may have a sudden onset in the central part of the cornea associated with keratitic precipitates and inflammatory cells in the anterior chamber (Fig. 15-9),

or it may occur at the margin of the graft and the host, with engorgement of blood vessels near the edematous area, accompanied by fine keratitic precipitates and inflammatory cells in the anterior chamber. The keratitic precipitates may form a line (Khodadoust line) on the endothelial surface. One should not wait for the appearance of a line to make a diagnosis of graft rejection, however, since this finding may be a late manifestation of the immunologic process that is destroying the endothelial cells. Any keratitic precipitates, engorgement of marginal blood vessels at the graft-host junction, or patches of corneal edema associated with inflammatory cells in the anterior chamber should be considered signs of a graft rejection. Therefore, any pa-

Girard, and Polack have suggested modifications of Cardona's implant [15].

tient who has undergone corneal transplantation should be encouraged to seek attention if symptoms of pain, redness, tearing, discomfort, or diminution of vision suddenly appear and persist for more than a few hours, since these symptoms may accompany the above signs.

Prognosis for reversal of a graft rejection is good if the symptoms are recognized and adequate treatment is undertaken immediately. The immediate instillation of topical steroids in copious amounts (one drop of 0.1% dexamethasone every hour around the clock) until the symptoms and signs abate is the treatment of choice. The tapering of the medication should be done gradually on the basis of the response to treatment, and even if the patient does not respond to treatment it is probably wise to continue this regimen for 3 weeks or so before it is deemed that the graft is irreversibly damaged. Some surgeons prefer to combine topical steroids with systemic steroids or even subconjunctival steroids, but it has yet to be proved that these treatments are any more successful than topical steroids alone. The responsibility for recognizing graft rejection must be borne by patient and surgeon alike, but even for those ophthalmologists who do not choose to perform their own grafts, it is mandatory that this reversible but potentially blinding complication of keratoplasty be clearly understood, and recognition and treatment should be in the province of all ophthalmologists.

KERATOPROSTHESES*

Since so many corneal diseases and injuries are followed by severe scarring and vascularization leading to graft failure, it is not surprising that the idea of replacing an opaque cornea with optically clear, nonbiologic material was envisioned many years ago. However, the use of synthetic materials as prosthetic implants was not investigated in detail until after World War II, when it was discovered that some plastics (e.g., Plexiglas) embedded in the cornea were well tolerated. Pioneering work in the field of keratoprosthesis was initiated by Cardona [7]. He used a variety of synthetic materials and designs and finally selected methyl methacrylate as the most efficacious and best tolerated material. Two designs for keratoprosthesis, the through-and-through and the nut-and-bolt, have become the most popular. Other surgeons such as Choyce,

*This section was written in collaboration with Calvin Roberts, M.D.

INDICATIONS
Careful selection of patients is critical. Only patients who are highly motivated and willing to accept the probable development of severe, sight-threatening complications should be considered for the procedure. Even in the absence of complications, frequent postoperative evaluation is necessary, obligating both the patient and the physician to periodic examinations for a long period. Therefore, the patient must be highly motivated and no longer able to function with his current vision.

Although differences of opinion exist as to the indications for keratoprosthesis, in general it is reserved for corneal opacification in which a penetrating keratoplasty would be unlikely to achieve visual improvement because of failure to heal or immunologic graft reaction. Nearly all proponents recommend keratoprosthesis only for patients with bilateral blindness, in whom the keratoprosthesis is the only method for achieving any useful vision. Obviously, keratoprosthesis is not indicated if noncorneal factors would preclude restoration of vision. Thus, glaucoma should be controlled, and ultrasound and retinal and optic nerve function testing should be done to rule out irremediable posterior pole disease before the use of a keratoprosthesis is considered.

In addition to patients with bilateral blindness for whom penetrating keratoplasty would be ineffective, a second group of patients who are candidates for keratoprosthesis are those who have had repeated penetrating keratoplasties with graft failure, regardless of the initial underlying disease. When a decision has been reached that further attempts at keratoplasty would be fruitless, particularly if there are complicating factors such as peripheral anterior synechiae or a shallow anterior chamber, a keratoprosthesis may offer some chance of rehabilitation [16].

Some surgeons offer keratoprosthesis as the primary mode of therapy for severe bullous keratopathy in elderly or totally disabled patients [8]. A keratoprosthesis can offer rapid visual rehabilitation in such cases. However, most surgeons feel that penetrating keratoplasty is just as successful, with fewer potential complications.

MATERIALS AND CONFIGURATIONS
The Cardona-type keratoprosthesis is constructed from methyl methacrylate. This material is not well tolerated by all patients, and other materials that may be more compatible with the surrounding fibrous tissue are being investigated. Polack and

Heimke [15] have used a keratoprosthesis made of silica oxide ceramic. They have shown that soft tissue adheres to the surface of this material, possibly preventing extrusion of the prosthesis and surface epithelial ingrowth. Strampelli [19] has proposed another alternative: A thin piece of bone and tooth is grafted to the surface of the cornea and becomes incorporated into the fibrous tissue. The acrylic optical cylinder then passes through the bone, through the stroma, and into the anterior chamber. The technique is called an *osteo-odontokeratoprosthesis*.

In most cases, the material is fabricated into a nut-and-bolt prosthesis (Fig. 15-10). The anterior and central optical portion are made in one piece and are threaded into a posterior disc. This tends to stabilize the prosthesis by clamping host tissue between the front and back portions. The through-and-through prosthesis does not have a supporting posterior disc and depends on support from sutures to the corneal tissue, augmented by cartilage or periosteum. In patients with thin corneas and poor conjunctivae (e.g., those with cicatricial pemphigoid, Stevens-Johnson syndrome, or chemical injury), additional support for the prosthesis is obtained by having the central optical portion pass through the upper lid as well (Fig. 15-11).

TECHNIQUES

Although the details of keratoprosthesis surgery are beyond the scope of this text, certain basic elements are shared by all of the methods. The first is penetration through the cornea and into the anterior chamber with a trephine, usually 3 mm in diameter. If lens extraction has not been done previously, it may be accomplished through an additional superior limbal incision. Partial vitrectomy and anterior membrane removal may also be done at this time. If a nut-and-bolt prosthesis is used, its posterior disc is inserted, and then the anterior portion of the prosthesis is threaded into it. The limbal incision is then closed. In the case of prosthesis without a posterior disc, it may not be necessary to open the eye at the superior limbus, depending upon the clarity of the anterior segment as viewed through the trephine opening. In all cases, care must be taken to assure adequate hemostosis, so that residual blood in the anterior segment will not interfere with vision and pressure control.

POSTOPERATIVE CARE

The use of topical antibiotics in the postoperative period is recommended. Gentamicin 0.3% three times daily for 14 days is the standard dosage. Atropine may also be used to reduce postoperative ciliary muscle spasm. The intraocular pressure can

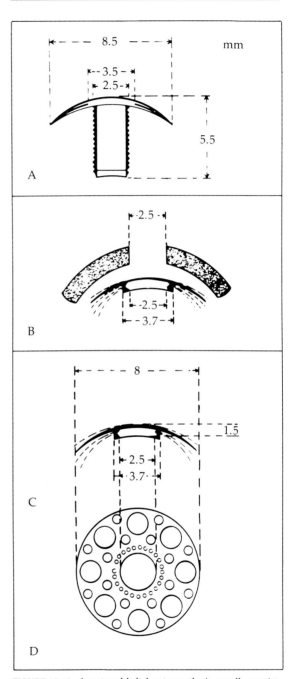

FIGURE 15-10. *A nut-and-bolt keratoprosthesis usually consists of an optically clear anterior and central portion (A) that is threaded into a posterior disc (B, C, and D), which may have holes drilled through it to facilitate proper nutrition of the anterior tissue. The back plate extends well onto the back of the cornea, with an 8-mm flange peripheral to the central 3.7-mm nut. (Courtesy Anthony Donn, M.D.)*

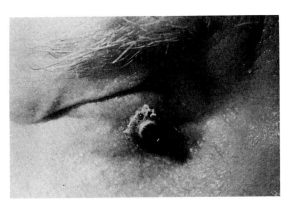

FIGURE 15-11. *Through-the-lid prostheses are useful in patients with thin corneas or poor conjunctivae.*

be estimated digitally, and oral carbonic anhydrase inhibitors (acetazolamide 250 mg 4 times daily) may be necessary to reduce it. Topical medication such as timolol maleate 0.5% twice daily can also be added if necessary. Topical corticosteroids are usually not indicated, since they may increase the likelihood of loss of corneal stroma surrounding the prosthesis. In conditions in which stromal loss has not been a problem earlier (e.g., repeated immunologic failure), topical steroids (0.01% dexamethasone 3 times daily) may be used to reduce postoperative inflammation.

COMPLICATIONS

Complications may occur at the time of surgery or in the early or late postoperative periods. Early complications include hemorrhage, wound leak, infection or uveitis, and glaucoma.

Hemorrhage is a likely possibility because of the rich vascular supply in the scarred cornea. If it occurs intraoperatively, bleeding must be controlled and residual blood must be washed out of the eye. Postoperatively, hemorrhage is a serious complication, although there is little that can be done about it. With adequate pressure control, hemorrhage may eventually clear, although fibrous organization of the anterior segment and vitreous may occur.

Wound leakage can occur because of the lack of healing around the prosthetic stem. Most such leaks will stop if aqueous production can be decreased. Pressure patching may be of some value in such leaks.

Sterile vitritis occurs in approximately half of all keratoprosthesis patients. It may be present even when topical steroids are given and should be treated vigorously with systemic steroids (e.g., 60

mg prednisone daily for 1 week) to prevent development of retroprosthetic membranes. Intraocular infection has been much less common than might be expected, in part because of the copious vascular supply of the scarred cornea.

Glaucoma is a very common complication of keratoprosthesis and is difficult to detect and treat because of the inability of the surgeon to assess the intraocular pressure postoperatively. These eyes are usually unresponsive to topical therapy and only moderately responsive to carbonic anhydrase inhibitors. Cyclocryotherapy can be done if all medical therapy fails.

The most common, as well as the most disastrous, late complication has been extrusion of the keratoprosthesis. However, recent procedures using the more modern style of nut-and-bolt and through-and-through keratoprostheses with autologous grafts have reduced the incidence of extrusion to below 20 percent. Although heroic attempts to replace the keratoprosthesis are usually attempted, visual recovery after extrusion is unlikely. In a patient in whom extrusion of the keratoprosthesis has occurred, enucleation of the eye is usually performed.

Even in the absence of early complication, subsequent anterior segment membrane formation, glaucoma, wound leak, or retinal detachment usually leads to marked loss of vision in a few years in most patients. It is virtually impossible to predict the duration of visual improvement in any patient. Despite that, many patients accept this uncertainty willingly in the hopes of regaining some of their previous vision and independence.

REFERENCES

1. Albrechtsen, D., et al. HLA-A,B,C,D, DR in clinical transplantation. *Transplant Proc.* 13:924, 1981.
2. Aldredge, O. C., and Krachmer, J. H. Clinical types of corneal transplant rejection: Their manifestations, frequency, preoperative correlates and treatment. *Arch. Ophthalmol.* 99:599, 1981.
3. Allansmith, M. R., Fine, M., and Payne, R. Histocompatibility typing and corneal transplantation. *Trans. Am. Acad. Ophthalmol. Otolaryngol.* 78:445, 1974.
4. Batchelor, J. R., et al. HLA matching and corneal grafting. *Lancet* 1:551, 1976.
5. Boruchoff, S. A. Corneal Surgery. In T. Duane (Ed.), *Clinical Ophthalmology.* Hagerstown, Md.: Harper & Row, 1976. Vol. 5, Chap. 6.
6. Capella, J. A., Kaufman, H. E., and Robbins, J. E. Preservation of viable corneal tissue. *Arch. Ophthalmol.* 74:669, 1965.
7. Cardona, H. Keratoprosthesis: Acrylic optical

cylinder with supporting interlamellar plate. *Am. J. Ophthalmol.* 54:284, 1962.

8. Donn, A. Aphakic bullous keratopathy treated with keratoprosthesis. *Arch. Ophthalmol.* 94:270, 1976.
9. Elschnig, A. On keratoplasty. *Prag. Med. Wochenschr.* 39:30, 1914.
10. McCarey, B., and Kaufman, H. E. Improved corneal storage. *Invest. Ophthalmol.* 13:165, 1974.
11. Miller, D., and Stegmann, R. Use of Na-hyaluronate in auto-corneal transplantation in rabbits. *Ophthalmic Surg.* 11:19, 1980.
12. Opelz, G., Mickey, M. R., and Terasaki, P. I. Calculations on long-term graft and patient survival in human kidney transplantation. *Transplant Proc.* 9:27, 1977.
13. Pape, L. G., and Balasz, E. A. The use of sodium hyaluronate (Healon) in human anterior segment surgery. *Ophthalmology* (Rochester) 87:699, 1980.
14. Paufique, L., Sourdille, G.-P., and Offret, G. *Les Greffes de la Cornée.* Paris: Masson, 1948.
15. Polack, F. M., and Heimke, G. Ceramic keratoprostheses. *Ophthalmology* (Rochester) 87:693, 1980.
16. Rao, G. N., Blatt, H. L., and Aquavella, J. V. Results of keratoprosthesis. *Am. J. Ophthalmol.* 88:190, 1979.
17. Stark, W. J. Transplantation immunology of penetrating keratoplasty. *Trans. Am. Ophthalmol. Soc.* 78:1079, 1980.
18. Stocker, F. W. Successful corneal graft in a case of endothelial and epithelial dystrophy. *Am. J. Ophthalmol.* 35:349, 1952.
19. Strampelli, B. Osteo-odonto-keratoprosthesis. *Ann. Ottal.* 89:1039, 1963.
20. Thoft, R. A. Indications for conjunctival transplantation. *Ophthalmology* (Rochester) 89:335, 1982.
21. Tudor Thomas, J. W. Corneal transplantation on an opaque cornea. *Proc. Roy. Soc. Med.* 1936.
22. Vannas, S., et al. HLA-compatible donor cornea for prevention of allograft reaction. *Albrecht Von Graefes Arch. Klin. Ophthalmol.* 198:217, 1976.
23. von Hippel, A. On Transplantation of the Cornea. Ber. Ophthalmol. Gel. Heidelberg, 18 (2nd meeting) 54, 1886.

Refractive Keratoplasty

David J. Schanzlin and Anthony B. Nesburn

The anterior corneal surface is the most powerful refracting interface of the eye. Therefore, small alterations in the curvature of this surface greatly alter the clinical refraction of the eye. Recently, many surgical techniques have utilized this principle to change the refractive state of the eye. These procedures range from the corneal incision techniques of radial keratotomy, corneal wedge resection, and corneal relaxing incisions, to the corneal lathing techniques of keratomileusis, keratophakia, and epikeratophakia. Still other procedures have applied localized heat to the cornea to cause shrinkage of the collagen matrices and thereby change the refractive power of the anterior corneal surface.

At present, all of these techniques, with perhaps the exception of corneal wedge resection and relaxing incisions for the correction of high postkeratoplasty astigmatism, are considered experimental. As such, patients undergoing these procedures for the correction of refractive errors should be advised of the experimental nature of the surgery, and the surgeon should perform these procedures only with the approval of an institutional review board.

With the growing interest in keratorefractive surgical techniques seen in the last 5 years, the next decade will undoubtedly provide major progress, including determining the answers to many of the questions about the safety and efficacy of the procedures and reproducibility and permanence of the results.

THERMOKERATOPLASTY

Cauterization of the cornea to correct keratoconus or severe astigmatism dates back at least 100 years. In 1900, Terrien [23] reported successful cautery treatment of severe astigmatism in a case of marginal degeneration. Knapp [15] in 1929 described a series of patients with keratoconus whose visual acuity improved after cauterization of the cornea. Unfortunately, in producing the effect, these thermal cautery techniques caused scarring, destruction, and dissolution of collagen fibers and occasionally even melting of the cornea.

Thermokeratoplasty for the treatment of keratoconus uses heat, which shrinks the cornea but does not cause melting of the stromal tissue [7, 8]. In 1975, Gasset and Kaufman [7] reported on 10 keratoconic eyes successfully treated by this method. Up to 2 years after the procedure, the majority of these patients maintained 20/30 visual acuity, and less than 5 percent of these eyes needed penetrating keratoplasty.

Others [A. B. Nesburn, unpublished data, 1980; 21] have not been as successful in using thermokeratoplasty to treat keratoconus. Their studies showed that the procedure is not predictable and the success rate is, at best, only 50 percent. Penetrating keratoplasty in thermokeratoplasty failures is complicated by stromal neovascularization induced by the original procedure as well as the marked tissue flaccidity of the peripheral recipient cornea, complicating wound closure and leading to extensive astigmatism. Because of these complications, thermokeratoplasty is used infrequently by corneal surgeons in this country.

In Japan, Itoi [10] recently reported low-temperature (75–90°C) thermokeratoplasty to be useful in treating mild to moderately advanced keratoconus.

Rowsey and Doss [18] are utilizing the Los Alamos radiofrequency probe to shrink corneal collagen in a selective, controlled procedure to induce refractive changes. The procedure, used in keratoconus, induces major scars and must be applied outside the visual axis. However, initial results are said to be promising.

LATHING PROCEDURES

TYPES

KERATOMILEUSIS
Keratomileusis (*kerato-* cornea + *mileus* carving) is a form of lamellar keratoplasty in which the patient's own cornea is lathed to correct spherical myopic or hyperopic refractive error. The technique has been developed by Jose Barraquer [1] over the last 25 years. At present, he and a handful of other surgeons are the only people using the technique. The principle of myopic and hyperopic keratomileusis involves changing the radius of curvature of the central anterior surface of the cornea by controlled lathing of the stromal side of a lamellar disc (lenticule) from the patient's own cornea. The lamellar disc is frozen and tooled by a specially modified contact lens lathe designed by Barraquer (Fig. 15-12). The cryolathe removes tissue under meticulous control until the desired power is achieved. The lenticule is then resutured onto the patient's cornea.

MYOPIC KERATOMILEUSIS
The keratomileusis technique for the correction of myopic refractive errors involves flattening of the

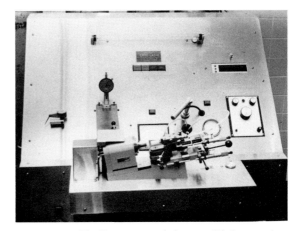

FIGURE 15-12. *The Barraquer cryolathe, a modified contact lens lathe used to cut various curves into a corneal lenticule while the tissue is frozen.*

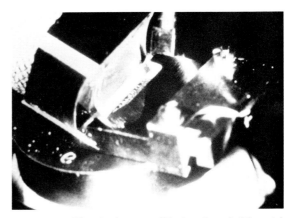

FIGURE 15-13. *The microkeratome slides in a channel of the metal ring that is apposed to the limbal region by suction. A thin disc of tissue can be seen emerging just in front of the cutting edge.*

central anterior corneal surface. To achieve this effect, a central corneal disc of uniform thickness is removed using the microkeratome (Fig. 15-13). A segment of the correct power is lathed from the posterior surface, making the center thinner than the periphery (Fig. 15-14). Resuturing this lenticule to the stromal surface results in a flatter central cornea, decreasing the refractive power of the cornea and correcting the myopic refractive error.

HYPEROPIC KERATOMILEUSIS
In hyperopic keratomileusis, a uniform lamellar disc from the patient's cornea is removed using the microkeratome and placed on the cryolathe. A convex lens is made by lathing the posterior surface of the cornea so that the periphery is thinner than the center. When the resulting lenticule is resutured, the radius of curvature of the central cornea increases, correcting hyperopic refractive errors (Fig. 15-15).

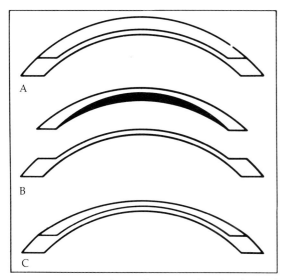

FIGURE 15-14. *Myopic keratomileusis. A. The original corneal cross section, showing the plane of separation of the stromal disc from the rest of the cornea. B. The lenticule is produced by removing a convex segment of tissue from the back of the disc, leaving a lens having minus power. C. Resuturing the minus-power lenticule back in its original position has the effect of reducing the power of the cornea.*

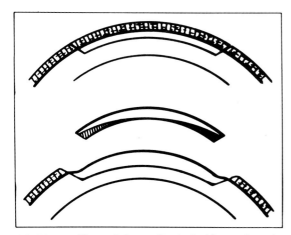

FIGURE 15-15. *Hyperopic keratomileusis. In this procedure, the lenticule produced on the lathe has plus power and increases the refractive power of the cornea when it is sutured in place.*

KERATOPHAKIA

Keratophakia is a lathing technique that uses donor corneal tissue to correct aphakic refractive errors. In keratophakia, the radius of curvature of the patient's cornea is steepened by placing an interlamellar plus-power lenticule in the host cornea.

A distinct advantage of keratophakia is that the plus-power lenticule can be lathed before surgery.

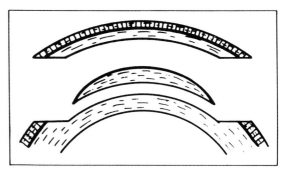

FIGURE 15-16. *Keratophakia. The anterior stromal disc is removed with a microkeratome, and a prelathed positive-power disc is placed between the disc and the underlying stromal bed, creating added positive refracting power.*

During surgery, the microkeratome is used to make a lamellar section in the host cornea (Fig. 15-16), forming an anterior disc having parallel faces. The disc is resutured using a double-running antitorque suture; just before the suture is tied, the prelathed donor lenticule is centered in the interlamellar space. The sutures are tightened and the knots buried.

The advantage of being able to prelathe the donor lenticule as well as the better surgical results have made keratophakia the most accepted of the Barraquer procedures among surgeons in the United States.

INDICATIONS FOR SURGERY

The Barraquer refractive surgery techniques should be performed only on normal eyes. The procedure is reserved for cases of typical spherical refractive correction when traditional forms of therapy, such as spectacle or contact lens therapy, do not solve the problem of ametropia. With the present state of the technology, patients should be advised that the surgery will decrease the amount of their refractive correction, but it is likely that they will still have some residual refractive error. Myopes who undergo myopic keratomileusis should be informed that, although the surgery modifies the anterior corneal refractive status, it does not affect the progression of their myopia. In addition, they must be told about the premature onset of presbyopia after the procedure.

The primary indication for these surgical procedures is monocular ametropia including myopic anisometropia, hyperopic anisometropia, monocular aphakia, aphakia in an eye the fellow eye of which has undergone refractive surgery, and monocular aphakia in those with poor tolerance to contact lenses who require cataract surgery on the fellow eye.

This surgery is not advisable for patients who have any evidence of external ocular disease, corneal disease, lacrimal gland hyposecretion, or glaucoma. Because of problems with microkeratome sections in eyes in which the corneal curvature is either too steep or too flat, patients with preoperative keratometry readings of less than 39 diopters or greater than 52 diopters should be excluded.

LATHING TECHNIQUE

Techniques of keratomileusis and keratophakia necessitate rapid and accurate mathematical calculations during the lathing procedure. The surgery cannot be performed accurately without computer technology. Early, less complicated programs for these procedures were carried out with programmable, hand-held calculators. However, in the last few years surgeons have switched to faster small computers to perform the tasks.

Computer technology is necessary because of the multiple variables involved with cryolathing procedures. These include (1) the thickness of the microkeratome-excised corneal disc, (2) the thickness of the remaining cornea, (3) the shrinkage of the lathing base with cooling, (4) the contraction of the lathing tool with cooling, (5) the swelling of the central corneal stroma with freezing, (6) the shrinkage of the corneal diameter with freezing, (7) the desired size of the central optical zone, and (8) the desired ultimate refraction.

RESULTS

KERATOMILEUSIS
The results of myopic keratomileusis and hyperopic keratomileusis for the correction of aphakia have recently been summarized by Barraquer [1]. A long-term analysis of myopic keratomileusis procedures performed in 1976 demonstrated less than optimal corrections. In these cases, corrections varied from an average of 58 percent of −9.37 diopters in monocular cases, to as little as 37.4 percent correction of −11.97 diopters in binocular cases. A careful analysis of his data allowed Barraquer to determine that there was greater stability in myopic keratomileusis when the corneal disc had a diameter under 7.5 mm and a thickness of under 0.30 mm and when the central thickness, after lathing, was near 0.1 mm. Using new parameters, he found greater stability of corrections, and on examining the data on 52 cases

performed in 1979, he reports ametropia visual acuities of better than 20/40 at 3, 6, and 12 months' follow-up.

The results of hyperopic keratomileusis, also reported by Barraquer [1], show between 78 and 85 percent of the desired correction using current programs. Neither hyperopic keratomileusis or myopic keratomileusis appeared to alter astigmatism, and best visual acuities were increased postoperatively to the 20/40 range.

Swinger and Barraquer [22] reported a random retrospective study of 159 of Barraquer's patients who underwent keratophakia and keratomileusis for correction of refractive errors. In patients who underwent myopic keratomileusis, the mean spherical flattening of the cornea, as determined by subjective refraction, was 5.92 diopters, and the maximum decrease was 15 diopters. Corrected visual acuities increased postoperatively in 67 percent of the patients by an average of 2.4 lines; the maximum improvement was only 6 lines. The acuity remained unchanged in 24.7 percent of the cases and decreased in 8.2 percent by an average of 2 lines. In this series, the accuracy of the procedure in obtaining the desired amount of correction was only 51.3 percent, with a range of −31.2 to 135 percent. The authors examined the stability of keratomileusis based on keratometry and refraction. They found that although the refraction changed at a rate of −0.30 diopters per year, this was not found to correlate with the change in the keratometry reading but most likely represented lenticular myopia or progressive axial elongation.

Friedlander and associates [4] have reported their success rate with hyperopic keratomileusis. All 7 patients in their series achieved 20/30 or better visual acuity. Eight of 11 patients who had homoplastic hyperopic keratomileusis using donor corneal tissue achieved 20/60 or better visual acuity. In this series, as well as in the series of Barraquer [1], it made little difference whether hyperopic keratomileusis was performed at the same time as intracapsular cataract extraction or as a secondary procedure.

KERATOPHAKIA
At present, keratophakia is the least complex and most practiced of the cryolathing refractive surgery techniques. Swinger and Barraquer [22] reported a randomized retrospective analysis of 41 keratophakia cases. The average power induced by this procedure was +10.27 diopters by keratometry, resulting in an average refractive change of 9.84 diopters. The astigmatism as shown by keratometry and refraction was increased on an average by 1.5 diopters with maximal astigmatic in-

duction of 5 diopters. No irregular astigmatism was noted. Postoperatively, the visual acuity was improved by 1 line or more in 39 percent of the patients, remained unchanged in 27 percent, and was decreased 1 line or more in 34 percent. The mean age of this group of patients was 16.14 years with a range of 2 to 56 years. Mild to moderate amblyopia was documented in 63 percent of these patients. All the patients who did show improvement of best corrected visual acuity of 2 lines or more were children who underwent orthoptic therapy postoperatively.

The accuracy of the keratophakia computer program was examined, and a percent of desired correction was calculated. By analysis of keratometric data, the mean correction was 93.5 percent (range 61.4–194 percent) of the desired correction. The keratometric readings stabilized by 6 months, and little change occurred thereafter.

Troutman and associates [24, 25] have reported their results with keratophakia. They achieved an average correction of 10 diopters with an average astigmatic error of 2.5 diopters. A change in their computer program increased the correction of refractive error up to 13 diopters with less than 2 diopters of astigmatism. Most of the patients in this series required spectacle correction to obtain maximal visual acuity; 16 of the 23 patients (70 percent) were correctable to 20/30 or better, and 91 percent were correctable to 20/60 or better. Four of the patients with 20/60 or less visual acuity had demonstrable macular disease.

Friedlander and associates [4] summarized their results with keratophakia between December 1977 and October 1979. Patient selection was based on stable visual acuity in the fellow eye of 20/40 or better and inability to wear contact lenses. All 13 patients who underwent keratophakia achieved 20/50 or better visual acuity, and 11 of the 13 had 20/40 or better visual acuity. A statistically significant average increase of 1.40 ± 0.48 diopters of astigmatism occurred postoperatively. Patients appeared to have stable refractions over the subsequent year of follow-up.

LIMITATIONS
Over the last several years, there have been many advances in the cryolathing of corneal tissue. There are still, however, inherent limitations that restrict the amount of refractive correction achievable with satisfactory and stable visual acuity.

The maximal corneal curvature considered stable is 59 diopters. Therefore, if the patient's preoperative central keratometry reading is 43 diopters, the maximal correction obtainable by any of the Barraquer techniques is 16 diopters. Similarly, the minimal corneal radius considered stable is 37 diop-

ters, and therefore a myope with a preoperative central keratometry reading of 47 diopters may only expect a maximum of 10 diopters of correction with myopic keratomileusis.

Another limitation of these lathing techniques is the thickness of the lathed tissue. Theoretically, for instance, in myopic keratomileusis, a concave lens could be of greater power if the optical zone could be made smaller. Optical zones, however, of less than 5.5 mm are undesirable because of the problems of glare that will develop.

COMPLICATIONS OF CRYOLATHING TECHNIQUES
With a technique as complex as the cryolathing of corneal tissue, errors can occur at any stage of the procedure. The most important complications seen with keratomileusis occur at the time of microkeratome section—if the section is made too thin, too thick, or irregular—and at the time of lathing—if the central area of the cornea is made too thin and perforation occurs.

Another complication encountered in any lamellar technique is the deposition of foreign bodies in the interfaces. Epithelial ingrowth into the lamellar space may occur. This is seen more frequently with keratomileusis than with keratophakia. Inaccurate centering of the donor disc is a major problem that leads to poor visual acuity and high postoperative astigmatism. Barraquer [1, 22] suggests that all of these complications are greatly reduced as one gains experience with the procedure.

EPIKERATOPHAKIA
Epikeratophakia represents a new and innovative approach to refractive corneal surgery. This technique, pioneered and developed by Werblin, Kaufman, and coworkers [13, 26], has been adapted and utilized for the correction of aphakic refractive error and keratoconus.

Epikeratophakia differs from the Barraquer techniques primarily because in the former the refractive correction is placed on the surface of the cornea rather than within a lamellar pouch. This surface "cap graft" or "living contact lens" adheres to a circumferential incision through Bowman's membrane, leaving the central cornea free of residual scarring [13]. A distinct advantage of this surgical approach is that the cap graft can be removed at any time, leaving the patient's central cornea clear.

INDICATIONS
The ultimate scope and acceptance of this form of refractive corneal surgery is not yet known. The ini-

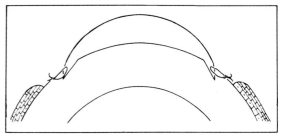

FIGURE 15-18. *Epikeratophakia. The donor lenticule is sutured to the cornea after the epithelium is removed with absolute alcohol. The wing of the lenticule is inserted into a groove cut into the patient's stroma inside an 8-mm trephine mark.*

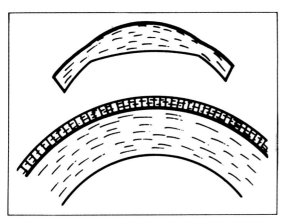

FIGURE 15-17. *Epikeratophakia. The donor stromal disc has been lathed to create a plus-power lenticule, with a thinner peripheral wing of tissue.*

tial favorable results reported by Werblin and co-workers [26] and Kaufman [13] for aphakic epikeratophakia make it an acceptable alternative in situations in which a secondary intraocular lens implant is contraindicated and contact lens fitting has failed after cataract surgery. Epikeratophakia for the correction of monocular aphakia after congenital cataract removal may prove to be another indication for this procedure. The distinct advantage of using this procedure in a congenital cataract case is that as the eye grows, the cap graft can be removed and a new one of the appropriate power can be placed.

Epikeratophakia cap grafts show promising early results for the treatment of mild to moderate cases of keratoconus in which there is no central scarring but there is extensive peripheral thinning of the cornea. In the latter situation, penetrating keratoplasty can be difficult and may result in high residual astigmatic errors.

TECHNIQUE

APHAKIA

The epikeratophakia procedure utilizes a donor corneal lenticule lathed in the form of a plus-power lens. The lathing technique is performed using the Barraquer cryolathe and computer programs designed specifically for epikeratophakia. With the lathing, a high central plus correction is possible. A thin peripheral wing is lathed for easy suturing to the host cornea (Fig. 15-17). The corneal lenticule is lathed to an ultimate diameter of 9 mm.

Vigorous debridement of the corneal epithelium is performed using cellulose sponges dipped in absolute alcohol. An 8-mm trephine is used to par-

tially incise the patient's cornea to a depth of 0.2 mm. Then, using Vannas scissors, a thin rim of epithelium and Bowman's membrane is excised from the inner diameter of the trephine mark. Meticulous irrigation and aspiration of the ocular surface is performed to remove all the residual epithelium and foreign particles from the operative field. The preground epikeratophakia lenticule is then sutured to the host cornea with the edges of the peripheral wing inserted into the groove that extends into Bowman's membrane and corneal stroma (Fig. 15-18). Using a donor lenticule 1 mm larger than the host trephine mark provides the most reliable refractive correction. After the lenticule is sutured, a soft contact lens that remains in place for at least 3 weeks to allow for re-epithelialization is placed on the cornea. Sutures are removed 4 to 6 weeks after surgery.

KERATOCONUS

The general epikeratophakia procedure for the correction of keratoconus is similar to that for aphakia. In the correction of the refractive error of keratoconus, however, the concept is to provide structural tectonic support to the ectatic cornea. Therefore, no myopic power is lathed into the donor cornea. The lenticule used for this procedure is 0.25 to 0.30 mm thick and has no refractive power. The lenticule is cut 0.5 mm larger than the trephine used to demarcate a central zone of the ectatic region of the cone. After vigorous debridement of the epithelium with absolute alcohol and irrigation, the cap graft is sutured in place with approximately 20 to 24 interrupted 10-0 nylon sutures that are tightened to produce the desired central corneal flattening. This technique produces marked flattening of the central cornea and reduction of corneal astigmatism [26]. Immediately after this procedure, the knots are buried superficially and a thin therapeutic soft contact lens is applied. The lens is left in place for 2 to 3 weeks to allow epithelialization of the cap graft. Ointment and lubricating drops are used frequently to protect the epithelium until suture removal takes place at 6 to 8 weeks.

RESULTS

A clinical study of the results of epikeratophakia has been reported by Werblin and coworkers [27]. This study included 42 patients who underwent aphakic hyperopic epikeratophakia. Preoperatively, all patients had stable visual acuities and were not candidates for either spectacle or contact lens correction. All had been aphakic for at least 3 months before the epikeratophakia procedure. Before and after operation, visual acuity, keratometry, pachometry, visual field, endothelial cell counts, and ultrasonography were measured carefully.

The authors reported the visual acuities in 32 patients followed for 4 to 12 months postoperatively. Five of the original 42 patients were eliminated from the tabulation because of loss of the graft from epithelial problems, three had non-graft related visual problems, one died, and one was lost to follow-up. The authors ascertained the role of surface irregularity in the slow visual recovery by measuring visual acuity with contact lens and pinhole acuities. These acuities were compared to spectacle correction at each postoperative examination. With contact lens or spectacle correction, the 32 patients had 20/50 or better average acuity at 4 months, the 29 patients followed 8 months had 20/40 or better average acuity, and the 16 patients followed 12 months had $20/30^{-2}$ average visual acuity.

LIMITATIONS

The primary drawback of epikeratophakia is the long convalescence. Generally, it takes 3 to 6 months before an optimal visual acuity is achieved, and it is 1 to 2 lines less than that theoretically achievable using contact lens refraction as a standard. Follow-up time has been short; however, once achieved, the visual acuity appears to be stable for at least 1½ years. The slow recovery of visual acuity appears to be related to opacities and irregularities within the lamellar cap graft. The rehabilitation time, in some instances, may be comparable to that in penetrating keratoplasty for keratoconus. However, in aphakia, when the technique is used in place of intraocular lens implantation, rehabilitation time is considerably longer than that for lens implantation.

Nevertheless, the concept of applying the refractive correction to the surface of the eye is very appealing. In the future, cap grafts may be available to correct astigmatism as well as hyperopic and myopic refractive errors. Certainly, the ease of this procedure and the possibility of readily available lyophilized prelathed tissue are extremely attractive. This will undoubtedly be an area of intense interest over the coming years.

COMPLICATIONS

The major complications of epikeratophakia include problems with epithelialization, dehiscence of the graft, infection, and persistent haziness of the lenticule.

Epikeratophakia is a new procedure, so all of the complications are not yet known. The most frequent complication is poor epithelialization of the acellular donor cap graft. The corneal epithelium that is not removed at the time of the surgery must slide, undergo mitosis, and attach solidly to the entire corneal surface. Because the cap graft protrudes, there is additional trauma from the lids that may impede healing. The role of delayed or abnormal innervation in epithelial healing is under investigation.

A rarer problem is dehiscence of the graft, which adheres to the host cornea only along the peripheral trephine site. The advantage of this peripheral adherence is that it allows easy graft removal and replacement with a graft of a different power if necessary. The disadvantage, however, is that blunt ocular trauma and early suture loss or removal can lead to graft dehiscence. In many cases, when this occurs, the graft must be replaced.

With a compromised epithelium and a nonviable donor cap, these patients are at risk of developing infections in the first few postoperative weeks. If infection occurs, it must be treated aggressively by identifying the infecting organism and eradicating it with appropriate antibiotic therapy. In some cases, this may necessitate removal of the graft to prevent the spread of the infection to the host cornea itself.

Another problem with epikeratophakia is a long-lasting haziness of the cap graft, which tends to clear with time. However, in some instances there are opacities or haze remaining even 3 to 6 months after surgery. What causes this persistent opacification is still unknown, but it is assumed to be a combination of increased corneal thickness, stress on the corneal endothelium, the slow repopulation of the donor tissue with host keratocytes, and possibly even stromal irregularities induced by the process of tissue lathing.

PENETRATING KERATOPLASTY

Although most penetrating keratoplasty is done for corneal opacity and thinning (c.f. Therapeutic Keratoplasty), the procedure has a major effect on the refractive state of the eye. For that reason, corneal transplantation should be considered a refractive surgical technique also. Certainly, microsurgery, finer sutures, better surgical technique, and improved antibiotic and corticosteroid therapy have greatly reduced chances of graft failure. With the improved potential of obtaining a clear graft, the major problem in penetrating keratoplasty today in many patients is high postoperative astigmatic errors.

High astigmatism results if either the donor or the recipient cornea is cut elliptically or if the sides of the donor button or the host wound are not perpendicular. Troutman and colleagues [24] have demonstrated that a 0.1 mm eccentricity causes as much as 1 diopter of postoperative astigmatism. Many groups are studying the surgical technique to prevent the development of postoperative astigmatism. To prevent this vision-limiting complication, the operating keratometer and various suture techniques are being examined closely to determine the optimal manner in which to perform penetrating keratoplasty. When high degrees of corneal astigmatism do occur after penetrating keratoplasty, corneal wedge resection or corneal relaxing incisions may be beneficial.

CORNEAL WEDGE RESECTION
Corneal wedge resections are especially useful in reducing high degrees of corneal astigmatism (10–20 diopters) seen after penetrating keratoplasty. High degrees of severe postcataract astigmatism are also correctable by wedge resection.

Corneal wedge resection [24] produces a steepening of the flatter corneal meridian. Removing a wedge from the flatter meridian also causes secondary flattening of the steeper meridian. Ideally this alteration leaves the cornea with a central spherical surface.

For correction of astigmatism following keratoplasty, a 90-degree crescentic triangular wedge of tissue centered on the axis of the flattest meridian is excised from the recipient cornea at the margin of the graft. The amount of tissue removed is approximately 0.1 mm per diopter of astigmatism [17]. Corneoscopy, which shows the topography of the peripheral cornea by the use of photography of reflected concentric circles, is helpful in deciding which of the two crescents of material in the flat meridian should be removed. Whichever appears flatter should be the section of the cornea chosen for the surgery.

The wedge of tissue is removed almost to Des-

cemet's membrane. Then 9-0 nylon sutures are placed, starting at the extremes of the surgical wound, with the central sutures placed last. Overcorrection of approximately 2 diopters is desired since this amount will be lost over the subsequent 3 to 6 months. Troutman (personal communication, September, 1981) has proposed the placement of two 10-0 nylon sutures in the previous graft wound on either side of the wedge excision, perpendicular to it. These sutures are tied using a slip knot under keratometric control to leave the cornea in a spherical state so that the effects of the desired postoperative overcorrection are not bothersome to the patient.

CORNEAL RELAXING INCISIONS
Another technique for altering postkeratoplasty astigmatism is a relaxing incision [24]. These incisions cause the cornea to gape and produce a resulting flattening of the steeper meridian and subsequent steepening of the opposite meridian.

After identifying the steepest meridian with a keratometer, corneoscope, or surgical keratometer, one or two deep vertical, linear 60- to 90-degree incisions centered along the steepest meridian are made. If the incision is made in the operative wound, care must be taken to be sure there is no posterior wound gape in this region. The surgery is most easily performed using a diamond knife. To exaggerate the slight gape of the incisions, two 10-0 monofilament nylon sutures are placed at 90 degrees to the axis of the relaxing incisions and tied tightly. This maintains the gaping of the wound until healing occurs. A soft contact lens can be fitted for the patient's comfort. Sutures are removed 4 to 6 weeks later.

Relaxing incisions can induce 5 to 10 diopters of change, are more easily performed than wedge resection, and result in earlier patient rehabilitation than wedge resection. In high postkeratoplasty astigmatism, many corneal surgeons feel that this is the procedure of choice unless the astigmatism is in excess of 15 diopters.

RADIAL KERATOTOMY
CLINICAL DEVELOPMENT AND APPLICATION
As first described by Sato and associates in 1953 [19], the radial keratotomy procedure called for radial partial-thickness incisions from both the endothelial and epithelial surfaces of the cornea. Any manipulation that causes damage to the corneal endothelium, such as incising the cornea from the anterior chamber, is not attractive because it can produce pronounced corneal decompensation. In fact, Kanai and colleagues [12] reported that of 80 of

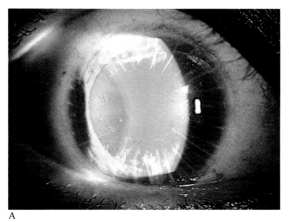

A

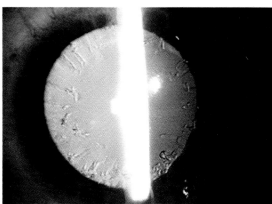

B

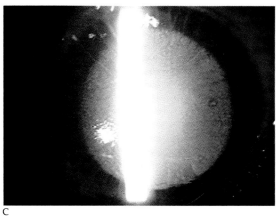

C

FIGURE 15-19. *Sato radial keratotomy procedure. A. Note multiple peripheral short cuts in the cornea. Scar associated with the incision does not extend into the visual axis. This patient underwent Sato procedure done 25 years earlier. B. Retroillumination shows the number of peripheral cuts. The endothelial incisions cannot be separated from those in the epithelium. The visual axis is relatively clear. C. Massive stromal and epithelial edema in the fellow eye. Vision was reduced to counting fingers.*

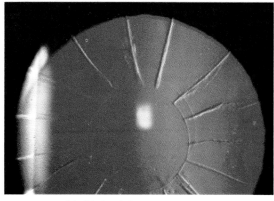

FIGURE 15-20. *Modified radial keratotomy procedure. Sixteen incisions are made from the limbus to the edge of the pupillary zone, from the epithelial side only. Cornea is edema-free 2 days after the procedure.*

Sato's original 281 cases, 60 (75 percent) needed penetrating keratoplasty by the age of 40 because of endothelial decompensation—an unusual finding since Fuchs' dystrophy is extremely rare in Japan (Fig. 15-19).

More recently, radial keratotomy has been limited to incision into the anterior stroma, avoiding the endothelial surface. Such incisions have been purported to be a safe and effective means of correcting mild to moderate degrees of myopia [3]. Investigators including Belyaev and Ilyina [2], Kio Tin [14], and, in particular, Fyodorov and Durnev [5, 6] have reported extensive experience with partial-thickness radial incisions of the cornea and limbal area for varying degrees of myopia. In early investigations, Fyodorov and Durnev [5, 6] employed keratometry to determine that considerable myopia may be reduced by making 16 partial-thickness incisions to approximately 80 percent of corneal depth (Fig. 15-20).

Fyodorov and Durnev believe that the change in corneal curvature and refractive power results from dissection of the circular ligament of the cornea. Originally described by Kokott [17], this structure's existence remains to be proved. As described by Fyodorov and Durnev, the dissection of these circular collagen fibers weakens the periphery of the cornea, which results in a slight bulging of the mid-periphery of the cornea and flattening of the central optical zone. This changes the overall profile of the cornea.

Knauss and coworkers [16] have suggested that the existence of the circular ligament of the cornea is not necessary to explain the results of radial keratotomy. Radial incisions are, in fact, capable of weakening the structure of the cornea itself, causing the periphery to bulge as a result of intraocular pressure. This peripheral bulge causes a secondary central flattening and myopia is decreased.

ANIMAL STUDIES

It is unfortunate that there are so few animal studies of radial keratotomy, because laboratory work is an important first step in the development of most surgical techniques. The safety and efficacy of new procedures, as well as their complications, variations, techniques, and the histopathologic alterations in affected tissues, may be determined in animals before human trials.

Radial keratotomy by Jester and colleagues [11] in monkeys showed that the corneal curvature tends to return to the preoperative readings by 6 months after surgery. Eight incisions produced 90 percent of the corneal flattening produced by 16 incisions. In addition, a 10 to 20 percent decrease in the central endothelial cell densities at 6 months after surgery was demonstrated.

In these animal procedures, 20 percent had clinically evident perforations at the time of surgery. Various degrees of corneal vascularization have been noted, particularly in those cases in which peripheral perforations occurred. In 2 cases that did not have any clinical signs of perforation, there was 360-degree neovascularization extending two-thirds of the way to the 3-mm central optical zone.

Another histopathologic finding was the inability to predict the exact depth of the incisions, even when a constant blade setting was used. Using a blade setting of 80 percent of the central corneal thickness, incision depth varied from 30 to 100 percent of the corneal thickness. This variability probably accounts for the unpredictability of this procedure that has been noted in both primates and humans. Probably, this particular factor can be minimized with future advances in microsurgery in instrumentation.

INDICATIONS

The indications for radial keratotomy are changing as the technique changes and evolves. The operation appears to be most beneficial to patients who have a refractive error of between −2 and −5 diopters. Most patients who have between −4 and −7 diopters of myopia, using current radial keratotomy techniques, appear to obtain between 2 and 4 diopters of correction, leaving them with some residual myopia. The procedure does not appear to be indi-

cated for patients who have refractive errors greater than 7 diopters because of the inherent limitations of the correction.

TECHNIQUE

The procedure is performed under local or topical anesthesia. Initially, 16 equally spaced radial incisions were made into the cornea, with the blade set at 80 percent of the central corneal thickness. A central optical zone varying in size from 3 to 5 mm was preserved, and the incisions were carried past the limbus in earlier methods.

Because a number of studies have shown that the major effects of radial keratotomy are achieved with only 8 incisions, 8-incision radial keratotomy is now the currently practiced procedure [11, 22]. The incisions are placed equally and radially, extending from the central clear zone to the corneal limbus. A variety of studies have shown that it is not necessary to carry the incisions past the limbus as originally described by Fyodorov and Durnev [5, 6].

Since it has been suggested that the smaller the diameter of the central clear zone, the greater the effect of the surgery, many surgeons alter the area of the central clear zone depending on the refractive error. For refractive errors between −2 and −3 diopters, a 4-mm central zone is used; for errors of −3.25 to −4 diopters, a 3.5-mm zone; and for errors greater than 4 diopters, a 3.0-mm zone.

The central clear zone is marked with a special dull trephine with central cross hairs. At this point in the procedure, if an ultrasonic pachometer is available, the central corneal thickness is measured. If no ultrasonic pachometer is available, the preoperative pachometry readings of the central cornea are used. The surgical blade is set at the desired depth of incision. Postoperative care need include only the use of topical antibiotics.

RESULTS

Recently, Fyodorov and Durnev [6] reported on 60 radial keratotomy patients with 6 months' to 3 years' follow-up. In this series, 4 patients had accidental perforation of the anterior chamber, but none had other complications. Fyodorov and Durnev stated that there were no visual acuity losses in any of the patients. In all cases, the keratometry measurements showed flattening of the corneal curvature in the optical zone, although this area was not involved in the incisions. Fyodorov and Durnev [6] also discussed 676 additional cases with a follow-up period of greater than 1 year. In patients with refractive errors between 0.75 and 3 diopters (130 patients), 70 percent obtained emmetropia, 13 percent had mild hyperopia, and 16 percent had mild myopia of between 0.25 and 0.75 diopters. Unaided visual acuity of 20/50 or better was claimed for all of these patients.

These results have generated a great deal of interest and controversy about radial keratotomy in the United States. Unfortunately, few objective, well-controlled studies of the clinical results of this surgery in this country have been reported [9]. Clearly, there are enormous gaps in our knowledge about the procedure, its mechanism, and its ultimate efficacy and safety.

COMPLICATIONS

The first and most serious complication of radial keratotomy is corneal perforation, which may occur during the surgery. Dangers of perforation include intraocular infection, endothelial damage, knife blade damage to the iris or lens, decreased intraocular pressure (making subsequent incisions more difficult), and the induction of astigmatism. Small perforations in which aqueous leak is confined to a drop or two may allow the surgeon to complete the operation. If aqueous leaks are larger, however, the eye becomes so soft that subsequent incisions cannot be carried out safely, and the operation must be canceled. If the perforation is extensive and involves a large tear in Descemet's membrane, it must be closed with interrupted 10-0 nylon sutures. One case of *Staphylococcus epidermidis* ophthalmitis has occurred after radial keratotomy in which no perforation had occurred (Culbertson, personal communication, November 1981).

Other possible complications of radial keratotomy include material such as blood, epithelium, lipid, or debris left in the wound, which causes scarring and influences wound healing; epithelial abrasion or recurrent erosion syndrome; eccentric position and irregularity of the incisions; vascularization of the incisions; ocular pain; flare; fluctuating vision; diminished quality of vision; regression of the initial postoperative effects; undercorrection; induction of astigmatism; poor centering of the optical zone; overcorrection, which produces hyperopia; precipitation of presbyopic symptoms; inability to wear spectacles; inability to wear standard contact lenses; and potential for damage to the corneal endothelium, which may result in decreased endothelial cell counts and possibly even endothelial cell dysfunction. As with the procedure of Sato and colleagues [19], the subclinical complications may not be observable acutely and may affect the cornea and other intraocular structures after many years [12].

Because of the many possible complications of this experimental procedure, radial keratotomy should be performed only under the aegis of an experimental protocol. The protocol should include a complete corneal evaluation, including preoperative specular microscopy and a postoperative repetition of these tests, to provide adequate information to document the safety and efficacy of the procedure.

REFERENCES

1. Barraquer, J. I. Keratomileusis for myopia and aphakia. *Ophthalmology* (Rochester) 88:701, 1981.
2. Belyaev, V. S., and Ilyina, T. S. Late results of scleroplasty in surgical treatment of progressive myopia. *Eye Ear Nose Throat Mon.* 54:109, 1975.
3. Bores, L. D., Myers, W., and Cowden, J. Radial keratotomy: An analysis of the American experience. *Ann. Ophthalmol.* 13:941, 1981.
4. Friedlander, M. H., et al. Clinical results of keratophakia and keratomileusis. *Ophthalmology* (Rochester) 88:716, 1981.
5. Fyodorov, S. N., and Durnev, V. V. The use of anterior keratotomy method with the purpose of surgical correction of myopia. In *Pressing Problems of Modern Ophthalmology.* Moscow, 1977. P. 47.
6. Fyodorov, S. N., and Durnev, V. V. Operation of dosaged dissection of cornea circular ligament in cases of myopia of mild degree. *Ann. Ophthalmol.* 11:1885, 1979.
7. Gasset, A. R., and Kaufman, H. Thermokeratoplasty in the treatment of keratoconus. *Am. J. Ophthalmol.* 79:226, 1975.
8. Gasset, A. R., et al. Thermokeratoplasty (TKP). *Trans. Am. Acad. Ophthalmol. Otolaryngol.* 77:441, 1973.
9. Hoffer, K., et al. UCLA clinical trial of radial keratotomy: Preliminary results. *Ophthalmology* (Rochester) 88:729, 1981.
10. Itoi, M. Computer Photokeratometry Changes Following Thermokeratoplasty in Refractive Modulation of the Cornea. In R. S. Schachar, N. S. Levy, and L. Schachar (Eds.), *Keratorefraction.* Denison, Tex.: L. A. L., 1981. Pp. 61–70.
11. Jester, J. V., et al. Radial keratotomy in nonhuman primate eyes. *Am. J. Ophthalmol.* 92:153, 1981.
12. Kanai, A., et al. The fine structure of bullous keratopathy after anteroposterior incision of the cornea for myopia. *Folia Ophthalmol. Jpn.* 30:841, 1979.
13. Kaufman, H. The correction of aphakia (36th Edward Jackson Memorial Lecture). *Am. J. Ophthalmol.* 89:1, 1980.
14. Kio Tin, M. Sclerokeratoplasty in treatment of progressive myopia. *Vestn. Oftalmol.* 3:24, 1976.
15. Knapp, A. Keratoconus: Etiology and treatment. *Arch. Ophthalmol.* 2:658, 1929.
16. Knauss, W. G., et al. Curvature changes in-

duced by radial keratotomy in solithane model of eye (abstract). *Invest. Ophthalmol. Vis. Sci.* 20(ARVO Suppl.):69, 1981.

17. Kokott, W. Über Mechanisch—Funktionelle Strukturen des Auges. *Arch. Ophthalmol.* 138: 424, 1938.

18. Rowsey, J. J., and Doss, J. D. Preliminary results of Los Alamos keratoplasty techniques. *Ophthalmology* (Rochester) 88:755, 1981.

19. Sato, T., Akiyama, K., and Shibata, H. A new surgical approach to myopia. *Am. J. Ophthalmol.* 36:823, 1953.

20. Schachar, R. A., Black, T. D., and Huang, T. A physicist's view of radial keratotomy with practical surgical implications. In R. A. Schachar, N. S. Levy, and L. Schachar (Eds.), *Keratorefraction.* Denison, Tex.: L. A. L., 1981. Pp. 195–220.

21. Stark, W. J. Audiodigest Ophthalmology, Vol. 13, August 1975.

22. Swinger, C. A., and Barraquer, J. I. Keratophakia and keratomileusis—clinical results. *Ophthalmology* (Rochester) 88:709, 1981.

23. Terrien, F. Dystrophie marginale symétrique des deux cornées avec astigmatism regular consécutif et guérison par la cautérisation ignée. *Arch. Ophtalmol.* (Paris) 20:12, 1900.

24. Troutman, B., Gaster, R., and Swinger, C. Refractive Keratoplasty. In *Symposium on Medical and Surgical Diseases of the Cornea* (Transactions of the American Academy of Ophthalmology). St. Louis: Mosby, 1980. Pp. 428–449.

25. Troutman, B., Swinger, C., and Kelly, R. J. Keratophakia: A preliminary evaluation. *Ophthalmology* (Rochester) 86:523, 1979.

26. Werblin, T., Kaufman, H. E., Friedlander, H. H., and Granet, H. Epikeratophakia: The surgical correction of aphakia. III. Preliminary results of a prospective clinical trial. *Arch. Ophthalmol.* 99:1957, 1981.

27. Werblin, T., et al. Epikeratophakia: The surgical correction of aphakia. *Ophthalmology* (Rochester) 89:916, 1982.

16. CONJUNCTIVAL SURGERY FOR CORNEAL DISEASE

Richard A. Thoft

CONJUNCTIVAL-CORNEAL RELATIONSHIPS

Although the conjunctiva surrounds the cornea and in many respects appears to be very different from it, there are a number of characteristics that the two epithelial layers have in common. For example, they are both highly innervated with sensory nerves, providing a very prompt and efficient sensory alert to trauma. Both epithelia also serve as efficient barriers to infection, aided in this role by being covered with a tear film that undergoes constant turnover, flushing the surface of bacteria and other noxious agents.

The differences in the conjunctival and corneal epithelial functions are appreciated easily also. The transparent and highly uniform refracting surface of the cornea contrasts with the vascular and mobile but relatively opaque conjunctival surface. In addition, the histologic and biochemical features of these two areas are distinct (c.f. Physiology of the Cornea: Metabolism and Biochemistry in Chapter 1, and Chapter 2, Morphology and Pathologic Responses of the Cornea to Disease). For example, the conjunctiva acts as an important source of tear mucins, with goblet cells making up 5 to 10 percent of the total number of its cells [31]. The corneal epithelial surface is, of course, devoid of such apparent mucin-producing cells but has mucin adsorbed to its plicate surface [15]. The corneal epithelium is 5 to 6 cell layers thick and has well-defined basal columnar cells, wing cells, and superficial squamous cells. Conjunctival epithelium, on the other hand, varies in thickness from 3 to 15 cell layers and lacks the orderly progression from basal columnar epithelium to superficial wing cells. Most important, the conjunctiva is characterized by a potentially voluminous subepithelial vascular network, with numerous inflammatory and immunologic cells present as permanent residents. In contrast, the corneal

Supported in part by research grants R01-EY01830 and R01-EY03061 from the National Institutes of Health.

epithelium rests upon the relatively uniform, avascular collagenous structure of the corneal stroma.

Biochemically, there are important differences related not only to the mucin production of the conjunctiva, but to the very different sources of epithelial nutrition. The conjunctival epithelium is at no time remote from blood vessels, so that carbohydrates, amino acids, and other nutrients readily diffuse from these vessels to the epithelium. The corneal epithelium receives most of its nutrition from the anterior chamber, and molecules must therefore diffuse across a relatively large distance. The corneal epithelium has a rich store of metabolic energy in the form of glycogen, which has been shown to be immediately available to respond to the needs imposed by trauma or anoxia (see Physiology of the Cornea: Metabolism and Biochemistry in Chapter 1). The conjunctival epithelium has only small amounts of glycogen [30] and depends less on that storehouse for metabolic needs. Other differences may exist in the basic metabolism. For example, histochemical data [4] and measurements of enzymes [30] in conjunctival biopsy specimens indicate that the conjunctiva is less dependent than the cornea on oxidative pathways, even though such pathways are more efficient in the production of high-energy molecules.

These kinds of histologic and biochemical differences become of greater interest when one considers circumstances under which conjunctival epithelium must cover the corneal stroma. Under conditions of extensive chemical or thermal trauma to the eye, all of the corneal epithelium is lost. Re-epithelialization of the corneal surface must then proceed from surrounding epithelium. There is considerable evidence that undamaged conjunctiva, given enough time, can transform into corneal epithelium when it (conjunctival epithelium) is forced to grow over a denuded corneal stroma [12, 21].

Corneal re-epithelialization from conjunctiva has been examined in detail in experimental animals [12, 21, 26, 30]. Resurfacing the cornea from conjunctiva proceeds at approximately 1 mm^2 per hour [13], so that epithelial closure of total cornea wounds would take 5 to 7 days. This re-epithelialization of the cornea from conjunctiva has been studied histologically to determine when the conjunctival attributes are lost [26]. One to 2 days after healing, the epithelium has one to two cell layers but is totally lacking in the goblet cells that are normally found in conjunctiva. The epithelium then thins down to one cell layer and assumes a more conjunctival appearance with many goblet cells 10 to 14 days after healing. The goblet cells then disappear, the epithelium thickens, and by 4 to 5 weeks after healing a characteristic corneal appearance is seen.

Biochemical and functional transformation lags considerably behind the morphologic transformation. Metabolite levels, enzyme activities, and protein profiles do not match those of corneal epithelium for several weeks. Even 2 to 3 months after conjunctival epithelium has healed over the cornea, the transformation seems incomplete, since vascularization (induced by wounding) results in reversion of some features of that epithelium to conjunctival (e.g., secretory IgA and goblet cells reappear). Also characteristic of re-epithelialization from conjunctiva are such problems as development of secondary defects and vascularization, especially in response to trauma. Thus, although it seems probable that complete transformation does occur eventually, it is important to realize that before transformation, the epithelium is not entirely equivalent to corneal epithelium [12, 20, 21, 26, 30, 32].

In addition, it seems likely that the peripheral ocular surface cells including conjunctival and limbal epithelium play an important role in the integrity of the corneal surface, even apart from the extreme case of total corneal epithelial loss. Several reports suggest that there is a constant movement of epithelial cells from the periphery toward the center of the cornea [1, 9, 16, 18, 26]. It has been demonstrated in animals that donor corneal epithelium is replaced after 6 to 12 months, leaving transplanted stroma of the donor covered by host epithelium [18]. In humans, it has been noted that there is centripetal movement of epithelium after keratoplasty [16] and that epithelial graft reactions do not occur after one year [1], presumably because all of the donor epithelium has been replaced by that time. These observations strengthen the thesis that central corneal epithelium is replenished in part from peripheral corneal cells, and these in turn may be derived from more peripheral limbal or conjunctival epithelium.

The concept that there may be a separate limbal epithelium that is not only anatomically different, but also biochemically and physiologically different from both corneal and conjunctival epithelium increases the complexity of our understanding of corneal resurfacing. The limbal epithelium, defined as a ½-mm zone just peripheral to the corneal epithelium and within the goblet cell–bearing conjunctival epithelium, may play a key role in re-epithelialization of the cornea in many total corneal epithelial defects [19].

THEORETICAL CONSIDERATIONS

Although the mechanisms involved in corneal re-epithelization from conjunctiva are occasionally called into play in the healing of corneal disease, by far the greatest utility served by the conjunctiva has been its use as a therapeutic apron for treating corneal lesions. This has been accomplished by surgically freeing the conjunctiva from its usual locus and positioning the resultant flap over the area of involved cornea. The healing in this case takes place not by proliferation and transformation of epithelial cells but by the application of the undersurface of the conjunctiva to the corneal lesion. There are different surgical procedures for elevating, moving, and securing conjunctival flaps, but all the methods have as their fundamental therapeutic goal the application of a raw vascularized surface of conjunctiva to an area of stromal melting or potential viral or fungal infection.

Other conjunctival surgery is done to resect a portion of conjunctiva thought to be responsible for the corneal disease. An example of such treatment is the excision of carcinomas, which show extensive involvement of the cornea occasionally. In a less obvious application, excision of conjunctiva has been done when it has been thought that conjunctiva was in part responsible for corneal ulceration, as in peripheral ulceration. This treatment has been employed in a variety of ways for a number of years but has never been thought uniformly successful [6, 10]. The theory was that the products of inflammation that build up in adjacent conjunctiva may be in part responsible for the ulceration and stromal loss seen in cornea. In fact, some evidence has been accumulated recently that implicates imflammatory and immune products (derived from conjunctival vessels) in the corneal ulcerative process [5, 6, 25]. It may therefore be useful to reduce the nidus of inflammatory products in peripheral corneal disease associated with stromal melting.

A related procedure is that of heparinization of areas of conjunctiva associated with corneal ulcerative lesions [2]. In these cases, the theory was that such ulceration is in part due to inadequate nutrition of peripheral cornea. The increased volume of blood presented to the limbus was thought to eliminate the ischemic area.

Resection has also been attempted in the treatment of inflammatory conditions that manifest themselves not only in the cornea but also in the conjunctiva. The most common example is superior limbic keratoconjunctivitis, in which excision of the superior conjunctiva has been associated with improvement [10]. The basis for conjunctival participation in corneal disease is not clear in this process either but may be related to the ongoing centripetal migration of epithelial cells onto the cornea from an area of abnormal conjunctiva.

Conjunctival transplantation is a procedure that relies on the transformation of conjunctival epithelium into corneal epithelium [27–29]. In this case, conjunctiva serves as a healthy source of ocular surface epithelial cells. The success of the procedure rests entirely on the complete transformation of conjunctival epithelium into corneal epithelium. It therefore does not act to heal by application of a rich vascular supply to the corneal lesion but by creating a new epithelial layer that tolerates an avascular environment. This procedure is not meant to be an alternative to a conjunctival flap, since the outcome of conjunctival transplantation is the restoration of a healthy, avascular surface. The indications for conjunctival transplantation are therefore quite different from those for conjunctival flap [29].

CONJUNCTIVAL FLAPS

INDICATIONS

Conjunctival flaps have been used as an effective treatment for recalcitrant corneal ulceration for many years. The procedure was first described in 1877 in the German literature [14, 24]. It was popularized in the early 1900s when conjunctiva was used primarily to reinforce cataract resections. The most widely quoted authority with regard to conjunctival flaps is Gundersen [14], who described a new technique of application in 1958. At that time, he described not only a new method for doing flaps but also a number of indications for their use. Prominent among the lesions described were herpetic ulcers of several types. Herpetic ulceration, with or without active viral proliferation, remains a serious complication of herpes infection. Stromal melting in herpes is usually halted with the use of a conjunctival flap, and a herpetic stromal ulcer rarely progresses to ulceration after such a flap has been applied.

Another important indication for conjunctival flapping is neuroparalytic keratitis, characterized by loss of sensation and epithelial integrity, with subsequent stromal ulceration. This condition frequently follows operations on the fifth nerve ganglion for trigeminal neuralgia and is seen occasionally after trauma or surgery for acoustic neuroma.

Keratitis sicca from a variety of causes can occasionally lead to desiccation and irritation so severe that even a tarsorrhaphy does not provide adequate comfort. When artificial tear solutions, punctal occlusion, tarsorrhaphy, and soft contact lenses are no longer effective in preventing drying, with subsequent epithelial loss and stromal ulceration, a conjunctival flap may be the only useful alternative.

Another use for conjunctival flaps is in severe peripheral marginal ulcerations. Since these can progress relentlessly toward the center of the cornea and can be associated with perforation, the application of a conjunctival flap may offer the only prospect for healing of the globe and resolution of the inflammation. Although recent evidence suggests that immunosuppression may be of value in some of these patients [11, 22], the course of the disease in others is still often relentless. Conjunctival flaps

may promote healing and improve comfort in such cases.

Another ocular condition that may be treated successfully with conjunctival flaps is ulceration associated with collagen vascular disease. In rheumatoid arthritis, the flap not only keeps the surface from drying but halts the progression of ulceration when other measures fail.

In general, conjunctival flaps are not used for unresponsive bacterial or fungal ulcers. Rarely, however, relentless progression may force one to consider a flap when all else fails.

PROCEDURE
Although each individual case will dictate the best method for applying a conjunctival flap, most methods rely upon the undermining of a large area of conjunctiva. This conjunctiva is subsequently mobilized, brought down over the denuded cornea, and sutured to paralimbal conjunctiva. The Gundersen flap [14], for example, is done as follows:

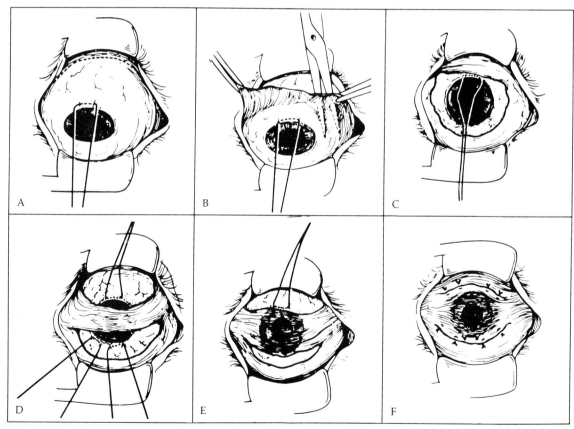

FIGURE 16-1. *Gundersen conjunctival flap—operative procedure. A. Exposure of bulbar conjunctiva by means of a traction suture placed through the upper limbus. B. Incision through the conjunctiva. C. Completion of peritomy. D. Bridge of conjunctiva lying over the cornea. E. Flap spread over cornea and sewn in position. F. Tenon's capsule sewn to the upper border of the conjunctival bridge. (From T. Gundersen, Conjunctival flaps in the treatment of corneal disease with reference to a new technique of application.* Arch. Ophthalmol. 60:880, 1958. Copyright 1958, American Medical Association.)

After general or local anesthesia, a silk traction suture is placed through the corneal limbus from 11:30 to 12:30 o'clock to control the globe and draw it strongly downward (Fig. 16-1A). This exposes the entire upper area of bulbar conjunctiva, a distance between the upper limbus and the upper fornix of 16 to 18 mm. Since the cornea is 12 mm in diameter, a bridge of at least this width must be available for adequate coverage. A subconjunctival injection elevates the conjunctiva from the globe. Great care must be taken not to perforate the portion of the conjunctiva that will eventually cover the cornea. With the conjunctiva ballooned up, a horizontal incision is made through it (Fig. 16-1B) following the reflection of the bulbar conjunctiva on the retrotarsal fold. The incision should be at least 3 mm long and should avoid the underlying Tenon's capsule. The dissection of the conjunctival bridge is begun from the fornix and carried down toward the upper limbus. The virtue of this dissection is that a thin flap is made, without incorporating a large amount of Tenon's capsule beneath it. The resultant flap is freed at the limbus superiorly, and is then ready to be applied to the cornea (Fig. 16-1C–F).

There are a number of opinions regarding the necessity for removing all of the corneal epithelium before the flap is brought down. All epithelium is absent in the area of the ulcerating lesion or infection, but the epithelium should be removed for a short distance peripheral to the lesion. Although it is not necessary to remove all of the corneal epithelium, total removal ensures a bond between the flap and the underlying cornea, and this will help prevent retraction. It is probably not desirable to remove the epithelium with chemical agents, since a mild chemical burn results in some cases, with destruction of the corneal epithelial basement membrane.

Once the flap is pulled down, it is sutured in place with 7-0 silk suture or other nonabsorbable suture. It is frequently useful to perform at least a small peritomy below, so that the raw edge of the flap can be apposed directly to the freshly cut edge of the inferior conjunctiva. Incorporating sclera at the limbus with the suture will ensure that the suture line does not migrate onto the cornea, producing potential gaps in the flap. The superior conjunctival area is left bare, since any attempt to cover it by mobilizing conjunctiva high in the fornix may lead to ptosis. The epithelium grows over the raw area with remarkable speed, rapidly reestablishing comfort.

The postoperative care need be nothing more than routine antibiotic ointment, although continued dilation of the pupil is desirable in most cases to prevent pain. There is no value in continuing the

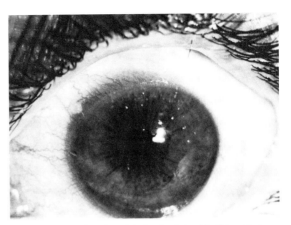

FIGURE 16-2. *Extirpation of the lacrimal gland in this patient was followed by recurrent epithelial breakdowns and filamentary keratitis. Chronic pain was alleviated only after a conjunctival flap was done.*

topical therapy for the underlying corneal disease since the flap is essentially impermeable to medication.

RESULTS

Conjunctival flaps have been used less and less frequently in recent years, in part because of better antibiotic, antiviral, and antifungal therapy. In addition, the use of corneal gluing and contact lenses has stopped the relentless progression of much stromal ulceration. Nevertheless, there are occasional conditions in which none of these measures seems to be effective. In Figure 16-2, for example, a case of severe keratoconjunctivitis sicca with filamentary keratitis as a result of extirpation of the lacrimal gland is shown. The patient was plagued by recurrent epithelial breakdown, with subsequent ulceration and chronic pain. Despite the frequent use of artificial tears, various kinds of soft contact lenses, and partial tarsorrhaphy, the desiccation, ulceration, and pain were controlled finally only with a conjunctival flap. As highly undesirable as the visual result was, the patient is now comfortable and able to work.

An example of the use of flaps in drying seen in Sjögren's syndrome is shown in Figure 16-3. In this patient, a partial bridge flap was done for chronic ulceration. Although originally applied as a total flap, it retracted over several weeks to cover just the area of ulceration. This has, however, been effective in maintaining corneal integrity, and the patient remains comfortable, although requiring frequent artificial tears.

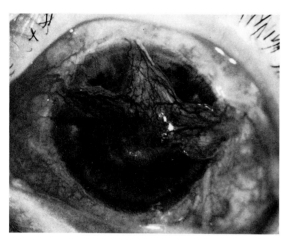

FIGURE 16-3. *Conjunctival flap in Sjögren's syndrome. A partial flap has been effective in maintaining corneal integrity in this patient who suffered from chronic ulceration.*

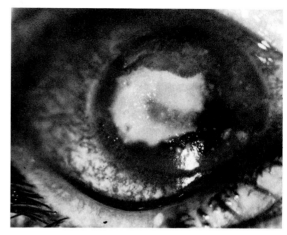

FIGURE 16-4. *Fungal ulceration following trauma was subsequently treated with a conjunctival flap, which promoted healing.*

The unusual case of a flap used for fungal ulcer is shown in Figure 16-4. This patient lost an eye some years earlier to a dynamite cap explosion. The remaining eye had many particles of debris remaining in the cornea and developed a progressive fungal infection by an organism characterized only as a dermatophyte. The topical therapy available was insufficient, and a conjunctival flap was done to promote healing. Figure 16-5 shows the results of the subsequent keratoplasty, done 9 months after the flap, which has remained clear for the last 10 years.

These results indicate that conjunctival flaps are useful for control of pain, infection, and stromal ulceration. After the corneal process appears to be arrested, flaps can be removed, frequently with vision restored by subsequent keratoplasty.

COMPLICATIONS

Few complications are associated with conjunctival flaps. Ptosis is a frequent occurrence but is usually slight. It results from too vigorous dissection high in the fornix in some cases. In cases in which the conjunctival fornix has been shortened, as in ocular surface diseases such as cicatricial pemphigoid or Stevens-Johnson syndrome, even the freeing up of 12 mm of conjunctiva may involve pronounced tension on the lid itself. Although ptosis is not a desirable feature, it is frequently a necessary trade-off for the benefits of a flap.

A second complication can be conjunctival cyst formation, which occasionally is severe enough to require marginal excision or unroofing of the cysts.

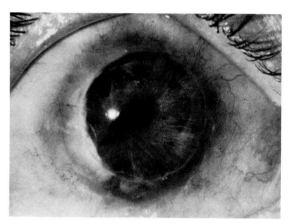

FIGURE 16-5. *Keratoplasty after conjunctival flap. Nine months after conjunctival flapping had promoted healing in the eye shown in Figure 16-4, a keratoplasty was done, which has remained clear for 10 years.*

These are the result of infolding of conjunctival edges during the procedure, with growth of the epithelium on the undersurface of the flap. Remnants of corneal epithelium may also proliferate to the back of the flap, which results in cysts lined with corneal epithelium. Cyst formation may require attention, but it is not a serious complication.

Although not a complication of flapping, perforation under conjunctival flaps can occur, but it is an unusual event. Even gross attempts to assess the pressure will usually indicate if this has occurred. Regardless of the underlying disease, persistent corneal perforation will lead to loss of the anterior chamber and severe secondary glaucoma. Even without perforation, it is not possible to follow with any degree of certainty the progress of any underlying inflammatory process. Complications of synechia formation and iritis cannot be readily observed.

CONJUNCTIVAL RESECTION

INDICATIONS

Conjunctival resection has been used most frequently in superior limbic keratoconjunctivitis [10]. This procedure has been proposed as a method of eliminating not only conjunctival reaction but also the inevitable superficial punctate keratitis seen as a component of the disease. The mechanism that makes such resections helpful is not clear but may be related to the drift of conjunctival cells across the limbus to the cornea in the normal centripetal motion. If such cells are abnormal, removing them may allow healthier conjunctiva to replenish the peripheral cornea, without subsequent epithelial abnormalities. Another explanation (c.f. Suspected Infectious Etiology in Chapter 5) suggests that excess movement of the superior bulbar conjunctiva may cause chronic irritation on a mechanical basis.

The method suggested is excision of a crescent of conjunctiva superiorly from approximately 10 to 2 o'clock, extending approximately 5 mm into the conjunctiva at its farthest point. The resection can be taken down to bare sclera, and the wound need not be closed. To some extent, the degree of resection depends upon the size of involved area and can be as broad as necessary to allow adjacent uninflamed conjunctiva to fill the gap. Topical antibiotics can be used until the area is re-epithelialized.

A second indication for conjunctival resection is that of peripheral marginal ulceration. Conjunctival resection may be tried as a desperate maneuver to halt the progression of Mooren's ulcer. In some cases, resection has produced at least transient epithelial healing and relief of pain [7].

Another use for conjunctival resection was suggested some decades ago, when it was thought that excision of acutely traumatized tissue after chemical or thermal injury would reduce subsequent inflammation and corneal ulceration [3]. Although the excision of conjunctiva during the acute phase of injury has been abandoned, it has been suggested that excision of conjunctiva may be important in the success of keratoplasty in healed chemical and thermal injury [8]. The basis for success in these cases is not clear but may rest in reducing inflammatory material in the limbal area as well as reducing the production of substances such as collagenase that have adverse effects on the cornea.

CONJUNCTIVAL TRANSPLANTATION

Conjunctival transplantation [27–29] was devised to permit the resurfacing of corneas damaged because

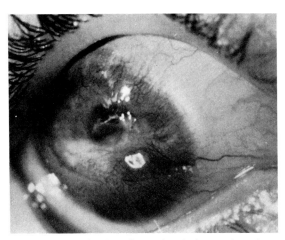

FIGURE 16-6. *Indications for conjunctival transplantation—chemical and thermal injury. In favorable cases, there is a dense layer of superficial scarring and vascularization, as in this cornea; the total thickness of the cornea is not involved.*

of chemical and thermal injury by epithelial cells drawn from healthy conjunctiva. As initially conceived, the procedure depended upon the transformation of conjunctival epithelium into corneal epithelium, as outlined above. The initial indications were limited to unilateral, relatively superficial chemical or thermal injury to the cornea. Recently, the indications have been extended to include recalcitrant epithelial defects associated with penetrating keratoplasty and herpes simplex.

There are two primary goals to be achieved by conjunctival transplantation. The first is stabilization of the ocular surface, with the elimination of repeated epithelial breakdowns. The second is clearing of the optical axis to permit better vision. Depending on which of these goals seems paramount, the procedure itself, particularly the depth of the initial keratectomy, must be modified to some degree.

INDICATIONS

Unilateral chemical and thermal injury is the most common indication for conjunctival transplantation. The most favorable cases are those in which there is a dense layer of superficial scarring and vascularization, without involvement of the total thickness of the cornea (Fig. 16-6). Although the procedure can be done on corneas that are scarred all the way through, the visual result is disappointing. Another potential problem is encountered in corneas with previous perforation or thinning. In these cases, the

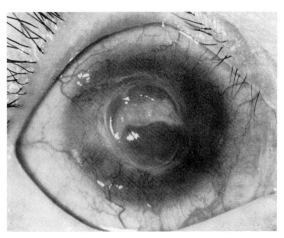

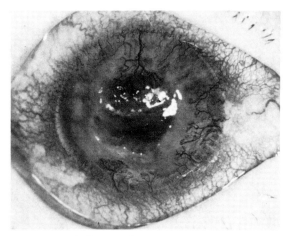

FIGURE 16-8. *Indications for conjunctival transplantation—chronic epithelial defect in herpes simplex. For approximately 18 months, this patient with herpes simplex had an epithelial defect that was unresponsive to contact lens or occlusive therapy.*

FIGURE 16-7. *Indications for conjunctival transplantation—ocular surface scarring after antiviral therapy. This patient had a persistent epithelial defect, surrounding conjunctival hyperemia, and superficial vascularization and scarring after prolonged antiviral treatment for an unconfirmed herpes infection.*

superficial keratectomy may be associated with surgical perforation.

A second indication for conjunctival transplantation is chronic, persistent, recurrent epithelial defects such as may occur for many years after chemical injury. In these cases, vision is frequently the least important goal. Rather, stabilization of the ocular surface, freeing the patient from repeated office visits and the use of contact lenses and antibiotic drops, is desirable. These cases may not have great visual potential but are a source of chronic discomfort for the patient and require constant care.

The third indication for conjunctival transplantation is persistent epithelial defect after penetrating keratoplasty. In many cases, these keratoplasties have been performed because of chemical trauma or herpes simplex. Such surface graft failures are frequently refractory to the use of soft contact lenses, and the inevitable scarring and vascularization of the surface ultimately destroys vision.

Another indication for conjunctival transplantation is the pseudopemphigoid seen after prolonged antiviral therapy (Fig. 16-7). The persistent epithelial defect, surrounding conjunctival hyperemia, and superficial vascularization and scarring seen in such cases are totally unresponsive to soft contact lens therapy and the use of topical steroids.

Even without antiviral toxicity, chronic epithelial defects may be seen in herpes simplex (Fig. 16-8). Conjunctival transplantation can be effective in stabilizing the corneal surface in such cases, and a

healthy fellow eye may be available for donation of conjunctiva. If endothelial damage from concurrent keratouveitis has occurred during the herpetic infection, restoration of surface integrity may lead to the formation of epithelial bullae. In such cases, one type of epithelial abnormality may be found after another (the defect) is treated. Therapy may then be directed to the less serious epithelial edema.

Other conditions in which conjunctival transplantation is still considered experimental are bilateral ocular disease such as cicatricial pemphigoid, Stevens-Johnson syndrome, or acne rosacea keratitis. In these cases, there is no certainty that healthy conjunctiva can be obtained from the patient, and donation must be from either heterologous cadaver tissue or from a family member who may or may not share HLA identity. Such cases require intensive immunosuppression for a short time and subject the patient to serious risk.

METHOD

Although modifications of the procedure for conjunctival transplantation have been suggested, my experience has been limited to a method that has changed very little over a 7-year period [27–29]. The procedure combines a number of different surgical procedures that are familiar to corneal surgeons. General anesthesia permits operation on both eyes and prevents the return of sensation prematurely during the operation. The first step (Fig. 16-9A) is resection of conjunctiva approximately 5 mm posterior to the limbus for 360 degrees, combined with a total superficial keratectomy that extends over the limbus, up over the convexity of the cornea, and across the opposite limbus (Fig. 16-9B). The purpose of this portion of the procedure is to resect whatever abnormal conjunctiva surrounds the limbus and to eliminate the superficial corneal scarring and vascularization that is responsible for poor vision. The depth of the keratectomy depends upon one's eventual goal for the patient. If stabilization of the ocular surface is the primary goal, the keratectomy need not be particularly deep. It is imperative, however, that all the subepithelial basement membrane be removed. Despite considerable evidence to the contrary in animals [17, 23], human corneal epithelium grows well over keratectomy sites. If a good visual result seems possible without a subsequent keratoplasty, a relatively deep keratectomy may be desirable. Such a keratectomy makes a subsequent keratoplasty more difficult because of the difficulty in apposing the thicker corneal graft onto the thinner peripheral corneal edge. The depth of the keratectomy depends in part on the variation and thickness of the cornea, and one must recognize the potential for perforation in thin areas.

The second step in the procedure is obtaining healthy conjunctiva from the fellow eye (Fig. 16-

9C). Because general anesthesia is used, subconjunctival anesthesia in the donor eye can be avoided. This prevents Tenon's capsule from being elevated and excised along with the more superficial layers. The best method for excising the conjunctiva employs smooth forceps to tent the conjunctiva, with amputation of the tissue with scissors (Fig. 16-10). Pieces no larger than 3 mm in diameter are large enough to provide adequate coverage of the host cornea. The excision sites are closed with nonabsorbable sutures to prevent granuloma formation.

The next step is to arrange the conjunctival grafts around the periphery of the keratectomized cornea (Fig. 16-9D). It is important to remember that the intent of the procedure is to provide epithelial cells for corneal re-epithelialization and not to provide total coverage of the raw stroma. Keeping the grafts peripheral prevents their extending so far toward the visual axis that they begin to cover the optical zone. It does not appear necessary to have the bases of the grafts meet at the limbus. The initial resection

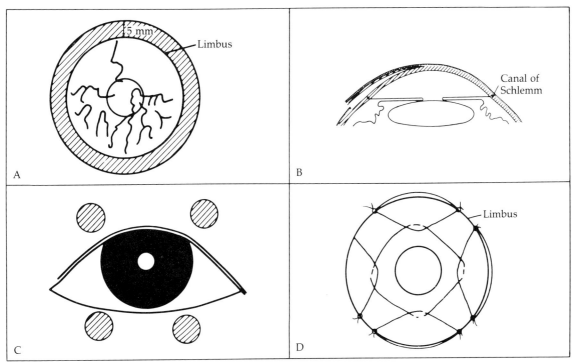

FIGURE 16-9. *Operative procedure for conjunctival transplantation. A. Conjunctival resection to bare sclera 5 mm outside the limbus. B. Lamellar keratectomy removing epithelial layer and superficial vessels and scarring. C. Source of conjunctival grafts. Grafts are taken from the uninjured fellow eye in four quadrants, from areas normally covered by the lids. D. Placement of conjunctival grafts. Monofilament nylon sutures anchor the grafts at the limbus. Continuous suture through the apices, but not into the corneal stroma, ensures apposition of the grafts to bare stroma. (From R. A. Thoft, Conjunctival transplantation. Arch. Ophthalmol. 95:1425, 1977. Copyright 1977, American Medical Association.)*

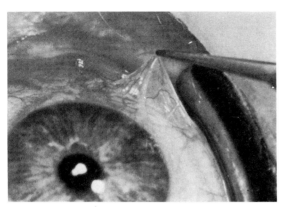

FIGURE 16-10. *Excision of conjunctival grafts. Conjunctiva of uninjured fellow eye is tented with smooth forceps and cut cleanly with scissors. Pieces approximately 3 mm in diameter are adequate to cover cornea.*

of conjunctiva gives the epithelium from the grafts an opportunity to meet peripherally before host epithelium can grow in. Care must be taken to see that the grafts are the right side up. The epithelial surface is shinier than the undersurface, and adherent Tenon's capsule usually appears white with irrigation.

The next step is anchoring the conjunctival grafts to the underlying sclera at the limbus, using 10-0 nylon suture (Fig. 16-9D). Sharp needles are ideal, so that the conjunctival pieces are not disturbed by the passage of the sutures. Since there is little tendency for the grafts to move, the bites can be small. Finally, a 10-0 nylon suture is passed through the apices of the conjunctival grafts to appose them to the raw stromal surface. Note that the suture does not go into the stroma itself but merely acts as a purse-string suture that keeps the tips from moving. A reasonably thick and stable soft contact lens is put over the cornea at the conclusion of the procedure to minimize disturbance of the grafts.

Postoperative care is limited to application of anti-

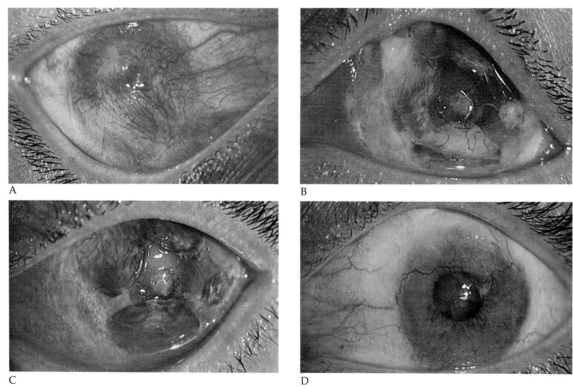

A

B

C

D

FIGURE 16-11. *Conjunctival transplantation. A. Preoperative alkali burn from hot radiator fluid 8 months after injury. Note the avascular island corresponding to the area of earlier persistent epithelial defect. The cornea has not perforated, although thin areas are present. B. Immediate postoperative appearance, showing pallor of the conjunctival grafts, whose apices are pulled toward, but not over, the visual axis. The encircling suture apposes the grafts to the stromal bed and a soft contact lens covers them. C. Vascularization of the grafts occurred on sixth day, with thickening and elevation. The epithelium is intact. D. After 25 months, atrophy of the surface vessels has occurred, the epithelial surface is smooth, and the visual axis is clear. (From R. A. Thoft, Conjunctival transplantation. Arch. Ophthalmol. 95:1425, 1977. Copyright 1977. American Medical Association.)*

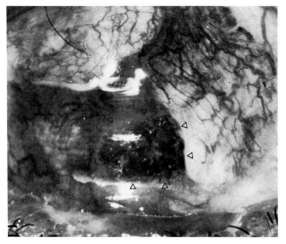

FIGURE 16-12. *Complications of conjunctival transplantation. Central corneal perforation, which occurred when the keratectomy was carried over an area of thin cornea, has been sealed with cyanoacrylate tissue glue, which is visible between the conjunctival grafts* (arrows).

biotics and mydriatics. Steroids are neither necessary nor desirable. After 2 days, the soft contact lens can be removed, although epithelialization is facilitated if the lens remains in place for as long as 3 weeks. The course of the re-epithelialization, which can be followed with a slit lamp, is generally concurrent with, although unrelated to, recanalization of the vessels in the conjunctival grafts. This recanalization makes the grafts somewhat edematous 1 week after the procedure, but this response regresses over the next several weeks.

RESULTS

The results of conjunctival transplantation are shown for 1 case (Fig. 16-11).

The average outcome of conjunctival transplantation is vision from 20/80 to 20/200. Poor in comparison to the normal vision in the opposite eye, it is usually sufficient to attain bilateral fixation and a satisfactory cosmetic result, even without the use of a contact lens. An occasional patient is motivated to wear a contact lens and can achieve vision in the 20/40 to 20/50 range. Such visual results are gratifying, and the results in such cases in general are far superior to those reported (after long-term follow-up) for penetrating keratoplasty in chemical and thermal injury.

Another important benefit is stabilization of the ocular surface after persistent defect. In these cases, conjunctival transplantation may be undertaken to relieve epithelial defects after keratoplasty. Although the visual results in such cases may not be particularly good, the healing of the surface and elimination of the need for frequent follow-up,

medication, and use of occlusion or contact lenses come as a welcome relief to both the patient and the physician.

COMPLICATIONS

The most serious complication of conjunctival transplantation is perforation of the cornea at the time of keratectomy (Fig. 16-12). The defect can be closed with glue; however, the glue acts as an inflammatory stimulus that has very adverse effects on subsequent epithelialization. Since perforation is so highly undesirable, the corneal thickness must be very carefully mapped, and particular care must be taken throughout the keratectomy.

Another serious complication is that of infection, which is not encountered except in cases in which the surface is particularly compromised, as in cicatricial pemphigoid or Stevens-Johnson syndrome. In 1 case of heterologous conjunctival transplantation to an eye with cicatricial pemphigoid, a severe corneal ulceration occurred 1 month after transplantation, despite apparent initial healing and establishment of epithelial integrity. This infection leads to loss of the eye and indicates that conjunctival transplantation further jeopardizes already compromised eyes. To date, no complications have been reported in donor eyes.

REFERENCES
1. Alldredge, O. C., and Krachmer, J. H. Clinical types of corneal transplant rejection. *Arch. Ophthalmol.* 99:599, 1981.
2. Aronson, S. B., et al. Pathogenic approach to therapy of peripheral corneal inflammatory disease. *Am. J. Ophthalmol.* 70:65, 1970.
3. Ballen, P. Mucous membrane grafts in chemical (lye) burns. *Am. J. Ophthalmol.* 55:302, 1963.
4. Baum, J. A histochemical study of corneal respiratory enzymes. *Arch. Ophthalmol.* 70:59, 1963.
5. Berman, M. B. Collagenase and Corneal Ulceration. In D. E. Wooley and J. M. Evanson (Eds.), *Collagenase in Normal and Pathological Connective Tissue.* New York: Wiley, 1980. P. 141.
6. Bloomfield, S. E., and Brown, S. I. Conjunctival collagenase: Partial purification. *Invest. Ophthalmol.* 13:546, 1974.
7. Brown, S. I., Mondino, B. J., and Rabin, B. S. Autoimmune phenomenon in Mooren's ulcer. *Am. J. Ophthalmol.* 82:835, 1976.
8. Brown, S. I., Tragakis, M. P., and Pearce, D. B. Corneal transplantation for severe alkali burns. *Trans. Am. Acad. Ophthalmol. Otolaryngol.* 76:1266, 1972.

9. Buck, R. C.   Cell migration in repair of mouse corneal epithelium. *Invest. Ophthalmol. Vis. Sci.* 18:767, 1979.

10. Donshik, P. C., et al.   Conjunctival resection treatment and ultrastructural histopathology of superior limbic keratoconjunctivitis. *Am. J. Ophthalmol.* 85:101, 1978.

11. Foster, C. S.   Immunosuppressive therapy for external ocular inflammatory disease. *Ophthalmology* (Rochester) 87:140, 1980.

12. Friedenwald, J. S.   Growth pressure and metaplasia of conjunctival and corneal epithelium. *Doc. Ophthalmol.* 5–6:184, 1951.

13. Friend, J., Kiorpes, T. C., and Thoft, R. A.   Diabetes mellitus and the rabbit corneal epithelium. *Invest. Ophthalmol. Vis. Sci.* 21:317, 1981.

14. Gundersen, T.   Conjunctival flaps in the treatment of corneal disease with reference to a new technique of application. *Arch. Ophthalmol.* 60:880, 1958.

15. Holly, F. J.   Tear film physiology and contact lens wear: I. Pertinent aspects of tear film physiology. *Am. J. Optom. Physiol. Opt.* 58:324, 1981.

16. Kaye, D. B.   Epithelial response in penetrating keratoplasty. *Am. J. Ophthalmol.* 89:381, 1980.

17. Khodadoust, A. A., et al.   Adhesion of regenerating corneal epithelium: The role of basement membrane. *Am. J. Ophthalmol.* 65:339, 1968.

18. Kinoshita, S., Friend, J., and Thoft, R. A.   Sex chromatin of the donor corneal epithelium in rabbits. *Invest. Ophthalmol. Vis. Sci.* 21:434, 1981.

19. Kinoshita, S., et al.   Limbal epithelium in ocular surface wound healing. *Invest. Ophthal. Vis. Sci.* 23:73, 1982.

20. Liu, S. H., et al.   Secretory component of IgA: A marker for differentiation of ocular epithelium. *Invest. Ophthalmol. Vis. Sci.* 20:100, 1981.

21. Maumanee, A. E.   Repair in the Cornea. In W. Montagne and R. E. Billingham (Eds.), *Advances in Biology of Skin.* New York: Pergamon, 1964. Vol. 5, *Wound Healing,* p. 268.

22. Mondino, B., Brown, S. I., and Rabin, B.   Cellular immunity in Mooren's ulcer. *Am. J. Ophthalmol.* 85:788, 1978.

23. Pfister, R. R., and Burstein, N.   The alkali burned cornea: I. Epithelial and stromal repair. *Exp. Eye Res.* 23:519, 1976.

24. Schöler, K. W.   *Jahresberichte über die Wirksamkeit der Augen-Klinik, in den Jahren 1874–1880.* Berlin: H. Peters, 1875–1881.

25. Seng, W. L., et al.   The effect of thermal burns on the release of collagenase from corneas of vitamin A–deficient and control rats. *Invest. Ophthalmol. Vis. Sci.* 19:1461, 1980.

26. Shapiro, M. S., Friend, J., and Thoft, R. A.   Corneal re-epithelialization from the conjunctiva. *Invest. Ophthalmol. Vis. Sci.* 21:135, 1981.

27. Thoft, R. A.   Conjunctival transplantation. *Arch. Ophthalmol.* 95:1425, 1977.

28. Thoft, R. A.   Conjunctival transplantation as an alternative to keratoplasty. *Ophthalmology* (Rochester) 86:1084, 1979.

29. Thoft, R. A.   Indications for conjunctival transplantation. *Ophthalmology* (Rochester) 89:335, 1982.

30. Thoft, R. A., and Friend, J.   Biochemical transformation of regenerating ocular surface epithelium. *Invest. Ophthalmol. Vis. Sci.* 16:14, 1977.

31. Thoft, R. A., and Friend, J.   Ocular Surface Evaluation. In J. Francois, S. I. Brown, and M. Itoi (Eds.), *Proceedings of the Symposium of the International Society for Corneal Research (Doc. Ophthalmol.* Proc. Series 20). The Hague: *Junk,* 1980. P. 201.

32. Thoft, R. A., Friend, J., and Murphy, H. S.   Ocular surface epithelium and corneal vascularization: I. The role of wounding. *Invest. Ophthalmol. Vis. Sci.* 18:85, 1979.

17. THERAPEUTIC SOFT CONTACT LENSES

Richard A. Thoft

The last decade has seen the use of soft contact lenses for therapeutic purposes emerge as one of the most important recent advances in the treatment of corneal disease. During this time, the goals to be achieved by lens wear, the characteristics of available lenses, the indications for their use, and the complications that may occur have been examined and defined, permitting increasingly successful use of therapeutic soft contact lenses.

GOALS OF THERAPEUTIC SOFT CONTACT LENS WEAR

Several specific goals may be achieved in the treatment of ocular surface abnormalities with soft contact lenses. The first of these is the reduction of pain. Patients with epithelial defects frequently have severe pain that is alleviated by soft lens wear. The mechanism for this relief may involve reduced cornea–palpebral conjunctiva apposition or, in edema patients, the physical limitation of epithelial swelling and bullae formation and rupture.

Second, lenses may provide mechanical protection for the surface. For example, aberrant lash or lid contact with the cornea is avoided when lenses are in place. Such protection is of value after chemical injury in which lid scarring is prominent or in cicatrizing ocular surface disease.

Third, lenses facilitate epithelial healing, thus contributing to stabilization of the surface. At least part of the improved healing is probably due to protection from the lids. Such protection prevents the dislodging of migrating epithelial cells that may have a very tenuous hold on the basement membrane.

Fourth, lenses may help maintain proper surface hydration, both by preventing evaporation of water from the surface and, in the case of high-water-content lenses, by providing a water reservoir for the surface.

In contrast to the cosmetic use of lenses, visual improvement is not a major therapeutic goal. Vision may be improved in some cases, however, as a result of smoothing of the refractive surface, since even a soft lens reduces small degrees of irregular astigmatism.

As is discussed in some detail below, the choice of lens is frequently determined by the goal to be reached. Thus, a lens with a high water content may be useful for a patient with dry eyes, whereas a thinner, less fragile lens with less water may be more desirable if mechanical protection is the major goal.

CHARACTERISTICS OF SOFT CONTACT LENSES

WATER CONTENT AND OXYGEN PERMEABILITY

The characteristics of the various soft contact lenses commonly used for therapeutic purposes are summarized in Table 17-1. The main characteristics to be considered are the nature of the polymer, the water content, and the thickness. These physical features define the gas permeability of the lenses. As shown by Refojo [13], oxygen transmission through lenses is directly related to the hydration and thickness of the lenses. In a closed eye, a lens that is 40 percent water can be only 0.05 mm thick for sufficient oxygen to reach the corneal surface (assuming all the oxygen reaches the surface through the lens). However, a lens that is 85 percent water, which presents a decreased barrier to diffusion, could be as thick as 0.23 mm. Thus, contact lens manufacturers, attempting to maximize the amount of oxygen available to the cornea, have made lenses that are very

thin (e.g., CSI, Hydrocurve II, and Ultrathin) or have a very high water content (e.g., Permalens, Sauflon, Softcon). Problems of fragility and spoilage have been associated with both types of lenses.

From the standpoint of corneal respiration, silicone is an attractive material for lenses because it is highly permeable to oxygen [14]. A silicone lens as thick as 0.4 mm still permits adequate oxygenation of the cornea. Unfortunately, silicone is strongly hydrophobic, which, because of breakup of tears on its surface, makes it a poor optical material and very uncomfortable to wear. In addition, silicone absorbs lipophilic substances such as cholesterol and cholesterol esters, which may alter the physical properties of the lens. Attempts by manufacturers to render the surface of silicone lenses less hydrophobic have resulted in the production of modified silicone lenses. Such lenses are currently undergoing clinical testing, and there is some evidence of progress in improving the wettability and patient tolerance of these lenses.

SIZE, BASE CURVE

The size and base curve are important in the actual fitting of a therapeutic lens. It is beyond the scope of this chapter to address fitting problems, except to note that some forms of corneal disease require special consideration. Larger lenses tend to be more stable on the eye and may be useful in cases of surface irregularity, e.g., recurrent stromal loss and subsequent healing in which the central cornea may not provide uniform support to the lens. A large lens increases the area of tissue that is depen-

TABLE 17-1. *Characteristics of Extended-Wear Soft Contact Lenses*

Lens	Water Content (%)	Polymer	Thickness (mm)	Base Curve (mm)	Diameter (mm)
High-water-content lenses					
Permalens (Cooper)	71	Poly(HEMA/vinyl pyrrolidone)	0.36–0.43	6.5–8.3	7.5–14.0
Sauflon (Sauflon International)	79	Poly(methyl methacrylate/ vinyl pyrrolidone)	0.22–0.45	7.5–9.6	13.0–15.5
Softcon (American Optical)	58	Poly(HEMA/vinyl pyrrolidone)	0.35–0.43	8.1, 8.4	14.5
Thin lenses					
CSI (Syntex)	39	Poly(glyceryl methacrylate/ methyl methacrylate)	0.05–0.20	9.0–9.7	13.6, 14.7, 15.1
Hydrocurve II (Soft Lenses)	55	HEMA/diacetone acrylamide	0.06–0.70	9.1–10.1	14.0–16.0
Ultrathin (Bausch & Lomb)	38	HEMA	0.05–0.07	8.6, 8.8	12.5
Intermediate lens					
Plano T (Bausch & Lomb)	39.6	HEMA	0.17	8.1	14.7
Silicone lens					
Silicon (Dow Corning)	0	Silicone rubber	0.10–1.50	7.4–8.2	11.3, 12.5

HEMA = 2-hydroxyethylmethacrylate

dent on translenticular exchange of nutrients, however, and may exaggerate relative anoxia, e.g., as in anterior segment necrosis.

The base curve variation can be used to modulate the amount of lens motion and, to a certain extent, the degree of tear exchange beneath the lens. For the most part, the bulk of oxygen and water exchange is across the lens and not beneath its edges [11], so that the size of the tear lake between the lens and the cornea is usually not directly related to the "tightness" of the lens. Ideally, the lens should not move against the epithelial surface unless it is cushioned by a layer of tears. Apposition of the lens at the limbus and on the conjunctiva creates metabolic demands that are easily met by the subjacent blood supply.

CHOICE OF LENS

Although all of the commonly used lenses will help in the treatment of surface disease, success is more likely if the choice of lens is related to the desired goal. For example, if the major goal is to prevent desiccation of the corneal surface, a thick lens with a high water content may be desirable. Thus, in the treatment of keratitis sicca or Sjögren's syndrome, lenses with a large water reservoir such as Permalens or Sauflon may be useful. However, these relatively thick, high-water-content lenses are more fragile, are more subject to spoilage, and have more variable optics (because of the variable amount of evaporation from them) than thinner lenses. On the other hand, if protection of the eye from mechanical damage by aberrant lashes is the primary goal, a thinner lens may be indicated. Thinner lenses have a lower water content but are easier to handle, are more rigid on the eye, and have more reliable optics. These lenses, e.g., CSI, Hydrocurve II, and Ultrathin, are also useful in treating persistent defects or recurrent erosion in eyes in which the tear film is normal. A third kind of lens in therapeutic use is the thick lens that does not have a high water content, e.g., Plano T. These lenses are considerably less flexible than either the very thin lenses or the high-water-content lenses and are useful in conditions in which there is a need to provide mechanical strength to alter changes in the ocular surface. For example, they may be used to ameliorate symblepharon formation after conjunctival trauma.

INDICATIONS

The wide variety of conditions for which soft lenses are used can be classified into a few major categories: primary corneal epithelial diseases, such as dystrophies; epithelial diseases secondary to trauma; viral disease; ocular surface disorders of presumed immunologic origin; keratitis sicca; and

epithelial disease secondary to endothelial failure. Each of these categories is discussed below, with illustrations of some of the more common disorders.

PRIMARY EPITHELIAL DISEASE

The dystrophies, or "anterior membrane" epithelial diseases (see Chapter 9, Dystrophies and Degenerations) can frequently produce intermittent epithelial breakdown severe enough to bring the patient to the ophthalmologist's attention. The most common of these in clinical practice is map-dot-fingerprint dystrophy (Cogan's syndrome). Occasionally, patients are seen with what appears to be a first attack of erosion, but the presence of multiple subepithelial changes indicates that the process has been going on for some time. It is useful to include patients with anterior membrane dystrophy in the larger group of patients who have recurrent erosion syndrome secondary to trauma, since the clinical management for both disorders is the same.

The decision regarding the application of a soft lens in recurrent erosion depends upon the severity, frequency, and duration of each attack. When the episodes of ocular irritation are limited to only a few minutes in the morning, a soft lens is probably not necessary. If, however, the symptoms last for several hours and are accompanied by pronounced tearing, pain, and photophobia that require cycloplegia and occlusion for relief, a soft lens may be useful. Although each practitioner will have his own rule of thumb regarding erosion frequency, most patients are troubled if a major attack occurs more often than once a month for 2 or 3 months. If there has been an antecedent injury, as is frequently the case in recurrent erosion, the longer the interval between the initial trauma and the subsequent breakdown, the less likely that a soft lens is necessary.

Usually, thin lenses of medium water content are used for erosive disorders. A lens without power is applied to permit customary vision. The duration of soft lens wear for these conditions is variable, but should be at least 3 or 4 months. This gives adequate time for the elaboration of hemidesmosomal attachments between basal cells and the underlying basement membrane. After the lens is discontinued, lubricating ointment is used at night for several more months.

Other specific epithelial dystrophic conditions may present with recurrent epithelial erosion. Prominent among these are Reis-Büchlers dystrophy and lattice dystrophy. These are rare conditions, but the patient is occasionally troubled by the erosive nature of the epithelial changes long before the dystrophies impinge seriously on vision. Chronic soft lens wear in such cases may be required, and success with lenses may have an important bearing on whether surgery is ever necessary.

Another erosive disorder is the epithelial abnormality in diabetes mellitus. Although decreased sensation has been recognized for some time [16], the particular vulnerability of the corneal epithelium after vitrectomy has been noted more recently [5, 10]. At the time of surgery, it is noted that the epithelium tends to come off the underlying stroma in sheets. Electron micrographs show that the basement membrane is frequently thickened and that the plane of disruption is between basement membrane and underlying stroma, rather than between basement membrane and basal cells [6, 18]. The resultant epithelial defects are recurrent. A soft contact lens in these cases stabilizes the epithelium and permits prompt healing. Again, the lens must be left in place for some weeks after surgery to assure firm epithelial adhesion.

TRAUMATIC EPITHELIAL ABNORMALITIES
In general, corneal abrasions secondary to trauma do not need soft contact lenses for adequate healing. Customarily, such abrasions are treated with antibiotics and pupillary dilation with a variable period of occlusion. Occasionally, however, the abrasion apparently disturbs the basement membrane to such an extent that epithelial cell adhesion is insufficient to permit healing of the defect. If a traumatic abrasion has not healed within 2 to 3 days, the patient may continue to have sufficient photophobia, tearing, and iritis to warrant a change in therapy. In these cases, a soft contact lens can be very beneficial. Although it may be difficult to fit the lens during the time of acute inflammatory response, once the lens is in place the patient generally reports immediate improvement in comfort and is able to do without occlusive bandaging. In these cases, as in erosive syndromes, the lens must be left in place for some time to assure firm adhesion of the epithelium to the underlying basement membrane and stroma. In most cases, cycloplegia must be continued for a number of days, at least until the epithelium is healed. The chronic use of antibiotic drops is controversial but is clearly indicated during the time of epithelial healing. Relatively few cases of traumatic abrasion require such therapy, but soft contact lenses can restore the patient's comfort and ability to work much sooner in severe cases.

Other forms of trauma include those that occur postoperatively after a cataract operation or a retinal detachment. An occasional occurrence after retinal detachment surgery, particularly when the epithelium has been removed for visualization of the fundus, is the persistence of an epithelial defect for many days. There is always the possibility that the epithelial failure may in part be due to anterior segment necrosis caused by sluggish aqueous humor turnover and reduced anterior segment circulation, particularly if many extraocular muscles have been removed during the procedure or if the ciliary arteries have been compromised. The differential diagnosis of mild anterior segment necrosis and pure traumatic erosion is usually not difficult. In anterior segment necrosis, not only is the epithelium sluggish in re-epithelializing, but there is usually pronounced stromal edema as a result of endothelial cell compromise. In addition, there may be fixation of the pupil, although this is difficult to determine postoperatively when cycloplegics have been instilled. Although not evident early, lenticular changes may occur if the ocular lens is in place. These findings are absent in delayed epithelial healing without anterior segment circulation problems. A soft contact lens may be applied in any case, particularly if the defect persists for more than 6 or 7 days postoperatively. In the case of anterior segment ischemia, application of the soft contact lens may be followed by an increase in the inflammatory response, which may take the form of a hypopyon. The appearance of a hypopyon under such circumstances is adequate reason to remove the lens, but the absence of corneal infiltration usually makes it possible to treat with antiinflammatory agents and to assume that no endophthalmitis or corneal ulcer is present.

Another category of traumatic epithelial defects is chemical and thermal trauma. Such trauma can occur after a variety of agents are accidentally splashed into the eyes (see Chemical Injuries in Chapter 14). Mild chemical injuries are frequently associated with partial corneal epithelial loss. In most cases, such epithelial defects heal as expected, with the conventional treatment of occlusion, antibiotics, and cycloplegics. Occasionally, however, the epithelial defect is quite persistent. Figure 17-1 shows an eye in which a mild chemical injury occurred. This eye did not heal well and had a persistent epithelial defect for some weeks after the injury. Healing was finally accompanied by superficial punctate keratitis and filamentary keratitis, which caused the patient considerable discomfort. A soft contact lens in this case was useful even after the period of epithelial healing and might have been useful during the period of healing. Soft contact lenses are not necessarily required in all

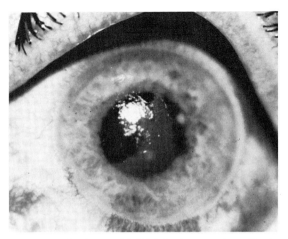

FIGURE 17-1. *Persistent epithelial defect in an eye that suffered a mild chemical injury.*

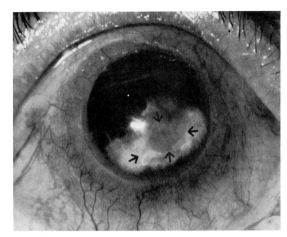

FIGURE 17-2. *Epithelial defect* (arrows) *following chemical injury. For 15 years after chemical injury, this eye had intermittent defects, which continued (as shown here) even after penetrating keratoplasty.*

chemical injuries, and an occasional patient finds the lens more uncomfortable than beneficial. If all of the corneal epithelium has not been lost, the transformation of conjunctiva does not play a role in re-epithelialization, which is usually speedy. Lenses should not be withheld if healing is poor, however, and in particular they may be considered early if the epithelial loss has been total.

Persistent epithelial defects that occur long after chemical injury are another indication for soft contact lens use. In these cases, however, soft contact lenses may not achieve the goal of epithelial healing. In Figure 17-2, a spontaneous epithelial defect that occurred 15 years after the initial chemical injury is shown after an intervening keratoplasty. In this case, the use of the soft contact lens made the patient more comfortable but did not achieve permanent healing of the defect. However, achieving comfort alone is an adequate reason to use contact lenses in persistent epithelial defects.

VIRAL DISEASE

The most common viral disease for which soft contact lenses are used is herpes simplex keratitis. Healing of the acute viral proliferative stage does not require the use of a contact lens because of the rapid clearing of the dendritic figure. However, the recurrence and persistence of an epithelial defect in herpes without apparent viral proliferation is a frequent finding. This stage of recurrent disease has been termed trophic, or "metaherpetic." The mechanism for trophic epithelial loss is not clear but may be related in part to decreased adhesion between the epithelium and the underlying stroma. Whatever the underlying cause, the defects can persist for weeks and months and may lead to stromal ulceration.

A soft contact lens is useful in many of these patients, perhaps by reducing the mechanical wiping off of the poorly adherent epithelium. The defect rarely persists for more than a few weeks after the lens is applied. Antivirals are usually not part of the therapy in persistent trophic defects; their use may in fact contribute to poor epithelial healing. Continued treatment with cycloplegics and prophylactic antibiotics can continue with the lens in place. If the lens has not been successful in closing the defect after several weeks, it probably will not have any further effect and may be removed. There is no particular contraindication to longer-term wear, although the complications of bacterial infection and lens-induced uveitis must be kept in mind.

In general, soft lenses are less effective when stromal ulceration accompanies the trophic defect. The same is true of ulcerative conditions secondary to other causes, in which the hoped-for effect of the soft contact lens is reestablishment of an intact epithelial layer. In the presence of active stromal dissolution, however, the epithelium appears slow to grow over and attach to the melting substrate.

The use of soft contact lenses for chronic defects in herpes zoster is also possible. Herpes zoster keratitis is much less common than herpes simplex keratitis, but the total corneal anesthesia found in herpes zoster makes epithelial breakdown common. Although the patient is not troubled by pain, the increased risk of infection in such devitalized tissue makes it desirable to facilitate epithelial closure.

Most other viral disorders are self-limited and evolve quickly enough so that soft contact lenses are not needed for their therapy. However, a recent study has shown that soft contact lenses produce some relief of symptoms and improved vision in patients with Thygeson's superficial punctate keratitis [17], a disease of possible viral origin.

OCULAR SURFACE DISORDERS OF PRESUMED IMMUNOLOGIC ORIGIN

Included in the category of ocular surface disorders that are presumed to be immunologic in origin are cicatricial pemphigoid, Stevens-Johnson syndrome, and rare syndromes such as Lyell's disease (see Suspected Infectious Etiology in Chapter 5). These conditions are characterized by chronic progressive involvement of the ocular surface. In general, there are accompanying systemic abnormalities, but these may appear considerably later than the ocular disorders. The ocular involvement usually starts with conjunctival hyperemia and may progress to symblepharon formation. Later in the course of the disease, keratitis sicca may be manifest. In many cases, the corneal epithelium shows marked superficial punctate keratitis and may start to show recurrent epithelial defects long before ocular drying or lid abnormalities are present. This is a characteristic feature of ocular surface disease in which both conjunctiva and cornea are involved. The conjunctival inflammation is chronic and, once tear flow has been interrupted, becomes quite severe. At the same time, the surface of the eye may tend to keratinize, producing, as an end-stage result, a leathery eye without useful vision.

The use of soft contact lenses in such patients is more complex than in those with erosive disorders without conjunctival or tear film abnormalities. In particular, the risk of infection is great, since not only is the tissue more vulnerable, but the tear supply and its resurfacing are frequently abnormal. The use of soft lenses in two major categories of patients with presumed autoimmune diseases—those with normal tear function and those with dry eyes—is discussed below.

NORMAL TEAR FUNCTION

When an early diagnosis of presumed immunologic ocular surface disorder has been made, the findings may be limited to mild symblepharon formation, conjunctival injection, and early superficial punctate keratitis. When the tear supply is normal, the patient may achieve increased comfort with contact lens application. In these cases, the potential for infection is no different from that for most patients. The use of prophylactic antibiotics seem reasonable, although no studies have demonstrated their value. Despite the fact that superficial pannus formation may be a complication of soft lens wear, in cicatricial pemphigoid and Stevens-Johnson syndrome pannus formation does not seem to be accelerated by the use of lenses.

DRY EYES

In patients who have a presumed autoimmune disease with ocular surface changes including keratitis sicca, the use of soft contact lenses is difficult. One should be certain that all measures to improve tear flow have been attempted before soft contact lenses are used. Specifically, punctal occlusion and the frequent use of artificial tears should be tried before soft contact lenses are introduced.

As in keratitis sicca patients in general, the success rate with low-water-content lenses is poor. These lenses have a tendency to dry because of their small water reservoir and are therefore uncomfortable and subject to folding and loss. High-water-content lenses, on the other hand, can be quite comfortable but require frequent replenishment of the water reservoir with saline solution. It may be important to use saline with no preservatives, since the required frequent application may lead to epithelial changes if the solution contains preservatives. The use of buffered, nonpreserved sterile saline has been a major advance in the care of high-water-content lenses in patients with keratitis sicca.

Since these eyes frequently have concurrent symblepharon formation, soft contact lenses may not remain in position because of shrinkage of the fornices. Regardless of size or base curve, soft lenses produce disappointing results if they are used in an attempt to maintain the depth of the fornices. Hard contact lenses or larger scleral shells may be more effective in retarding symblepharon formation. However, the metabolic load added because of poor tear exchange may aggravate the underlying epithelial disease, leading to defect formation and additional vascularization.

Silicone lenses have found some usefulness in healing epithelial defects in these ocular surface diseases. Not only are these lenses somewhat more rigid and therefore more useful in preventing symblepharon to the limbus; their high degree of oxygen permeability may reduce the tendency toward pannus formation.

KERATITIS SICCA

Patients with keratitis sicca occasionally benefit from soft contact lenses [9]. These patients are similar to the group of patients with dry eyes discussed above, except that conjunctival changes are absent. Before soft lenses are tried, other therapeutic modalities, including frequent use of artificial tears and ointment, should be attempted. Even with a soft lens, artificial tears (or saline) must be applied frequently to keep the lens from drying. Failure is usually due to lens irritation or loss because of the drying. In addition, patients with a poor tear flow have a somewhat higher incidence of infection [2].

EPITHELIAL DISEASE SECONDARY TO ENDOTHELIAL FAILURE

There are three major conditions in which epithelial changes result from endothelial abnormalities: Fuchs' dystrophy, aphakic or pseudophakic bullous keratopathy, and keratoconus with hydrops. The final result of all three is epithelial edema and bullae formation, the symptoms of which are frequently best relieved by the use of soft lenses.

Fuchs' dystrophy is not associated with enough endothelial failure to produce bullous keratopathy until late in the course of the disease. When bullous keratopathy does occur, the patient may be acutely uncomfortable (as in other forms of bullous keratopathy) and may suffer serious visual decrease because of the epithelial irregularity. The use of a soft lens in Fuchs' dystrophy (as in all sorts of epithelial edema) adds an additional metabolic burden to the epithelium [19], which may in turn increase the degree of stromal edema. For that reason, it is difficult in some mild cases of Fuchs' dystrophy to be certain that the lens is useful. Since no harm is done, however, with its application, a soft contact lens certainly can be tried if the patient is symptomatic. As in most cases of gross epithelial edema, the use of the soft lens does not necessarily greatly improve vision.

The use of soft contact lenses in aphakic bullous keratopathy has been perhaps the most gratifying clinical application. In the past, aphakic bullous keratopathy produced not only poor vision in many postoperative cataract patients, but also a high degree of disability as a result of pain. Before corneal grafting became useful for bullous keratopathy, a number of procedures, including cauterization and conjunctival flaps, were used to treat the epithelial bullae. Even though corneal grafting is now quite successful in aphakic bullous keratopathy, it is frequently difficult to justify the procedure when the patient has one good eye. The ability to use soft lenses to treat the aphakic bullous keratopathy has permitted penetrating keratoplasty to be deferred in many such cases.

For the most part, the choice of soft contact lens is not highly critical in aphakic bullous keratopathy. Since the condition is already characterized by mas-

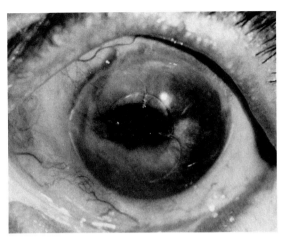

FIGURE 17-3. *Pseudophakic bullous keratopathy as a result of diminished endothelial function coincident with implantation of an intraocular lens. The area of edema is inferior to the visual axis. This patient did not wish to have the intraocular lens removed or to undergo penetrating keratoplasty. A soft contact lens was used to alleviate discomfort.*

sive degrees of stromal and epithelial edema, the additional edema that may be caused by the continuous-wear lens is not important. The patient's increased comfort is the primary goal of the use of the lens and is immediately apparent. Most patients are able to tolerate lenses for prolonged periods and usually do not develop the complications of lens deposits and vascularization that might be expected in view of the complications seen with extended-wear aphakic lenses for visual purposes. The use of prophylactic antibiotics is controversial but is probably indicated in view of the vulnerability of the underlying epithelium.

Patients with pseudophakic bullous keratopathy, in whom endothelial function has diminished coincident with implantation of an intraocular lens, are another group for whom soft contact lenses are useful. These patients may not desire further surgery but may have all of the symptoms of the more usual bullous keratopathy (Fig. 17-3). In such cases, patients may be able to obtain comfort with a soft contact lens.

The use of contact lenses in the hydrops seen in keratoconus is an unusual application. In most cases, the acute edema seen with rupture of Descemet's membrane neither lasts long enough nor is severe enough to require treatment other than occlusion and cycloplegia for 2 or 3 weeks. Occasionally, however, the rent is large enough and the area of edema broad enough to create extensive epithelial edema and disabling photophobia (Fig. 17-4).

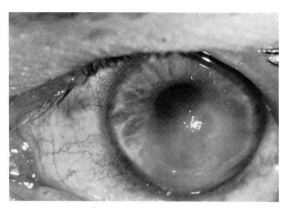

FIGURE 17-4. *Epithelial edema and severe photophobia secondary to hydrops in keratoconus. This 21-year-old patient, who was unable to work because of the hydrops, was restored to full activity by the use of a contact lens. The hydrops healed within 3 months, and the lens was discontinued.*

With the application of a contact lens, the hydrops usually heals within 2 to 3 months. The lens can be discontinued before all of the stromal edema is resolved. Superficial vascularization may occur rarely but does not persist after the lens is removed.

COMPLICATIONS

In general, the underlying disease overshadows the adverse effects of soft lenses, so that subtle complications may well be overlooked. Three such changes are epithelial edema, stromal edema, and vascularization. These, coupled with their attendant redness and irritation, can be categorized as minor complications, as can lens deposits. Major complications that area easily diagnosed regardless of the nature of the underlying disease include sterile infiltrates, sterile hypopyon, and bacterial ulcer.

MINOR COMPLICATIONS

The minor complications of therapeutic contact lenses result in no major long-term adverse effects.

REDNESS AND IRRITATION

When enough time (2–4 hours) is taken for the initial fitting of a soft lens, redness and irritation will usually be observed before the patient leaves the office. The use of lenses of different sizes, base curves, and water content will allow selection of the one type that is most comfortable. Occasionally, however, redness and irritation may become apparent only after a few weeks. In these cases, these findings are frequently associated with early vascularization and a minor anterior chamber reaction.

Photophobia may become marked, and in some cases there can be abrasion of the epithelium. In general, the lens must be removed for a few days. Such a complication does not preclude refitting at a later date with a different lens [2].

EDEMA

Pronounced transient edema is seen in 20 to 30 percent of lenses fitted for extended-wear refractive purposes but is frequently overlooked in therapeutic cases. It is probably not possible, nor necessary, to detect this complication in cases in which stromal and epithelial edema are already prominent features of the disease, e.g., bullous keratopathy, herpetic defects with disciform edema, or anterior segment necrosis.

EPITHELIAL EDEMA

The epithelial edema seen with therapeutic contact lenses is of two types, intercellular and intracellular. Intercellular edema is a result of endothelial failure, which leads to bulk flow across the stroma of extracellular fluid that pushes between the epithelial cells, elevating some of them from the basement membrane to form fluid-filled bullae. Intracellular edema, on the other hand, is the accumulation of fluid within the cells, probably because of alterations in cation and water pumping. This type of edema may be the result of trauma that leads to increased cellular permeability and water influx or of a decrease in the amount of energy available for cation pumping. Both the increased trauma from the soft lens wear and the anoxia produced tend to create intracellular edema. These problems are superimposed on all diseases in which soft lenses are used. Epithelial edema also is associated with decreases in epithelial glycogen levels [19]. Since there is evidence that epithelial glycogen plays a role in epithelial migration [8], the finding of major epithelial edema, in a condition not showing edema before the lens was applied, indicates that the epithelium may not adhere or heal as desired beneath the lens.

STROMAL EDEMA

In humans, nearly all chronic stromal edema develops as the result of inadequate endothelial function. The endothelial function may be inadequate because the endothelium is nutritionally deprived (as in anterior segment necrosis), of insufficient quantity (because of endothelial cell loss after cataract extraction), or overloaded by fluid (because of tears in Descemet's membrane, e.g., in acute hydrops in keratoconus).

Stromal edema and attendant folds in Descemet's membrane have been associated with the use of soft

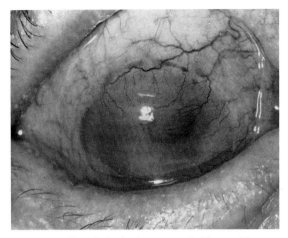

FIGURE 17-5. *Vascularization in a cornea of a 70-year-old woman who wore soft lenses for several years for bullous keratopathy. (From R. A. Thoft and E. F. Mobilia, Complications with therapeutic extended wear soft contact lenses.* Int. Ophthalmol. Clin. *21(2):197, 1981.)*

lenses for several years [12, 15]. Earlier observers postulated that soft lenses produce stromal edema by producing endothelial anoxia and resultant decreased corneal deturgescence, but the fact that the endothelium can derive its total oxygen supply from the aqueous humor [4] cast doubt on that explanation. The production of increased quantities of lactate by an anoxic epithelium, however, does seem to be a likely cause of stromal edema. Increased lactate would cause an increased osmotic pressure in the stroma [7], resulting in stromal edema. As discussed above, such lens-induced edema might not be recognized in the evaluation of a soft lens used for bullous keratopathy or for an epithelial defect in the presence of underlying herpetic disciform edema. However, since stromal edema is frequently reversible and usually not harmful, increased edema is usually not a major complication in the therapeutic use of soft lenses.

VASCULARIZATION

The mechanism responsible for vascularization under soft lenses has not yet been elucidated. Usually, the vessels are quite superficial rather than deep, which suggests a relationship to the epithelium. Although an angiogenic factor has been postulated in both normal and abnormal corneal epithelium [3, 20], the circumstances responsible for production and release of such a factor are not known. Anoxia seems a reasonable stimulus; so, in fact, does trauma.

Figure 17-5 shows the type of vessels associated with contact lens intolerance. The vessels most often originate at the superior limbus, although they also can originate at the limbus closest to areas of stromal pathologic changes. They are superficial and regress when the soft lens is removed, unless they extend to an area of active disease such as a herpetic stromal ulcer. In some cases, vessels are not considered a complication but are desirable for healing the underlying disease. In chemical burns, stromal ulceration, or ocular surface disease such as cicatricial pemphigoid, for example, vascularization appears to be an obligate component of surface healing [1] and may be one of the goals sought by the use of soft lenses.

In the treatment of epithelial defects without stromal involvement, however, such vessels not only are undesirable in themselves, but signal the presence of epithelial distress. A soft lens that is otherwise well tolerated, however, need not be removed if its use is actually associated with epithelial healing, and the vessels do not encroach on the visual axis. Superficial vascularization is slow to develop, and the underlying disease may be healed before the lens has to be removed.

LENS DEPOSITS

Continuous wear of the lenses common in therapeutic use leads to the buildup of white or gray elevated or sheetlike deposits in some patients. Although deposits on soft contact lenses are not harmful, they frequently lead to sufficient irritation to cause the patient considerable discomfort.

Lens changes need not be frequent, but chronic use of therapeutic lenses may be inconvenient and relatively costly in patients with long-term problems such as bullous keratopathy. Lenses used in dry eye patients seem more likely to develop deposits. In any case, once a patient begins to show deposit formation, deposits are likely to occur with each new lens.

MAJOR COMPLICATIONS

Complications such as sterile infiltrates, sterile hypopyons, and bacterial ulcers cause alarm when seen and may cause serious, permanent abnormalities. Although sterile infiltrates and hypopons resolve without sequelae after lens removal, they are not easily distinguished from infectious processes. In all such cases, the lenses must be removed and cultured for bacteria and fungi if at all possible. Microbiologic evaluation of infiltrates and ulcers must be performed immediately, utilizing smears for Gram's and Giemsa stains and cultures inoculated on blood medium, Sabouraud agar, and meat broth. An anaerobic culture should also be

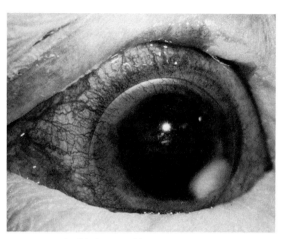

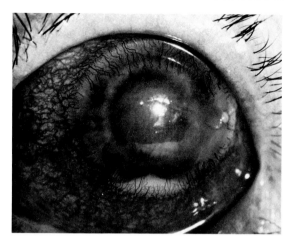

FIGURE 17-7. *This patient with herpes simplex developed a trophic defect. Subsequent treatment with a thin soft lens resulted in the development of the hypopyon seen inferiorly. (From R. A. Thoft and E. F. Mobilia, Complications with extended wear soft contact lenses.* Int. Ophthalmol. Clin. *21(2):197, 1981.)*

FIGURE 17-6. *In this 65-year-old woman with bilateral cicatricial pemphigoid, a silicone lens was placed for an epithelial defect. Recurrent, nonspecific infiltrates were associated with continuous use of the therapeutic lens. (From R. A. Thoft and E. F. Mobilia, Complications with extended wear soft contact lenses.* Int. Ophthalmol. Clin. *21(2):197, 1981.)*

started, if possible. Hypopyon without apparent infiltrate does not warrant anterior chamber tap, since it is nearly always a manifestation of lens intolerance without infection.

Despite the necessity to view every infiltrate and inflammatory reaction as secondary to infection, most of them are not. Specific characteristics of each of these conditions are discussed in more detail below.

STERILE INFILTRATES

Sterile infiltrates follow the application of lenses by days or weeks. Such infiltrates usually occur in relatively asymptomatic eyes. There is little photophobia, injection, or discharge, and the anterior chamber reaction is slight. The infiltrate is likely to be peripheral rather than central. Once the lens is removed, the infiltrate clears within a few days even without intensive antibiotic therapy. The cause may involve localized epithelial necrosis from either trauma or anoxia. Refitting the patient with a flatter lens after the infiltrate clears may prevent the problem in the future.

Sterile infiltrates are not uncommon in cicatricial pemphigoid with or without lenses, and their occurrence with silicone lenses is even more common (Fig. 17-6). Although the initial clinical response to such ulcers is appropriate bacteriologic workup and therapy, repeated occurrences in a patient may be less worrisome. Soft lens therapy may even be con-

tinued in the presence of the infiltrate if epithelialization and surface vascularization seem to be contributing to healing.

STERILE HYPOPYON

The occurrence of uveitis sufficient to cause layering of white cells in the anterior chamber is an unusual complication of therapeutic soft lens use. The hypopyon is not necessarily associated with a corneal infiltrate (Fig. 17-7). When such an infiltrate is present as a result of the underlying disease (e.g., herpes simplex), it is not possible to rule out infection, and the usual diagnostic and therapeutic measures must be taken. When a corneal infiltrate is absent or of long duration, and the hypopyon follows the application of the lens by only 48 to 72 hours, it is safe to assume that the hypopyon is noninfectious. Treatment then consists of removal of the lens and mydriasis. The reaction resolves in a few days.

The pathogenesis of this uveitis is not known. It appears with greater frequency in conditions such as anterior segment necrosis or after extensive retinal detachment procedures, which suggests some relationship to reduced aqueous turnover. Epithelial defects in such cases are often treated with less difficulty by routine patching and antibiotics rather than a soft lens.

BACTERIAL ULCERS

Bacterial ulcers are rare in cosmetic wear of soft lenses but are seen occasionally with therapeutic lenses. As described earlier, the inevitable effects of

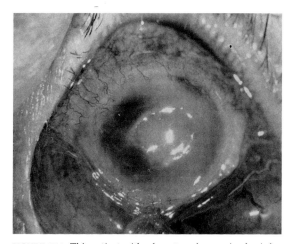

FIGURE 17-8. *This patient with a long-term herpes simplex infection had a corneal graft that performed well for several years until a recent rejection episode. The rejection was treated with high-dose corticosteroids, which cleared the stromal edema but may have led to herpes in the graft. Antivirals were given, and a soft lens was applied to treat the epithelial defect. The* Serratia marcescens *bacterial infection shown here occurred 2 weeks after application of the lens. (From R. A. Thoft and E. F. Mobilia, Complications with extended wear soft contact lenses.* Int. Ophthalmol. Clin. 21(2):197, 1981.)

soft lenses include some degree of epithelial anoxia and trauma. In addition, there is a markedly reduced flow of tears beneath soft lenses, which tends to decrease the cleansing function of the tear film and lids. When these factors are coupled with the increased vulnerability of a cornea involved in a disease and with the use of medication such as corticosteroids that may reduce tissue defenses, it is remarkable that there are not more infections. Such a combination of problems is shown in Figure 17-8.

Such cases serve to emphasize the fact that soft contact lenses further compromise corneal resistance to infection. The possibility of secondary bacterial or fungal infection is greatest when other abnormalities are present. The clinician should be aware that reduced tear flow, stromal ulceration, and local or systemic immunosuppression increase the hazards associated with soft lens therapy. Even the constant use of routine antibiotics may not prevent secondary infection, and frequent patient visits may be necessary to manage not only the primary disease but the useful, but potentially hazardous, use of the soft lens.

REFERENCES

1. Conn, H., et al. Stromal vascularization prevents corneal ulceration. *Invest. Ophthalmol. Vis. Sci.* 19:362, 1980.
2. Dohlman, C. H., Boruchoff, S. A., and Mobilia, E. Complications in use of soft contact lenses in corneal disease. *Arch. Ophthalmol.* 90:367, 1973.
3. Eliason, J. A. Leukocytes and experimental corneal vascularization. *Invest. Ophthalmol. Vis. Sci.* 17:1087, 1978.
4. Fatt, I., Freeman, R. D., and Lin, D. Oxygen tension distributions in the cornea: A re-examination. *Exp. Eye Res.* 18:357, 1974.
5. Foulks, G. N., et al. Factors related to corneal epithelial complications after closed vitrectomy in diabetes. *Arch. Ophthalmol.* 97:1076, 1979.
6. Kenyon, K. R. Recurrent corneal erosion: Pathogenesis and therapy. *Int. Ophthalmol. Clin.* 19(2):169, 1979.
7. Klyce, S. D., and Bernegger, O. Epithelial hypoxia, lactate production and stromal edema. *Invest. Ophthalmol. Vis. Sci.* 17:277, 1978.
8. Kuwabara, T., Perkins, D. G., and Cogan, D. G. Sliding of the epithelium in experimental corneal wounds. *Invest. Ophthalmol.* 15:4, 1976.
9. Mobilia, E., Dohlman, C. H., and Holly, F. A comparison of various soft contact lenses for therapeutic purposes. *Contact Intraocular Lens Med. J.* 3:9, 1977.
10. Perry, H. D., et al. Corneal complications following closed vitrectomy through the pars plana. *Arch. Ophthalmol.* 96:1401, 1978.
11. Polse, K. A. Tear flow under hydrogel contact lenses. *Invest. Ophthalmol. Vis. Sci.* 18:409, 1979.
12. Polse, K. A., and Mandell, R. B. Etiology of corneal striae accompanying hydrogel lens wear. *Invest. Ophthalmol.* 15:553, 1976.
13. Refojo, M. F. Materials in bandage lenses. *Contact Intraocular Lens Med. J.* 5:34, 1979.
14. Refojo, M. F. Contact Lenses. In Kirk and Othmer (Eds.), *Encyclopedia of Chemical Technology* (3rd ed.), Vol. 6. New York: Wiley, 1979. P. 720.
15. Sarver, M. D. Striate corneal lines among patients wearing hydrophilic contact lenses. *Am. J. Optom.* 48:762, 1971.
16. Schwartz, D. E. Corneal sensitivity in diabetes. *Arch. Ophthalmol.* 91:174, 1974.
17. Tabbara, K. F., et al. Thygeson's superficial punctate keratitis. *Ophthalmology* (Rochester) 88:75, 1981.
18. Taylor, H. R., and Kimsey, R. A. Corneal epithelial basement membrane changes in diabetes. *Invest. Ophthalmol. Vis. Sci.* 20:548, 1981.
19. Thoft, R. A., and Friend, J. Biochemical aspects of contact lens wear. *Am. J. Ophthalmol.* 80:139, 1975.
20. Thoft, R. A., Friend, J., and Murphy, H. S. Ocular surface epithelium and corneal vascularization in rabbits: I. The role of wounding. *Invest. Ophthalmol. Vis. Sci.* 18:85, 1979.

INDEX

INDEX

Ablepheron, 356
Abrasion, corneal
  antibiotics in, 415
  soft contact lens in, 480
Acetic acid, 431. *See also* Chemical injuries, acid
Acetylcysteine
  in dry eye syndrome, 305
  in therapy of trophic postherpetic ulcers, 187
  use as collagenase inhibitor, 427
Acid injuries, 430–433. *See also* Chemical injuries, acid
Acremonium, 128–129
Acyclovir
  antiviral action of, 122
  in herpes ocular infection, 184–185
Adenovirus ocular infections, 196–197, 201–204
  epidemic keratoconjunctivitis, 196–197, 201–204
  nonspecific follicular conjunctivitis, 204
  pharyngoconjunctival fever, 203–204
Adenyl cyclase, role in anaphylaxis, 89–90
Adherent cells. *See* Macrophages
Adhesive, surgical
  in corneal trauma, 418–419
  in corneal ulcer, 165–166
  role in stromal ulceration, 61–62
  in trophic postherpetic ulcers, 187, 191
Adjuvant, 77
Adrenergic system, in corneal epithelium, 19
Aflatoxin, 130
Agenesis of the cornea, 355–356
Aging
  corneal degenerations due to, 330, 334–336
  physiologic corneal changes due to, 330
Alcoholism, nutritional disorders in, 408
Alkali injuries, 422–430. *See also* Chemical injuries
Alkaptonuria, 375–376
Allergy. *See also* Atopy; Hypersensitivity
  immunologic mechanisms of, 89–90

Allergy—*Continued*
  ocular, 231–242
    atopic keratoconjunctivitis, 234–236
    definition of atopy, 231
    giant papillary conjunctivitis in contact lens wearers, 239–242
    hay fever reactions, 232–234
    vernal keratoconjunctivitis, 236–239
Alpha-2-macroglobulin, collagenase inhibition by, 27
Amantadine, antiviral action of, 122
Amino acids, metabolism in corneal epithelium, 18
Aminoglycosides, 159, 161
Ammonia, eye toxicity of, 422. *See also* Chemical injuries, alkali
AMP, cyclic. *See* Cyclic AMP
Amphotericin B, 131. *See also* Polyenes
  in fungal keratitis, 173–174
Ampicillin, 161
Amyloid
  in lattice dystrophy, 340–341
  properties of, 376, 377
  protein of, 331–332
Amyloidosis, 376–378
Anaphylaxis, ocular manifestations, 90
Ankyloblepharon, 356
Anomalies. *See* Congenital anomalies, corneal
Anoxia, effect on corneal epithelium, 20
Antagonism, antibiotic, 137
Anterior chamber
  cleavage syndrome, 359–364
  immunologic aspects of, 98
Anterior segment
  herpes zoster ophthalmicus of, 190
  keratoplasty combined with reconstruction of, 445
  soft contact lens in necrosis of, 480
Antibiotics, 134–141
  in alkali injuries, 427
  categories according to mechanism of action, 136
  in corneal trauma, 415, 420
  in corneal ulcer, 157–165
  in inclusion conjunctivitis, 218–219

491

Antibiotics—*Continued*
  mechanism of action, 136–137
  in neonatal inclusion blennorrhea,
    219
  in penetrating keratoplasty, 445
  peptides, 163
  pharmacokinetics of, 137–141
  resistance of bacteria to, 134–136
  topical, subconjunctival administra-
    tion of, 138–141
  in trachoma, 217–218
Antibody. *See also* Immunoglobulins
  antigen combination with, 78
  B-lymphocyte production of, 78–80
  in complement activation, 82–83
  cytotoxic, 91
  in herpesvirus infections, 118–119
  in immune complex disease, 92
  and immunologic enhancement, 86
  production in eye, 98–99
  role in immunity to infection, 94
  in tears, 34
  to tumors, 95
Antifungal agents. *See also* Polyenes
  combined treatment with, 175
  flucytosine, 175
  in fungal keratitis, 173–175
  imidazole compounds, 174–175
  mechanism of action of, 131, 173–
    174
Antigens
  antibody combination with, 78
  classification of, 78
  in cornea, 97
  and corneal graft rejection, 95–97
  in corneal stromal inflammation, 59
  in immune complex disease, 92
  in immune response, 77–78
  tumor-specific transplantation, 94–
    95
Antihistamines, and tear secretion, 36
Antilymphocyte serum (ALS), 87
Antimalarials, ocular side effects of,
    252
Antimetabolites, 136
Antineoplastic agents, effect on im-
    mune response, 87–88
Antiviral chemotherapy, 121–123,
    184–186
  acyclovir, 122
  amantadine, 122
  5-(2-bromovinyl)-2'-deoxyuridine,
    122–123
  cytarabine, 122
  2-deoxy-D-glucose, 123
  in herpes zoster ophthalmicus,
    191–192
  idoxuridine, 122
  mechanisms of action in, 121
  phosphonoacetic acid, 123
  polyanions in, 121–122
  ribavirin, 123
  rifampin, 123
  thiosemicarbazones, 123

Antiviral chemotherapy—*Continued*
  trifluridine, 122
  vidarabine, 122
Aphakia, epikeratophakia in, 458
Aphakic bullous keratopathy, 69, 70,
    72
Appositional suturing, 417–418
Aqueous humor
  in acid burns, 432
  in alkali burns, 423
Ara-A. *See* Vidarabine
Arcus juvenilis, 367
Arcus senilis, 334
Arlt's line, 214
Arthritis
  in lupus erythematosus, 268
  in progressive systemic sclerosis,
    281
  rheumatoid. *See* Rheumatoid ar-
    thritis
Ascher, partial limbal coloboma of,
    360
Ascorbate
  role in collagen synthesis, 423
  use in alkali injuries, 428
Aspergillus, 128–129
Aspirin, in rheumatoid arthritis, 252
Astigmatism
  corneal, 359
  corneal wedge resection for, 460
  after keratoplasty, 460
Atopic dermatitis, ocular manifesta-
    tions, 234–236
Atopy, 231–232. *See also* Allergy
Autoantigen, 77
Autoimmune disease. *See also* Im-
    munologic diseases
  cicatricial pemphigoid, 288
  erythema multiforme, 289–290
  lupus erythematosus, 264
  in Mooren's ulcer, 245
  pemphigus foliaceus, 286–287
  pemphigus vulgaris, 285
  Sjögren's syndrome, 310
  Stevens-Johnson syndrome. *See*
    Erythema multiforme
  viral infections role in, 94
Autoimmunity, 86
Autonomic nervous system
  and corneal wound healing, 49
  innervation of eye, 317
  in tear film formation, 35
Autoplaquing, 109
Axenfeld's anomaly and syndrome,
    363

B cells
  and immunologic tolerance, 85–86
  role in immune response, 78–80
Bacitracin, 163
Bacteria, 105–112
  classification of, 105–106
  cultural characteristics, 108–110
  eye vulnerability to, 93–94
  infections due to
    clinical features in cornea, 150–
      153

Bacteria, infections due to—*Continued*
  histopathology and stages of
    corneal ulcers, 153–156
  organism role in, 148–150
  treatment of corneal ulcers, 156–
    166
  morphology and staining character-
    istics, 106–108
  pathogenicity of, 111–112
  resistance to antibiotics, 134–136
  role in corneal infection, 148–150
  tests for identification, 110–111
Bacterial conjunctivitis, trachoma
    and, 215
Bacterial ulcer, soft contact lens use
    complicated by, 486–487
Bactericidal, 136
Bacteriostatic, 136
Band keratopathy, 259
  calcium deposition in, 330–331,
    383–385
  disorders associated with, 384–385
  in dry eye syndrome, 306–307
Bandage contact lens
  in corneal ulcer, 165
  in dry eye syndrome, 304
Bare sclera technique, 393
Base curve variation, 478–479
Basement membrane. *See also* Des-
    cemet's membrane;
    Epithelium, corneal
  corneal erosion due to disorders of,
    55–57
  dystrophy involving, 337–338
  morphology of, 43–45
Basophils, 80
Battery acid injuries, 430
Bell's palsy, 318. *See also* Facial nerve,
    palsy
Bell's phenomenon, 318–319
Benzalkonium chloride, danger as ir-
    rigating solution, 433
Biber-Haab-Dimmer dystrophy, 340–
    341
Birth trauma, corneal edema due to,
    366
Bitot's spots, 406
Blepharitis, in dry eye syndrome,
    306
Blinking, tear film dynamics during,
    38
Blood agar plates, 108
Bowen's disease, 396
Bowman's layer
  calcification in, 259, 330–331, 384
  collagen in, 25
  dystrophies involving, 336–338
  morphology of, 45
Breakup time, 38–39
Bromhexine hydrochloride, and tear
    secretion, 36
5-(2-bromovinyl)-2'-deoxyuridine
    (BVDU)
  antiviral action of, 122–123
  in herpes simplex ocular infection,
    185
  in herpes zoster ophthalmicus,
    191–192

Bullous diseases, corneal manifestations, 284–291
Bullous keratopathy
  in disciform keratitis, 183–184
  soft contact lens in, 483
Burns. *See also* Chemical injuries
  corneal response to limited surface injury, 49, 51

Calcific band keratopathy, 330–331
Calciphylaxis, 331
Calcium
  deposition in Bowman's layer, 259, 330–331, 384
  deposition in cornea, 383–385
  dietary causes of excess of, 384
  in hyperparathyroidism, 384
Calcium hydroxide, eye toxicity of, 422. *See also* Chemical injuries, alkali
Candida, 127–130
  treatment of keratitis due to, 176
Cap graft, 457–458. *See also* Epikeratophakia
Carbenicillin, 161
Carotene, 403. *See also* Vitamin A
Cataract
  in atopic keratoconjunctivitis, 234
  corneal edema after removal of, 10
  with iridogoniodysgenesis, 363
  keratoplasty combined with extraction of, 445
  management in juvenile rheumatoid arthritis, 260
Cauterization
  in corneal edema, 14
  for refractive error, 453–454
Cazenave's disease, 286–287
Cell transformation, in viral infections, 116–117
Cell wall inhibitors, 136
Cell-mediated immunity, 92–93
  in atopic keratoconjunctivitis, 235
  in contact dermatitis, 97
  in corneal graft rejection, 95–97
  diseases with defect in, 93
  factors required in, 81
  in infection, 94
  in neoplastic disease, 94–95
  role in Mooren's ulcer, 245
  T-cell role in, 81
Central cloudy dystrophy, 343
Central crystalline dystrophy, 341–342
Cephalosporins, 161–162
Chandler's syndrome, 9
Chemical injuries, 422–433
  acid, 430–433
  alkali, 422–430
    clinical features, 423–426
    toxic effects, 422–423
    treatment, 426–430
Chickenpox. *See also* Herpes zoster ophthalmicus
  ocular complications of, 189
Chlamydia, characteristics of organism, 210–214
  feline pneumonitis, 219–220

Chlamydia, characteristics of organism—*Continued*
  ocular infections, 210–220. *See also* Trachoma
    inclusion conjunctivitis, 218–219
    neonatal inclusion blennorrhea, 219
    trachoma, 215–218
    psittacosis, 220
Chloramphenicol, 162
Cholesterol, corneal deposits, 342
Cholinergic system
  in corneal epithelium, 18–19
  in corneal ulcer, 165
Chondroitin sulfate proteoglycan, 22–23
Choristomas, 364
Choroid
  hemorrhage in eye trauma, 420
  in lupus erythematosus, 267
  in progressive systemic sclerosis, 280
  vasculitis in polyarteritis nodosa, 273
Chromic acid, 431. *See also* Chemical injuries, acid
Chromosomal aberrations, in viral infections, 116
Cicatricial pemphigoid. *See* Pemphigoid, cicatricial
Climatic droplet keratopathy, 336
Clindamycin, 163
Clostridia, corneal ulcers due to, 153
Clotrimazole, 174–175
Coagulase, 110, 111
Coat's white rings, 333
Cogan's microcystic epithelial dystrophy, 337–338
Cogan's syndrome, 324–326
Collagen, 23–25
  defects in synthesis
    in acid injuries, 432
    and corneal ulcer, 423
Collagen diseases. *See also* Rheumatoid diseases
  lupus erythematosus, 264–270
  polyarteritis nodosa, 270–275
  scleroderma, 279–281
  Wegener's granulomatosis, 275–279
Collagenase, 26–27
  in alkali burns, 423
Collagenase inhibitors, 27
  in alkali injuries, 427–428
  in corneal ulcer, 165
Commotio retinae, 421
Complement
  activation of, 82–83
  in corneal stromal inflammation, 59
  role in immune reaction, 82–85
  in tears, 34
Complement fixation test, for chlamydia, 213
Computers, in lathing techniques, 456
Congenital anomalies, corneal, 355–368
  absence, 355–356
  curvature abnormalities, 358–359

Congenital anomalies, corneal—*Continued*
  mass lesions, 364–365
    choristomas, 364
    dermoids, 364–365
    metaplasias, 364
  megalocornea, 356–357
  mesodermal dysgenesis, 359–364
  microcornea, 357–358
  transparency abnormalities, 365–367
Congenital hereditary endothelial dystrophy, 66, 68, 70, 345, 365–366
Congenital hereditary stromal dystrophy, 344
Conjunctiva
  corneal relationships to, 465–466
  cysts after conjunctival flap, 470
  epithelium of, 465–466. *See also* Epithelium, conjunctival
  goblet cell counts in, 302
  lymphatics in, 97
  neoplasms of. *See* Conjunctival tumors
  in porphyria, 372
  surgical procedures involving, 465–475
  xerosis of, 406
Conjunctival flap, 467–471
  in alkali injuries, 428–429
  in corneal edema, 14
  in corneal trauma, 419
  in corneal ulcer, 166
  in fungal keratitis, 176
Conjunctival resection, 471
Conjunctival transplantation, 471–475. *See also* Transplantation, conjunctival
Conjunctival tumors
  melanoma, 394–396
  papillomas, 393–394
  pterygium, 391–393
  squamous cell carcinoma, 396–398
Conjunctivitis
  acute follicular, 196
  adenoviral infections, 196–197, 202–204
  atopic type, 90
  bacterial, and trachoma, 215
  in corneal ulcers, 150
  differential diagnosis of, 196
  in dry eye syndrome, 306
  episcleritis distinguished from, 253
  giant papillary, 239–242
  hay fever, 232–234
  herpes zoster causing, 190
  inclusion. *See* Inclusion conjunctivitis
  nonspecific follicular, 204
  papillary, 297
  superior limbic keratoconjunctivitis, 221–224
Contact dermatitis
  cell-mediated immunity in, 97
  hay fever differentiated from, 234
  sensitizers in, 97

Contact lens
    in alkali injuries, 428
    bandage. *See* Bandage contact lens
    biochemistry of wear, 20–21
    in corneal trauma, 416
    effect on corneal immunity, 148
    in epithelial basement membrane
        dystrophy, 338
    giant papillary conjunctivitis associ-
        ated with, 239–242. *See also*
        Conjunctivitis, giant papil-
        lary
    in keratoconus, 348
    in Mooren's ulcer, 247
    papain cleaner for, 242
    soft, 477–487
        in corneal edema, 13
        size, base curve, 478–479
        water content and oxygen per-
            meability, 478
    soft versus hard, effect on papillae,
        240
    in superficial punctate keratitis, 226
    therapeutic use of soft lens, 477–
        487
        choice of lens, 479
        complications, 484–487
        goals of wear, 477–478
        indications for, 479–484
    in therapy of trophic postinfectious
        ulcers, 186–187
    in trigeminal palsy, 322
Copper
    abnormal metabolism. *See* Wilson's
        disease
    deposition in eye, 385–386
Cornea farinata, 330
Cornea guttata. *See* Guttata
Cornea, horizontally oval, 358
Cornea plana, 358
Cornea, vertically oval, 358
Corneal arcus, 334
Corneal astigmatism, 359
Corneal erosion. *See* Erosion, corneal
Corneal relaxing incisions, 460
Corneal wedge resection, 460
Corneal wetting time. *See* Tear
        breakup time
Corneoscopy, 460
Corticosteroids
    in alkali injuries, 427
    in atopic keratoconjunctivitis, 235
    in cicatricial pemphigoid, 289
    in Cogan's syndrome, 325–326
    in contact lens–associated giant
        papillary conjunctivitis,
        242
    in corneal inflammation, 12, 87
    in corneal ulcer, 27, 165
    in disciform keratitis, 188
    in epidemic keratoconjunctivitis,
        202
    in erythema multiforme, 291
    in fungal keratitis, 176

Corticosteroids—*Continued*
    in graft rejection, 450
    in hay fever, 234
    in herpes zoster ophthalmicus,
        192–193
    in immune complex-mediated her-
        petic disease, 187
    immunologic effects in eye tissue,
        87, 94, 185
    in iridocyclitis of juvenile
        rheumatoid arthritis, 260
    in keratoprosthesis, 452
    in lupus erythematosus, 270
    in Mooren's ulcer, 247
    in nummular keratitis, 228–229
    in pemphigus foliaceus, 287
    in pemphigus vulgaris, 286
    in penetrating keratoplasty, 445
    in polyarteritis nodosa, 275
    positive and negative factors in
        herpes keratitis, 94
    postoperative use in lamellar kera-
        toplasty, 440
    pros and cons in herpes simplex
        ocular infection, 185–186
    in rheumatoid arthritis, 252
    in Sjögren's syndrome, 313
    in superficial punctate keratitis,
        224–226
    in vernal keratoconjunctivitis, 238–
        239
Cranial nerves
    corneal manifestations of disorders,
        315, 317–323
    facial palsy, 317–319
    trigeminal palsy, 319–323
    herpes zoster involvement of, 190
    innervation of eye by, 315–317
Cromoglycate, 238
Cryotherapy, in melanoma, 395–396
Cryptophthalmos, 356
Crystalline dystrophy, 341–342
Cultures
    for bacteria, 108–110
    for chlamydia, 212–213
    in corneal ulcer, 156–157
    in eye trauma, 414
    for fungi, 128–129, 172
    for herpes simplex, 180
Cyanoacrylate glue. *See also* Adhe-
        sive, surgical
    in therapy of trophic postherpetic
        ulcers, 187, 191
Cyclic AMP
    in anaphylactic hypersensitivity,
        89–90
    factors affecting level of, 90
    in hay fever, 233
Cyclophosphamide, in Wegener's
        granulomatosis, 279
Cycloplegics
    in alkali injuries, 427
    in corneal ulcer, 165
Cystinosis, 374–375
Cystoid macular edema, 421
Cytarabine, antiviral action of, 122
Cytomegalovirus infection, ocular in-
        volvement, 204

Dapsone, in ocular cicatricial pem-
        phigoid, 289
Degenerations, 329–336
    aging causing, 330, 334–336
    amyloidosis, 331–332
    arcus senilis, 334
    calcific band keratopathy, 330–331
    central, 330–334
    classification of, 330
    climatic droplet keratopathy, 336
    Coat's white rings, 333
    cornea farinata, 330
    dellen, 334
    dystrophies distinguished from
        329–330
    Hassall-Henle bodies, 334–335
    hyaline, 333
    keloid formation, 333
    lipid, 333
    mosaic shagreen of Vogt, 330
    pellucid marginal, 335
    peripheral, 334–336
    pigmentary, 333–334
    Salzmann's nodular, 332–333
    Terrien's marginal, 335
    white limbal girdle of Vogt, 334
Dellen, 294, 295, 334
Denervation, of corneal epithelium,
        19–20
2-Deoxy-D-glucose, antiviral action of,
        123
Depositions
    amyloidosis, 376–378
    calcium, 383–385. *See also* Band
        keratopathy
    copper, 385–386
    corneal, 367
    cystinosis, 375
    in familial plasma cholesterol ester
        deficiency, 380
    gold, 386
    mucopolysaccharidoses, 380–383
    silver, 386
    uric acid, 374
Dermoid, corneal, limbal and epibul-
        bar, 364–365
Descemet's membrane. *See also* En-
        dothelium, corneal
    collagen in, 25
    in Fuchs' dystrophy, 346
    Hassall-Henle bodies in, 334–335
    morphology of, 46
    wound healing in, 62, 64, 68
Diabetes mellitus
    primary corneal basement mem-
        brane disorder in, 55, 57
    soft contact lens for erosions in,
        480
Dietary deficiency, 401–409. *See also*
        Nutritional disorders
Disciform keratitis, 183–184
    treatment of, 188
Disodium cromoglycate, in vernal
        keratoconjunctivitis, 238
Donor
    in conjunctival transplantation, 473
    material used in lamellar kerato-
        plasty, 438

Donor—*Continued*
material used in penetrating keratoplasty, 441–443
methods of preparation of material,
443
in penetrating keratoplasty, 442
in lamellar keratoplasty, 440
Dopamine-beta-hydroxylase
deficiency, 326
Drugs
effect on tear flow, 35–37
and erythema multiforme, 289–290
immunoenhancement, 86–87
immunosuppression, 87–88
role in lupus erythematosus, 265
Dry eye. *See also* Sjögren's syndrome
band keratopathy in, 385
categories of syndromes, 293–295
aqueous tear deficiency, 293
lipid abnormalities, 294
mucin deficiency, 294
clinical features, 295–297
complications of, 306–307
conjunctival flap for, 469–470
diagnostic tests for, 297–301
rose bengal stain, 298–299
Schirmer test, 300–301
tear breakup time, 299–300
filaments in, 296–298
keratoconjunctivitis sicca syndrome, 293–307
laboratory tests in, 301–302
and loss of transparency, 367
Sjögren's syndrome, 309–313. *See
also* Sjögren's syndrome
soft contact lens in, 482–483
tear increase in, 296
treatment, 303–306
Dysautonomia, familial, 326–327
Dyskeratosis, 224
Dystrophy, corneal
anterior keratoconus, 347–348
basement membrane, 337–338
bleblike, 338
Bowman's layer, 338–339
central cloudy, 343
central crystalline, 341–342
cornea guttata, 345
congenital hereditary, 344, 345
congenital hereditary endothelial,
68, 70, 365–366
congenital hereditary stromal, 366
degenerations distinguished from,
329–330
endothelial, 344–349
epithelial, 336–338
fleck, 342–343
Fuchs', 346–346. *See also* Fuchs'
dystrophy
gelatinous drop-like, 332
granular, 339–340
juvenile hereditary, 336–337
lattice, 340–341. *See also* Lattice dystrophy
macular, 341
map-dot-fingerprint, 55–57, 337–338
Meesman's, 336–337
polymorphic, 343

Dystrophy, corneal—*Continued*
posterior amorphous corneal, 343–
344
posterior keratoconus, 348–349
posterior polymorphous, 72, 344–
345
pre-Descemet's, 343
Reis-Bücklers, 338, 339
soft contact lens for, 479–480
stromal, 339–344
vortex, 338

Echothiophate iodide, use in alkali
burns, 428
Edema, corneal, 3–15
birth trauma causing, 366
clinical evaluation of, 10–12
in congenital glaucoma, 366
in congenital hereditary endothelial
dystrophy, 345, 365–366
development of, 6–8
disciform keratitis causing, 183–184
effect on visual acuity, 7
elevated intraocular pressure causing, 10
endothelial dystrophies causing,
8–9
Chandler's syndrome, 9
congenital hereditary, 9
Fuchs' dystrophy, 8–9
epithelial, 6–7
soft contact lens use complicated
by, 484
in Fuchs' dystrophy, 346
in graft rejection, 8, 449
in herpes simplex infection, 8
inflammation causing, 7–8
intraocular surgery causing, 10
keratoconus causing, 9–10
medical treatment of, 12–13
pathologic processes leading to,
7–10
regulation of stromal hydration
and, 3–6, 28
soft contact lens use complicated
by, 484–485
stromal, 6
soft contact lens use complicated
by, 484–485
surgical treatment of, 13–15
trauma causing, 10
types of, 6–7
uveitis and, 8
EDTA
in band keratopathy, 260, 331
collagenase inhibition by, 27
Eledoisin, and tear secretion, 36
Elschnig spots, 273, 274
Embryotoxon
anterior, 367
posterior, 360
Endophthalmitis, after trauma, 421
Endothelial dystrophy, 344–349
congenital hereditary, 9
corneal edema due to, 8–9
Endothelial pump, and stromal hydration, 5

Endothelium, corneal
in aphakic bullous keratopathy, 69,
70, 72
clinical evaluation of, 10–12
congenital dystrophy of, edema in,
365–366
dystrophies involving, 336–338
functions of, 27–28
in graft rejection, 96, 449–450
in guttata and Fuchs' dystrophy,
67, 70
importance in penetrating keratoplasty, 442
metabolism of, 28
morphology of, 46
in Peters' anomaly, 66, 68
in posterior polymorphous dystrophy, 72
and stromal hydration, 5, 28
wound healing in, 62, 64, 68 118
Enterovirus ocular infection, 206–207
Enzymes
in alkali burns, 423
bacterial, role in pathogenicity,
148–149
of *Moraxella*, 112
of pneumococcus, 112
of *Pseudomonas*, 112
role in bacterial resistance to antibiotics, 134–135
staphylococcal, 111
of *Streptococcus pyogenes*, 111–112
Eosinophils, role in anaphylaxis, 90
Epibulbar dermoids, 364–365
Epidemic keratoconjunctivitis, 196–
197, 201–203. *See also under*
Adenovirus ocular infections
Epidermal growth factor (EGF), and
corneal wound healing, 49
Epikeratophakia, 457–459
Episcleritis, 253–256
Epitheliopathy, dry eye syndrome
due to, 295
Epithelium
conjunctival, 465–466
corneal
abnormalities in trigeminal palsy,
320–321
as barrier against viral infection, 118
basement membrane of, 25
denervation effects on, 19–20
dystrophies involving, 336–338
endothelial failure causing, soft
contact lens in, 483–484
in eye immunity, 147–148
function of, 17
and graft rejection, 449
herpes simplex-induced ulcerations of, 181–182
treatment, 186
metabolism of, 17–19
morphology of, 43–45
response to extensive surface injury, 49–51

Epithelium, corneal—*Continued*
  response to limited surface injury, 49–51
  role in collagenase production, 26
  and stromal hydration, 5
  surface disorders, soft contact lens in, 482
  trophic (metaherpetic) ulcerations of, 182
    treatment, 186–187, 191
  vitamin A action in, 405
  wound healing in, 46–49
  limbal, 466
Epstein-Barr virus infection, ocular involvement, 204
Erosion, corneal
  in diabetes mellitus, 55, 57
  pathologic reaction in recurrent disorders, 55–57
  primary and secondary basement membrane disorders causing, 55–57
  recurrent after tauma, 419–420
  soft contact lens for, 479–480
Erythema multiforme, 289–291
Erythrogenic toxin, 111
Erythromycin, 162–163
Evaporation, 5–7
Exotoxin A, 112
Eye
  antibody production in, 98–99
  defense mechanisms of, 147–166
  and immune response, 97–99
    antibody production and, 98–99
    blood vessels role in, 97
    lymphatics and, 97–98
    tear film role,98
  innervation of
    autonomic, 317
    motor, 316–317
    sensory, 315–316
  lymphatics in, 97–98
  viral infections of
    laboratory diagnosis of, 123–125
    direct examination of clinical materials, 123–124
    isolation and examination from clinical specimens, 124
    serologic diagnosis, 125
    viruses causing, 123
  vulnerability to bacteria, 93–94
Eye drops, pharmacokinetics of, 137–139
Eyelid
  abnormalities in dry eye syndrome, 294–295
  taping in facial palsy, 319

Fabry's disease, 379–380
Facial nerve
  anatomy of, 316–317
  palsy, 315, 317–319
Familial plasma cholesterol ester deficiency, 380

Fanconi's syndrome, 374–375
Feline pneumonitis, 219–220
Filaments, 296–298
Fistula, after corneal trauma, 420
Flat cornea. *See* Cornea plana
Fleck dystrophy, 342–343
Fleischer ring, 347
Floaters, in dry eye, 297
Flucytosine, 175
Fluorescein
  in tear breakup time test, 299–300
  in tear secretion studies, 37
Fluorescein dilution test, in dry eye, 301–302
Fluorescent antibody test, for chlamydia, 212
Fluorophotometry, corneal epithelium evaluated by, 12
Folic acid antagonists, effect on immune responses, 88
Foreign body, removal of, 415–416
Fuchs' dystrophy, 8–9, 346–347
  clinical features, 346
  corneal edema in, 9
  corneal endothelium in, 67, 70
  guttata in, 8–9
  pathologic changes, 346
  soft contact lens in, 483
  treatment, 347
Fungi, 127–131
  in corneal infections, 127
  cultural characteristics of, 128–129
  habitat of, 127
  immunologic aspects, 130–131
  keratitis due to, 168–176. *See also* Keratitis, fungal
  conjunctival flap for, 470
  mechanism of agents against, 131
  morphology of, 127–128
  pathogenicity of, 130
  tests for identification of, 129–130
Furrows
  in rheumatoid arthritis, 255–256
  treatment, 257
Fusarium
  antifungal treatment of, 175
  cultural characteristics of, 128
  morphology of, 127–128

Gelatinous drop–like dystrophy, 332
Giant papillary conjunctivitis. *See* Conjunctivitis, giant papillary
Giemsa stain, for chlamydia, 211
Glaucoma. *See also* Intraocular pressure
  corneal edema due to, 10, 366
  goniodysgenesis with, 363
  in herpes zoster ophthalmicus, 191
  after keratoprosthesis, 452
  microcornea and, 357–358
  in Scheie's syndrome, 382
Glucose
  metabolism in corneal endothelium, 28
  metabolism in corneal epithelium, 17–18
  in tear film, 33

Glucose 6-phosphatase deficiency, 383
Beta-glucuronidase deficiency, 383
Glue. *See* Adhesive, surgical
Glutathione, metabolism in corneal endothelium, 28
Glycocalyx, role in eye immunity, 147–148
Glycogen
  contact lens wear effect on, 20
  metabolism in corneal epithelium, 17–18
Glycoproteins, 21–22
  vitamin A action on, 405
Glycosaminoglycan
  in cornea, 22
  corneal deposits in macular dystrophy, 341
  evaporation and, 5–6
  intraocular pressure and, 5
  and stromal swelling pressure, 5
Goblet cells
  in conjunctiva of dry eye patient, 302
  role in corneal response to surface injury, 51
Gold, deposition in eye, 386
Goldenhar's syndrome, 365
Goniodysgenesis with glaucoma, 363
Gougerot-Sjögren syndrome, 309. *See also* Sjögren's syndrome
Gout, 373–374
Graft. *See also* Rejection, graft
  failure after penetrating keratoplasty, 448
  rejection
    cell-mediated immunity in, 95–96
    after penetrating keratoplasty, 448–450
    treatment of, 96–97
Gram stain, in corneal ulcer, 157
Granular dystrophy, 339–340
Groenouw I dystrophy, 339–340
Groenouw II dystrophy, 341
Gundersen flap, 468–469
Guttata
  cornea, 345
    congenital, 361
    corneal endothelium in, 70
  in Fuchs' dystrophy, 8–9

Hapten, 77
Hassall-Henle bodies, 334–335
Hay fever reactions, 232–234
  ocular manifestations, 90
Heart, in lupus erythematosus, 269
Heerfordt's syndrome, 318. *See also* Facial nerve, palsy
Helminths, role in Mooren's ulcer, 244
Helper T cells, 81
Hemorrhage, subchoroidal, 420
Heparin
  antiviral action of, 122
  subconjunctival injection in alkali injuries, 428
Hepatitis B, role in polyarteritis nodosa, 271

Hepatolenticular degeneration. *See* Wilson's disease

Herbert's pits, 214

Herpes simplex infections, 178–189
  acyclovir in, 122
  BVDU in, 122–123
  chromosomal aberrations in, 116
  conjunctival transplantation after, 472
  corticosteroids in, 94
  2-deoxy-D-glucose in, 123
  dissemination in newborn, 120
  epidemiology, 178
  idoxuridine in, 122
  immunoglobulins role against, 118–119
  incidence, 178
  latent, 121
  ocular infection
    antiviral drugs against, 184–186
    clinical features, 180–184
    congenital and neonatal, 180
    corneal basement membrane disorder in, 57
    corneal edema in, 8
    diagnostic tests, 180
    disciform keratitis, 183–184
      treatment, 188
    epidemiology, 178
    immune defense mechanisms in, 179–180
    immune rings, 183
      treatment, 187
    interstitial keratitis, 182
    laboratory diagnosis of, 124
    latency and trigger mechanisms for reactivation, 178–179
    limbal vasculitis, 183
      treatment, 187
    nummular keratitis differentiated from, 228
    primary, 180–181
    recurrent, 181–184
      epithelial infectious ulceration, 181–182
      epithelial trophic ulceration, 182
      iridocyclitis and trabeculitis, 184
      stromal disease, 182–184
      treatment, 188–189
  soft contact lens in, 481
  treatment of, 186–189
    combined epithelial and stromal disease, 188
    immune rings, 187
    interstitial keratitis, 187–188
    iridocyclitis and trabeculitis, 188–189
    keratoplasty in, 189
    limbal vasculitis, 187
    primary infection, 186
    recurrent epithelial ulcer, 186
    stromal disease, 188
    trophic postinfectious ulcer, 186–187, 191
  phosphonoacetic acid in, 123
  serodiagnosis of, 124, 125

Herpes simplex infections—*Continued*
  treatment of periocular infection, 186
  trifluridine in, 122
  vidarabine in, 122

Herpes zoster ophthalmicus, 189–193
  anterior segment disease, 190–191
  iritis in trigeminal palsy of, 321
  pathogenesis of, 189
  relation between neuronal patterns and disease, 190
  soft contact lens in, 481–482
  treatment, 191–193
  trigeminal palsy in, 321, 322

Herpesvirus ocular infections, 204. *See also* Herpes simplex infections; Herpes zoster ophthalmicus
  cytomegalovirus, 204
  Epstein-Barr virus, 204

Hexosamine, in tears, 302

Hexose monophosphate shunt, in corneal epithelium, 18

Histamine
  role in allergy, 90
  role in hay fever, 233
  tear levels in vernal keratoconjunctivitis, 238

Histocompatibility antigens, 78
  diseases associated with, 78
  and graft rejection, 449
  matching in corneal transplantation, 96–97
  in penetrating keratoplasty, 442
  in Sjögren's syndrome, 312

History-taking, in dry eye syndrome, 295–296

Homing, 79–80

Homogentisic acid. *See* Alkaptonuria

Hormones
  and corneal wound healing, 49
  role in lupus erythematosus, 265–266

Hunter's syndrome, 382

Hurler's syndrome, 381

Hyaline degeneration of cornea, 333

Hydration, corneal, 3–6, 28. *See also* Stromal hydration (H)

Hydrochloric acid, 431. *See also* Chemical injuries, acid

Hydrofluoric acid, 431. *See also* Chemical injuries, acid

Hyperlipidemia, central crystalline dystrophy and, 342

Hyperlipoproteinemias, 380

Hyperopia, keratomileusis in, 454–455

Hyperparathyroidism, 384

Hypersensitivity, 89–93. *See also* Allergy
  in hay fever, 232
  in nummular keratitis, 227
  type I: anaphylactic response, 89–90
  type II: cytotoxic response, 91
  type III: immune complex response, 91–92
  type IV: cell-mediated immune response, 92–93

Hypertonic solutions
  corneal edema treated by, 13
  in epithelial basement membrane dystrophy, 338

Hypophosphatasia, 384

Hypopyon, soft contact lens use complicated by, 486

Hypotears, 303

I-cell disease, 379

Idoxuridine (IDU)
  antiviral action of, 122
  in herpes simplex ocular infection, 184–185
  in herpes zoster ophthalmicus, 191
  in superficial punctate keratitis, 226

IgA, 79–80

IgD, 80

IgE, 80
  in anaphylaxis, 89–90
  in atopic keratoconjunctivitis, 234–235
  in atopy, 231
  in hay fever, 232–233

IgG, 79

IgM, 80

Imidazole antifungal agents, 174–175

Immune complexes, 91–92
  in erythema multiforme, 290
  in herpes simplex-induced stromal disease, 182–183
  in lupus erythematosus, 264
  mechanism of response, 92
  in peripheral corneal melting, 255–256
  in polyarteritis nodosa, 271
  in rheumatoid arthritis, 253
  scleritis and episcleritis due to, 253
  in Wegener's granulomatosis, 276

Immune reaction
  anaphylaxis, 89–90
  cell-mediated, 92–93. *See also* Cell-mediated immunity
  components of, 77–85
    antigens, 77–78
    B-lymphocytes, 78–80
    complement, 82–85
    killer and natural killer lymphocytes, 81–82
    macrophages, 82
    T-lymphocytes, 80–81
  corticosteroids effect on, 94
  cytotoxic, 91
  drug effects on, 86–88
  hypersensitivity responses, 89–93
  immune complex, 91–92
  ocular considerations affecting, 97–99
  testing for, 88–89
  viral disease mediated through, 120

Immune rings, 183

Immunity
  cell-mediated. *See* Cell-mediated immunity
  compromising factors interfering with, 148

Immunity—*Continued*
  corticosteroid effects in eye tissue, 185
  defense mechanisms of eye, 147–148
  in eye infection, 94
  and fungal infection, 130–131
  in herpes simplex ocular infection, 179–180
  and neoplastic disease, 95
  and viral infection, 117–120
Immunofluorescence, chlamydia identification by, 213
Immunoglobulins, 78–80. *See also* Antibody
  in tears, 34
  in viral infection, 118–119
Immunologic diseases. *See also* Autoimmune disease
  cicatricial pemphigoid, 287–289
  corneal manifestations of dermatologic disorders, 284–291
  erythema multiforme, 289–291
  Mooren's ulceration, 244–248
  ocular allergies, 231–242. *See also* Allergy, ocular
  pemphigus, 284–287
  polyarteritis nodosa, 270–275
  rheumatoid diseases, 249–261. *See also* Rheumatoid diseases
  scleroderma, 279–281
  Stevens-Johnson syndrome. *See* Erythema multiforme
  systemic lupus erythematosus, 264–270
  Wegener's granulomatosis, 275–279
Immunologic enhancement, 86–87
Immunologic tolerance, 85–86
Immunology, 77–99. *See also* Immune reaction
  cell alteration in, 85–88
  components of immune reaction, 77–85
  and contact dermatitis, 97
  of corneal graft rejection, 95–97
  hypersensitivity reactions, 89–93
  infection and, 93–94
  inflammation related to, 85
  ocular considerations of, 97–99
    antibody production, 98–99
    blood vessel factors, 97
    lymphatics, 97–98
    tear film, 98
  testing of, 88–89
  tumors and, 94–95
Immunosuppression
  drugs causing, 87–88
  in Sjögren's syndrome, 312–313
Immunotherapy, in anaphylaxis, 90
Inclusion blennorrhea, neonatal, 214–215, 219
Inclusion bodies, 116, 119
Inclusion conjunctivitis, 218–219

Infants, keratoplasty in, 368
Infections
  bacterial, 147–166. *See also* Bacteria, infections due to cell-mediated immunity in, 93–94
  chlamydial, 210–220
  conditions suspected as, 221–229
    nummular keratitis, 226–229
    superficial punctate keratitis, 224–226
    superior limbic keratoconjunctivitis, 221–224
  after conjunctival transplantation, 475
  of cornea, bacteria causing, 105
  after corneal trauma, 420
  fungal, 168–176. *See also* Fungi
  latent, 121
  mechanism of virulence in, 93
  organisms causing. *See* Infectious agents
  soft contact lens use complicated by, 486–487
  viral, 178–193, 196–207. *See also* Viral infections
Infectious agents
  bacteria, 105–112
  fungi, 127–131
  viruses, 115–125. *See also* Viruses
Infectious mononucleosis, ocular involvement in, 204
Inflammation, corneal. *See also* Keratitis
  corneal edema due to, 7–8
  corticosteroids effect on, 87
  in immune response, 85
  neurogenic and nonneurogenic control of, 85
  role in ocular immune response, 97
  of stroma, 58–59
  suppression of, 12
Injuries, corneal
  chemical, 422–433. *See also* Chemical injuries
  extensive ocular surface, 51–53
  limited ocular surface, 49–51
  trauma, 413–421
    complications, 419–421
    diagnosis, 413–414
    soft contact lens in, 480–481
    treatment techniques, 414–419
      observation, 415
      patching, 415
      removal of foreign bodies, 415–416
      soft contact lens, 416
      surgical adhesive, 418–419
Interferon, role in viral infections, 119
Interleukin-2, 81
Intraocular pressure. *See also* Glaucoma
  in alkali burns, 425–427
  and corneal epithelial edema, 6
  and corneal hydration, 5
  elevated
    corneal edema in, 10
    in penetrating keratoplasty, 445

Intraocular pressure—*Continued*
  and indications for keratoplasty, 441
  prostaglandin inhibitors effect on, 88
  reduction in corneal edema, 12–13
Iodine, as stain for chlamydia, 212
Iridocyclitis
  band keratopathy in, 385
  of herpes simplex disease, 184
    treatment, 188–189
  in herpes zoster ophthalmicus, 191
  in juvenile rheumatoid arthritis, 258–259
    treatment, 260
Iridogoniodysgenesis with cataract, 363
Iris
  in amyloidosis, 378
  essential atrophy of, 346
  mesodermal dysgenesis of, 361
  prolapsed, 417
  after penetrating keratoplasty, 446
  prominent processes of, 360–361
Iron, deposits in cornea, 333
Irrigation
  in acid injuries, 432–433
  in alkali injuries, 426

Joints. *See* Arthritis
Juvenile hereditary epithelial dystrophy, 336–337
Juvenile rheumatoid arthritis, 258–260

K cells. *See* Killer cells; Lymphocytes
Kayser-Fleischer ring, 324, 385
Keloid
  corneal, 364
  formation in cornea, 333
Keratan sulfate, 22–23
Keratectasia, 359
Keratinization
  in dry eye syndrome, 307
  xerophthalmia, 53, 54
Keratitic precipitates, 183
Keratitis. *See also* Ulcer, corneal
  bacterial
    causes of, 149, 150
    clinical features, 150–153
    histopathology and stages of, 153–156
    treatment of, 156–166
  chlamydial, 214–219
  congenital, 367
  in corneal response to injury, 58–59
  disciform, 183–184
    treatment of, 188
  exposure, 315, 318. *See also* Facial nerve, palsy
  fungal, 168–176
    clinical features, 169–171
    etiology, 168–169
    histopathology, 173
    incidence, 168
    laboratory diagnosis, 171–173
    secondary to bacterial infection, 172–173
    treatment, 173–176

Keratitis—*Continued*
  herpes simplex, 178–189. *See also*
    Herpes simplex infections,
    ocular infection
  herpes zoster causing, 190–191
    with trigeminal palsy, 321
  interstitial, 182–183, 325. *See also*
    Cogan's syndrome
    in lupus erythematosus, 266
    in measles, 206
  metaherpetic, 321
    in mumps, 206
  neuroparalytic, 315. *See also* Cranial
    nerves, corneal manifesta-
    tions of disorders
    conjunctival flap for, 467
  neurotrophic, 315. *See also* Trigemi-
    nal nerve, palsy
  nummular, 226–229
  in rheumatoid arthritis, 254–255
  rubella, 367
  scleritis associated with, 254–255
  sclerosing, 254–256
  striate, 6
  superficial punctate, 224–226
  syphillis, 367
  in vernal keratoconjunctivitis, 237
  viral, 178–193, 196–207. *See also*
    Herpes simplex infections,
    ocular infection; Herpes zos-
    ter ophthalmicus
    adenovirus disease, 196–197,
      201–204
    cytomegalovirus disease, 204
    differential diagnosis of, 198–200
    Epstein-Barr virus disease, 204
    herpes simplex, 178–189
    herpes zoster, 189–193
    paramyxovirus disease, 206
    picornavirus disease, 206–207
    poxvirus disease, 205–206
    togavirus disease, 207
Keratitis sicca. *See also* Dry eye
  conjunctival flap for, 468
  hay fever differentiated from, 234
  soft contact lens in, 482–483
Keratoconjunctivitis
  atopic, 234–236
  atopic type, 90
  epidemic, 196–197, 201–203. *See
    also* Adenovirus ocular in-
    fections
  superior limbic, 221–224
    conjunctival resection for, 471
  vernal, 236–239
Keratoconjunctivitis sicca, 293–307.
  See also Dry eye
  conjunctival flap for, 469
  in rheumatoid arthritis, 252
  treatment, 256
Keratoconus
  anterior, 347–348, 358
  comparison of various types, 360
  corneal edema in, 9–10
  endothelial wound healing in, 65,
    68
  epikeratophakia in, 458–459
  generalized posterior, 358–359

Keratoconus—*Continued*
  posterior, 348–349
    circumscribed, 361–362
  soft contact lens in, 483–484
  thermokeratoplasty for, 453–454
Keratocytes
  morphology of, 45
  role in stromal ulceration, 61
  in wound healing, 57–58, 60–61
Keratoglobus, 348, 349, 358
Keratolysis, 256, 258
Keratomalacia, 405–406, 408
Keratomileusis, 454–456
Keratopathy
  aphakic bullous. *See* Aphakic bul-
    lous keratopathy
  band, 259–260
  bullous, after trauma, 421
  climatic droplet, 336
Keratophakia, 455–457
Keratoplasty
  in amyloidosis, 332
  in chemically injured eye, 429
  conjunctival transplantation after,
    472
  in corneal edema, 13–14
  in corneal trauma, 419
  in Fuchs' dystrophy, 346
  after fungal keratitis, 175–176
  in granular dystrophy, 340
  for herpes simplex–scarred cornea,
    189
  for herpes zoster ophthalmicus, 193
  history of, 437
  increasing performances of, 437–
    438
  in infants, 368
  in keratoconus, 348
  keratoprosthesis, 450–452. *See also*
    Keratoprosthesis
  lamellar, 438–440
  penetrating, 441–450
    for refractive errors, 459–460
    tectonic, 441
  postoperative management, 14
  in pterygia, 393
  refractive, 453–463
    corneal relaxing incisions, 460
    corneal wedge resection, 460
    epikeratophakia, 457–459. *See
      also* Epikeratophakia
    lathing procedure, 454–457. *See
      also* Lathing procedures
    penetrating keratoplasty, 459–
      460
    radial keratotomy, 460–463. *See
      also* Radial keratotomy
    thermokeratoplasty, 453–454
  therapeutic use, 437–452
  types of procedures, 438
Keratoprosthesis, 450–452
  in chemically injured eye, 429–430
  complications, 452
Keratotomy, radial, 460–463. *See also*
    Radial keratotomy
Keratitis urica, 374
Ketoconazole, 174–175
Khodadoust line, 449

Kidney
  calcium deposition in failure, 384
  in lupus erythematosus, 268–269
  in polyarteritis nodosa, 274
  in progressive systemic sclerosis, 281
Killer cells, 81–82
  role in viral infections, 120
Kinins, in inflammation, 85
Kirby-Bauer test, 134
Kwashiorkor, 402

Lacerations. *See* Injuries, corneal
Lacrimal glands. *See also* Tear film;
    Tears
  IgA secretion in, 80
  secretion rate of, 37
  stimulation of, 305
Lamellar keratoplasty. *See* Kerato-
    plasty, lamellar
Latex test, for rheumatoid factor, 251
Lathing procedures, 454–457
  keratomileusis, 454–455
  keratophakia, 455
Lattice dystrophy, 340–341, 378
  corneal erosion in, 57
Lavage, in corneal ulcer, 165
Lecithin cholesterol acyltransferase
    deficiency, 380
Lens
  autoantibodies to, 97
  bandage. *See* Bandage contact lens
  contact. *See* Contact lens
  rupture of, 418
Lens deposits, soft contact lens use
    complicated by, 485
Lethal midline granuloma, 278
Leukocytes. *See* Neutrophils
Leukotrienes, 85, 89, 90
Levamisole, 87
Lids. *See* Eyelid
Lignac-Fanconi syndrome, 374–375
Limbal vasculitis, 183
Limbus, epithelium of, 466
Lime, eye toxicity of, 422. *See also*
    Chemical injuries, alkali
Limulus lysate assay, in corneal ulcer,
    157
Lipid
  abnormalities in dry eye syndrome,
    294
  degeneration of cornea due to de-
    posits of, 333
  in tear film, 31–32, 37–38
Loeffler medium, 109, 110
Lungs
  in lupus erythematosus, 269
  in Wegener's granulomatosis, 277,
    278
Lupus erythematosus, 264–270
  diagnosis of, 269, 270
  ocular involvement, 266–267
  pathogenesis, 264–265
  systemic involvement, 267–270
  treatment, 270

Lye, eye toxicity of, 422. *See also*
  Chemical injuries, alkali
Lymphatics, in cornea, 97–98
Lymphocytes, 80–81
  B cells. *See* B cells
  corticosteroids effect on, 87
  T cells. *See* T cells
  testing for immune reactions in-
    volving, 8
Lysozyme
  staphylococci producing, 111
  tear levels in dry eye, 302
  in tears, 33–34
  techniques of measuring, 302

M. fortuitum, corneal ulcers due to, 153
Macrophages
  in corneal stromal inflammation, 59
  corticosteroids effect on, 87
  role in immune reaction, 82
  role in viral infections, 119–120
Macular dystrophy, 341
Macular hole, 421
Magnesium hydroxide, eye toxicity
    of, 422. *See also* Chemical in-
    juries, alkali
Malnutrition, 401–403. *See also* Nutri-
    tional disorders
  and alcoholism, 408
Mannitol salt agar medium, 108
Map-dot-fingerprint dystrophy, 55–
    57
Marasmus, 401–402
Maroteaux-Lamy syndrome, 383
Mast cells
  in contact lens–associated giant
    papillary conjunctivitis, 240
  and immune response, 80
  role in hay fever, 232–233
  in vernal keratoconjunctivitis, 237–
    238
Maxwell-Lyons sign, 236
Measles, eye involvement, 206
Mediators, in hay fever, 233
Medroxyprogesterone
  use as collagenase inhibitor, 427–
    428
  use in herpes ocular infection, 185
Meesmann's epithelial dystrophy,
    336–337
Megalocornea, 356–357
Melanin, deposits in cornea, 333–334
Melanokeratosis, striate, 336
Melanoma, corneal, 394–396
Melting, 61. *See also* Ulcer, corneal
Meniscus floaters, in dry eye, 297
Meniscus height, in dry eye, 297
Mercurial compounds, band
    keratopathy associated with,
    385
Mesodermal dysgenesis, 359–364
  circumscribed posterior
    keratoconus, 361–362
  congenital cornea guttata, 361

Mesodermal dysgenesis—*Continued*
  of iris, 361
  posterior embryotoxon, 360
  posterior polymorphous dys-
    trophy, 361
  prominent iris processes, 360–361
  recurring combinations of, 363–364
  sclerocornea, 362–363
Metabolic diseases, 371–386
  alkaptonuria, 375–376
  amyloidosis, 376–378
  calcium, 383–385
  copper, 385–386. *See also* Wilson's
    disease
  cystinosis, 374–375
  Fabry's disease, 379–380
  familial plasma cholesterol ester
    deficiency, 380
  glucose 6-phosphatase deficiency,
    383
  gout, 373–374
  hyperlipoproteinemia, 380
  mucolipidoses, 378–379
  mucopolysaccharidoses, 380–383
  poryphyria, 371–373
  Tangier disease, 380
Metals, deposits in cornea, 334
Metaplasias, corneal, 364
Methicillin resistance, 135–136
Methotrexate, effect on immune re-
    sponses, 88
Methylcellulose drops, 303
Miconazole, 174–176
Microbiology
  antibiotic mechanisms, 134–141
  diagnosis of corneal ulcer, 156–157
  infectious agents
    bacteria, 105–112
    fungi, 127–131
    viruses, 115–125
Microcornea, 357–358
Microphthalmos, 357
Microtiter indirect immunofluores-
    cence, 213
Mikulicz's disease, 309. *See also* Sjö-
    gren's syndrome
Millard-Gubler syndrome, 318
Moisture chamber, use in facial palsy,
    319
Molluscum contagiosum, eye involve-
    ment, 205–206
Monocytes, role in fungal infection,
    131
Mooren's ulcer, 244–248
  clinical course in, 335–336
  conjunctival resection for, 471
  polyarteritis nodosa distinguished
    from, 273
  Terrien's marginal degeneration
    differentiated from, 335–336
  Wegener's granulomatosis distin-
    guished from, 277
Moraxella, 106
  corneal ulcer due to, 149
  cultural characteristics, 109–110
  enzymes of, 112
  morphology and staining character-
    istics, 107, 108

Moraxella—*Continued*
  pathogenicity of, 112
  tests for identification, 110–111
  toxins of, 112
Morquio's syndrome, 383
Mosaic shagreen of Vogt, 330
Mucin
  deficiency in tears, 294, 295
  role in tear film, 38
  in tears of dry eye patient, 302
Mucolipidoses, 378–379
Mucomyst. *See* Acetylcysteine
Mucopolysaccharide, corneal deposits
    in macular dystrophy, 341
Mucopolysaccharidoses, 380–383
  beta-glucuronidase deficiency, 383
  Hunter's syndrome, 382
  Hurler's syndrome, 381
  Maroteaux-Lamy syndrome, 383
  Morquio's syndrome, 383
  ocular manifestations, 381
  Sanfilippo's syndrome, 382–383
  Scheie's syndrome, 381–382
Mucus
  in giant papillary conjunctivitis,
    239–240
  strands in dry eye, 297
  in tear film, 34–35, 38
  in vernal keratoconjunctivitis,
    236
Mumps, eye involvement, 206
Munson's sign, 347
Muramidase. *See* Lysozyme
Myopia, keratomileusis in, 454, 455

Nanophthalmos, 357
Nasociliary nerve, herpes zoster in-
    volvement of, 190
Natamycin, 131. *See also* Polyenes
  in fungal keratitis, 173, 176
Natural killer cells, 81–82
  role in viral infections, 120
Neonatal inclusion blennorrhea. *See*
    Inclusion blennorrhea,
    neonatal
Neoplasms
  calcium deposition in cornea in,
    384–385
  cell-mediated immunity in, 94–95
  conjunctival, 391–398
  corneal, 391–398
    benign, 391–394
    malignant, 394–398
    melanoma, 394–396
    papillomas, 393–394
    pterygium, 391–393
    squamous cell carcinoma, 396–
      398
  variety, 391
Nervous system
  Cogan's syndrome, 324–326
  cornea manifestations of diseases
    of, 31–327
  facial nerve palsy, 317–319
  familial dysautonomia, 326–327
  in lupus erythematosus, 269
  trigeminal nerve palsy, 319–323
  Wilson's disease, 323–324

Neurotrophic changes and drying of the cornea, 367
Neutrophils
   in corneal ulcers, 153–155
   in eye immunity, 148
   in fungal infection, 131
   in viral infections, 120
Newborn
   herpes keratitis in, 180
   inclusion blennorrhea in, 214–215, 219
Newcastle disease, eye involvement, 206
Night blindness, 408. *See also* Vitamin A, deficiency of
Nikolsky's sign, 285
Nitric acid, 431. *See also* Chemical injuries, acid
Nocardia, corneal ulcers due to, 153
Nonspecific follicular conjunctivitis, 204
Nosocomial infections, epidemic keratoconjunctivitis, 196–197
Nummular keratitis, 226–229. *See also* Keratitis, nummular
Nutrition, of corneal and conjunctival epithelium, 466
Nutritional disorders, 401–409
   in alcoholism, 408
   kwashiorkor, 402
   marasmus, 401–402
   protein-energy malnutrition, 402–403
   vitamin A deficiency, 405–408. *See also* Vitamin A, deficiency of
Nystatin, in fungal keratitis, 176

Ochronosis, 375
Ocular cicatricial pemphigoid. *See* Pemphigoid, cicatricial
Oral contraceptives, and tear secretion, 36
Osmolality, tear, 39
   in dry eye, 302
Osteo-odonto-keratoprosthesis, 451
Oxygen
   contact lens effect on, 21
   in corneal epithelium, 18
   metabolism in corneal endothelium, 28
   permeability through soft contact lens, 478
   in tear film metabolism, 33
Oxyphenbutazone, in episcleritis and scleritis, 256

Pachometry, corneal epithelium evaluated by, 11–12
Pain, soft contact lens in reduction of, 477
Papain contact lens cleaner, 242
Papillary conjunctivitis. *See* Conjunctivitis, giant papillary
Papillomas, 393–394
Paramyxovirus ocular infections, 206
   measles, 206
   mumps, 206
   Newcastle disease, 206

Parasympathetic nervous system
   and corneal wound healing, 49
   innervation of eye, 317
   in tear film formation, 35
Parotid flow rate, 311
Patching, in corneal trauma, 415
Pathogenicity
   of bacteria, 111–112
   bacterial characteristics affecting, 148–150
   of fungi, 130
   of viruses, 115–120
Pathogens. *See* Infectious agents
Pellucid marginal degeneration, 335
Pemphigoid, 287–289
   bullous, 287
   cicatricial, 53–55, 287–289
   soft contact lens in, 482
Pemphigus, 284–287
   foliaceus, 286–287
   vulgaris, 285–286
Penetrating keratoplasty. *See* Keratoplasty, penetrating
D-Penicillamine, in Wilson's disease, 324
Penicillin, 161
   resistance, 161
Peptide antibiotics, 163
Permeability, antibiotics increasing, 136
Peters' anomaly, 363–364
pH, and alkali toxicity to eye, 422–423
Phagocytosis, 82
Pharmacokinetics
   of eye drops, 138–139
   of eye ointment, 139
Pharyngoconjunctival fever, 203–204
Phosphonoacetic acid, antiviral action of, 123
Physalaemin, and tear secretion, 36
Physical examination
   in dry eye, 296–297
   after eye trauma, 413–414
Picornavirus ocular infection, 206–207
Plasmapheresis, in pemphigus vulgaris, 286
Plasmin, 85
   role in injured corneal epithelium, 26
Platelet activating factor, 90
Pneumococcus, 106–107, 112
   corneal ulcers due to, 150
Pneumonia, feline, 219–220
Polyanions, antiviral action of, 121–122
Polyarteritis nodosa, 270–275
   ocular involvement, 273–274
   systemic involvement, 274–275
Polychondritis, relapsing, 260–261
Polyenes, 173–174
Polymorphic stromal dystrophy, 343
Polymorphonuclear leukocytes. *See* Neutrophils
Polymyxin, 163
Porphyria, 371–373
Posterior amorphous corneal dystrophy, 343–344
Posterior embryotoxon, 360

Posterior polymorphous dystrophy, 72, 344–345, 361
Potassium hydroxide, eye toxicity of, 422. *See also* Chemical injuries, alkali
Poxvirus ocular infections, 205–206
   molluscum contagiosum, 205–206
   vaccinia, 205
   variola, 205
Prausnitz-Küstner reaction, 231
Prausnitz-Küstner test, 89–90
Pre-Descemet's dystrophy, 343
Procollagen, 23–25
Progressive systemic sclerosis, 279–281. *See also* Scleroderma
Prolapse, intraocular, 416–417
Properdin system, 83
Prostaglandins
   in corneal vascularization, 59
   in inflammation, 85
   inhibitors effect on immune response, 88
Prosthesis. *See* Keratoprosthesis
Protein
   antibiotic inhibitors of synthesis, 136
   metaboism in corneal epithelium, 18
Protein-energy malnutrition, 402–403
Proteoglycans, corneal, 22–23
   and corneal hydration, 4
   functions of, 23
Provera. *See* Medroxyprogesterone
Pruritus, in vernal keratoconjunctivitis, 236
Pseudogerontotoxon, in vernal keratoconjunctivitis, 237
Pseudomonas, 106–107, 110, 112
   corneal ulcer due to, 149, 151–152
   corticosteroids effect on, 165
   fungal keratitis compared with, 170–171
Psittacosis, 219
Psychological disorders, in dry eye syndrome, 307
Pterygium, 391–393
Ptosis, after conjunctival flap, 470
Punctal occlusion, 304–305

Radial keratotomy, 460–463
Radiation therapy, for melanoma, 395
Ramsey Hunt syndrome, 318
Raynaud's phenomenon, in progressive systemic sclerosis, 280
Refractive keratoplasty, 453–463. *See also* Keratoplasty, refractive
Rehabilitation, of chemically injured eye, 429–430
Reis-Bücklers dystrophy, 338–339
Rejection, graft, 448–450
   corneal edema due to, 8
   definition, 448
   endothelial, 449–450
   epithelial, 449

Rejection, graft—*Continued*
  immunology of, 449
  treatment, 96–97
Relapsing polychondritis, 260–261
Relaxing incisions, 460
Resistance, antibiotic, 134–136
Retina
  in lupus erythematosus, 267
  in polyarteritis nodosa, 273–274
  in progressive systemic sclerosis, 280
  vasculitis of, 267
Retinol, 403. *See also* Vitamin A
Rheumatoid arthritis, 249–258
  juvenile. *See* Juvenile rheumatoid
      arthritis
  ocular manifestations, 252–258
  systemic manifestations, 250–252
Rheumatoid diseases, 249–261
  juvenile rheumatoid arthritis, 258–
      260
  relapsing polychondritis, 260–261
  rheumatoid arthritis, 249–258
Rheumatoid factor, 249
  presence in various diseases, 252
  tests for, 251
Ribavirin, antiviral action of, 123
Rieger's anomaly and syndrome, 363
Rifampin, 163
  antiviral action of, 123
Riley-Day syndrome, 326–327. *See
      also* Dysautonomia, familial
Rose bengal dye
  in dry eye, 298–299
  in facial palsy, 319
  for tear function, 39
Rubella
  eye involvement, 207
  keratitis at birth due to, 367
Rubeosis iridis, 421

Sabouraud medium, 171
Salicylate, 252
Salivary glands, biopsy of accessory
      glands in Sjögren's syn-
      drome, 311
Salzmann's nodular degeneration,
      332–333
Sanfilippo's syndrome, 382–383
Scars
  in corneal response to injury, 59, 61
  stromal, 59, 61
  in vitamin A deficiency, 408
Scheie's syndrome, 381–382
Schirmer test, 38
  anesthesia in, 301
  in dry eye, 300–301
  type I versus type II, 301
Schnyder's crystalline dystrophy,
      341–342
Schwalbe's ring, 360
Sclera. *See also* Episcleritis; Scleritis
  classification of diseases of, 253
  laceration of, 420–421
  in porphyria, 372–373

Scleritis
  herpes zoster causing, 190
  immune complexes role in, 253
  in lupus erythematosus, 266
  in polyarteritis nodosa, 273
  in rheumatoid arthritis, 253–254
  sclerosing keratitis complicating,
      254–255
  treatment, 256
  in Wegener's granulomatosis, 277
Sclerocornea, 362–363
Scleroderma, 279–281
Scleromalacia perforans, 253–254, 373
Seanear-Usher syndrome, 284
Seidel's test, 413, 414
Sexually transmitted disease, inclu-
      sion conjunctivitis, 218
Sicca syndrome. *See also* Dry eye;
      Sjögren's syndrome
  in lupus erythematosus, 266
Silver, deposition in eye, 386
Silver nitrate, in superior limbic
      keratoconjunctivitis, 224
Sjögren's syndrome, 309–313. *See also*
      Dry eye
  bromhexine hydrochloride in, 36
  conjunctival flap for, 469–470
  in rheumatoid arthritis, 252
Skin
  in lupus erythematosus, 268
  in polyarteritis nodosa, 274
  in progressive systemic sclerosis, 280
Skin tests
  for chlamydia, 213–214
  in hay fever, 233
  for immune responsiveness, 88
Slow virus, role in superficial punc-
      tate keratitis, 224–225
Smallpox, eye involvement, 205
Sodium hyaluronate, in corneal
      trauma, 417
Sodium hydroxide, eye toxicity of,
      422. *See also* Chemical in-
      juries, alkali
Sorbitol pathway, in corneal
      epithelium, 18
Speckled dystrophy, 342–343
Spectinomycin, 163
Specular microscopy, corneal
      epithelium evaluated by, 11
Squamous cell tumor of conjunctiva,
      396–398
Stains
  of bacteria, 106–108
  for chlamydia, 211–212
  in corneal ulcer diagnosis, 157
  for fungal keratitis, 171–172
Staphylococcus, 105–106, 108, 110–111
  corneal ulcer due to, 149, 151
Staphyloma, congenital anterior, 359
Sterile infiltrates, soft contact lens use
      complicated by, 486
Steroids. *See* Corticosteroids
Stevens-Johnson syndrome. *See*
      Erythema multiforme
Still's disease, 258
Streptococcus, 106–107, 108–112
  corneal ulcers due to, 150–151

Streptococcus—*Continued*
  pneumoniae. *See* Pneumococcus
      pyogenes
    enzymes of, 111–112
    toxins of, 111
Streptokinase, role in pathogenicity,
      112
Streptolysin O, 111
Striate keratitis, 6
  contact lens wear causing, 20
Striate melanokeratosis, 336
Stroma
  cellular metabolism in, 27
  collagen in, 23–27
  congenital hereditary dystrophy of,
      366
  dystrophies involving, 336–338
  glycoproteins in, 21–22
  herpes simplex disease of, 182–184
    treatment of, 187–188
  herpes zoster disease of, 191
  inflammation of, 58–59
  morphology of, 45
  proteoglycans in, 22–23
  scarring of, 59, 61
  surface proteins in, 27
  terminology of macromolecules
      contained in, 21–23
  ulceration of, 61–62
  vascularization of, 59
  wound healing of, 57–58, 60–61
Stromal hydration (H), 3–5
  regulation of, 4–6, 28
Stromal swelling pressure, 4
Stromal ulcer. *See* Ulcer, stromal
Subchoroidal hemorrhage, 420
Subconjunctival antibiotic injections,
      139–141
Sulfonamides, 163
  in trachoma, 217–218
Sulfur dioxide, 430–431. *See also*
      Chemical injuries, acid
Sulfuric acid, 430. *See also* Chemical
      injuries, acid
Sulfurous acid, 430–431. *See also*
      Chemical injuries, acid
Sunglasses, in pterygia, 392
Superficial punctate keratitis, 224–226
Superior limbic keratoconjunctivitis,
      221–224
Suppressor T cells, 81
  and autoimmunity, 86
Surface proteins, 27
Surgical adhesive. *See* Adhesive, sur-
      gical
Suturing
  appositional, 417–418
  in corneal trauma, 417–418
  in lamellar keratoplasty, 440
  in penetrating keratoplasty, 444, 447
Swimmers' goggles, 304
Symblepharon
  after alkali burns, 426
  prevention in alkali burns, 428
Sympathetic nervous system. *See also*
      Autonomic nervous system
  innervation of eye, 317
  in tear film formation, 35

Synechiae, after penetrating kerato-
plasty, 446
Synergism, antibiotic, 136–137
Syphilis, keratitis at birth due to, 367

T cells, 80–81
in anaphylaxis, 90
in atopic keratoconjunctivitis, 235
in cell-mediated immunity, 92–93
and immunologic tolerance, 85–86
in lupus erythematosus, 264–265
in prevention of corneal graft rejection, 97
in viral infections, 119
Tangier disease, 380
Tarsorrhaphy
in dry eye syndrome, 305–306
in facial palsy, 319
in trigeminal palsy, 322–323
Tear breakup time, 38–39
in dry eye, 299–300
Tear film, 31–39
after alkali burn, 426
epitheliopathy causing irregularity
in, 295
immunologic function of, 98
in vitamin A deficiency, 406
Tear osmolality, 39
in dry eye, 302
Tears, 33–39. See also Dry eye
aqueous deficiency, 293, 294. See
also Sjögren's syndrome
artificial drops, 303
chlamydiae isolated from, 212
in hay fever, 233
hexosamine in, 302
histamine levels in vernal
keratoconjunctivitis, 238
IgA in, 80
increase in dry eye, 296
inserts as substitutes, 303–304
insufficiency in progressive systemic sclerosis, 280
low osmolality drops, 303
lysozyme levels in dry eye, 302
mucin deficiency, 294, 295
mucin levels in dry eye patient,
302
and pharmacokinetics of antibiotic
eye drops, 138–139
preservation in dry eye syndrome,
304–305
in sleep, 295
stimulation in dry eye syndrome,
305
supplementation in dry eye syndrome, 304–305
Terrien's marginal degeneration, 335
Tetracycline, 162
Thermokeratoplasty, 453–454
in keratoconus, 348
Thiosemicarbazones, antiviral action
of, 123
Thyroid disease, superior limbic
keratoconjunctivitis and,
221
Ticarcillin disodium, 161

Tissue adhesives. See Adhesive, sur-
gical
Tissue culture, for chlamydia, 212
Togavirus ocular infection, 207
Tolerance, immunologic, 85–86
Tonometer, spread of epidemic
keratoconjunctivitis by, 202
Toxins, bacterial, 111–112
role in pathogenicity, 149
fungal, 130
Trabeculitis, of herpes simplex dis-
ease, 184, 188–189
Trachoma, 210, 215–218
Transduction, 134
Transfer factor, 87
Transformation, in viral infections,
116–117
Transparency abnormalities of the
cornea, 365–367. See also
specific entry
Transplantation
conjunctival, 471–475
corneal. See Keratoplasty
Transplantation antigens. See also Histocompatibility antigens
tumor-specific, 94–95
Trauma
corneal edema due to, 10
effect on corneal epithelium, 20
Tricarboxylic acid cycle, in corneal
epithelium, 18
Trichothecenes, 130
Triethylenethiophosphoramide, for
pterygia, 393
Trifluridine (F_3T)
antiviral action of, 122
in epidemic keratoconjunctivitis,
203
in herpes ocular infection, 184–
185
Trigeminal nerve
anatomy of, 315–316
palsy, 315, 319–323
Tumors. See Neoplasms
Tumor-specific transplantation antigens, 94–95
viral, 95

Ulcer
corneal, 25–26. See also Keratitis
in acid injuries, 432
in alkali burns, 423, 425
in anesthetic eye, 323
causes of, 26, 149, 150
clinical features, 150–153
collagenase and, 26–27
conjunctival flap for, 467, 468
conjunctival resection for, 471
course of bacterial causes of, 149–
150
in erythema multiforme, 290
eye drops versus subconjunctival
antibiotic injection in,
139–141
fungi causing, 168–169
gold deposition causing, 386
herpes simplex–induced epithelial eruptions, 181–182

Ulcer, corneal—Continued
histopathology and stages of,
153–156
inhibition of collagenase in treatment of, 27
location of, 149
microbiologic diagnosis of, 156–
157
Mooren's, 244–248. See also
Mooren's ulcer
after penetrating keratoplasty,
446–447
in polyarteritis nodosa, 273
in rheumatoid arthritis, 255–256
soft contact lens use complicated
by, 486–487
after trauma, 420
treatment of, 157–166
adjunctive therapy, 165–166
aminoglycosides, 159–161
cephalosporins, 161–162
chloramphenicol, 162
choice of antibiotic, 157–159
choice of antibiotic route, 163–
165
clindamycin, 163
erythromycin, 162–163
penicillins, 161
peptide antibiotics, 163
rifampin, 163
spectinomycin, 163
sulfonamides, 163
tetracycline, 162
topical versus subconjunctival
antibiotics in, 164
vancomycin, 162
trophic (metaherpetic) epithelial
lesions, 182
treatment, 186–187, 191
in vernal keratoconjunctivitis,
237
von Hippel's posterior, 362, 364
in Wegener's granulomatosis,
277
with xerosis, 407–408
Mooren's, 244–248. See also
Mooren's ulcer
stromal, 61–62
in dry eye syndrome, 306
in trigeminal palsy, 321
Ultraviolet irradiation, role in lupus
erythematosus, 265
Uric acid. See Gout
Uveitis
and corneal edema, 8
of herpes simplex diseases, 184
treatment of, 188–189
immune complex role in, 92
in lupus erythematosus, 266
Uveoparotid fever, 318. See also Facial
nerve, palsy

Vaccinia, 205
Vancomycin, 162

Varicella infection. *See* Herpes zoster ophthalmicus
Variola, 205
Vascularization
  in corneal response to injury, 59
  soft contact lens use complicated by, 485
Vasculitis
  classification of, 272
  in Cogan's syndrome, 324–325
  limbal, 183
  in polyarteritis nodosa, 271–272
  retinal, 267
  systemic. *See also* Polyarteritis nodosa
  in Wegener's granulomatosis, 275–279
Vasoconstricting agents, in hay fever, 234
Vidarabine
  antiviral action of, 122
  in herpes infection, 184–185
Viral infections, 115–125
  and autoimmune disease, 94
  chemotherapy against, 121–123. *See also* Antiviral chemotherapy
  laboratory diagnosis in eye, 123–125
  pathogenesis of, 115–120
  pattern of disease in, 120–121
Virulence, 93
Viruses, 115–125. *See also* Viral infections
  classification of, 115, 117
  and induced autoimmunity, 86

Viruses—*Continued*
  keratitis due to, 178–193, 196–207. *See also* Herpes simplex infections; Herpes zoster ophthalmicus
  adenovirus disease, 196–197, 201–204
  differential diagnosis of, 198–200
  herpes simplex, 178–189
  herpes zoster, 189–193
  pathogenesis of, 115–120
  possible role in nummular keratitis, 227
  possible role in superficial punctate keratitis, 224
  role in lupus erythematosus, 265
  slow, 224–225
  structure of, 115
  tumor-specific transplantation antigens of, 95
Vision, corneal edema effect on, 7
Vitamin A, 403–409
  action in eye, 405
  deficiency of
    causes, 405
    ocular changes in, 406
    in peripheral tissue, 405
  immunologic effects of, 87
Vitrectomy, keratoplasty combined with, 445
Vitreous
  complications after corneal trauma, 420
  corneal edema due to contact of, 10
Vitritis, after keratoprosthesis, 452
Vogt-Koyanagi-Harada disease, 325
von Gierke's disease, 383

von Hippel's posterior corneal ulcer, 362, 364
Vortex dystrophy, 338

Waaler-Rose test, 251
Water, corneal, 3–6, 28. *See also* Edema, corneal
Wedge resection, 460
Wegener's granulomatosis, 275–279
  ocular involvement, 277
  systemic involvement, 277–278
Wessley rings, 183
White limbal girdle of Vogt, 334
Wilson's disease, 232–324
Wound healing
  in corneal ulcers, 155–156
  in epithelium, 46–49
  keratocytes in, 57–58, 60–61
  after penetrating keratoplasty, 447–448
  proteoglycans role in, 23
  soft contact lens and, 477
  in stroma, 57–58, 60–61

Xerophthalmia, 53, 405
  pathologic reaction in cornea, 53, 54
Xerophthalmic fundus, 408
Xerosis
  conjunctival, 406
  corneal, 406–407
Xerostomia, 309. *See also* Sjögren's syndrome

Yeast. *See Candida*

Zoster. *See* Herpes zoster ophthalmicus